Practical Otology for the Otolaryngologist

Practical Otology for the Otolaryngologist

Seilesh Babu, MD

PLURAL PUBLISHING
INC.
SAN DIEGO
OXFORD
MELBOURNE

PLURAL PUBLISHING
INC.

5521 Ruffin Road
San Diego, CA 92123

e-mail: info@pluralpublishing.com
Web site: http://www.pluralpublishing.com

Typeset in 10½/13 Palatino by Flanagan's Publishing Services, Inc.
Printed in Malaysia by Four Colour Print Group

NOTICE TO THE READER
Care has been taken to confirm the accuracy of the indications, procedures, drug dosages, and diagnosis and remediation protocols presented in this book and to ensure that they conform to the practices of the general medical and health services communities. However, the authors, editors, and publisher are not responsible for errors or omissions or for any consequences from application of the information in this book and make no warranty, expressed or implied, with respect to the currency, completeness, or accuracy of the contents of the publication. The diagnostic and remediation protocols and the medications described do not necessarily have specific approval by the Food and Drug administration for use in the disorders and/or diseases and dosages for which they are recommended. Application of this information in a particular situation remains the professional responsibility of the practitioner. Because standards of practice and usage change, it is the responsibility of the practitioner to keep abreast of revised recommendations, dosages, and procedures.

Library of Congress Cataloging-in-Publication Data

Practical otology for the otolaryngologist / edited by Seilesh Babu.
p. ; cm.
Includes bibliographical references and index.
ISBN-13: 978-1-59756-254-6 (alk. paper)
ISBN-10: 1-59756-254-8 (alk. paper)
I. Babu, Seilesh.
[DNLM: 1. Ear Diseases. WV 200]
LC Classification not assigned
617.8--dc23

2012043308

Contents

Foreword

In 1986, the Michigan Ear Institute was established. Dr. T. Manford McGee had been in otologic practice in the greater Detroit area for over twenty years and it was during these years that he established a very strong and loyal relationship with Providence Hospital in Southfield, Michigan.

My otologic career had taken me from a solo private practice in Victoria, British Columbia, Canada, to membership in the House Ear Clinic in Los Angeles, California, and then to faculty membership in the Department of Otolaryngology/Head and Neck Surgery at the University of Michigan in Ann Arbor. I had the privilege to practice in both private practice and academic sections of otology and witnessed the strengths and weaknesses of both.

As time passed, both Dr. McGee and I had envisioned the concept of an "Ear Institute" with all the resources and services appropriate for such a preeminent center. This "proposal" included a medical office building, fully equipped with audiologic and vestibular evaluation capabilities. At the hospital, three operating rooms dedicated to otologic, neurotologic, and skull base surgery, with specialized, dedicated surgical nurses, appropriate otologic surgical instruments, intraoperative monitoring equipment, surgical microscopes, and audiovisual equipment was designed. Providence Hospital would also fund a fellowship program in otology, neurotology, and skull base surgery, as well as provide a temporal bone surgical dissection laboratory and complete audiologic and vestibular testing facilities; this truly provided a unique opportunity.

We jointly decided to proceed, and in 1986 the Michigan Ear Institute was established. While Dr. McGee had a career in otosclerosis and stapes surgery, it was decided with the rapid emergence of neurotologic diagnosis and surgery that the practice would be devoted to otology, neurotology, and skull base surgery, and future associates would be young, fellowship-trained individuals in this broader field.

Thus, in rapid succession doctors Jack Kartush, Dennis Bojrab, and Michael LaRouere joined the original faculty. Later, several Michigan Ear Institute fellows remained on faculty as well: doctors John Zappia, Eric Sargent, and Seilesh Babu.

It is with great pride that I introduce this book (and its companion, *Practical Neurotology and Skull Base Surgery*), edited by Dr. Seilesh Babu and contributed to by many other members of the Michigan Ear Institute and their former fellows. This book reflects 25 years of experience in clinical otology, neurotology, and skull base surgery, an experience rich in contributions in diagnosis, evaluations, electrophysiologic monitoring, and surgical technique innovations and modifications.

As I reflect upon the past 50 years of clinical otology, the changes that have occurred during those decades are nothing less than amazing.

In otosclerosis surgery, the fenestration operation had just given way to the stapes mobilization procedure. Soon refixation of the stapes became apparent and the total stapedectomy operation became popular. With time this has been replaced generally by the small footplate fenestra techniques.

In chronic ear and cholesteatoma surgery, canal wall-down techniques were standard when the intact canal wall procedure was proposed. The controversy that ensued was clearly apparent every four years when proponents of each technique shared their views at the Shanbaugh-Shea workshops, often in heated exchanges of opinion. Now surgeons are equally adept at either procedure as dictated by the disease process at hand.

In 1957, vestibular surgery was limited to the oval window labyrinthectomy, and later, transmastoid labyrinthectomy provided complete unilateral ablation.

Facial nerve surgery at this earlier time was limited to transmastoid decompression. It was believed that one should not incise the facial nerve sheath for fear of disturbing the endoneural fluid compartments. With increasing surgical exposures within the temporal bone we have learned that facial nerve decompression and mobilization from the geniculate ganglion and even more proximally, into the parotid gland, is possible, often without paresis of the facial nerve.

Glomus tumors of the temporal bone, while described earlier by Rosenwasser, were not clearly differentiated into glomus tympanicum or glomus jugulare, a distinction of great importance when surgical removal is entertained.

Transtemporal acoustic tumor surgery was in its infancy in the 1960s. Dr. William House of Los Angeles, California, was evolving the surgical approaches that we routinely use today. In these early days, operative morbidity and mortality were still high. Now mortality rates are less than 1% and postoperative cerebrospinal fluid leaks, meningitis, and facial paralysis are markedly reduced. The concepts of planned subtotal tumor removal, staged removal of large tumors, and leaving a minute fragment of tumor on the facial nerve to preserve function have all evolved. The routine use of facial nerve monitoring in acoustic tumor surgery as pioneered by Dr. Jack Kartush has revolutionized dissection and manipulation of the facial nerve during acoustic tumor surgery.

Cochlear implant surgery is now regularly performed upon the profoundly deafened individual. Surgery is performed as young as 1 year of age, and this age continues to become younger. The implant devices are multiple-channeled and reliable. Speech and language acquisition in these early implanted infants are most impressive.

Bone-anchored hearing systems (BAHA) pioneered in Sweden have assumed a useful place in hearing amplification. These devices were not available several decades ago.

Finally, mention must be made concerning temporal bone and cranial imaging techniques, now so crucial in the diagnosis of many otologic and neurotologic conditions. Prior to 1974, the only temporal bone imaging available were plain x-rays. To evaluate the posterior fossa and internal auditory canal, pantopaque had to be introduced into the lumbar subarachnoid space and with fluroscopic assistance guided into posterior cranial fossa.

In 1974, the EMI scan, the predecessor of the CT scan, was introduced. Early designs were crude—we now have elegant image capabilities of the temporal bone. However, even with the addition of contrast material, resolution for acoustic tumors is limited to those lesions larger than one centimeter.

However, in the early 1980s the MRI scan was introduced. Initially, this was not a great benefit without contrast. Soon, gadolinium was introduced to MRI imaging, and now allows the greatest resolution of even the smallest lesions, a truly invaluable evaluation tool for the inner ear and adjacent structures.

In summary, I congratulate most sincerely Dr. Babu and his collaborators as they present these most contemporary surgical and practical texts in the field of otology, neurotology, and skull base surgery. It is my hope that by highlighting (be it even so briefly) the state of our otologic subspecialty some 50 years ago, the reader will truly appreciate the progress and advances summarized in these volumes.

Malcolm D. Graham, MD
Department of Otolaryngology—
Head and Neck Surgery
Emory University, Atlanta, Georgia

Preface

The field of otology is evolving from the treatment of potential life-threatening infections over a century ago to now providing quality of life improvements by treating dizziness, improving hearing, and resecting tumors with less morbidity. The management of dizziness has improved with surgical options and experience with treatment of superior canal dehiscence. Success with cochlear implantation has become commonplace, and now temporal bone implants and middle ear implants are expanding the benefit received by those with hearing loss. Soon stem cell research and intratympanic therapy improvements may revolutionize inner ear pathology and its treatment. Improvements in microscopic and endoscopic dissection as well as intraoperative monitoring have reduced operative morbidity.

Despite these changes, many residents note that their otologic experience in the office and the operating room lacks modern updates, techniques, and management procedures. This book was developed with this in mind: to provide the practicing otolaryngologist, resident, and student with a diagnostic and management book describing the practical application of knowledge for patients suffering from otologic pathology. Our goal was to have the reader be able to use this book to capitalize on the breadth of experience and knowledge from experts in the field and apply their experience in an approach that would benefit them on a day-to-day manner.

Introduction

This book is designed for you! Whether a practicing otolaryngologist, ENT resident, medical student, physician assistant, nurse practitioner, or physical therapist dealing with dizziness, this book is for you. Otology as a branch of general otolaryngology deals with symptoms that are commonly seen in many practices such as hearing loss, balance issues and dizziness, cholesteatoma, and ear infections, and these topics are covered in great detail in this book.

Graduating residents seem to have less comfort with otologic procedures than in the past. Also, our own ENT residents and neurotology fellows continually ask for a recommendation for a concise book covering the disorders of the temporal bone that is up-to-date and clinically and surgically oriented. Thus, this book was created to attempt to improve residents' comfort with diseases and surgeries involving the temporal bone. With this in mind, a practical approach to the clinical management of diseases affecting the temporal bone was devised. It is the culmination of countless hours of hard work by numerous authors who are clinically as well as surgically experienced.

Covering the pertinent details for daily practice, this book discusses topics ranging from basic history and physical examination skills necessary in evaluating patients with dizziness to the surgical details of procedures involving the temporal bone. Clinical and surgical pearls abound in this text that all practitioners will find beneficial, from authors known for large clinical volume of experience and surgical acumen.

Chapters are organized in parts, starting with Part I, which covers audiologic and vestibular testing. Part II covers diseases affecting the external ear and middle ear. Part III discusses facial nerve testing in an in-depth yet pragmatic manner, with a chapter on facial nerve pathology as well. Part IV covers inner ear pathology, such as congenital hearing loss, dizziness, and specific diseases such as Ménière's disease, superior canal dehiscence, and benign positional vertigo. The final chapter is placed as an addendum, a surgical dissection guide or manual to allow readers to practice in the temporal bone laboratory.

The hope for this book is to provide an easy-to-understand format that blends the complexity of diseases of the temporal bone so that history, physical examination, testing and interpretation, and imaging can be combined in a practical way for all levels of expertise. The large clinical practice of the authors has created numerous teaching pearls that can be assimilated into the reader's practice, assisting them in daily rounds, patient care, and board preparation.

Acknowledgments

This book required numerous dedicated authors from around the country who devoted a great amount of time and effort to make this a success. It would not be possible without their guidance and assistance and I am deeply appreciative. I also would like to thank my gifted teachers, mentors, friends, and associates who have guided me throughout my medical journey, especially at Northeastern Ohio Universities College of Medicine (NEOUCOM), Henry Ford Health System, and the Michigan Ear Institute (MEI). My colleagues, office staff, and operating room personnel at MEI make it truly enjoyable to come to work and care for patients in a comfortable, caring, and educational manner. I thank them for this as they make it a joy to come to work every day.

I must acknowledge my parents and siblings for their continuous support. My parents (Lakshman and Renuka Babu) sacrificed immensely in order to provide the gift of opportunity through education for my siblings (Niharika Wunnava and Mayukh Babu) and myself. Their dedication has guided each of us to success with our careers and with our families. I would also like to extend my gratitude to my in-laws (Mark and Jan Crooks) for adding to my life and for their generous support.

Of course, I must thank my loving and extraordinary wife, Abbey, who provided support and guidance throughout this project. Even my three sons (Kavan, Kethan, and Karun) and daughter (Kareena) helped by asking when my "story was going to be done?"—thus making sure I would stay on task! I love my children for providing the fun, excitement, and laughter that shows us what makes life so enjoyable and extraordinary on a daily basis.

I would personally like to extend sincere thanks to Cheryl Thrushman at Providence Hospital and Alison Devine at MEI. Their tireless effort and early morning meetings allowed many of the images and text to be created for the book. Their attention to detail and prompt response on project deadlines allowed things to be done in a timely fashion.

Contributors

Nouha Alammar, DO
Henry Ford Macomb Hospital, MI
Otolaryngology & Facial Plastic Surgery Residency
Post Graduate Year 5 (PGY-5)
Michigan State College of Osteopathic Medicine, 2004
Chapter 7

Patrick Antonelli, MD, FACS
George T. Singleton Professor and Chair
University of Florida Deptartment of Otolaryngology
Chapter 5

Gregory J. Artz, MD
Assistant Professor
Department of Otolaryngology—Head and Neck Surgery
Division of Neurotology/Skull Base Surgery
Thomas Jefferson University
Philadelphia, Pennsylvania
Chapter 4

Seilesh Babu, MD
Division of Otology/Neurotology/Skull Base Surgery
Michigan Ear Institute
Farmington Hills, Michigan
Assistant Professor of Otolaryngology
Wayne State University
Detroit, Michigan
Chapters 6, 7, 12, 14, 15, and 23

Ben Balough
Captain, Medical Corps, USN
Naval Medical Center San Diego
Associate Professor of Surgery
Uniformed Services University of the Health Sciences
Chapter 20

Dennis Bojrab
Michigan Ear Institute
Chief, Dept. of Otolaryngology
Wm Beaumont Hospital
Chief, Department of Skull Base Surgery
Providence Hospital
Clinical Professor, Department of Otolaryngology and Neurosurgery
Wayne State University
Chapter 8

Brian Duff, MD
Chief, Deptartment of Otolaryngology
Rhode Island Hospital/Nasbro Children's Hospital
Associate Professor, Warren G. Alpert School of Medicine
Brown University
Chapter 6

Gerard J. Gianoli, MD, FACS
Vice President, The Ear and Balance Institute,
Baton Rouge, Louisiana
Clinical Associate Professor, Dept. of Otolaryngology
and Dept. of Pediatrics, Tulane University School of Medicine
New Orleans, Louisiana
Chapters 21 and 22

Jewel Greywoode, MD
Chief Resident
Otolaryngology–Head and Neck Surgery
Thomas Jefferson University
Philadelphia, Pennsylvania
Chapter 4

Yoav Hahn, MD
Fellow, Otology, Neurotology, Skull Base Surgery
Michigan Ear Institute
Chapter 9

David Healy, Jr., MD
CDR MC USN
Department of Otolaryngology
Tripler Army Medical Center
Honolulu, Hawaii
Chapter 20

Michael Hoa, MD
Chief Resident
Department of Otolaryngology
Wayne State University School of Medicine
Chapter 16

Michael Hoffer, MD
Department of Otolaryngology
Naval Medical Center
San Diego, California
Chapter 20

Jack Kartush, MD
President—Michigan Ear Institute
Clinical Professor—Wayne State University, Dept. of Otolaryngology
Chief Medical Officer—Biotronic NeuroNetwork
Chapter 9

Matthew Kircher, MD
Neurotology Fellow
Michigan Ear Institute
Chapter 10

Michael LaRouere, MD
Attending Neurotologist Michigan Ear Institute
Chair, Department of Neurotology, Providence Hospital
Clinical Associate Professor, Wayne State University
Chapter 19

Chris Linstrom, MD
Professor of Otolaryngology—Head and Neck Surgery
Professor of Neurological Surgery
The New York Medical College
Valhalla, New York
Surgeon Director, Otology and Neurotology
The New York Eye & Ear Infirmary
New York, New York
Adjunct Professor of Audiology
The Graduate Center/ Health Sciences Doctoral Program
City University of the City of New York
New York, New York
Chapters 11 and 13

Paulette McDonald, MA
Director of Audiology
Michigan Ear Institute
Chapter 15

William McFeely, Jr., MD
President, North Alabama ENT Associates, PC
Staff Surgeon, Huntsville Hospital
Staff Surgeon, Crestwood Hospital
Huntsville, Alabama
Chapter 1

Raj Murali, MD, FRCSE, FACS, FRCSC
Professor and Chairman
Department of Neurosurgery
The New York Medical College,
Valhalla, New York
Chapter 11

Vincent Ostrowski, MD
Midwest Ear Institute
Indianapolis, Indiana
Chapter 3

Aftab Patni, MD, FACS
The Ear, Nose, Throat, and Plastic Surgery Associates
Medical Director, Vestibular Rehabilitation Center at Florida Hospital
Winter Park, Florida
Chapter 10

Travis Pfannenstiel, MD
Otology & Neurotology Section Chief
Department of Otolaryngology
San Antonio Military Medical Center
Ft Sam Houston, Texas
Assistant Professor of Surgery
F. Edward Hébert School of Medicine
Uniformed Services University of the Health Sciences
Bethesda, Maryland
Chapter 8

Sandra Porps
Doctor of Audiology
Clinical Audiologist at the Michigan Ear Institute

Certificate of Clinical Competence in Audiology
Chapter 2

Howard Sander, MD
Chairman of Neurology Division
New York University
New York, New York
Chapter 12

Eric Sargent, MD, FACS
Attending Physician, Michigan Ear Institute
Clinical Associate Professor, Wayne State University School of Medicine
Department of Otolaryngology—Head and Neck Surgery
Chapters 15 and 18

Dan Sdrulla, MD, PhD
Neurotology Fellow
Michigan Ear Institute
Chapter 14

Robert Standring, MD
Henry Ford Health System
Chapter 6

Eloy Villasuso III, MD
Professional Staff
Department of Otolaryngology
Otology, Neurotology & Skull Base Surgery
Cleveland Clinic Florida
Weston, Florida
Chapter 17

Sean Wise, MD
Neurotology Fellow
Michigan Ear Institute
Chapter 17

John Zappia, MD
Michigan Ear Institute
Chapters 2 and 16

This book is dedicated to the mentors and teachers that have come before us and led the way to the formation of the Michigan Ear Institute, especially Dr. T. Manford McGee and Dr. Malcolm Graham. They have provided insight and experience that has been passed down to training otologists for decades. Dr. McGee completed tens of thousands of stapedectomies, providing an immense knowledge base about otosclerosis and its surgical treatments. Dr. Graham, having been with the great Drs. William House and Howard House in Los Angeles, California, for many years, brought many of the teachings from the House Ear Institute to the Midwest. Here, it continued to be fostered, cultivated, and expanded.

Much of our current success can be directly attributed to these great doctors and their wonderful contributions to the field of otology and skull base surgery, which has been passed on from one generation to the next with participation in preceptorships and fellowships.

All of us in our current field owe our otologic forefathers a great deal of gratitude for their exquisite teachings and hope that we too will learn the ability to teach effectively and to share experiences with others in a similar fashion, so as to continue to share and expand on our knowledge base for the betterment of patient care.

PART I

Evaluating Patients with Otologic Disease

CHAPTER 1

History and Physical: Dizzy Evaluation

William McFeely, Jr.

INTRODUCTION

Evaluation of the dizzy patient presents a diagnostic challenge. The physician must take an accurate history, and perform a thorough detailed examination. To facilitate this, the physician must demonstrate a systematic approach. After executing a careful history and physical examination, an appropriate diagnosis may be made in the majority of dizzy patients. The history alone is often very suggestive of a diagnosis. Expensive laboratory, radiographic, and other testing frequently can be avoided. Specific symptoms guide the examination and additional workup as necessary.

OBTAINING THE DIZZINESS HISTORY

Patients with dizziness should be asked to fill out a dizziness questionnaire prior to the evaluation. An example of a questionnaire used by some otologists is demonstrated in Table 1–1. The questionnaire preferably is done at home with no time restraints; it allows the patient to begin to characterize their symptoms in an orderly fashion. The questionnaire itself includes many categories: chief complaint, history of present illness, past medical history, past surgical history, medications, allergies, family history, social history, and review of systems. As noted by Rubin[1] and Singleton,[2] there is a very broad differential diagnosis with respect to the dizzy patient. The questionnaire can help greatly in terms of narrowing down this differential to a working diagnosis.

The first step in taking the history is to understand what the patient means by "dizziness." Dizziness may represent a variety of feelings. It is critical that the otologist understands the exact sensation that the patient is experiencing. It is best to ask the patient what is meant by dizziness, without actually using that specific term. Table 1–2 outlines many of the common responses. Based on the terminology used, the physician can classify the sensation. Once the sensation has been described, it must then be further characterized. It is important to determine if the dizziness is episodic (ie, comes in attacks or spells), or constant. Table 1–3 shows how to characterize dizziness in more detail. It is important to learn about the very first spell, and determine whether that spell was different than symptoms currently being experienced. Timing, duration, severity, frequency, alleviating factors, exacerbating factors, and associated symptoms must be elicited.

ASSOCIATED SYMPTOMS

After characterizing what a patient means by the word dizziness, it is necessary to identify any associated symptoms. Sensations that began at the same time as the dizziness need to be investigated. These associated symptoms are either synchronous with the spell, asynchronous with the spell, or continuous while the dizziness occurs. The associated symptoms must be differentiated as either otologic (ear) or nonotologic (other). Although it might be obvious that patients with presumed inner ear malfunction have ear symptoms, nonotologic associated symptoms must not be overlooked. They frequently suggest a particular diagnosis.

Table 1–1. History and Dizziness Intake Questionnaire

I. What best describes your dizziness? Put an X in the appropriate box.

YES	NO	
☐	☐	1. Sensation that you are turning or spinning inside
☐	☐	2. Visual blurring or jumping with focusing problems during head motion.
☐	☐	3. Objects spin or whirl around you with your eyes opened.
☐	☐	4. Objects spin or whirl around you with your eyes closed.
☐	☐	5. Loss of balance when walking:
☐	☐	a. Fall to right
☐	☐	b. Fall to left
☐	☐	6. Tendency to fall:
☐	☐	a. To the right?
☐	☐	b. To the left?
☐	☐	c. Fall Forward?
☐	☐	d. Fall Backward?
☐	☐	7. Spinning / turning sensation when:
☐	☐	a. Lie Down?
☐	☐	b. Roll to right?
☐	☐	c. Roll to left?
☐	☐	d. When look down or bend over?
☐	☐	8. Swimming sensation in your head.
☐	☐	9. Spinning sensation in your head.
☐	☐	10. Lightheadedness or faint feeling.
☐	☐	11. Loss of equilibrium, imbalance, or unsteadiness.
☐	☐	12. Blacking out or actual fainting.
☐	☐	13. Loss of consciousness, or passing out.
☐	☐	14. Headache, head pressure, eye pressure.
☐	☐	15. Nausea with or without vomiting.

II. Please check either YES or NO and fill in the boxes.

YES	NO	
☐	☐	1. My dizziness is constant.
☐	☐	2. My dizziness comes in attacks or spells
☐	☐	3. When did dizziness first happen?
☐	☐	4. If in attacks, how often do they happen?
☐	☐	5. If in attacks, how long do they last?
☐	☐	6. Do you have any warning that the attack is about to begin?
☐	☐	7. Are you completely free of dizziness in between attacks?
☐	☐	8. Does dizziness occur only with certain body positions?
☐	☐	9. Do you have trouble walking in the dark?
☐	☐	10. When you are dizzy, do you have to hold onto something when standing?
☐	☐	11. Do you know of any possible cause or trigger of your dizziness?
☐	☐	12. What triggers your dizziness?
☐	☐	13. Does anything stop the dizziness or make it better?
☐	☐	14. What makes your dizziness worse?
☐	☐	15. Were you exposed to any irritating chemicals, fumes at the onset of dizziness?
☐	☐	16. Do you have any allergies to medications?
☐	☐	17. Did you ever injure your head severely?
☐	☐	18. Do you take any medications regularly? If so, what are they?
☐	☐	19. Do you use tobacco in any form? How much
☐	☐	20. Do you use alcohol? How much?
☐	☐	21. How many cups of coffee, tea, or colas do you drink each day?
☐	☐	22. Have you ever had ear surgery?

Table 1–1. *continued*

III. Do you have any of the following ear symptoms? Put an X in the appropriate box, and circle ear					
YES	NO				
☐	☐	1. Difficulty in hearing?	Both ears	Right	Left
☐	☐	2. When did this hearing problem start?	Both ears	Right	Left
☐	☐	3. Is it changing? Is it getting better or worse?	Both ears	Right	Left
☐	☐	4. Does your hearing fluctuate or go up and down?	Both ears	Right	Left
☐	☐	5. Do you wear hearing aids	Both ears	Right	Left
☐	☐	6. Noise in your ears?	Both ears	Right	Left
☐	☐	7. Describe the noise?	Both ears	Right	Left
☐	☐	8. Does ear noise change with the dizzy spell? How?	Both ears	Right	Left
☐	☐	9. Ear fullness or stuffiness?	Both ears	Right	Left
☐	☐	10. Does this change during the dizzy spell?	Both ears	Right	Left
☐	☐	11. Pain in your ears?	Both ears	Right	Left
☐	☐	12. Drainage from your ears?	Both ears	Right	Left
☐	☐	13. Distortion of sound?	Both ears	Right	Left
☐	☐	14. Sensitivity to sound?	Both ears	Right	Left
☐	☐	15. Fluttering sound in ears?	Both ears	Right	Left
☐	☐	16. Pulsing sound in ears?	Both ears	Right	Left

IV. Have you ever experienced any of the following symptoms? Put an X in the appropriate box, and circle if constant or if in episodes.				
YES	NO			
☐	☐	1. Double vision:	Constant	In Episodes
☐	☐	2. Spots before the eyes:	Constant	In Episodes
☐	☐	3. Cloudiness of vision:	Constant	In Episodes
☐	☐	4. Numbness:	Constant	In Episodes
☐	☐	5. Blurred vision or blindness:	Constant	In Episodes
☐	☐	6. Weakness or clumsiness:	Constant	In Episodes
☐	☐	7. Difficulty with speech:	Constant	In Episodes
☐	☐	8. Difficulty with swallowing:	Constant	In Episodes
☐	☐	9. Tingling around the mouth:	Constant	In Episodes
☐	☐	10. Visual distortion with head motion:	Constant	In Episodes

V. Please check either YES or NO in the appropriate box.		
YES	NO	
☐	☐	1. Do you get dizzy after exertion or working too hard?
☐	☐	2. Did you get new glasses recently?
☐	☐	3. Do you tend to get upset or anxious easily?
☐	☐	4. Do you get dizzy when you have not eaten for a long time?
☐	☐	5. Is your dizziness connected with your menstrual period?
☐	☐	6. Have you ever had a severe neck injury?
☐	☐	7. Are you a diabetic?
☐	☐	8. Do you have high or low blood pressure?
☐	☐	9. Do you have a heart condition?
☐	☐	10. Did you recently start a new diet?
☐	☐	11. Did you recently start a new medicine?

Table 1–2. Characterizing Dizziness

Medical Term	Self-Description
Dizziness	Spatial disorientation
Vertigo	Sensation of movement, motion, or rotation
Disequilibrium	Off balance, imbalance, giddiness
Oscillopsia	Difficulty walking or riding, horizon moving, unable to focus on objects
Physiologic dizziness	Motion sickness, space sickness, height vertigo, blacking out, constant motion sensation after travel
Pre-syncope	Lightheadedness or almost fainting, hyperventilation
Psychophysiologic dizziness	Panic attacks, hyperventilation, phobias, anxious
Ocular dizziness	Trouble focusing eyes, vision distortion
Multisensory dizziness	Imbalance, unsteadiness, off-balance feeling
Central dizziness	Spinning sensation inside the head

Table 1–3. Classifying the Dizziness Sensation

Type of Spells	One Type of Feeling, Multiple Sensations
Initial spell	Length, timing, nature of spell
Last spell	Length, timing, nature of spell
Frequency of spells	Number of times per day, week, month, or year
Duration of spell	Seconds, minutes, hours, days, weeks or longer
Alleviating factors	Change in position, medications, relation to meals
Exacerbating factors	Causal event, position change, exertion, weather
Associated symptoms	Nausea and vomiting, ear fullness, hearing loss, tinnitus, sensation change, weakness, syncope, lightheadedness, headaches, heart racing

As depicted in Table 1–4, otologic associated symptoms include hearing loss, tinnitus, aural fullness, otalgia, otorrhea, hyperacusis, and diplacusis (the perception of a single auditory stimulus as two separate sounds). Each of these may be characterized more completely in terms of quality, timing, and duration. Documentation must also be made as to whether one or both ears are involved. Subclassification can lead toward the correct diagnosis in many instances. Most vestibular sources of dizziness will manifest with one or more of these.

Table 1–4. Otologic Associated Symptoms

Tinnitus	Intermittent, constant, pulsing
Hearing loss	Progressive, sudden, fluctuating
Aural fullness	Pressure, popping
Otalgia	Quality, timing, duration, severity
Otorrhea	Waxy, clear, or purulent drainage
Hyperacusis	Hypersensitivity or pain with hearing
Dyplacusis	Distortion or double-sound with hearing

Neurologic Associated Symptoms

Specific neurologic symptoms may be related to an abnormality within the central or peripheral nervous systems. Symptoms may include headache, gait ataxia, visual disturbances (such as blurring or photophobia), and change in nerve function. As seen in Table 1–5, various symptoms are associated with specific neurologic abnormalities.

Headaches are very important to consider in the evaluation of the dizzy patient. In those patients with migraines, there is a significant incidence of migraine-associated dizziness. Migraines may occur with or without a visual, gustatory or auditory aura; they frequently are associated with photophobia. Dizziness can occur as part of the aura. Migraine headaches are not always temporally related to the dizziness. According to Dieterich and Brandt[3] migraine patients may experience both true spinning vertigo and episodic, nonvertiginous dizziness with imbalance.

Migraine-associated vertigo can occur in spells, and is sometimes triggered by a position change. Benign positional vertigo of childhood is commonly

Table 1–5. Neurologic Associated Symptoms with Dizziness

Visual disturbances, diplopia, photophobia
Headaches, migraines, head pressure
Paresis, paralysis, numbness, hemiparesis
Taste distortion, smell distortion
Tremors, shaking, gait ataxia
Concentration or memory problems
Dysphagia, dysphonia, dysarthria
Urinary or bowel incontinence
Loss of consciousness
Cranial nerve palsy
Neck stiffness or pain

thought to be linked to migraines. As noted by Eggers,[4] migraine-related vertigo has been statistically related to other etiologies which themselves cause dizziness: benign paroxysmal positional vertigo (BPPV), Ménière's disease, orthostatic hypotension, and anxiety disorders. Physicians should keep these in mind when treating a patient with both headaches and dizziness.

When a dizzy patient describes associated neurologic symptoms, consideration should be given towards radiographic imaging. Cranial nerve abnormalities, decrease in sensation and strength, or seizure activity may suggest a defect within the cortex or brain stem. Visual dysfunction such as diplopia, visual field defects, and abducens paralysis may suggest a diagnosis of pseudotumor cerebri (benign intracranial hypertension). Vague feelings of blacking out during dizzy episodes or confusion afterward may indicate underlying seizures. Other symptoms such as auditory hallucinations, automatisms, and absences suggest temporal lobe epilepsy. Dizziness is a common initial symptom in those with multiple sclerosis or other central degenerative diseases. Selective scanning with high resolution computed tomography (CT) scanning with contrast or enhanced magnetic resonance imaging (MRI) typically is diagnostic for mass lesions as well as other central pathology. The otologist should have a low threshold with respect to ordering these tests in certain patients.

Psychiatric Associated Symptoms

People with psychophysiologic dizziness often describe a relatively constant disequilibrium. As noted by Clark et al[5] and Furman and Jacob,[6] the dizzy sensation is most often not usually described as spinning quality vertigo; it frequently occurs in those who are anxious or phobic. It is often a diagnosis of exclusion once other diagnostic possibilities have been ruled out. Chronic or repeated episodes of dizziness from any cause can lead to a secondary anxiety or depression disorder. Sklare et al[7] have noted the association of panic disorder and dizziness. Symptoms that suggest psychiatric illness include: depression, anxious feeling, pallor, dyspnea, hot flashes or chills, excessive sweating, frequent diarrhea, agitation, restlessness, irritability, a spacey feeling, and the sensation of brain fogginess. Referral for psychological counseling, behavioral therapy and possibly vestibular rehabilitation may be beneficial.

As documented by Evans,[8] hyperventilation syndrome produces a variety of somatic symptoms which are induced by physiologically inappropriate hyperventilation. Dizziness, faint feeling, or lightheadedness symptoms can usually be reproduced with voluntary hyperventilation in the physician's office. Voluntary hyperventilation should thus be attempted in those with possible psychiatric symptoms or anxiety. Reassurance and education are helpful treatment options. Other options could include: pharmaceutical management, biofeedback, breathing exercises, and ultimately psychiatric referral may be necessary.

Autonomic Associated Symptoms

As noted by Nakagawa et al,[9] disturbance of the autonomic nervous system (dysautonomia) is associated with dizziness and balance problems. Vertigo and unsteadiness may be described by those with dysautonomia. Dizziness is often noted upon rapid changes from sitting or supine to upright. Orthostatic (or postural) hypotension is defined as a drop in systolic or diastolic blood pressure by 20 mm Hg after standing for 60 seconds. This disorder is very common in elderly patients that are on numerous medications for a variety of medical conditions. It sometimes is caused by a circulatory disturbance, fluid imbalance, or medication side effect.

There are some forms of autonomic dysregulation that demonstrate persistent or recurrent disequilibrium (not vertigo) or a foggy headed sensation. Staab and Ruckenstein[10] report that this disorder is frequently a diagnosis of exclusion. Referral to an autonomic specialist may be reasonable in many cases. Tilt table and hyperventilation tests may be used to evaluate for dysautonomia.

Other Associated Symptoms

Many other metabolic or systemic disorders can be associated with dizziness. Symptoms to look for include: palpitations, chest discomfort, breathing problems, temperature intolerance, fever, chills, unexplained change in weight, nausea or vomiting, and sinus congestion or drainage. These symptoms can suggest myriad underlying conditions. Examples of these include: cardiac rhythm problems, hypoglycemia, hyperglycemia, hypotension, hypertension, hypothyroidism, hyperthyroidism, immunologic abnormalities, allergic problems, and asthma.

Infectious diseases including Lyme disease and syphilis have a variety of consequences on the human body. The doctor treating dizzy patients must consider all these. A cardiac source of dizziness should be suspected when there is a lightheaded or faint feeing described. Rhythm abnormalities can produce paroxysmal collapses and dizziness. Cardiac evaluation should be encouraged in those with suspicious heart symptoms. Medications frequently produce the side effect of dizziness. Nonvertiginous dizziness and imbalance is the most common presentation of this. The physician should always inquire about timing of dizziness relative to medication dosing; care should be taken to identify new medications that were started around the time of dizziness onset.

OFFICE EXAMINATION OF THE DIZZY PATIENT

Although the history alone may suggest a possible diagnosis, confirmation with office examination typically is necessary. A thorough head and neck as well as neurotologic examination is critical. This should include examination of the ears with otoscopy; it may demonstrate an obvious problem such as middle ear effusion or cholesteatoma. One should also carefully observe for the presence of spontaneous, gaze-evoked, or headshake-evoked nystagmus. Systematic assessment of posture and gait is then performed. A considerable amount of information can obtained through clinical posture and gait testing. Although many of these clinical balance tests are nonspecific, they can indicate an underlying vestibular abnormality. Most of these tests can be performed in the office without any expensive equipment. Positional testing is also a useful part of the examination that frequently leads to a diagnosis. The thorough physician incorporates additional eye movement and clinical cerebellar examinations to help clarify the underlying pathology.

Postural and gait tests are based on a simple principle. There are three main peripheral components (or inputs) to balance: labyrinthine, visual, and proprioceptive. When one or more are removed, the other(s) must be relied on to maintain equilibrium. The brain must also analyze all the information provided through peripheral inputs. Clinical office-based tests cannot measure the separate relative value of vision or proprioception alone, but can give some idea if there is a problem with either of these peripheral components. Ataxia may be seen with underlying central nervous system abnormalities. Abnormal central processing leads to poor performance on all of the clinical posture and gait tests. There are a variety of very useful clinical tests to evaluate gait and posture as shown in Table 1–6.

Gait Testing

Observation of ambulation or simple gait is the least complicated of all posture and gait tests to perform. This can be done upon arrival of the patient to the office, or on the way back to an exam room. A keen physician may learn a great deal about the dizzy patient before taking the history. Gait should be reassessed during the actual examination as well to assess for changes. An inconsistency between the initial entrance gait and ensuing reevaluation could indicate malingering or nonorganic pathology.

Table 1–6. Office Examination of Gait, Posture, and Positioning

Simple walking gait
Tandem gait
Figure of eight tandem gait
Classic Romberg
Quix gait testing
Sharpened Romberg
Turning gait testing
Unterberger (Fukuda) stepping test
Sensory conflict postural testing
Orthostatic testing
Potentiated Valsalva maneuver
Dix-Hallpike maneuver

Patient ambulation during simple gait must be carefully observed. Common abnormalities include: broad-based gait, shuffling, veering, and ataxia. It should be noted if the patient requires assistance to ambulate, stand, or transfer. Documentation is needed when the subject requires a walker, cane, or person in order to ambulate. Requiring frequent touch during ambulation often indicates vestibular weakness. An ataxic or broad-based gait frequently implies an underlying central disorder. Striking objects or walls could also indicate a primary visual or somatosensory disturbance such as neuropathy. Exaggerated dizziness could indicate malingering, especially if inconsistency is noted.

Having the patient close the eyes, and walk in a straight line may also assess gait. A cerebellar disorder or vestibular weakness may produce veering towards the affected side. Cerebellar abnormalities can sometimes lead to the feet advancing while the torso does not. Additional investigation of the cerebellum can be done using a variety of coordination tests. With asynergia testing, the subject stands upright with the eyes closed, and then bends over backwards. The normal patient will flex the knees to gain postural control. Cerebellar dysfunction is associated with minimal or no knee flexion. According to Catena et al,[11] a continuous sequential question and answer task while walking is a good way to evaluate for the effect of concussion and traumatic brain injury. Patients with a history of traumatic brain injury usually demonstrate instability during the question and answer assignment.

Tandem gait testing is an easily performed test to assess cerebellar function. Stepping one foot in front of the other (in tandem) with the eyes open allows for evaluation of cerebellar function because vision compensates for vestibular and proprioceptive weakness. An acute vestibular injury or weakness, however, can affect the results. Eyes-closed tandem gait provides a better evaluation of vestibular function alone. This is especially true when cerebellar and proprioceptive components are intact. If abnormal, either of these inputs can affect results. Patients with acute or longstanding vestibular weakness typically perform poorly on this test.

The tandem gait test is quite nonspecific and frequently nonlocalizing; many feel that falling to one particular side does not consistently indicate the side of weakness. Walking on a rail that is raised a few inches off the ground can increase test sensitivity. The test may be somewhat nonspecific in that some normal individuals may have difficulty with this as well.

Figure of eight tandem gait walking is another variation that requires functioning cerebellar and vestibulospinal systems. The vestibulospinal system involves complex reflexes that continuously regulate muscle tone to preserve stability. Subjects with vestibular weakness frequently fail this test.

The standard Romberg test is a test of both proprioception and vestibular components. The subject must stand with both feet close together with the arms at the sides or folded in front. Having the arms extended can sometimes help maintain balance (ie, like a balancing pole of a circus entertainer). The physician first observes with the eyes open, and subsequently with the eyes closed. The patient attempts to maintain balance. The clinician or other office personnel must be ready to prevent potential injury from a fall. Those with an acute peripheral vestibular injury will most often veer toward the side of the weakness. Chronic vestibular weakness with partial compensation may or may not produce abnormalities on this test.

As described by Hart,[12] the Quix test is similar to the standard Romberg test. With feet together, the subject points at the physician with arms extended at shoulder level. This is again done with eyes open and then closed. Listing or veering to one side indicates an underlying vestibular problem. As with the original Romberg test, it is relatively nonspecific. Some patients are able to use the extended arms to help maintain balance, by this means passing the test.

The sharpened or tandem Romberg test is a variation of the original standard test. The only difference is that the feet are placed with one directly in front of the other in tandem fashion. Again vision is allowed in the beginning, and consequently excluded for at least 10 seconds. Many older and very obese patients may not be able to perform this test because of difficulty maintaining the necessary stance. All variations of the Romberg test examine proprioception and the vestibulospinal system to some degree. Most authors feel that the sharpened test may be a more sensitive indicator of vestibular impairment specifically.

According to Singleton,[2] the turning test is another good way to assess gait. With the eyes closed, the subject is asked to walk straight, and then turn quickly 180 degrees to the right or left. He or she then stops at a point of attention. Substantial sway or listing signifies a positive test. Patients tend to veer or fall toward the weak vestibular side. Many believe that this test can demonstrate the side of the weakness, and can help diagnose an inner ear fluid leak (perilymph fistula).

Tests of Posture

The Unterberger postural test is commonly performed to assess posture. Fukuda later modified it as a specialized stepping test. The patient must march in place with the arms extended straight out at shoulder level. Just as with the Romberg test, it is done initially with eyes open, then with eyes closed. At least 50 steps are required to make a true evaluation. As with other balance tests, the clinician should be nearby to make sure that the subject does not fall. Normal patients remain consistently in place, go forward no more than 50 cm, and turn less than 30 degrees of midline. If the patient drifts outside of the normal ranges, this test is considered positive; it typically indicates unilateral or bilateral vestibular weakness. Typically, the patient gradually marches toward the side of the greater vestibular weakness. One study by Moffat et al[13] found that 71% of patients with an acoustic neuroma had a positive test result. The vast majority of those undergoing this test are not aware of movement from the starting position, although some might try to compensate for it when it is noted. Patients must not be allowed to open their eyes during the test as this will affect results. The amount of stray can be quite dramatic and patients and family members are often astonished by the amount of stray noted.

Platform posturography certainly would be considered to be one of the most valuable tools to a doctor treating dizzy patients. When this expensive equipment is unavailable, sensory conflict posture tests (aka "poor man's posturography" or foam and dome testing) may be utilized. These tests can be performed in clinic during the initial examination, as the equipment required is minimal. The test involves six test conditions; they mimic those done during platform posturography sensory organization testing. For all conditions, the patient is instructed to maintain stability. The first three test conditions are performed on a hard level surface whereas conditions four through six are done with the subject standing on a thick foam surface. The foam prevents proprioceptive clues from the joints, and increases resting body sway. The eyes are open during conditions one and three, closed on conditions two and four, and finally vision is confused on conditions three and six. A visual conflict dome can be constructed out of a paper lantern that surrounds the head. This lantern produces abnormal visual clues, and confuses vision during conditions three and six. When taken together, these six conditions help to discover the source of imbalance. The tests helps clarify which of the three peripheral components (visual, vestibular, and proprioceptive) are malfunctioning.

Normal subjects will have little difficulty during any of the six test conditions. As noted by Gianoli et al,[14] malingering patients typically have more difficulty with the easiest test conditions (one and four) since they would rather not fall when they cannot see. Condition number two is essentially the standard Romberg test. Sensory conflict posture testing is felt to be a practical alternative to formal platform posturography for those that do not have easy access to it. There is little doubt that computerized dynamic platform posturography testing can objectively assess balance during a variety of conditions; objective deficit quantification is possible. Results over time are frequently used by physicians, physical therapists, and insurance companies to track response to vestibular rehabilitation physical therapy or other forms of therapy.

A rapid change in body posture or position may impact blood pressure. Orthostatic hypo- or hypertension may be the principal source of a subject's imbalance, particularly in the elderly population. It is usually worth checking orthostatic blood pressure and pulse on all patients with complaints of unsteadiness and/or presyncope (sensation of fainting or loss of consciousness). Presyncope can also be due to etiologies such as metabolic disorders such as hypoglycemia or possibly cerebral ischemia. Orthostatic blood pressure readings are typically taken first while supine, then while standing. Orthostatic hypotension is defined as drop of at least 20 mm Hg systolic or diastolic blood pressure and a simultaneous rise in pulse. The patient should be asked if the dizziness experienced during orthostatic testing matches the dizziness noted subjectively at home. Cardiology referral is usually indicated if blood pressure readings change dramatically. Dysautonomia must also be considered.

According to Benarroch et al,[15] the potentiated Valsalva maneuver represents another postural test that can confirm presyncope or faint feeling. The patient is asked to squat for approximately 30 seconds, and then rapidly stand while straining into a closed glottis. Alternatively, the patient could blow air into a sphygmomanometer at 40 mm Hg for 15 seconds instead of straining into the closed glottis. A faint feeling may be noted which correlates to the patient's usual subjective dizziness sensation. The test produces a reduction of venous blood return to the heart; it may further help categorize dizziness. Cardiology referral may also be helpful in this instance.

Dix-Hallpike Positioning Test

Positional testing is useful portion of the office exam. As originally described by Dix and Hallpike,[16] positional testing can confirm a diagnosis of BPPV (benign paroxysmal positional vertigo). Symptoms include vertigo with change in head position, lightheadedness, imbalance, and nausea.

During the Dix-Hallpike test, the subject is brought rapidly from a sitting to a supine position, with the head turned 45 degrees to one side and extended approximately 20 degrees backward. A burst of rotary nystagmus is classically noted after a brief delay that is geotropically rotational. It will typically fatigue out within a few minutes or less. Once supine, the eyes are usually observed for about 30 to 45 seconds. If no gross nystagmus is observed on one side, the other side is tested with the opposite ear going toward the floor. Sensitivity of the Dix-Hallpike maneuver can be increased with the regular use of Frenzel lenses. These allow for more accurate visualization of subtle eye movements.

Anterior-canal BPPV nystagmus, which is rare, is rotary, with its vertical component beating downward. With horizontal-canal involvement, nystagmus is ageotropic.

Other diagnoses involving the labyrinth can also be made based on specific eye movements during positional testing. Atypical, long-lasting, or otherwise abnormal eye movements during testing might indicate the need for a more complete examination of the vestibular system. Some of these findings suggest the possibility of central pathology. Electronystagmography and/or rotary chair testing might be clinically warranted in these cases.

Additional Vestibular, Cerebellar, and Miscellaneous Testing

Eye movements must be assessed during the examination of the dizzy patient. Careful observation can distinguish between a peripheral or central source for the symptoms. Spontaneous nystagmus, gaze-evoked nystagmus, headshake-evoked nystagmus, smooth pursuit testing, and saccade testing all are critical portions of the otology exam. Cerebellar limb tests can rule out a cerebellar source. Miscellaneous tests include the aural pressure and sound tests; these can indicate specific unusual abnormalities within the temporal bone itself.

Asking a patient to fix the gaze on a specific target allows for the identification of spontaneous nystagmus. As with other eye examinations, the application of Frenzel lenses can augment the sensitivity of this evaluation. Visual acuity also can affect all eye exam results. The normal patient shows no excessive saccadic movement or nystagmus when asked to perform target fixation. A pendular type of nystagmus usually is due to a congenital central source. Direction-changing nystagmus also typically is consistent with a central source. On the other hand, a jerking direction-fixed nystagmus most often occurs with a peripheral abnormality.

When a subject holds an eccentric gaze about 30 degrees for 10 seconds in both the horizontal and vertical planes, an assessment can be made for gaze-evoked nystagmus. Many normal individuals have a mild nystagmus at end gaze that is physiologic. Most normal patients show little or no nystagmus at all. A jerking nystagmus in the direction of gaze typically indicates a central phenomenon. Some common causes of this are medications, drugs that can have an effect on the flocculus in particular. Lateral gaze down-beating nystagmus often indicates a midline cerebellar problem, or sometimes underlying Arnold Chiari malformation.

The examiner should test for eye pursuit by asking the patient to follow a finger through a 60 degree arc in both the horizontal and vertical planes. The normal subject demonstrates smooth pursuit with the eyes. Irregular, sporadic tracking can be due to a number of sources including medication effect and level of alertness. Elderly people often show irregular pursuit primarily due to advancing age. A saccadic pursuit can indicate a central process involving brainstem, cerebellum, or other areas in the brain such as the parietal lobe.

To assess for saccades, the patient is asked to alternate gaze between two fixed points (typically the examiner's fingers). The normal response is an accurate and rapid eye movement with a conjugate appearance. Disconjugate, slow, or late saccades indicate a central abnormality within the brainstem or sometimes the frontal lobe. Parkinson's patients often fail on saccade testing. Undershooting or overshooting the target consistently also is consistent with a central source in the cerebellum or brainstem.

Another way to differentiate between central and peripheral pathology is the headshake test. The subject is asked to shake the head for 20 seconds in both the horizontal and vertical planes. The examiner can do the shaking for the patient if he or she is unable to do it at about 2 Hz. The normal response to this test is no obvious nystagmus. Vertical nystagmus typically points to a central source. Unidirectional nystagmus in the plane of the headshake implies a peripheral source. The nystagmus observed is frequently opposite to the affected peripheral system; this is not always the case in Ménière's disease, however.

A brief check of cerebellar limb tests is usually worthwhile when examining the dizzy patient. In a span of less than a minute, the practitioner can clinically rule out a cerebellar source for dizziness. Commonly employed tests include finger-to-nose, rapid alternating movements, and heel-to-shin. Inaccurate movements with dysdiadochokinesia or dysmetria typically reflect underlying cerebellar weakness or dysfunction.

Other miscellaneous tests include aural pressure and sound testing. By stimulating the ear with a positive pressure, strong vibration or loud sound, a few specific abnormalities in the ear can be demonstrated. A horizontal nystagmus can be consistent with a leakage of inner ear fluid, or perilymph fistula. Vertical nystagmus has been seen in those with an anatomical dehiscence of the superior semicircular canal.

CONCLUSIONS

A carefully obtained medical history is most important when evaluating a dizzy patient. Many clues about the underlying disorder can be obtained from the history of present illness and past medical history. It is important that the physician focus on all associated symptoms, and not simply dwell on the dizziness complaint itself. These associated symptoms must not be overlooked as the correct diagnosis may be missed without recognizing them. A wide variety of nonotologic associated symptoms occur in dizzy patients; numerous organ systems can be the culprit. The dedicated physician considers neurologic, psychogenic, cardiac, autonomic, systemic, and metabolic disorders within the differential diagnosis. Abnormalities within these systems generally can be ruled in or ruled out with appropriate questioning. More than one system may be contributing to the symptoms experienced by the dizzy patient.

Posture, gait, positioning, eye movement, and cerebellar tests have become extremely valuable tools in the clinician's armamentarium for evaluating the dizzy subject. Most of these inexpensive tests can be done easily and rapidly in the office. Essential information can often be obtained, both specific and nonspecific. The posture and gait tests are thought to reaffirm the patient's reason for seeking assistance with their problem as most normal individuals have little difficulty performing these. Careful assessment of eye movement, posture, gait and positioning is of paramount importance when evaluating a patient with dizziness. When taken in conjunction with a good history, a thorough exam can often pinpoint the underlying abnormality.

REFERENCES

1. Rubin W. Differential diagnosis of disorders causing dizziness. *Amer J Otology.* 1993;14(3):309–312.
2. Singleton GT. Evaluation of the dizzy patient. In: Bailey BJ, ed., *Head and Neck Surgery—Otolaryngology.* Philadelphia, PA: JB Lippincott Co; 1993:1870–1876.
3. Dieterich M, Brandt T. Episodic vertigo related to migraine (90 cases): vestibular migraine? *J Neurol.* 1999; 246(10):883–892.
4. Eggers SD. Migraine-related vertigo: diagnosis and treatment. *Curr Pain Headache Rep.* 2007;11(3):217–226.
5. Clark MR, Sullivan MD, Katon WJ, et al. Psychiatric and medical factors associated with disability in patients with dizziness. *Psychosomatics.* 1993;34(5):409–415.
6. Furman JM, Jacob RG. Psychiatric dizziness. *Neurology.* 1997;48:1161–1166.
7. Sklare DA, Stein MB, Pikus AM, Uhde TW. Dysequilibrium and audiovestibular function in panic disorder: symptom profiles and test findings. *Amer J Otology.* 1990; 11(5):338–341.
8. Evans RW. Neurologic aspects of hyperventilation syndrome. *Sem Neurol.* 1995;15(2):115–125.
9. Nakagawa H, Ohashi N, Kanda K, Watanbe Y. Autonomic nervous system disturbances as etiological background of vertigo and dizziness. *Acta Otolaryngol (Stockh) Suppl.* 1993;504:130–133.
10. Staab JP, Ruckenstein MJ. Expanding the differential diagnosis of chronic dizziness. *Arch Otolaryngol Head Neck Surg.* 2007;133(2):170–176.
11. Catena RD, van Donkelaar P, Chou LS. Altered balance control following concussion is better detected with an attention test during gait. *Gait Posture.* 2007;25(3):406–411.
12. Hart CW. The Quix test. *Laryngoscope.* 1983;93:1160–1161.
13. Moffat DA, Harries MLL, Bagulley DM, Hardy DG. Unterberger's stepping test in acoustic neuroma. *J Laryngol Otol.* 1989;103:839–841.
14. Gianoli G, McWilliams S, Soileau J, et al. Posturographic performance in patients with the potential for secondary gain. *Otolaryngol Head Neck Surg.* 2000;122:11–18.
15. Benarroch E, Sandroni P, Low P. The Valsalva maneuver. In: Low P, ed., *Clinical Autonomic Disorders.* Boston, MA: Little Brown & Co; 1993:209–215.
16. Dix R, Hallpike CS. The pathology, symtomatology and diagnosis of certain common disorders of the vestibular system. *Proc R Soc Med.* 1952;45:341–354.

CHAPTER 2

Audiologic Testing and Interpretation

Sandra Porps and John Zappia

INTRODUCTION

Assessment of the auditory system is an important part of the evaluation of the otologic/neurotologic patient in addition to the history and physical examination. The role of the auditory system and various auditory tests is discussed, including the audiogram, immitance testing, otoacoustic emissions, electrocochleography, and audiometric brainstem response testing.

SOUND

Sound has a physical and psychoacoustical definition. Physically, sound is a mechanical vibration transmitted through an elastic medium. At sea level, sound travels through air at approximately 331 m/s (1087 ft/s, 760 mph). Sound is transmitted much more efficiently in liquids and even better in solids. For example, sound travels at about 1482 m/s in water.[1] In bone, the speed of a sound wave is 3780 m/s.[2] This efficiency in solids/bone is useful in portions of testing and in bone conduction amplification.

Waves, in this case sound, have two fundamental physical features: amplitude and frequency. The amplitude refers to the size or displacement of the wave and is related to intensity. The decibel (dB) is the unit for sound amplitude and is described in more detail below. The frequency refers to the cycles per unit of time, typically hertz (Hz) or cycles per second.

Psychoacoustically, sound is related to the perception of the sound wave through the sense of hearing. The perceptual correlate of amplitude is loudness which does have a unit: the sone. One sone equals the loudness of a 1000-Hz tone at 40 dB SPL.[3] The perceptual correlate of frequency is pitch.

HUMAN EAR

Animals have varying degrees of hearing ability. The healthy human ear can generally detect sound waves in the frequency range of 20 to 20,000 Hz. The loudness (or dynamic) range extends from the average threshold for hearing of 0 dB HL to the uncomfortable level of approximately 110 dB HL.[3] The human ear is not equally acute in all frequencies and is generally most sensitive from 1000 to 4000 Hz.[3] There are two basic parts of the peripheral auditory system. The conductive portion is made up of the auricle, external auditory canal, tympanic membrane, and the middle ear including the ossicles. The sensorineural portion consists of the cochlea and the cochlear portion of the VIIIth nerve. Hearing loss is classified as sensorineural, conductive, or mixed based on which of these anatomic areas is involved (Table 2–1). Hearing loss is also classified based on the severity, with mild suggesting 25 to 40 dB, moderate suggesting 40 to 55 dB, moderate/severe suggesting 55 to 70 dB, severe suggesting 70 to 90 dB, and profound being greater than 90 dB.[3]

Table 2–1. Hearing Loss Classification

Normal Hearing	0–25 dB HL
Mild Hearing Loss	25–40 dB HL
Moderate Hearing Loss	40–55 dB HL
Moderate/ Severe Hearing Loss	55–70 dB HL
Severe Hearing Loss	70–90 dB HL
Profound Hearing Loss	90+ dB HL

DECIBEL

The decibel is the unit reflecting the loudness of sound. The initial work with sound led to the discovery that the approximate threshold for hearing in the human ear was 20 μPa (micropascals) of pressure and the upper level of tolerance was about 20,000,000 μPa. This awkward 1,000,000 fold scale was reduced to 6 with the use of the base 10 logarithmic scale. The unit, originally called the transmission unit and later renamed the bel in honor of Alexander Graham Bell, was conversely felt to be awkwardly small. Dividing this bel by 10 resulted in the more useful unit, commonly referred to as the decibel (dB).

The original and most basic type of decibel is dB SPL (sound pressure level). This was based on the standard of 20 μPa. To create a unit that is more useful in audiometry, the variable frequency sensitivity of the human ear was taken into account in the dB HL (hearing level). The human ear sensitivity in healthy young adults in dB SPL at different frequencies is shown in Table 2–2. Each of these is then set to 0 dB in the new hearing level (HL) scale. This scale is used is all audiometers. Currently the data are based on the 2004 information from the American National Standards Institute, a private nonprofit organization that oversees the voluntary standardization and assessment of US products.[4]

For a given individual, a third type of decibel is recognized that uses that individual's threshold as zero. This is the dB SL (sensation level). Either the pure-tone average or the speech reception threshold (see below) can be used to define an individual's threshold. For example, if a patient has a pure-tone threshold at 1000 Hz at 25 db HL and a 1000-Hz tone is presented at 65 dB HL, the tone is actually being presented at 40 dB SL.

Table 2–2. Reference Equivalent Threshold Sound Pressure Levels (dB re 20 μPa)

Frequency (Hz)	TDH 39 Earphones
250	25.5
500	11.5
1000	7.0
2000	9.0
3000	10.0
4000	9.5
6000	15.5
8000	13.0

Source: Data from Martin and Clark, 2000, p. 43.[3]

A concept to understand in this logarithmic scale is that a 10 dB increase signifies a tenfold increase in intensity whether going from 10 to 20 dB or 90 to 100 dB. A 20 dB increase signifies a 100-fold increase in intensity. The decibel unit always signifies the same quantity but the SPL, HL, and SL designation determine where 0 dB is on the scale.

INTERAURAL ATTENUATION

The final concept necessary in understanding basic audiograms is that of interaural attenuation, which is defined as the reduction of sound intensity in the ear opposite to its presentation. Because of the efficiency of sound transmission through solids, interaural attenuation of sound during bone conduction testing is 0 to 10 dB. When sound is presented in one ear through air (with supra-aural headphones) interaural attenuation is in the range of 40 to 50 dB.[5] It is thought that perhaps this is the presentation level at which bone conduction is induced and that, in fact, the sound reaches the contralateral ear via bone conduction. The more isolated the presentation, such as with inserts, the greater the attenuation.[3] Frequency can also influence interaural attenuation with higher frequencies having greater attenuation than lower frequencies. Generally audiologists consider interaural attenuation of supra-aural headphones to be 40 dB, insert earphones to be 60 dB, and bone conduction to be 0 dB.[6]

BASIC AUDIOMETRY

Pure-Tone Audiometry

The pure-tone audiogram is shown in Figure 2–1. The horizontal axis is frequency in hertz (Hz) and the vertical axis is loudness in dB HL. The test symbols

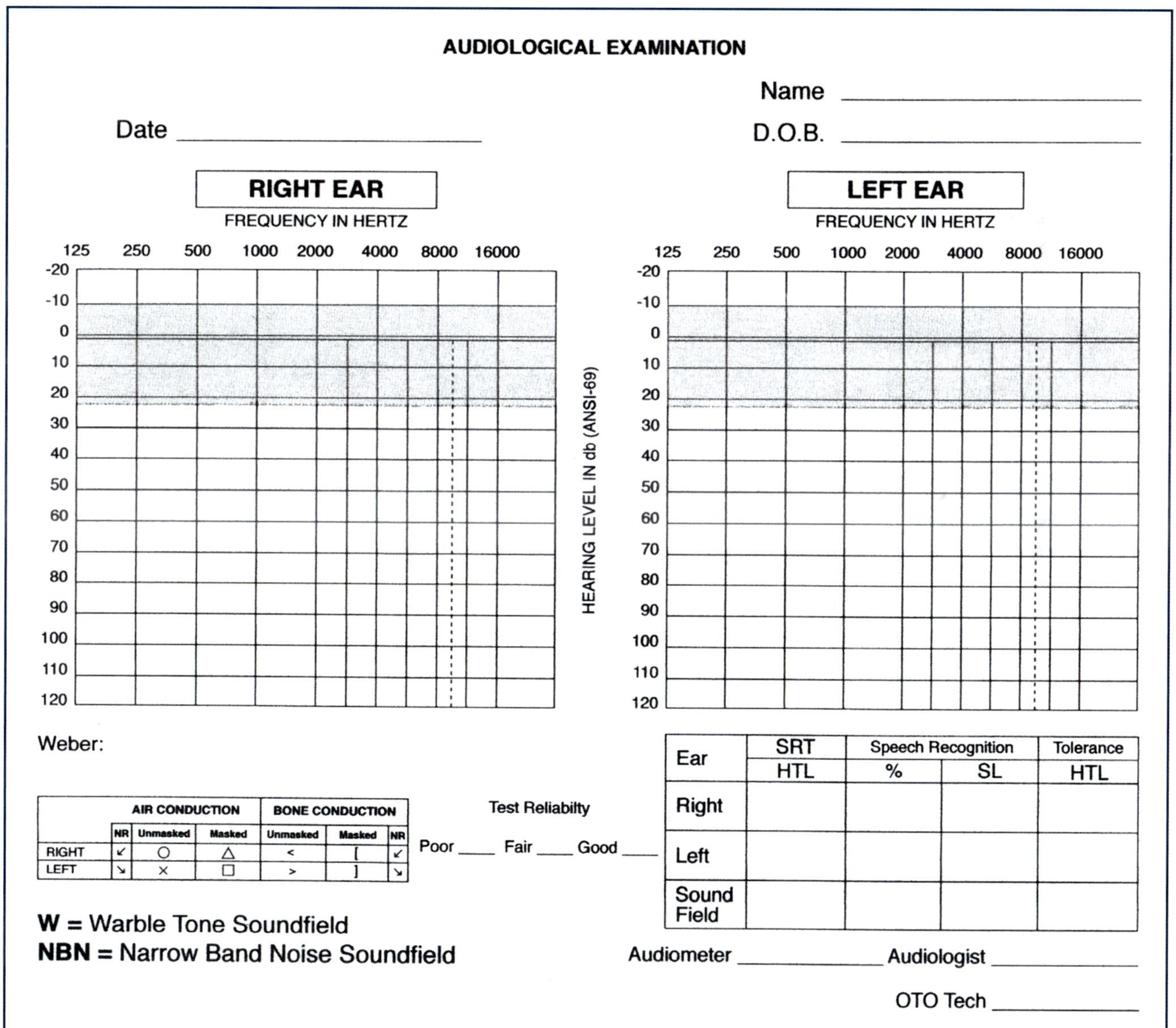

Figure 2–1. Audiogram.

are seen in the key at the bottom left of Figure 2–1. The common symbols depend on whether the tone is presented to the left or right ear, via air or bone, and if masking is used. If there is no response to the presented tone at the loudest presentation level then the appropriate symbol is placed at the level of presentation and the downward arrow is attached.

Air Conduction

Although less formal and screening techniques are available, the standard audiogram is typically performed in a soundproof booth. Conventionally one will test air pure-tones from 250 to 8000 Hz at octave intervals with 3000 and 6000 Hz occasionally being used. Presentation is either via headphones or soft ear inserts. The headphones can be simpler but the inserts are generally better as they can prevent canal collapse, maximize interaural attenuation, and are disposable. The maximum presentation levels vary slightly depending on frequency and audiometer, but are in the range of 100 to 120 dB HL. Lower frequency presentations frequently stimulate vibrotactile sensation that can confuse test results. During testing in a person with a significant low frequency hearing loss, the tester must determine if the tone was heard by bone conduction or perceived by vibrotactile sensation. Frequencies higher than 8000 Hz can be done with a basic audiometer but require special headphones.

Bone Conduction

For bone conduction, testing is completed in the 250 to 4000 Hz range. Because bone conduction vibrators require greater energy than air conduction receivers to generate a level high enough to stimulate normal hearing, the maximum presentation levels are in the 50 to 80 dB range.[3] Lower pitch bone pure tones are particularly likely to be perceived by vibrotactile sensation, especially at the commonly tested lower frequencies of 250 and 500 Hz. During testing it must be understood whether perception is aural or vibrotactile. In cases where the patient perceives the tone through vibrotactile sensation, the tester may place the initials "VT" above the frequency in question. The reason that bone pure tones are not tested above 4000 Hz is that the sound radiating from the bone conduction vibrator may be heard by the non-test ear resulting in artificially low bone conduction thresholds.[7]

Test Procedure

Whether testing air conduction or bone conduction, the tester typically begins by presenting a tone that the patient will likely hear. This is determined based on case history, interaction with the patient, and previous audiograms, if available. The patient will indicate to the tester if the particular tone is heard either by a signaling device (pushing a button) or by raising his hand. If the patient hears the initial tone, the tester reduces the tone by 10 dB and presents again. This continues until the patient stops responding. The tester then raises the tone by 5 dB until the patient responds. The tester will reduce the tone by 10 dB once again and repeat the process.[3] The threshold is determined when the patient responds two out of three times at the same level. Although there are different methods of testing for specific situations such as a patient with nonorganic hearing loss, the "down 10, up 5" method is the most common.

Pure-Tone Average

A common entity based on the pure-tone results is the pure-tone average (PTA). This is the average of the 500, 1000, and 2000 Hz (and sometimes 3000 Hz) in decibels. Because these frequencies are in the middle of speech range, the PTA generally correlates with the speech reception threshold discussed below.

Masking

Ensuring that the test ear is the ear detecting the presented sound is important. This is most likely to occur when the hearing is different between ears. The better ear will possibly detect the tested sound when presented to the poorer ear. Understanding the dB levels of interaural attenuation for bone and air conduction help predict when this problem may occur.

Figure 2–2 is the audiogram of a person with no hearing in their left ear where no masking is used

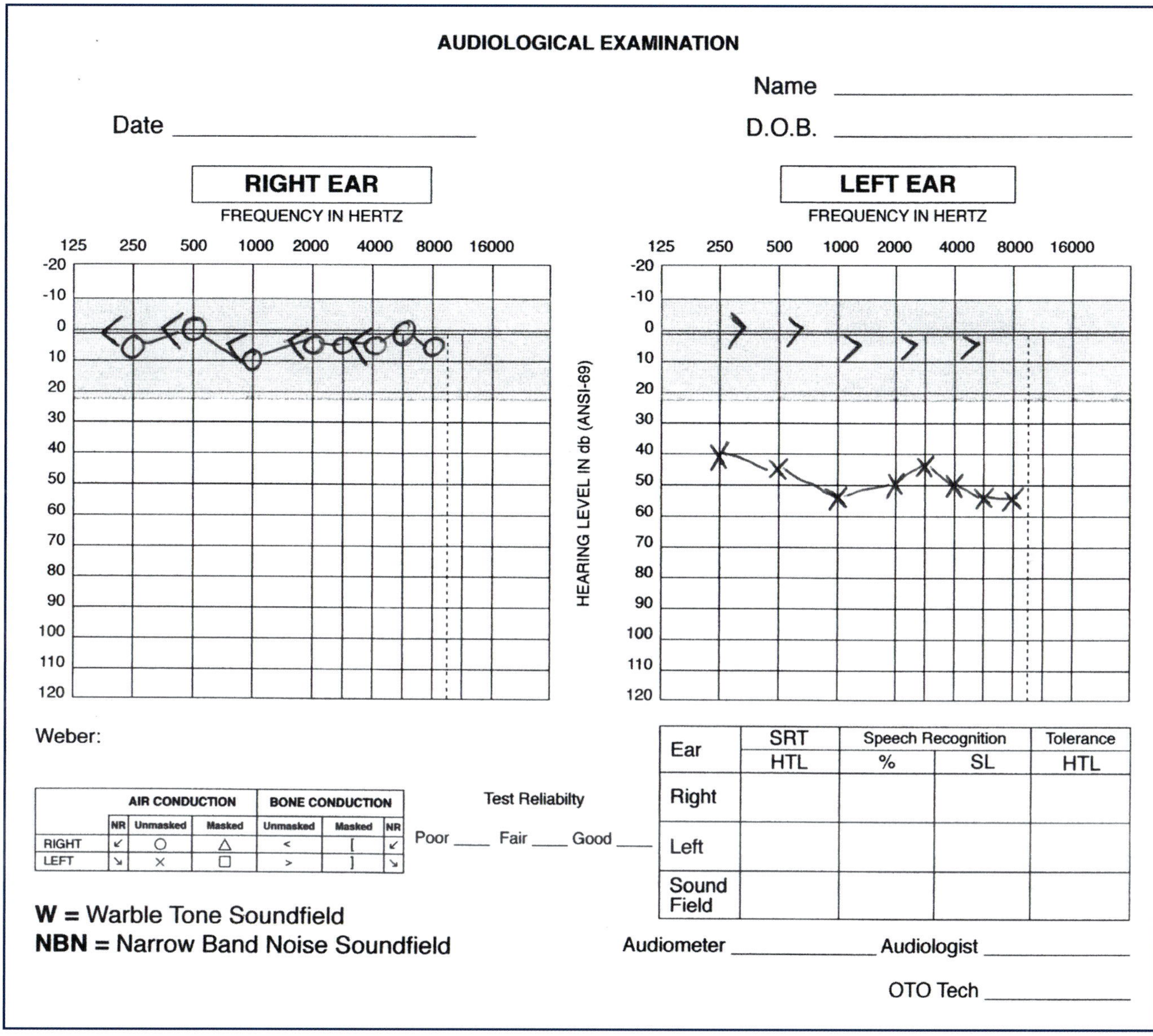

Figure 2–2. Unmasked audiogram in patient with complete left ear hearing loss.

during testing. Normal bone and air levels are seen in the right ear. In the left ear an apparently normal bone level is seen at all frequencies. This is expected remembering that interaural attenuation for bone is 0 to 10 dB. The air pure-tone level suggests a 50 to 60 dB hearing loss throughout the measured frequencies. This should also be expected knowing that interaural attenuation for air is in the 40 to 50 dB range. The result is commonly referred to as a shadow audiogram. The only way to accurately assess the poorer hearing left ear is to prevent the right ear from detecting the sound.

This is where masking is used. When necessary in pure-tone testing, a narrow frequency band of sound, centered on the test frequency, is presented via air to the nontest ear.

One of the more difficult testing situations arises when trying to test a person with bilateral hearing loss where at least one of the sides is conductive. It is possible in this situation to experience a masking dilemma. This occurs when testing the conductive hearing loss side for bone hearing level, in a person with contralateral hearing loss. The problem arises because masking is presented via air conduction. In the bilateral conductive hearing loss seen in Figure 2–3, the problem can be illustrated when testing for the bone level at 500 Hz in the right ear indicated by the circle. Appropriate masking will be needed in the nontest left ear. This narrowband sound centered on 500 Hz presented via air conduction must be >60 dB HL for the contralateral left ear to detect it. The dilemma arises now because interaural attenuation for air is 40 to 50 dB, meaning that the masking tone could possibly be heard by the right (test) ear

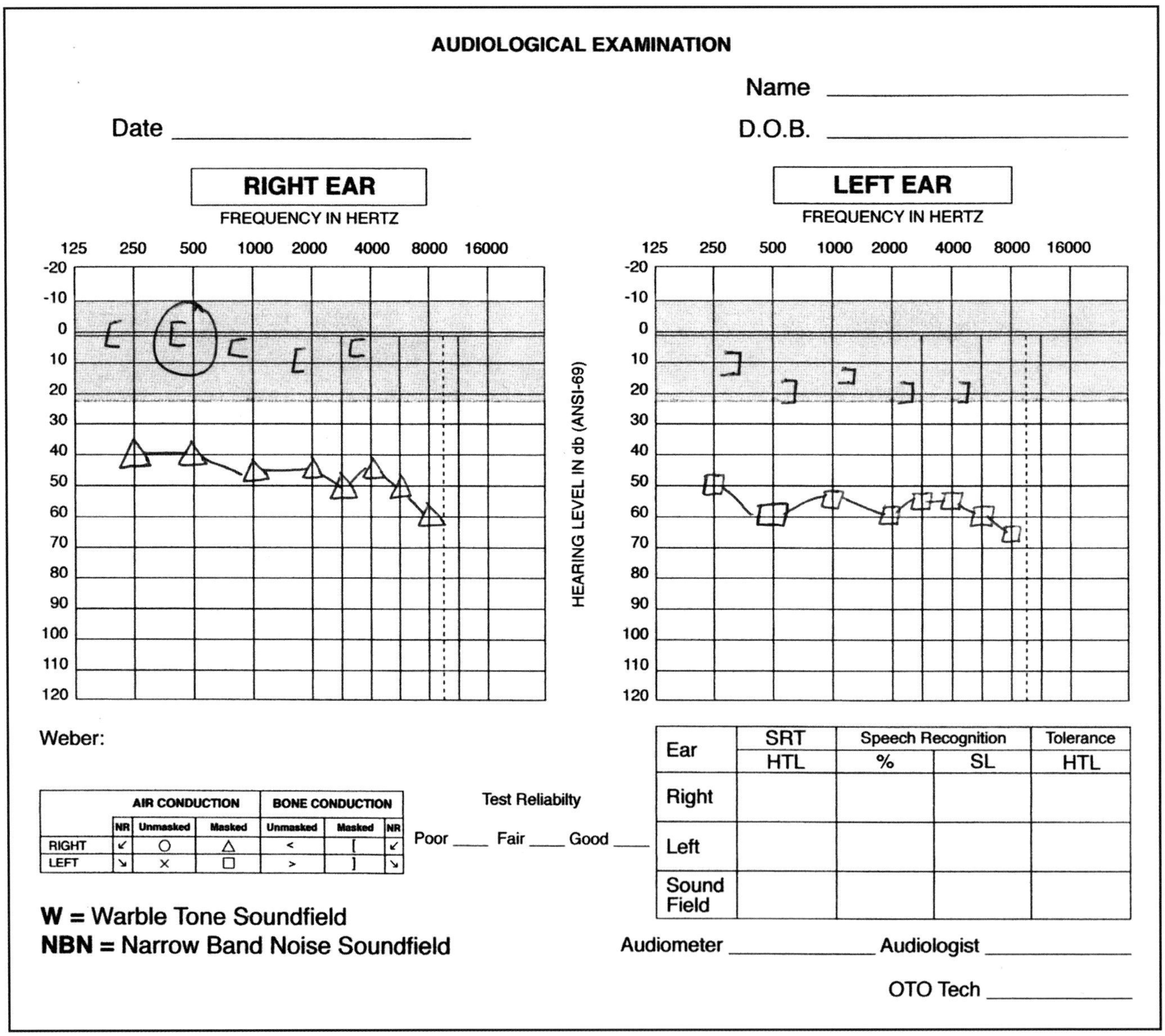

Figure 2–3. Bilateral conductive hearing loss audiogram.

literally masking the presentation 500 Hz bone pure tone. If this is the case, then the test tone will need to be presented louder for detection. When this occurs, it may not be possible to accurately determine the bone level resulting in the masking dilemma. If one increases the masking presentation level then the test tone will need to be increased appropriately to overcome it. When the test tone and the opposite masking tone move together like this it suggests a masking dilemma has been encountered.

Speech Reception Threshold

The second part of the basic audiogram is the speech reception threshold (SRT). The SRT is the level (in dB HL) at which one can reliably repeat 50% of the spondee words presented. Spondee words are those with equal emphasis on each of their two syllables (ie, cowboy, baseball). This can be completed either with live or recorded voice. Live voice can be performed quicker but it is less uniform than recorded voice. The results are usually recorded in a box somewhere on the audiogram (see bottom right of Figure 2–1). Because interaural attention for air is 40 to 50 dB, one must consider speech masking, which uses a broader band (than pure-tone) speech noise, when there is a significant difference between the ears. Its use is usually indicated by a circled small letter "m" next to the result.

Other speech thresholds include speech awareness threshold (SAT) or speech detection threshold (SDT) both of which are the softest level a person is aware that speech is present. Although the SRT is the preferred measurement, there are several situations in which the SDT may be the only speech measurement obtained. Nonnative English speakers may be unable to repeat English words. Patients with certain types of hearing loss may have no ability to understand speech or have profound hearing with little or no ability to present words above thresholds. Also, young children may be unable or unwilling to repeat words.

The SRT usually correlates with the PTA. Variance from this can be seen in pseudohypoacusis or in steeply sloping hearing losses where the SRT may be closer to the best tone(s) in the PTA than the average of the .5, 1, and 2 kHz (Figure 2–4).

Word Recognition Score

Word recognition score (WRS), speech recognition, and speech discrimination are all synonyms for the quantitative measurement of the ability to understand phonetically balanced words presented above an individual's threshold defined by the SRT. Phonetically balanced words are single syllable words marked by a consonant-vowel-consonant structure (ie, ball, rat, pool). Word understanding increases up to 30 to 40 dB above an individual's hearing threshold. As a result, WRS is most commonly obtained 30 to 40 dB above SRT or 30 to 40 dB SL.[7] The results are reported in percentages with anything above 88% being accepted as normal.

The level of presentation is determined by the tester and can depend on various factors. Reasons to choose a presentation level greater than 40 dB SL include someone with a steeply down sloping pure-tone hearing result like that depicted in Figure 2–4. One can assume that this patient would have a reduced WRS simply because the majority of the high pitched tones are not heard and not necessarily because there is a true discrimination or retrocochlear problem. Increasing the presentation level should result in increased WRS in this situation if there is no other problem. If the WRS decreases with increased presentation level, then rollover is present, which can be an indication of a retrocochlear problem.

The situations where phonetically balanced words might be presented below 30 dB SL include the person with a severe or profound hearing loss where 30 dB SL may be intolerably loud or beyond the limits of the audiometer. Also there are people with sound sensitivity who will not tolerate sounds significantly above their thresholds. Clinically, this represents hyperacusis and can occur in disorders such as Ménière's disease. The physiological phenomenon is called recruitment.

ACOUSTIC IMMITTANCE

Indirectly, through measurement of reflected sound levels, the size of the ear canal as well as the status of the tympanic membrane and the middle ear can be assessed. To do this, the ear canal is sealed with

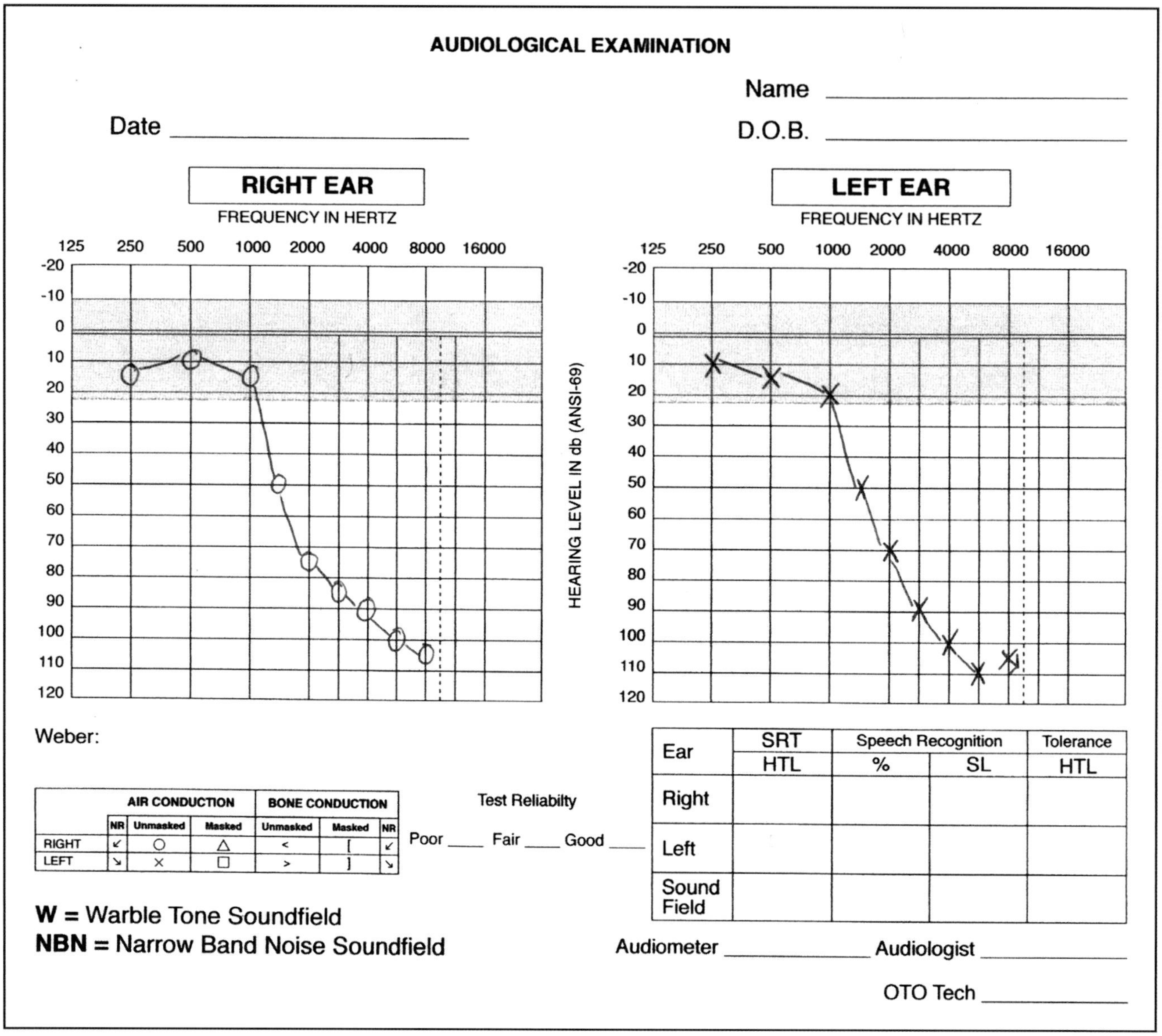

Figure 2–4. Audiogram of a steeply sloping hearing loss. For this patient, the SRT of the left ear would be approximately 20 dB HL whereas the PTA is 35 dB HL. This is an instance in which the SRT and PTA do not correlate.

a probe that contains three ports (Figure 2–5). One of the ports is a speaker that presents a continuous 226-Hz tone into the ear canal. A second port is a microphone that records the level of the tone in the sealed ear canal. The third port alters and controls the pressure in the enclosed ear canal. Inability to seal the ear canal, excessive cerumen, or inappropriate placement of the tip of the probe will either alter results or prevent any information from being obtained.

When the probe is placed in the ear canal and a seal is obtained, the space is pressurized to 200 daPa (decapascals). The larger the ear canal, or connecting space, the lower the amplitude of sound that the microphone records. A volume in milliliters is calculated from this information. A typical ear canal will

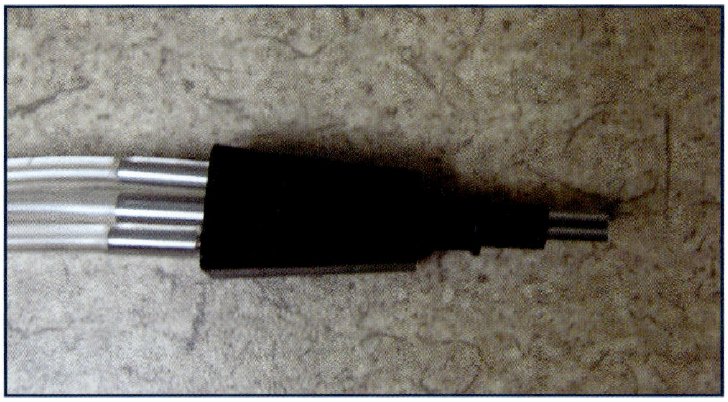

Figure 2–5. Impedance bridge probe for immittance testing.

be 0.63 to 1.46 mL.[7] An abnormally large ear canal, a mastoid cavity, or a tympanic membrane perforation will result in a large ear canal volume estimate.

Tympanometry

The flexibility or compliance of the tympanic membrane can be measured with immitance audiometry. After the canal volume measurement, the pressure is gradually lowered from 200 daPa to –400 daPa. Again, there is ongoing measurement of the loudness of the 226-Hz tone. The sound is loudest when the tympanic membrane is under pressure (ie, least mobile). This occurs when the pressure difference on either side is greatest, as much of the sound is reflected off the stiff surface. When the pressure is equal on both sides of the tympanic membrane, it becomes relatively flaccid and absorbs much of the sound energy resulting in much less sound reaching the microphone. This low point in the amplitude of the sound recorded by the microphone results in the "peak" seen in the typical tympanogram (Figure 2–6). In a normal ear the peak typically is present between –100 and 100 daPa and is classified as type A.

The height of the peak can vary outside an expected range. In patients with ossicular fixation or tympanosclerosis, the peak will be small and is classified as type A_s, where "s" represents shallow. A type A_d tympanogram occurs in those with ossicular discontinuity or an excessively flaccid drum where the amplitude of the peak will be greater than normal, where "d" represents deep.

If the pressure in the middle ear is low, as in eustachian tube dysfunction, the corresponding peak on the tympanogram will be shifted. If the peak occurs at less than –100 daPa it is considered abnormal with –100 to –200 daPa classified as type C as shown in Figure 2–6C. When there is fluid behind the tympanic membrane or extreme negative pressure, there will be very little variation in the amplitude of the 226-Hz tone recorded and the tracing will appear relatively flat. If the peak occurs at less than –200 daPa, or the tracing is flat, they are classified as type B as in Figure 2–6B. A tympanic membrane perforation or the presence of tympanostomy tubes will result in a similar type B tracing as the pressure is being applied to the bony walls of the ear canal and middle ear, which respond little to the pressure variance. The physical exam and the ear canal volume estimate should clue one in to the possible cause of this tympanometric finding.

Stapedial Reflex

The acoustic or stapedial reflex is the reflexive contraction of the middle ear muscles in response to sound stimulation. The tensor tympani and stapedius muscles can act to dampen the motion of the malleus and stapes respectively to protect the cochlea from intense sounds. In humans, the reflex involves primarily the stapedius muscle unless the sound is sufficiently intense and unexpected to create a startle reflex which activates the tensor tympani.[7]

The reflex is bilateral with both stapedius muscles activated with unilateral input. The cochlear nerve carries the information to the ventral cochlear nucleus then to the superior olivary complex bilaterally. There the reflex is completed when the facial nuclei receive the information and transmit the efferent response through the facial nerve to the stapedius muscles bilaterally.

The reflex occurs within 10ms of the stimulus and is recorded with a probe (identical to that used in tympanometry). The response can be determined by a change in the recorded 226-Hz tone loudness as the eardrum becomes less "compliant" with the muscle contraction. The ear receiving the stimulus is called the stimulus ear and the one being monitored (either ipsilateral or contralateral) for the reflex is

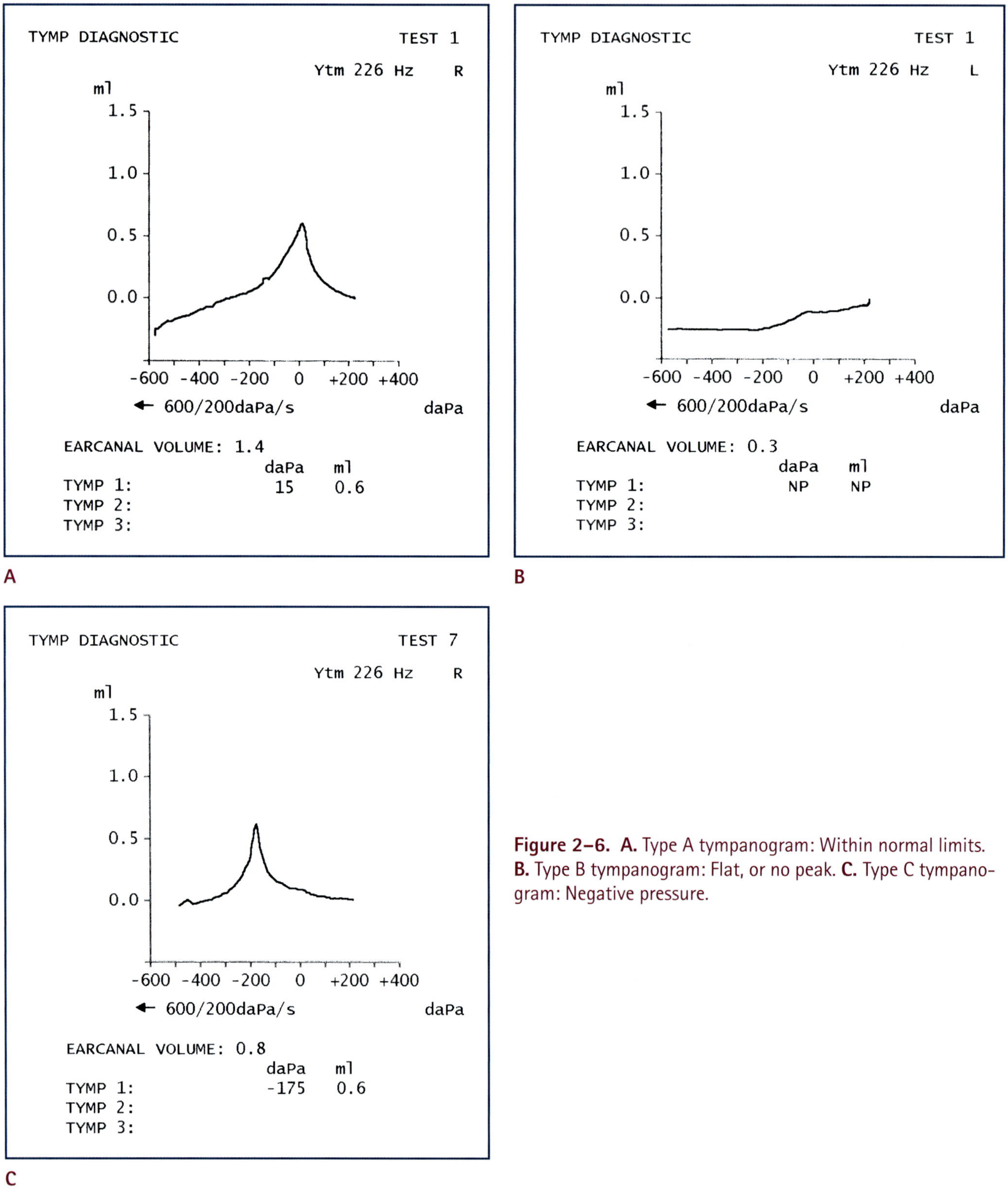

Figure 2–6. A. Type A tympanogram: Within normal limits. **B.** Type B tympanogram: Flat, or no peak. **C.** Type C tympanogram: Negative pressure.

the probe ear. The stimulus can be either pure-tone (.5, 1, 2, 4 kHz) or click sounds. Thresholds for pure-tones are typically 70 to 90 dB SL and 20 dB lower for clicks. Routinely the stimulus is presented at 80 to 110 dB HL.

A normal reflex is seen in Figure 2–7. In a normal individual, the response threshold will be maintained as long as the stimulus is presented. On the afferent side, lack of response or elevated thresholds can be a result of hearing loss, retrocochlear problems, or brainstem abnormalities. On the efferent side, facial nerve abnormalities, ossicular problems (fixation or discontinuities), or transection/absence of the stapedius muscle can be reasons for lack of response. Occasionally, the threshold can be reduced in cochlear problems due to recruitment. Reflex decay is the situation where the response amplitude lessens over time and can be indicative of a retrocochlear problem.

OTOACOUSTIC EMISSIONS

Although the inner ear is more known for its ability to detect sound, it is also capable of producing low amplitude acoustic signals that can be recorded and utilized in a variety of situations. Otoacoustic emissions (OAEs) are sounds that originate in the cochlea and traverse the middle ear into the external ear canal where they can be measured. They are felt to be related to the efferent amplification function of the inner ear with the likely source being the outer hair cells.

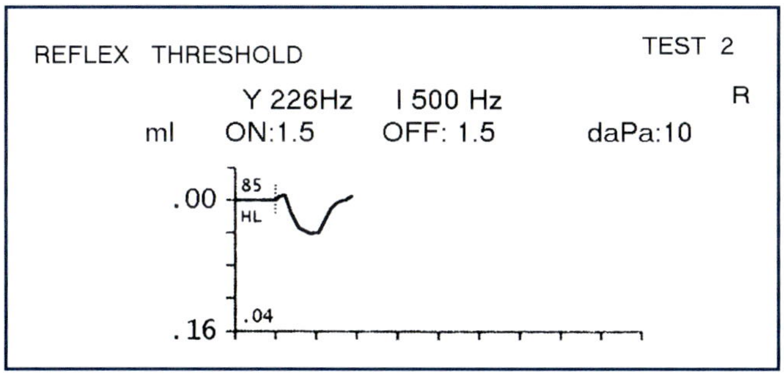

Figure 2–7. Normal stapedial reflex test tracing.

OAEs are not affected by level of consciousness. They are affected by external noise levels which can obscure these low amplitude signals. Testing should be performed in a quiet or soundproof room in order to minimize environmental noise. Fluid, cerumen, or moderate hearing loss will affect the results of the testing. The state of the patient can also be a limitation. Crying, talking, or excessive muscular activity can make testing difficult or impossible. Under difficult conditions, more averages may be necessary to obtain accurate results. The signal can be undetectable in many of these instances.

There are two classes: spontaneous and evoked. Spontaneous otoacoustic emissions (SOAEs) can be recorded by inserting a sensitive miniature microphone in the ear canal and amplifying the output. SOAEs appear as pure-tone-like signals. It is estimated that 50% of normal hearing individuals will have SOAEs. Although it was initially thought that there might be a correlation of SOAEs and tinnitus, this has not proven to be the case.[8] SOAEs have not proven clinically useful.

The more measurable and useful are the evoked responses: transient evoked (TEOAE) and distortion product (DPOAE). Because the OAEs are low amplitude, signal averaging linking the recording period to the stimulus presentation with multiple (hundreds) presentations is necessary. TEOAEs can be generated by either a brief click or a tone-burst stimulus. In general, TEOAEs are larger amplitude and elicited at lower thresholds in those with SOAEs. They can be used in infant screening and in difficult to test populations. TEOAEs are measurable in nearly all ears with normal hearing sensitivity and normal middle ear function.[8] TEOAEs cannot be measured if a person's auditory thresholds exceed 30 dB HL.[9]

In DPOAEs, two different frequency tones are presented simultaneously resulting in an emitted tone from the cochlea. The two pure-tone stimuli frequencies are designated "f1" and "f2." The presentation levels of the two tones are designated "L1" and L2." The resultant DPOAEs occur at predictable frequencies mathematically related to the primary frequencies (f2–f1, 2f1–f2, 3f1–2f2, and 2f2–f1). Typically, the 2f1–f2 DPOAE has the largest amplitude in humans. As a result it has been the most extensively investigated so that DPOAE typically refers to the 2f1–f2 frequency.

DPOAEs, like TEOAEs, can be measured in nearly 100% of normal hearing ears with normal middle ear function.[8] Figure 2–8 is a DPOAE in a normal-hearing individual. DPOAEs are present in individuals whose auditory thresholds are less than 50 dB HL.[9] Testing protocols will usually include 5 to 8 test frequency combinations. They are most commonly utilized in infant screening protocols, inner ear integrity testing, and in gross verification of hearing thresholds obtained in other ways. They can be particularly useful in identifying auditory neuropathy where a subject will have variable peripheral hearing levels, an absent ABR and a normal DPOAE.

ELECTROCOCHLEOGRAPHY

Electrocochleography (ECoG or ECochG) is the technique of recording electrical impulses from the cochlea and the cochlear nerve. There are three entities observed in an ECoG: the cochlear microphonic,

BIO-LOGIC OTOACOUSTIC EMISSIONS (OAE) REPORT - Page 1 of 1

Patient: test,
Birthdate: Ear: Left
ID:
Comment:

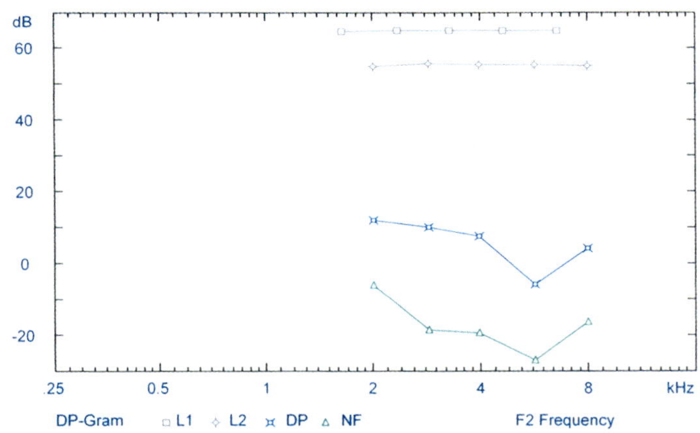

Left: 10-Sep-08: -: 2-8 kHz Diagnostic Test: 08I10D00.OAE

L1(dB)	L2(dB)	F1(Hz)	F2(Hz)	GM(Hz)	DP(dB)	NF(dB)	DP-NF(dB)
64.8	55.1	6563	8016	7253	4.0	-16.4	20.4
64.8	55.4	4641	5672	5130	-6.0	-27.0	21.0
65.0	55.5	3281	3984	3616	7.6	-19.6	27.2
65.0	55.6	2344	2859	2589	9.9	-18.8	28.7
64.5	54.7	1641	2016	1818	11.8	-6.3	18.1

Figure 2–8. Normal DPOAE test results from 2000 to 8000 Hz. GM (Hz)-geometric mean of the test frequencies. GM is the frequency of interest in the cochlea that the measured DPOAE in the ear canal (usually 2f1–f2) represents. DP (dB)—amplitude of the resultant DPOAE. NF (dB)—amplitude of the background noise. DP–NF (dB)—amplitude difference between DP and NF. Criteria vary for different test equipment but for this test there must be a difference (DP–NF) of 6 dB in order to be valid.

the summating potential, and the action potential. The cochlear microphonic (CM) is an alternating current potential that resembles the waveform of the acoustic stimulus and is present as long as there is a stimulus. It can be obtained with a click stimulus but is generally best seen with a tone-burst stimulus. The hair cells are felt to be the source of this electrical entity. The summating potential (SP) is a direct current (DC) potential that appears as a baseline shift of the CM and is also felt to originate from the hair cells. It is most clearly seen with tone-burst stimuli, but can be seen as a hump or shoulder on the initial side of the large amplitude action potential (AP) with a click stimulus. As the CM and SP are generated in the cochlea they occur slightly before the AP in the recordings. They also persist as long as the stimulus is present. The AP is the third measurable entity and is the equivalent of the first wave of the ABR originating in the first portion of the VIIIth nerve. As with the ABR, this is best seen with a click stimulus.

The responses can be recorded from the external canal, the tympanic membrane or with a needle electrode on the promontory. In the ear canal, recordings can be obtained with a gold foil electrode placed in contact with the skin. Transtympanic needle electrodes in contact with the promontory give the most robust responses requiring little signal averaging. Unfortunately this is relatively invasive, generally requires a physician's presence, and can be uncomfortable. As a result they are less commonly used. A generally more acceptable option is a gel-tipped electrode placed against the tympanic membrane. There are some technical issues with the placement of these electrodes that are usually overcome with experience. There can be some discomfort but the tympanic membrane electrode is generally well tolerated. These recordings from the tympanic membrane provide an adequate compromise between quality of recording, comfort to patient, and ease of use. This electrode contact with the tympanic membrane can be verified by measuring the impedance prior to beginning the testing. The electrode is held in place with a standard foam insert transducer tip. The secondary electrode can be placed on the forehead, scalp, contralateral earlobe, or mastoid. The common electrode can be placed on the nasion, either earlobe, or mastoid.

The stimulus is a click or tone-burst generally presented at 85–95 dB HL or greater depending on the patient's hearing thresholds. The click stimulus is 100 μs duration.[7] The tone-bursts have a 5- to 10-ms plateau with a 2-ms rise and fall time. Typically, the stimulus presentation rate is 7.1/s or 11.1/s for clicks and 27.7/s for tone-bursts. Responses are recorded for 10 ms after initiation of stimulus. Transtympanic recording will usually require 100 presentations whereas approximately 1,000 repetitions are necessary in tympanic membrane recordings to get a good waveform for analysis.

The primary clinical application of ECoG is identification of endolymphatic hydrops. It is thought that the presence of endolymphatic hydrops alters the characteristics of the basilar membrane leading to an elevation of the SP.[10] A generally more reproducible entity than the SP alone is the ratio of the SP to the AP amplitude.[11] The click evoked ECoG usually gives a more robust and easier to interpret response. The cutoff for the SP/AP amplitude ratio varies with different techniques and facilities but is generally in the range of .4 to .6 with anything above this considered suspicious for endolymphatic hydrops. The reported sensitivity and specificity of ECoG vary but in general it is felt that an elevated SP/AP ratio is strongly suspicious for hydrops but a normal ratio does not necessarily eliminate it from consideration.

Figure 2–9 displays a patient with a normal ECoG for the left ear and an abnormal ECoG for the right ear. The left ear waveform is robust, has good morphology, and an SP/AP ratio of .232. The right ear waveform has fair morphology and an SP/AP ratio of .432. The right ear was suspected of having endolymphatic hydrops due to the elevated SP/AP ratio.

AUDIOMETRIC BRAINSTEM RESPONSE TESTING

The audiometric brainstem response (ABR) is a series of far-field electrical waveform obtained in response to a sound stimulus. These low-amplitude electrical signals were not able to be identified until the response could be time locked to the stimulus and repeated enough times to average out the myriad of

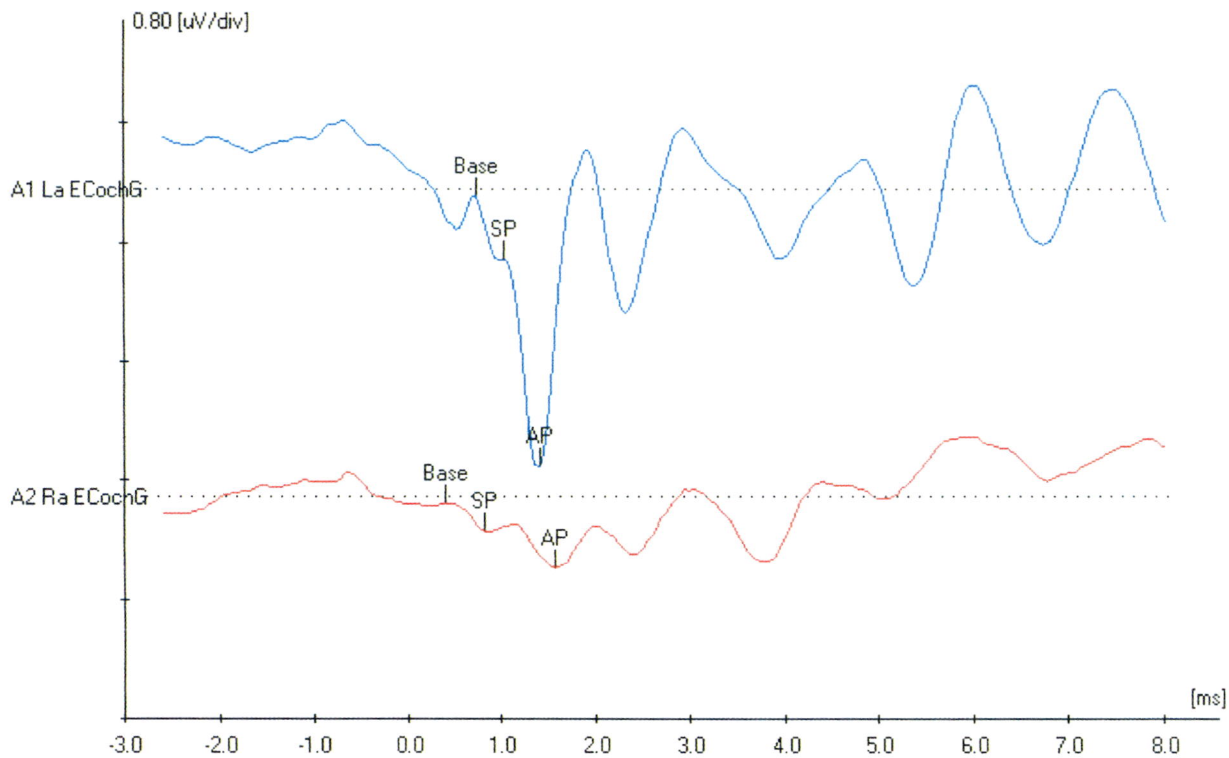

Latencies (ms)

Label Index	*Base*	*SP*	*AP*
A1	**0.74**	**1.03**	**1.41**
A2	**0.41**	**0.82**	**1.57**

Interamplitudes (uV)

Label Index	*SP-Base*	*AP-Base*	*SP/AP Ratio*
A1	**-0.420**	**-1.810**	**0.232**
A2	**-0.190**	**-0.440**	**0.432**

Figure 2–9. Normal ECOG study for the left ear. Abnormal ECOG study for the right ear. The left ear tracing shows a robust response with an SP/AP amplitude ratio of .23. The right ear tracing shows a less robust response compared to the left ear with an SP/AP amplitude ratio of .43 suggesting endolymphatic hydrops.

background electrical activity and allow the desired signal to be "seen." The ABR in not affected by level of consciousness but can be affected by motion or activity. In younger or uncooperative subjects, sedation may be necessary. The ABR can be seen as early as 27 to 28 weeks gestation and generally reaches adult form by about 18 months to 2 years of age.[12]

There are generally five repeatable and useful waves generated within the first 10ms after appropriate stimulation of the cochlea. The waves are generated as the information traverses the cochlear nerve, the cochlear nucleus, the superior olivary complex, the lateral lemniscus as the information ascends to the inferior colliculus and then to the temporal lobe. Waves I and II are most likely generated along the cochlear nerve. Wave III probably is initiated in the cochlear nucleus. Waves IV and V are theorized to originate in the superior olivary complex and the lateral lemniscus respectively.[13] Waves I, III, and V are the most identifiable and as a result, useful clinically. Table 2–3 shows the normal latencies of the ABR waveform.

For recording, a ground electrode is placed on the forehead, an inverting electrode is placed around the ear, and a non-inverting electrode is placed on the scalp. The stimulus is generally presented through an ear canal insert. There are several commercial devices available to record auditory evoked data. They typically consist of electrodes, a transducer, an amplifier, and a signal averager usually controlled by a computer program.

The stimulus most commonly used is a click stimulus of 100-µs duration in the 2000 to 4000-Hz frequency range. These clicks are able to generate a robust response from the cochlea to initiate the electrical transmission in the VIIIth nerve. The presentation rate varies but is chosen to not in any way resemble the 60 Hz signal that is present in many electrical systems. It needs to be fast enough to perform an adequate number of repetitions in a reasonable amount of time but cannot be so fast so that the stimulus of one presentation might interfere with the recording of the previous waveform. Rates do vary to balance the above issues but 11.1, 13.3, and 27.7/s are some of the more commonly reported ones. Generally, 1500–2000 repetitions are necessary to obtain a reliably repeatable waveform. Tone-bursts can also be used in certain instances but the responses are not always as robust or repeatable. The higher pitched tone-bursts tend to give larger amplitude responses likely because there is less diffusion of the signal near the basal cochlea.

Table 2–3. Average ABR Latencies for Waves I–V

Wave	Average Latency
I	1.5 msec
II	2.5 msec
III	3.5 msec
IV	4.5 msec
V	5.5 msec

Source: Data from Hall, 1992, p. 17.12

The ABR is frequently used to identify retrocochlear problems. For this the click stimulus is generally presented at 90 to 95 dB HL. The stimulus needs to be adequately above the threshold of hearing to obtain an appropriate response. Therefore the subject's hearing in the 2 to 4 kHz range must be known. Hearing levels worse than 55 dB in this higher frequency range can interfere with the results and interpretation. Figure 2–10 is an ABR of a patient with a retrocochlear problem.

The latencies of the waves are the most commonly used pieces of information. The absolute latencies are informative but most commonly the comparison bilaterally is used. The interaural latency difference of wave V has been discussed most frequently. Interaural latency difference limits of .2 or .4 ms are most commonly used. The sensitivity, the percentage of abnormalities detected (true positives), and the specificity, the percentage of normals detected (true negatives), are affected with choice of cutoffs. In the era before MRI, sensitivities of 96 to 100% were reported. Since the introduction of the MRI, lower results have been observed.[14] The accuracy of MRI has obviously had an effect. The quality of the equipment and the cutoff parameters can also affect the results. Because ABR is simpler and less expensive than MRI, it continues to be an important tool in evaluating retrocochlear pathology.

ABR is also valuable in threshold testing. Clicks can be used to assess hearing levels in the 2- to 4-kHz range. Pure tones can also be used but are more difficult to obtain due to noise levels impacting the recordings. ABR threshold testing can be used to approximate hearing levels in infants or other patients who are unable to perform traditional air conduction testing. Using the standard ABR setup, wave V is identified, usually at 90 dB nHL (0 dB nHL is the stimulus level that is expected to correlate with 0 dB HL). From there, the stimulus is lowered by 20 dB increments until wave V disappears. Then the stimulus is increased and decreased in 5 dB increments until the softest level at which wave V reliably

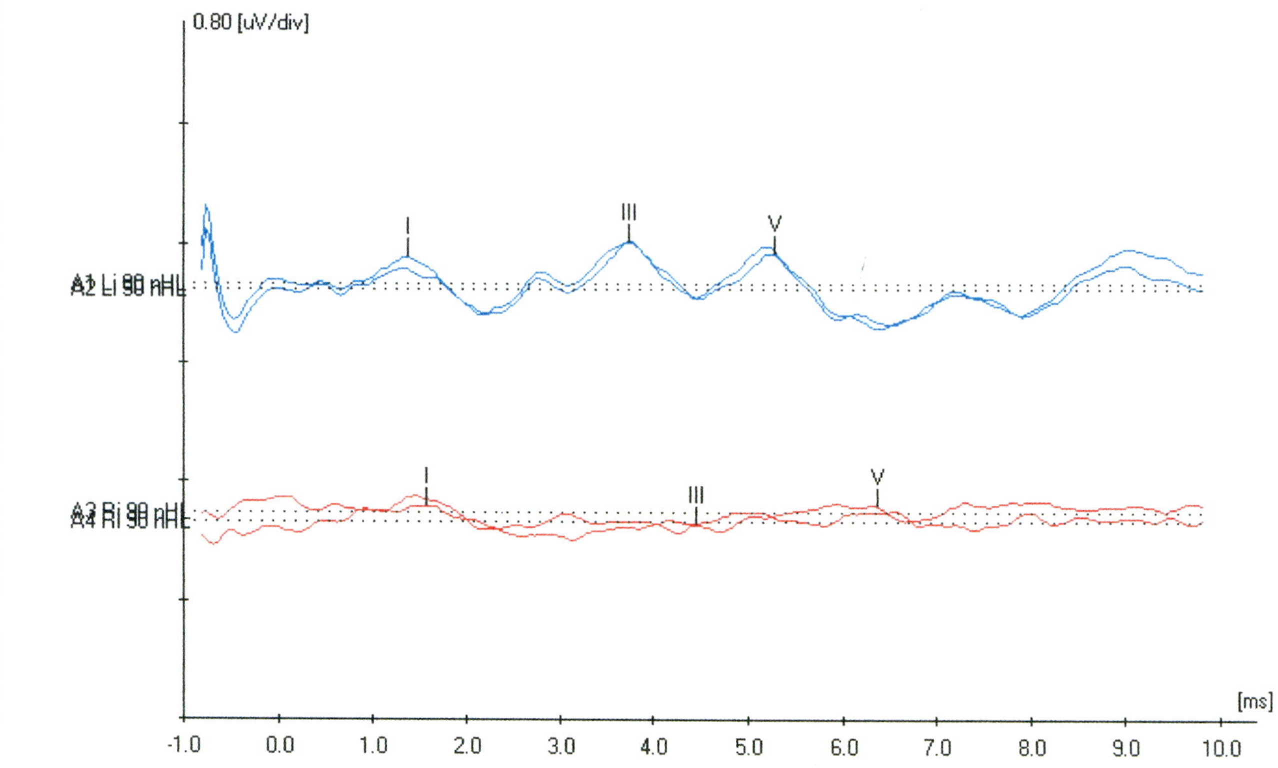

Latencies (ms)

Label Index	*I*	*II*	*III*	*IV*	*V*
A1	**1.37**		**3.74**		**5.28**
A3	**1.57**		**4.45**		**6.36**

Interlatencies (ms)

Label Index	*I-III*	*III-V*	*I-V*
A1	**2.37**	**1.54**	**3.91**
A3	**2.87**	**1.92**	**4.79**

Figure 2–10. ABR study. The upper waveform indicates a left ear with good retrocochlear function. The lower waveform with poor morphology and delayed wave V indicates a right ear with poor retrocochlear function, in this case an acoustic neuroma.

repeats is identified. Depending on the equipment used, the hearing level in dB HL is usually 10 to 20 dB better than the threshold in dB nHL. For example, if the ABR threshold is at 40 db nHL, the threshold for traditional air conduction testing would be between 20 and 30 dB HL. It is important to remember that ABR click stimuli can only approximate hearing between 2 and 4 kHz and that tone-burst testing is necessary if you wish to approximate hearing in the lower frequency range.

CONCLUSION

Audiologic testing is an important part of evaluation of the patient with otologic/neurotologic complaints. Understanding the basic concepts of sound, the human ear's capabilities, the decibel and interaural attenuation are important in test interpretation. Comfort with the basic audiogram, which consists of pure-tone thresholds, SRT, and WRS, is necessary in any clinician evaluating patients with ear related problems. Although less commonly utilized, more advanced testing includes acoustic immitance, OAEs, ECoG, and ABR. Understanding the role and techniques of these entities is important in care of these patients.

REFERENCES

1. Cutnell JD, Johnson KW. Speed of sound in water. *Physics*. New York, NY: Wiley; 1997:468.
2. Hatakeyama R, Yoshizawa M, Moriya T. A method for the measurement of acoustic impedance and speed of sound in a small region of bone using a fused quartz rod as a transmission line. *Jap J Appl Physics*. 2000;39(11): 6449–6454.
3. Martin FN, Clark JG. *Introduction to Audiology*. 7th ed. Needham Heights, MA: Allyn and Bacon; 2000.
4. American National Standards Institute. *American National Standard Specification for Audiometers*. ANSI S3.6-2004. New York, NY: Author, 1996.
5. Katz J. *Handbook of Clinical Audiology*. Baltimore, MD: Williams and Wilkins; 1972.
6. Beyer C. Preventing clinical errors in hearing care. *Audiology Online*. 2006.
7. Katz J. *Handbook of Clinical Audiology*. 5th ed. Baltimore, MD: Lippincott Williams and Wilkins; 2002.
8. Glattke TJ, Kujawa SG. Otoacoustic emissions. *Amer J Audiol*. 1991;1(1):29–40.
9. Alpiner J, McCarthy P. *Rehabilitative Audiology Children and Adults*. 3rd ed. Baltimore, MD: Lippincott Williams & Wilkins; 2000.
10. Dauman R, Aran JM, Charlet de Sauvage R, Portmann M. Clinical significance of the summating potential in Ménière's disease. *Am J Otol*. 1988;9:31–38.
11. Eggermont JJ. Analysis of compound action potential responses to tone bursts in the human and guinea pig cochlea. *J Acoust Soc Am*. 1976;60(5):1132–1139.
12. Hall III JW. *Handbook of Auditory Evoked Responses*. Needham Heights, MA: Allyn and Bacon; 1992.
13. Hood L. *Clinical Applications of the Auditory Brainstem Response*. San Diego, CA: Singular; 1998.
14. Zappia JJ, O'Connor CA, Wiet RJ, Dinces EA. Rethinking the use of auditory brainstem response in acoustic neuroma screening. *Laryngoscope*. 1997;107(10):1388–1392.

CHAPTER 3

Vestibular Testing

Vincent Ostrowski

INTRODUCTION

A careful and thorough bedside history and neurotologic examination is essential for making an accurate clinical diagnosis in the patient with dizziness. Electronystagmography (ENG), rotary chair test (RCT), and computerized dynamic posturography (CDP) should be considered an important adjunct in the evaluation and management of these patients. The physician must couple the results of the clinical evaluation with the results of vestibular tests to solidify a diagnosis and help to direct treatment. Test results should not be considered alone without the clinical history. Testing often quantifies a clinical diagnosis but can also help to rule in or rule out a diagnosis. However, it is also important to remember that not every patient with dizziness needs vestibular testing.

Symptoms of a peripheral vestibular hypofunction are commonly related to the resulting disturbance in the vestibulo-ocular reflex (VOR). The VOR provides the ability to maintain clear vision during locomotion to prevent slip of a visual image that is focused on the retina. Assessing the integrity of the vestibulo-ocular reflex (VOR) is an integral part of vestibular testing. Quantifying the degree of vestibular loss and level of vestibular compensation are the most common applications of ENG and RCT. Quantifying and differentiating among the wide variety of possible sensory, motor, and central adaptive impairments to balance control is the most common application of CDP. Vestibular testing will be described in this chapter. Vestibular evoked myogenic potential (VEMP) and Electrocochleography (EcoG) are discussed further in Chapter 17.

ELECTRONYSTAGMOGRAPHY (ENG)

Patients with peripheral or central balance disorders often exhibit abnormal eye movements that can be measured and recorded. Electronystagmography (ENG) is a method of monitoring eye movements. For nearly 40 years, it has been widely used in the diagnostic evaluation of patients with dizziness or unsteadiness. The examination consists of a battery of tests that are collectively referred to as the ENG. The battery includes Calibration, Spontaneous Nystagmus, Gaze Test, Saccades, Sinusoidal Tracking, Optokinetic Nystagmus, Position Tests, and Caloric Tests. This battery of tests is designed to reveal vestibular and nonvestibular origins of eye movement abnormalities. A variety of eye movement recording equipment is currently available. The most common techniques used are videonystagmography (VNG) and the traditional electro-oculography (EOG). It is important to have patients abstain from vestibular suppressant medications (eg, diazepam) for at least 48 to 72 hours prior to ENG, as this can also be a cause of a "false-negative" test.

Electro-oculography (EOG)

Electro-oculography is the traditional technique of monitoring eye movements during the ENG and is based on the fact that there are steady direct current (DC) potentials, corneoretinal potentials, between the corneas and retinas of the eyeballs. These potentials create an electric field in the front of the head that rotates as the eyes rotate in their orbits. The cornea is relatively positively charged in comparison to the retina; thus an electric potential exists between the two.[1] This potential is generated by the metabolic activity of the retinal pigment epithelium. The retina is negatively charged relative to the cornea and therefore electrical potential can be measured between the two by means of skin surface electrodes. In neutral position the average potential measured is about 1 mV. Movement of the eyes causes potential changes relative to the skin electrodes. Movement of this electric field produces a roughly linear change in the voltage between electrodes attached to the skin on either side of the eyes. Electrodes placed on the patient's temples monitor horizontal eye position. Vertical eye position is monitored by electrodes placed above and below one of the patient's eyes. Some benefits of the EOG surface electrodes are that they are simple and relatively inexpensive. Disadvantages include the inability to monitor ocular torsion, being subject to bioelectric noise from facial muscles and a resolution of about 1 degree/second while monitoring eye movements.

Video-oculography (VNG)

Video-oculography is a technique that has recently become commercially available which utilizes digital video recorded eye movements. VNG is a computer-based system that records eye movement under test situations. The computer locates the eye position by detecting the pupil and tracking its center. The internal computer program plots, measures, and analyzes the eye movements under a battery of tests. This technique is easier and quicker than using electrodes with minimal patient preparation and only one calibration is necessary speeding up test time (Figure 3–1). Depending on the system, ocular torsion can be monitored by video, unlike EOG. Without the bioelectric interference from facial

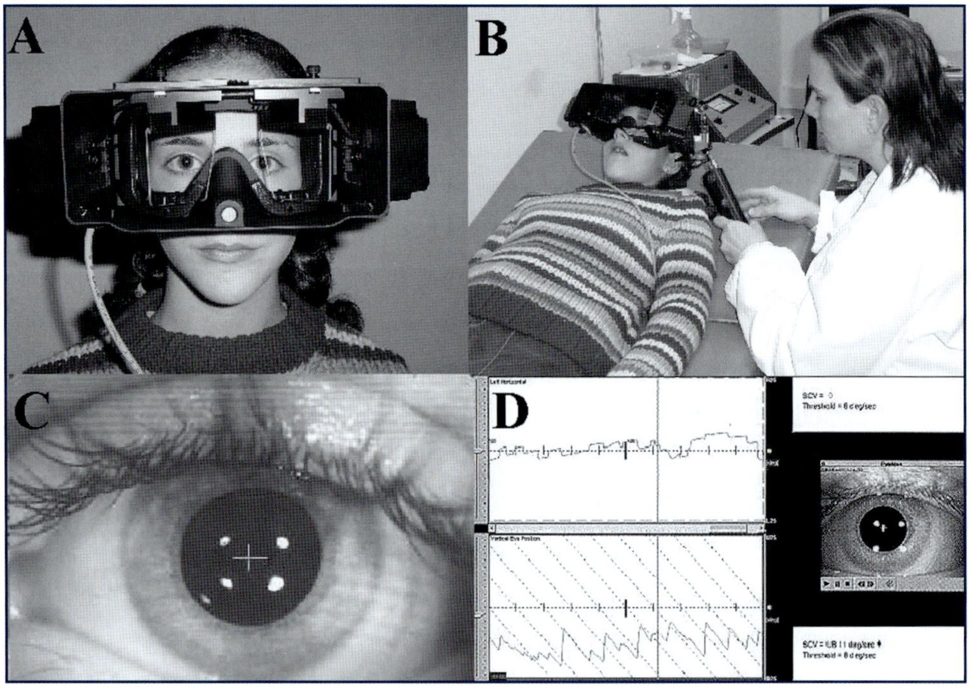

Figure 3–1. A. Infrared videonystagmography goggles (visual fixation blocking screen removed). **B.** Typical caloric application setup with video goggle monitoring. **C.** Infrared papillary tracking to monitor nystagmus. **D.** Digitized video output monitoring both horizontal and vertical nystagmus components.

muscles, tracings are clean with no drift as seen with traditional EOG tracings. Monitoring resolution can detect 0.1 degree per second movements. Blink artifact can be an issue as the eyes must be kept open during testing and some patients experience claustrophobia and may not tolerate the sensation of confinement. The testing equipment is expensive.

Routine Components of Electronystagmography

The ENG test battery generally consists of several tests. Testing can be grouped into oculomotor tests, position tests, and caloric tests. Testing nystagmus involves measurement of the slow phase of nystagmus as it is generated by the vestibuloocular reflex. Oculomotor test abnormalities usually give poor lesion site localization but are useful and commonly related to central nervous system dysfunction. In the gaze test, the patient's eye movements are monitored as he fixates while gazing 30 degrees to the right, 30 degrees to the left, 30 degrees up, and 30 degrees down. Young normal individuals rarely have any nystagmus while fixating at any of these gaze positions, but many elderly individuals have endpoint nystagmus. The gaze test detects nystagmus from vestibular origin as well as central nervous system origin. Upbeat nystagmus occurs most commonly as a result of medullary lesions involving vertical vestibular pathways.[2] The gaze test may also detect spontaneous nystagmus caused by a unilateral vestibular lesion.

Smooth pursuit requires the patient to smoothly track a target moving back and forth in the horizontal or vertical plane in a sinusoidal fashion. This involves central oculomotor pathways usually related to the vestibulocerebellar region. Saccade testing requires the patient to track a target in a horizontal or vertical plane to random locations. This is usually a light "dot" controlled by the computer. Saccade responses involve mainly brainstem and cerebellar pathways. Abnormally slow saccades velocities are characteristic of several degenerative and metabolic diseases of the central nervous system. Patients may also show abnormalities of saccade accuracy, making saccades that are too small or too large, indicating a lesion of the cerebellar nodulus. They may also show abnormally long saccade latencies, which have been associated with lesion of the frontoparietal cortex.[2] Optokinetic nystagmus (OKN) is generated as the patient follows a series of visual targets rapidly moving right then rapidly moving to the left. This nystagmus is a retinal reflex response and usually has a central nervous system origin in cases of abnormal OKN (Figure 3–2).

Position tests are performed by slowly moving the patient into various static head positions. Common examples would be supine with head turned left and then right. Visual fixation should be avoided. Nystagmus may be direction-fixed or direction-changing in the various positions. In the presence of previously identified abnormal oculomotor test results, definitive peripheral versus central etiology is not able to be determined. Nystagmus is described by the direction of the fast-phase, whether geotropic or ageotropic, whether it fatigues and if there is any torsional component involved. Positional nystagmus can be produced by either central or peripheral lesions. Results of positional testing are usually thought to be peripheral as long as the oculomotor testing was normal, there is no fixation, spontaneous nystagmus is absent, slow phase velocity is 6 degrees per/second or greater and there is no change in nystagmus direction within a given head position. Exact localization of the peripheral lesion may not be possible.[3]

The most common abnormality seen in the positional test is spontaneous nystagmus. It is suppressed by visual fixation and often suppression is so strong that spontaneous nystagmus is abolished by fixation. If fixation suppression is poor, it is an indication of a central nervous system lesion involving the pathways responsible for VOR cancellation. Spontaneous nystagmus is a reflection of tonic left-right vestibular asymmetry. It typically is seen after a recent unilateral peripheral vestibular lesion and has fast phases away from the side of the lesion.

Positioning tests are commonly performed to detect Benign Paroxysmal Positional Vertigo (BPPV). BPPV is discussed in greater detail in Chapter 21 but is included here as the Dix-Hallpike test is commonly and routinely included on most ENG/VNG tests. The patient is subjected to two brisk movements, both beginning with the patient in the sitting

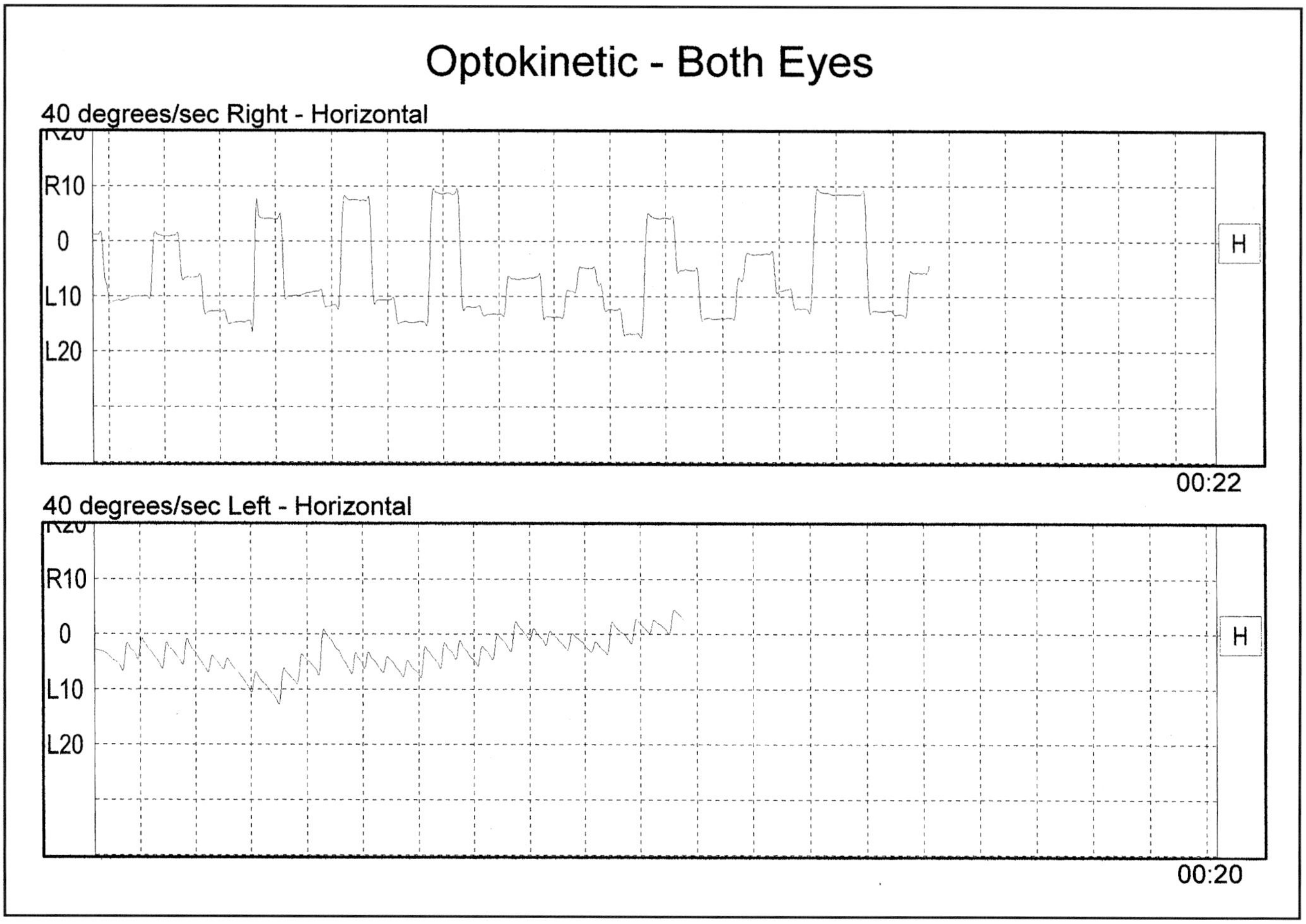

Figure 3–2. VNG tracing of abnormal right optokinetic nystagmus.

position. The patient's head is first turned 45 degrees toward one side. Then the examiner, standing to the side or behind the patient, pulls him briskly backward so that he is lying supine with his head still turned to that side and hanging over the end of the examining table. The examiner holds the patient's head in that position for at least 20 seconds and monitors his eye movements. Then he returns the patient to the sitting position. If a response was elicited, the examiner repeats the same maneuver to determine if it fatigues. Then he performs the maneuver with the patient's head turned 45 degrees to the other side, and if a response is elicited, repeats the maneuver to determine if it fatigues. The classic nystagmus found in posterior semicircular canal BPPV will be a geotropic torsional nystagmus with a horizontal nystagmus component toward the dependent ear. With the patient's symptomatic right ear down, the examiner will see a horizontal component toward the floor, and the superior poles of the eye rotate counterclockwise toward the ground from the examiner's viewpoint.

Typical findings of classic posterior canalithiasis BPPV will be a delayed onset of nystagmus of between 2 to 20 seconds after the patient reaches the head-hanging position before the nystagmus begins. Nystagmus is always transient; that is, it rapidly builds in intensity (crescendos), slowly abates (decrescendos) and finally disappears (within 45 seconds) as the head remains in position. Nystagmus is always accompanied by vertigo, usually intense, that follows the same time course of the nystagmus.

Nystagmus is usually fatigable; that is, it progressively diminishes in intensity with repetition of the Dix-Hallpike maneuver. Typical of ENG technology is the inability to record torsional nystagmus. Video capture will allow visualization of torsional nystagmus. Other types of nystagmus response, generally of central nervous system origin, are rarely provoked by the Hallpike maneuver. Usually, this nystagmus is strictly down beating without any torsional component. If so, it may be due to Chiari malformation, cerebellar degeneration, or a selective lesion of the cerebellar flocculus.[4]

Bithermal Caloric Test

The bithermal caloric test is the most likely vestibular test to lateralize a peripheral vestibular lesion as it specifically tests the integrity of the horizontal semicircular canals and their afferent pathways. Other vestibular test procedures, such as rotation testing and posturography, necessarily involve stimulation of both labyrinths together and therefore permit masking of abnormal responses from one labyrinth by normal responses from the opposite ear.

The patient is placed in the supine position with his head elevated by 30 degrees to place the horizontal canal in the vertical plane. The standard caloric stimulus consists of 250 mL of water irrigated into the external ear canal within 30 sec. The temperature of the water is 30 degrees C for the cool irrigation and 44 degrees C for the warm irrigation. Some examiners use air (8 L at 24 degrees C and 50 degrees C within 60 seconds) instead of water as the caloric stimuli. The basic assumption of the caloric test is that, for a given individual, the two ears receive equal caloric stimuli. If both vestibular systems are normal, they should produce responses of approximately equal intensity. Therefore the strength of the caloric responses from the two ears is compared. Most examiners use the formula for Unilateral Weakness (UW):

$$\frac{(RW + RC) - (LW + LC)}{RW + RC + LW + LC} \times 100 = UW$$

RW, RC, LW, and LC are peak slow phase velocities of the responses to right warm, right cool, left warm, and left cool responses, respectively, and UW is unilateral weakness. The normal limit of ±20% to 25% for UW is widely accepted (Figure 3–3).

Where the bithermal caloric test is highly sensitive to unilateral peripheral vestibular lesions, it is relatively insensitive to bilateral lesions. The usual rule of thumb is that a bilateral weakness exists if caloric responses (warm response plus cool response) of both ears fall below 12 degrees per/sec. Patients with labyrinthine hypofunction may demonstrate reduced or absent caloric responses to the initial bithermal stimuli. In this case, the test is repeated with ice water (approximately 0 degrees C) irrigations. However, one should keep in mind that the absence of a caloric response does not always imply absent peripheral function, as the stimulus levels are below the level within which the vestibulo-ocular reflex generally functions. Caloric stimulation is a low-frequency stimulus whereas the vestibular system has the capacity to function well over a wide variety of frequency stimuli. This has been compared to the analogy of performing an audiogram testing only one frequency. Aside from not being able to test the full dynamic range of the vestibular system, the caloric test only tests the lateral semicircular canal while the superior and posterior canals and utricle and saccule are not tested.

ENG testing is an important tool in the management of the patient with dizziness. It is by no means a substitute for a thorough neurotologic history and physical examination, and results should be interpreted in light of the clinical evaluation. Those who utilize ENG testing should have a thorough understanding of how the test is performed, what its components are, and the significance of the results. The clinician with a critical eye should always evaluate ENG reports. When used properly, ENG is arguably the single most valuable test currently available in the vestibular laboratory.

ROTATIONAL CHAIR TEST

Caloric testing has been and remains the primary method of evaluating vestibular function in patients complaining of dizziness. Despite its usefulness, caloric testing has a number of limitations. The caloric stimulus is difficult to control, is poorly tol-

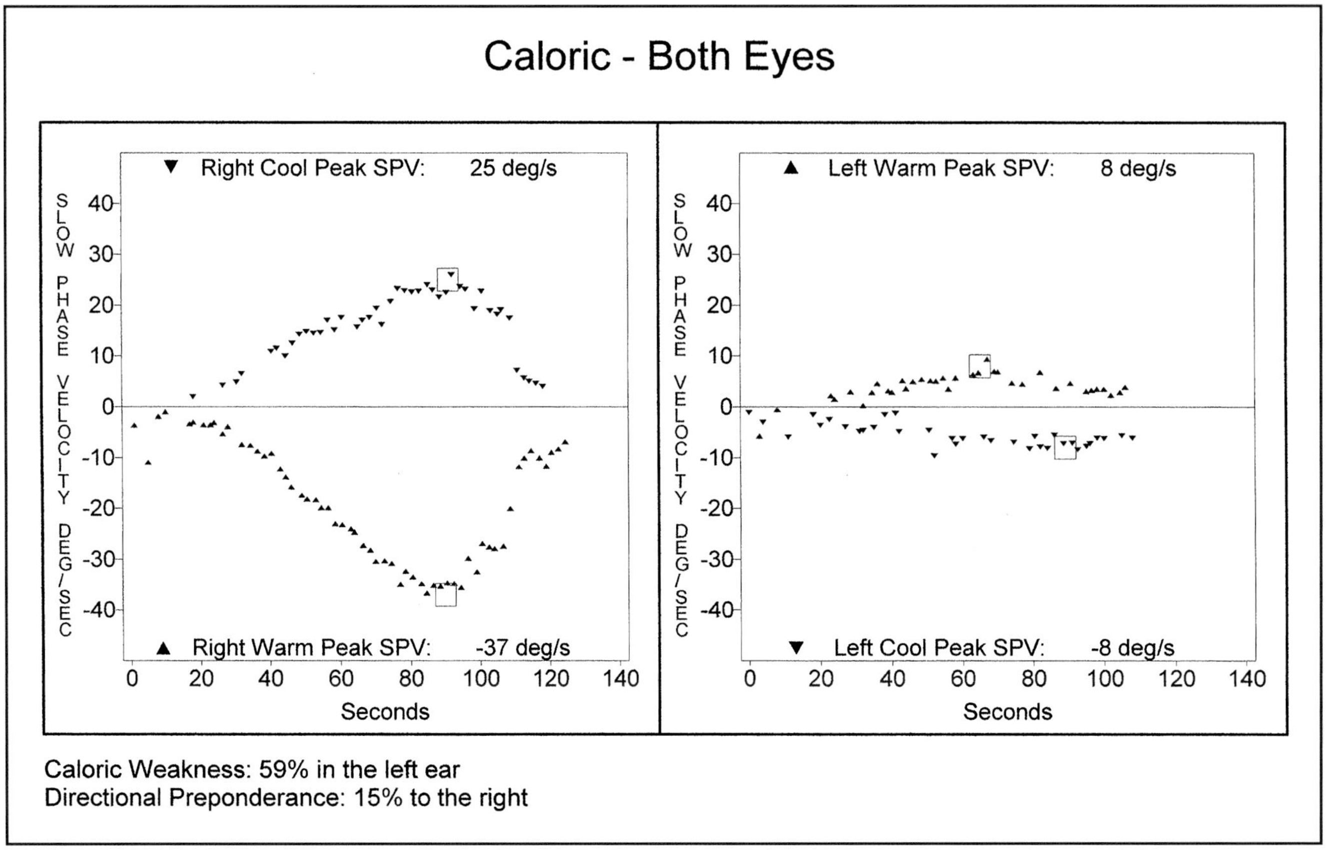

Figure 3–3. Caloric data tracing for right and left ears. A reduced vestibular response of 59% is seen in the left ear.

erated, and measures only the relative function of one ear with respect to the opposite ear. The caloric stimulus is considered to be a very low frequency test of vestibular function compared to the dynamic range of the vestibulo-ocular reflex (VOR). Unlike caloric testing, rotational tests allow multifrequency stimulation of the vestibular system.[5] Furthermore, the stimulus is well tolerated and independent of anatomical features of the ear. Rotational tests have been used to evaluate vestibular function for nearly a century. Over the years, various testing methods have been tried, but the one that has proven most useful involves positioning the patient so that the rotational axis is vertical and passes through the center of the head, thus stimulating only his horizontal semicircular canals.

The most widely used rotation test is the so-called slow harmonic acceleration test in which the patient is rotated sinusoidally at different frequencies.[6] The patient is seated in a chair mounted on a servo-controlled torque motor enclosed within a lightproof, sound-attenuating booth (Figure 3–4). The horizontal semicircular canals are in the plane of rotation and horizontal eye movements are monitored by electro-oculography (EOG) or video oculography, the same methods used in ENG testing. The patient is tested in total darkness with eyes open while performing mental arithmetic. He undergoes sinusoidal oscillation about a vertical axis at several different frequencies. The exact test protocol varies somewhat among laboratories, but a commonly used procedure employs oscillation frequencies of 0.01, 0.02, 0.04, 0.08, 0.16, 0.32, and 0.64 Hz, with peak angular velocities of 50 deg per/s at each frequency.[5] The patient undergoes multiple cycles of oscillation at each frequency.

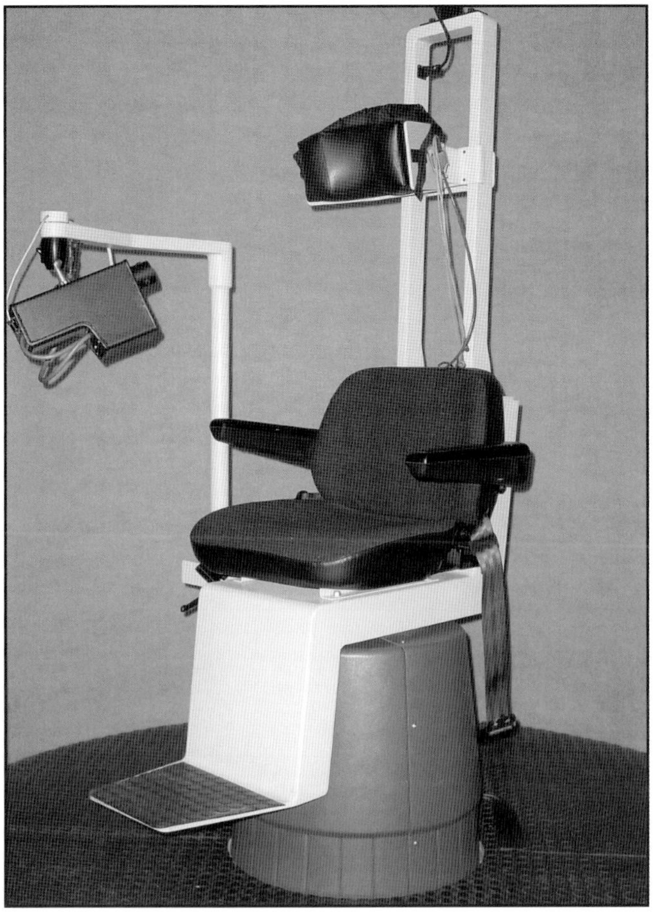

Figure 3–4. Computer controlled rotational chair as seen inside a light-tight testing booth. Head stabilization brace and infrared camera also shown.

The purpose of the vestibulo-ocular reflex is to produce eye movements that compensate for head movements. When the VOR operates in its optimal range, the eye movements exactly mimic the head movements in the opposite direction. If the reflex performs perfectly, the slow phase eye velocity plot would have the mirror image of the head velocity plot. However, compensation is less than perfect. The gain of slow phase eye velocity signal with respect to head velocity is only about 0.6. In other words, the eyes do not move quite fast enough during the nystagmus slow phases to compensate entirely for head movements. The computer then compares the head velocity and slow-phase eye velocity and calculates three measurements: phase, gain, and symmetry for each of the test frequencies.

The phase angle is the timing difference between the head and eye velocities and is presented as an angular unit of degrees rather than a unit of time. If the direction of slow phase eye velocity is exactly opposite the direction of head velocity at all times, the phase angle is 180°. Gain is defined as the ratio of peak eye velocity to peak head velocity. For perfect compensatory eye movements, the gain is 1. Asymmetry is defined as the difference between rightward and leftward eye velocities. For perfect compensatory eye movements, asymmetry is 0° (Figure 3–5). Although other causes are possible, the main reason for the presence of significant asymmetry is spontaneous or positional nystagmus in the sitting position.

Phase and gain values show progressive phase lead and gain reduction as oscillation frequency decreases. Symmetry values are approximately zero at all frequencies. At the higher frequency of 0.64 Hz, these relationships are about the same as they are at 0.16 Hz, but when the person is oscillated at progressively lower frequencies of 0.04, and finally 0.01 Hz, these relationships show progressive change. Slow phase eye velocities exhibit progressively lower gains, and they are no longer exactly opposite in phase, but rather displayed progressively larger phase leads.[5] In other words, changes in slow phase eye velocity occur more and more in advance of head velocity.

The slow harmonic acceleration test shows abnormalities primarily at the lowest and at the highest oscillation frequencies. Low frequencies reveal abnormal phase leads and gain reductions. High frequencies reveal asymmetries. Patients with acute unilateral peripheral lesions show the most severe abnormalities (Figure 3–6). ENG performed at the same time as rotation testing showed right-beating spontaneous nystagmus as well as weak caloric responses from the left ear. At the lower oscillation frequencies, this patient displayed progressively greater than normal phase leads, which is thought to be caused by a loss of velocity storage that is normally provided by the central vestibular system to enhance the low-frequency response of the vestibulo-ocular system.[7] Loss of velocity storage

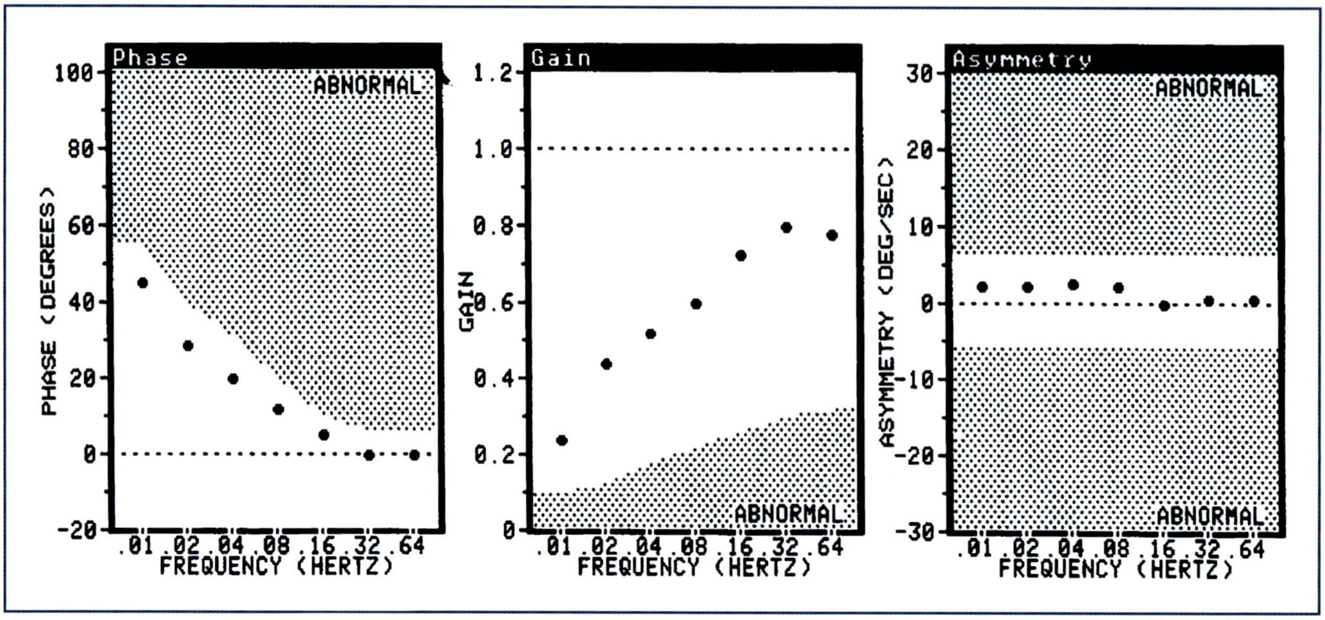

Figure 3–5. RCT data for normative subject. Averaged phase, gain, and asymmetry values are all outside the abnormal shaded data regions.

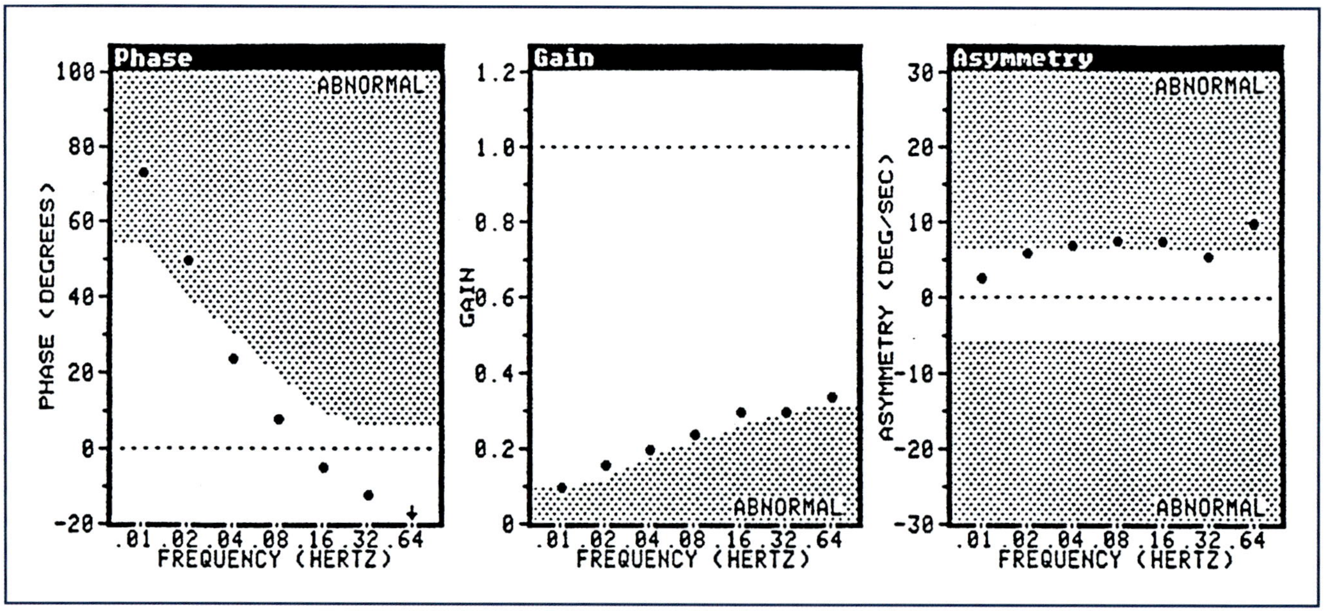

Figure 3–6. RCT data for a patient with an acute unilateral vestibular loss. Low frequencies reveal abnormal phase leads and gain reductions. High frequencies reveal asymmetries.

seems to represent habituation to the strong tonic asymmetry produced by the unilateral peripheral vestibular lesion.[8] Loss of velocity storage is not an exclusive feature of unilateral peripheral vestibular lesions. It is seen in a variety of vestibular disorders, both peripheral and central, and has also been observed in normal individuals who have undergone prolonged rotation.[9]

This patient also has a rightward asymmetry. That is, nystagmus with leftward slow phases is stronger than nystagmus with rightward slow phases. At low oscillation frequencies, the asymmetry is about equal to the slow phase velocities of the patient's spontaneous nystagmus with eyes closed; but at higher frequencies, the asymmetry is greater than could be accounted for by the spontaneous nystagmus. This additional asymmetry is thought to be due either to saturation of inhibitory responses of the intact labyrinth during rotation toward the side of the lesion or to an asymmetric loss of velocity storage.[8] This response pattern: abnormal low-frequency phase leads and high frequency asymmetry, is routinely observed in patients with acute unilateral peripheral vestibular loss.[6]

Abnormal low-frequency phase lead is the most common abnormality seen in the slow sinusoidal rotation test. This is a typical response in a patient who has undergone vestibular compensation to a unilateral loss (Figure 3–7). The caloric weaknesses in such a patient would usually be greater than 50%.

The slow harmonic acceleration test also shows abnormalities in patients with bilateral loss of vestibular function. The patient in Figure 3–8 is a patient with total bilateral absence of caloric response of unknown etiology. Rotation chair testing confirms bilateral caloric loss (see Figure 3–8). The patient failed to show a clear nystagmus response at any oscillation frequency. Most patients with bilateral absence of caloric response show absent responses or reduced response gains at the lower oscillation frequencies, but normal gains at the highest frequencies. Baloh et al[10] reported rotation testing often demonstrates normal vestibular function at high frequencies even when ice water irrigations have failed to provoke a response from either ear. In these cases, the results of caloric and rotation tests are not contradictory, since the caloric response is a response to a low-frequency stimulus and therefore should be similar to responses to low-frequency rotational stimuli. However, in other cases, rotation testing shows normal response gains at all frequencies despite absent caloric responses, indicating a false positive caloric test result. Clearly, the slow harmonic acceleration test is the procedure of choice in evaluating patients suspected of having bilateral loss of vestibular function. The caloric test, even with ice water, does not define the extent of the loss and sometimes yields false positive results.

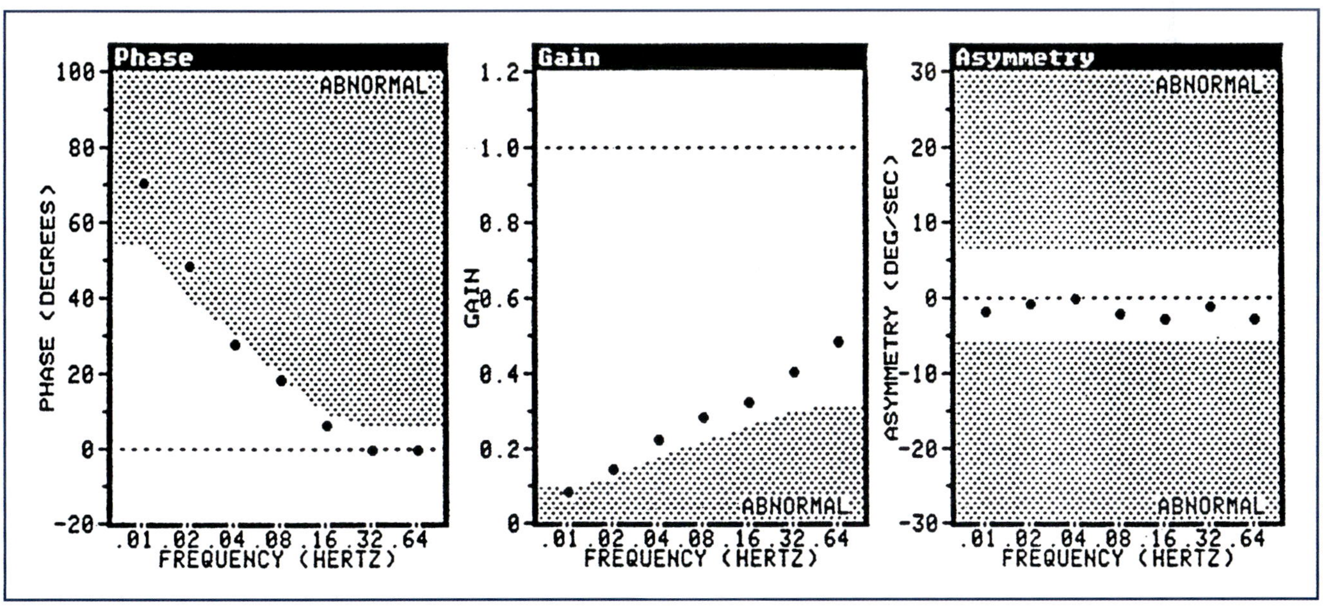

Figure 3–7. RCT data for a patient who has undergone vestibular compensation to a unilateral loss. Abnormal low-frequency phase lead is the most common abnormality seen in the slow sinusoidal rotation test.

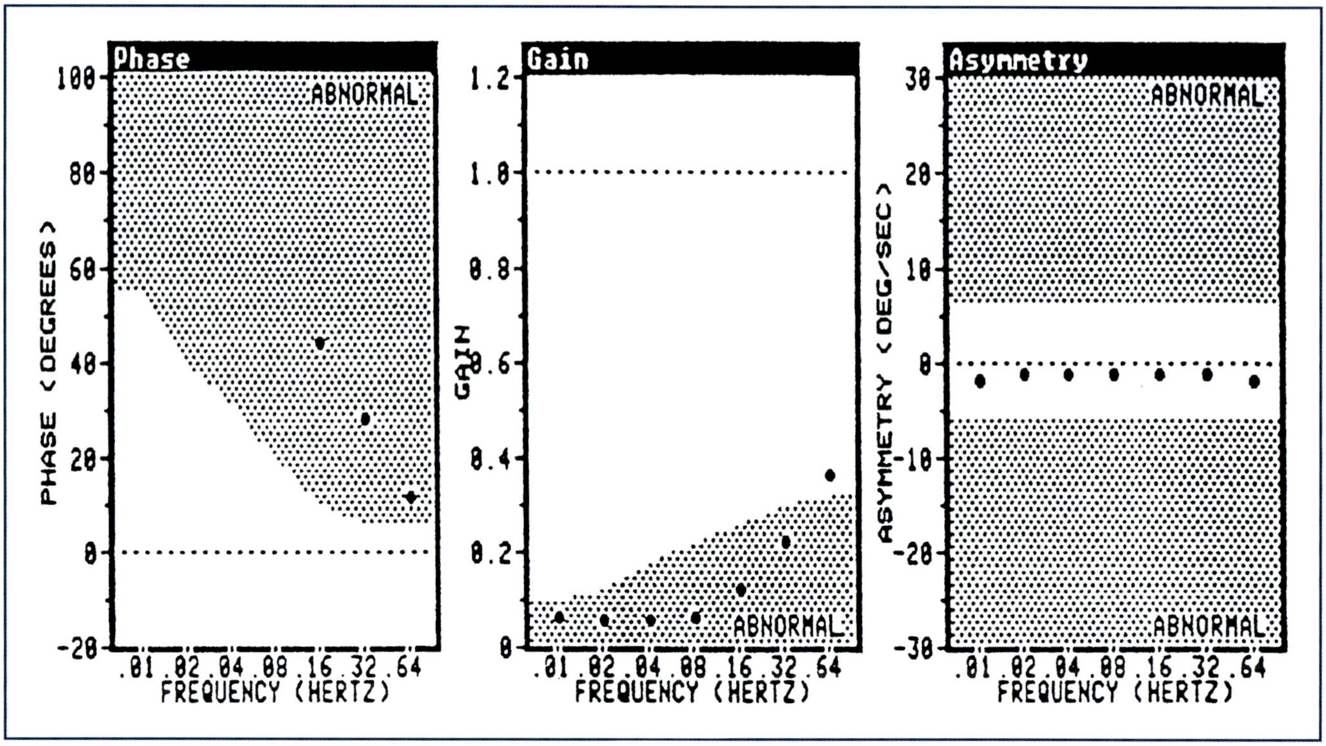

Figure 3–8. RCT data for a patient who has suffered a bilateral peripheral vestibular loss. Phase lead and depressed gain is seen in all but the highest rotational frequencies.

Advantages and Disadvantages of Rotational Chair Testing

RCT determines vestibular response over a spectrum of different frequencies of stimulation, not just the low-frequency tested by caloric stimulus. The degree of vestibular compensation can be assessed over time to evaluate improvement in vestibular performance or decline in VOR due to vestibulotoxic agents. RCT is valid when the caloric irrigations are below 10 degrees per/second bilaterally, when caloric irrigations cannot be performed, or when results in the two ears may not be compared reliably because of anatomic variability. Rotation testing can distinguish between true bilateral vestibular lesions and false positive caloric reduction caused by poor irrigations. RCT is the gold standard test to determine presence of bilateral vestibular loss. Last, RCT can be used to assess pediatric vestibular function when caloric testing is not tolerated.

Despite the applications described above, rotation testing remains mostly insensitive to common vestibular abnormalities, namely, unilateral vestibular lesions. In most cases, the level of unilateral loss must be substantial before any rotational abnormalities become apparent. Frequently, the sidedness of pathology remains undetermined and RCT cannot determine peripheral versus central pathologies. Last, like caloric testing, RCT only assesses the lateral semicircular canal and RCT technology is expensive and thus not commonly available.

VESTIBULAR EVOKED MYOGENIC POTENTIAL (VEMP)

The VEMP test is an evoked potential test of the saccule and inferior vestibular nerve response to sound stimulus. The VEMP tests the inferior vestibular nerve, rather than the superior vestibular nerve tested in the ENG, and may serve a complimentary role in the evaluation of the patient's vestibular system. Sound stimulates the saccule, travels along the inferior vestibular nerve to the vestibular nucleus in the brainstem. From there, the reflex response are sent to the neck muscles via the medial vestibulospinal tract. The net effect of stimulation of the saccule is inhibition with relaxation of the neck muscles noted on tracings.

The saccular response to sound is typically measured with a cervical muscle electrode though other sites are possible. The VEMP response will be present even with advanced sensorineural hearing loss but are typically reduced or absent if conductive hearing loss is present. Further studies are being done on variations of VEMP testing for oculomotor responses (oVEMP) and bone conduction VEMP.

For the the more common cervical VEMP, a sound tone burst is delivered to the ear and the sternocleidomastoid muscle response is monitored via surface EMG electrodes while the patient tenses the neck muscle, usually by having the supine patient elevate their head. When inferior vestibular nerve dysfunction is present the thresholds may be elevated or the amplitude of the response may be depressed such as with aminoglycoside ototoxicity. In the condition of superior canal dehiscence, the thresholds are reduced as it takes less sound intensity to stimulate a response. VEMP may be helpful in bilateral vestibular disease, Ménière's disease, and superior canal dehiscence. This is further discussed in Chapters 17 and 22.

COMPUTERIZED DYNAMIC POSTUROGRAPHY (CDP)

Computerized dynamic posturography (CDP) is a quantitative balance test that assesses standing balance function under a variety of conditions. It is based on a computerized testing device, called the SMART EquiTest® (NeuroCom® International, Inc., Clackamas, Oregon) The CDP consists of a platform that is capable of moving back and forth and tilting in the pitch plane about an axis colinear with the patient's ankle joints. During the test, the patient stands independently on the platform, wearing a harness for safety, facing a visual screen that is capable of tilting about the same axis as the platform. As the patient sways on the platform, a built-in force plate measures the changes in the position of the patient's center of gravity. These data are transmitted to the computer, which calculates the angle of the body sway in the pitch plane (Figure 3–9).

CDP is used to objectively quantify and differentiate among the wide variety of possible sensory, motor, and central adaptive impairments to balance control. CDP cannot diagnose pathology of site-of-lesion but can identify and differentiate the functional impairments associated with the pathological processes. Because of the complex interactions among sensory, motor, and central adapting processes, CDP requires separate protocols to adequately differentiate among impairments. CDP exposes the patient to a variety of controlled visual and support surface conditions to better quantify the failure of adaptive mechanisms.[11]

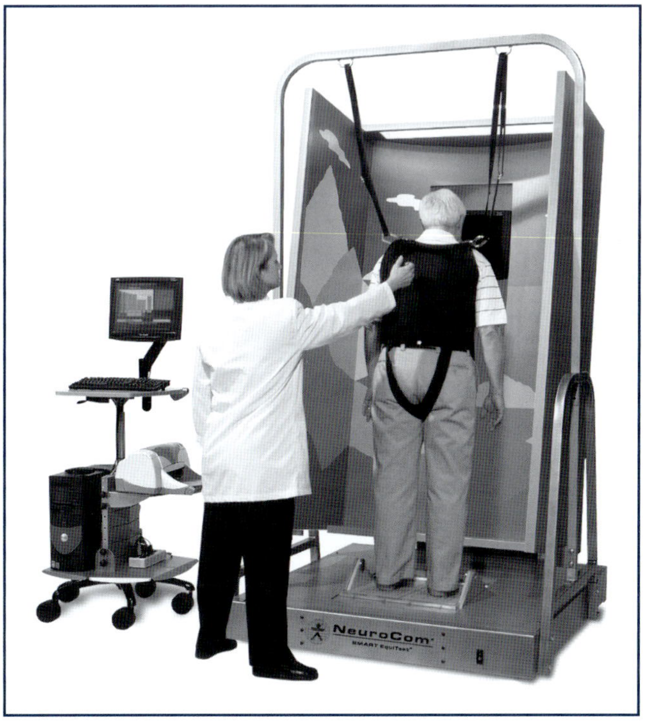

Figure 3–9. The SMART EquiTest® Dynamic Platform Posturography device. (Courtesy of NeuroCom® International, Inc)

CDP includes isolation and quantification of several features. These include: orientation inputs from the visual, vestibular and somatosensory systems, central integrating mechanisms for selecting functionally appropriate orientation senses, functionally appropriate movement strategy in a variety of controlled task conditions, and isolation and quantification of motor output mechanisms for generating timely and effective postural movements. Standardized test protocols include Sensory Organization Test (SOT), Motor Control Test (MCT), and Adaptation Tests (ADT). During the SOT, the utility of visual, vestibular, and proprioceptive inputs in controlling spontaneous sway is eliminated without provoking motor reactions by moving the support surface and the visual enclosure in response to the patient's postural movements. During the MCT and ADT, reactions are provoked by unexpected abrupt movements of the support surface. Because the measures of postural stability, as well as the motions of the support surface and visual surround, are precisely controlled and calibrated relative to the patient's height and weight, standardized graphical summaries can compare the patient's results to those of age-matched asymptomatic individuals.

The Sensory Organization Test (SOT)

SOT objectively identifies problems with postural control by assessing the patient's ability to make effective use of (or suppress inappropriate) visual, vestibular, and proprioceptive information. During the sensory organization test, the patient's postural stability is evaluated under six conditions in which either visual or proprioceptive cues (or both) are denied. Normally, patients maintain their balance by integrating visual, vestibular and somatosensory cues. The visual cues can be disrupted in one of two ways: visual input can be denied (by blindfolding the patient), or visual cues can be disrupted by sway-referencing the surroundings. Normal subjects will ignore inaccurate sway-referenced visual input, relying on other information to maintain their balance.[12]

Patients may display either an inability to make effective use of individual sensory systems, or inappropriate adaptive responses, resulting in the use of inaccurate sense(s). The six test conditions in the sensory organization test are as follows:

1. Support fixed, eyes open, visual fixed
2. Support fixed, eyes closed, visual fixed
3. Support fixed, eyes open, visual sway-referenced
4. Support swayed, eyes open, visual fixed
5. Support swayed, eyes closed, visual fixed
6. Support swayed, eyes open, visual sway-referenced.

The patient is subjected to each test condition three times, and an equilibrium score is calculated for each condition. The equilibrium score compares the patient's sway in the antero-posterior (AP) direction, compared to the theoretical limits of AP sway. A score of 100% implies little sway, and lower scores correspond to greater amounts of sway. The differences in scores for the six conditions are then analyzed to determine the specific nature of the patient's balance disorder (Figure 3–10). Of particular interest is the Vestibular Ratio, which compares conditions 1 and 5 and delineates the reduction in stability when the visual and somatosensory inputs are disrupted. Although healthy subjects will have some sway in condition 5, those with vestibular disease score poorer than average.

In addition to the Equilibrium Score during SOT Sensory Analysis, Strategy Analysis and Center of Gravity Alignment data are also displayed. Separate ratios of Condition 2 to the baseline average yield the somatosensory (SOM) ratio, Condition 4 to the baseline average yield the visual (VIS) ratio, Condition 5 to the baseline average yield the vestibular (VEST) ratio and the sum of conditions 3 and 6 to the sum of conditions 2 and 5 yield the vision preference (PREF) ratio. A low SOM ratio signifies impaired ability to use somatosensory information. A low VIS ratio signifies impaired ability to use visual information. A low VEST ratio signifies impaired ability to use vestibular information and a low PREF ratio implies visual dependence to maintain balance.

The Strategy Analysis is a graphical representation of how a patient maintains their balance in the face of an unsteady support surface. Flexion and Extension of both the ankle and hip joints are common means to remain upright and thus preventing

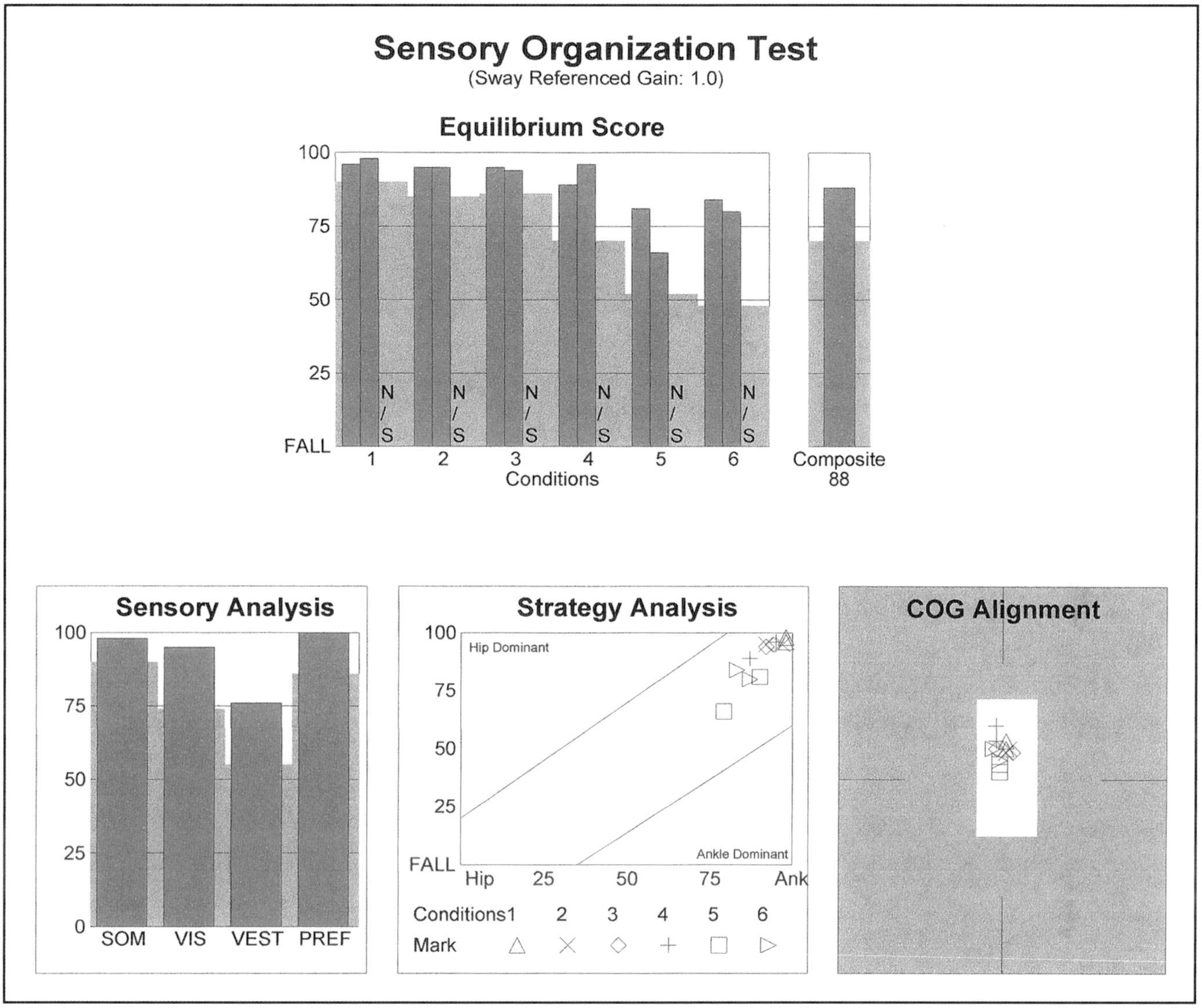

Figure 3–10. Normal balance pattern. (Courtesy of NeuroCom® International, Inc)

a fall. Ankle strategy is used appropriately to correct small body deviations and hip strategy is used to correct larger upper body deviations in fall prevention. Appropriate scores fall in the diagonal region of the plot. Upper left values are seen in patients using inappropriate hip strategy to correct small body position deviations. Lower right values are seen in patients using inappropriate ankle strategies to correct large body position deviations. The Center of Gravity (COG) plot shows the patient's COG at the start of each trial. The most common examples of Sensory Organization Tests are the Vestibular Loss Pattern (Figure 3–11), Visual Dependence Pattern (Figure 3–12), Somatosensory Dependence Pattern (Figure 3–13), and last the Aphysiologic (Malingering) Pattern (Figure 3–14).

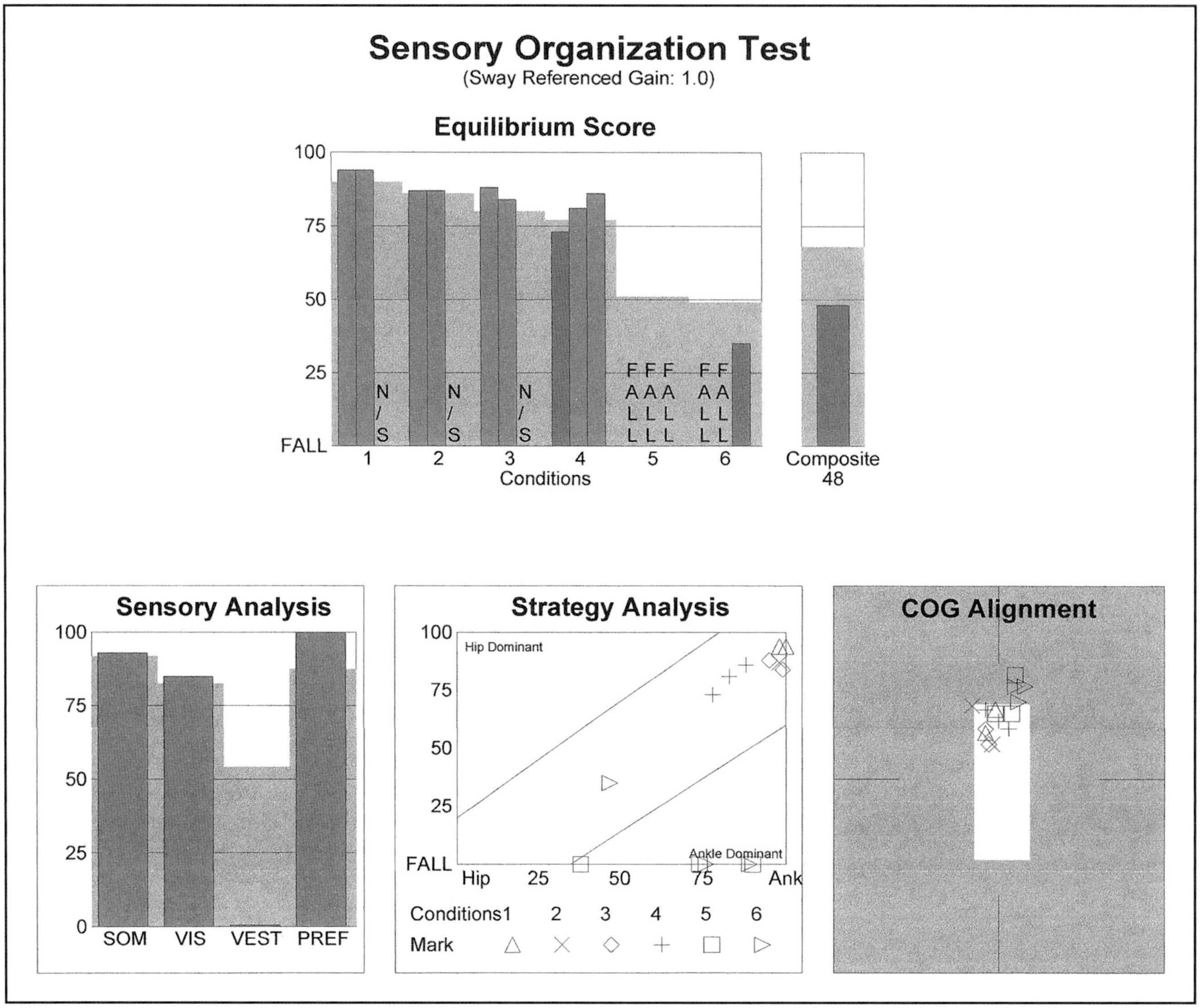

Figure 3–11. Vestibular loss pattern. (Courtesy of NeuroCom® International, Inc)

The Motor Control Test (MCT)

The motor control test assesses the patient's ability to quickly and automatically recover from unexpected external provocations. Sequences of small, medium, or large (scaled to the patient's height) translations in forward and backward directions elicit automatic postural responses. Measurements include onset timing, strength and lateral symmetry of responses. Aphysiologic MCT is very obvious with widely variable responses, delayed (volitional) responses and excessive, rhythmic or circular responses to small perturbations. Aphysiologic patterns will also be seen in the SOT testing, specifically in the setting of grossly abnormal SOT and normal MCT values.[13]

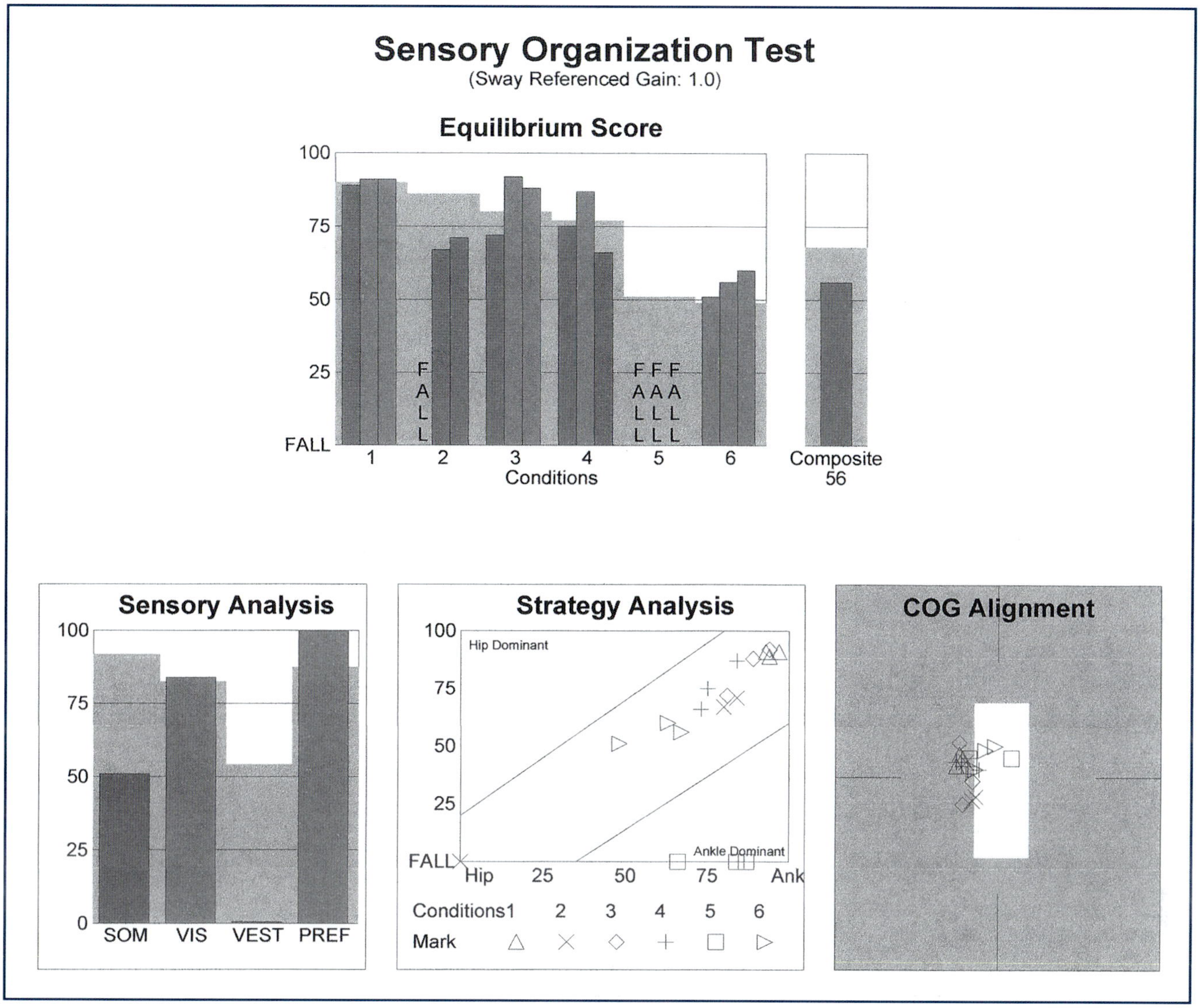

Figure 3–12. Visual dependence pattern. (Courtesy of NeuroCom® International, Inc)

The Adaptation Test (ADT)

The adaptation test assesses the patient's ability to modify motor reactions and minimize sway when the support moves unpredictably in the toes-up or toes-down direction. For each platform rotation, a sway energy score quantifies the magnitude of the force response required to overcome induced postural instability. This adaptive test simulates daily life conditions such as irregular support surfaces.

Although other vestibular testing will localize pathology and quantitate impairment, posturography will demonstrate a patient's functional impairment as it pertains to the sensory and motor impairments caused by the balance deficit. Identifying maladaptive compensatory mechanisms provides the clinician the best information as to how to best direct a patient's therapy and also to how evaluate success in treatment.

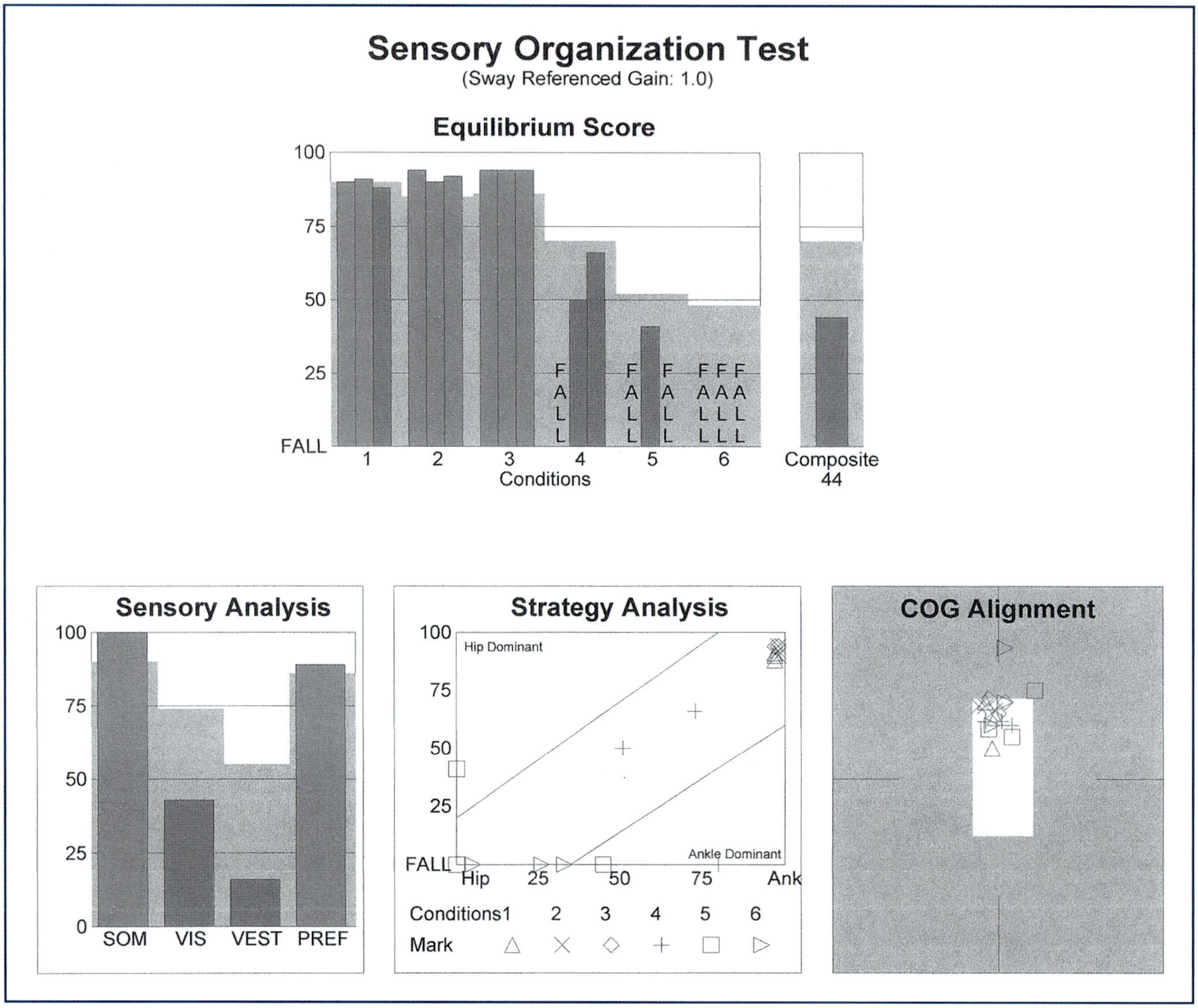

Figure 3–13. Somatosensory dependence pattern. (Courtesy of NeuroCom® International, Inc)

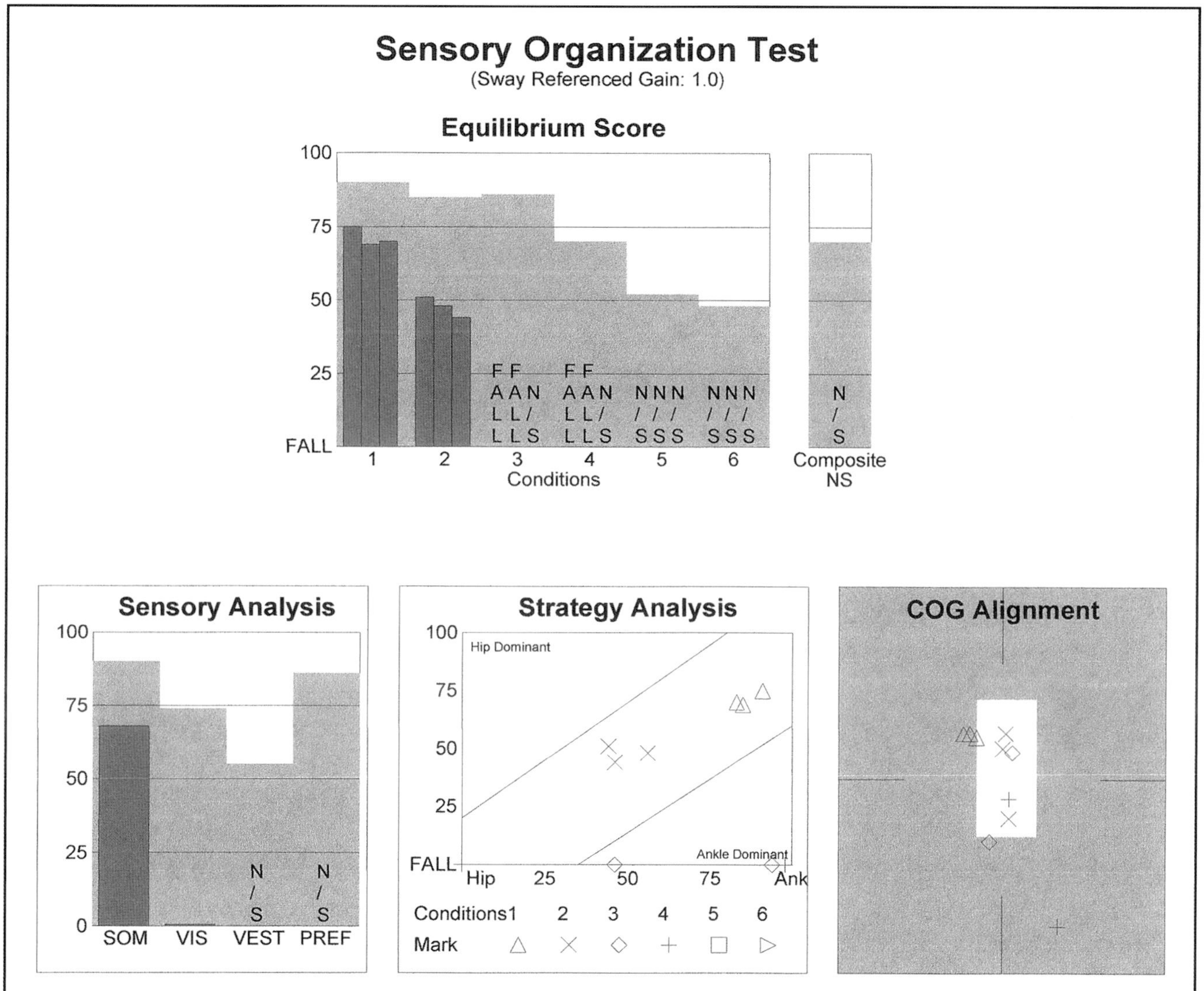

Figure 3–14. Aphysiologic (malingering) pattern. (Courtesy of NeuroCom® International, Inc)

REFERENCES

1. Leigh RJ, Zee DS. *The Neurology of Eye Movements,* 2nd ed. Philadelphia, PA: FA Davis; 1999.
2. Fisher A, Gresty M, Chambers BR, Rudge P. Primary position up beating nystagmus: a variety of central positional nystagmus. *Brain*. 1983;106:949–964.
3. Shepherd NT. Electronystagmography (ENG) testing. In: Goebel J, ed. *Practical Management of the Dizzy Patient*. Philadelphia, PA: Lippincott Williams & Wilkins; 2001:113–127.
4. Brandt T. Positional and positioning vertigo and nystagmus. *J Neurol Sci*. 1990;95:3–28.
5. Baloh RW, Sills AW, Honrubia V. Impulsive and sinusoidal rotatory testing: a comparison with results of caloric testing. *Laryngoscope*. 1979;89:646–654.
6. Stockwell CW, Bojrab DI. Interpretation and usefulness of rotational testing. In: Jacobson GP, Newman CW, Kartush JM, eds. *Handbook of Balance Function Testing*. St. Louis, MO: Mosby Year Book, Inc; 1993:237–248.
7. Raphan T, Matsuo V, Cohen B. Velocity storage in the vestibulo-ocular reflex arc (VOR). *Exp Brain Res*. 1979; 35:229–248.
8. Honrubia V. Vestibulo-ocular reflexes in peripheral labyrinthine lesions: I. unilateral dysfunction. *Am J Otolaryngol*. 1984;5:15–26.
9. Baloh RW, Henn V, Jager J. Habituation of the human vestibulo-ocular reflex by low frequency harmonic acceleration. *Am J Otolaryngol*. 1982;3:235–241.
10. Baloh RW. Changes in the human vestibulo-ocular reflex after loss of peripheral sensitivity. *Ann Neurol*. 1984;16: 222–228.
11. Nasher LM. Computerized dynamic posturography: Clinical applications. In: Jacobson DP, Newman CW, Kartush JM, eds. *Handbook of Balance Function Testing*. Chicago, IL: Mosby-Year Book; 1993.
12. Schieppati M, Hugon M, Grasso M. The limits of equilibrium in young and elderly normal subjects and in parkinsonians. *Electoencephalogr Clin Neurophysiol*. New York, NY: Elsevier Science; 1994.
13. Gianoli G, McWilliams S. Posturographic performance in patients with the potential for secondary gain. *Otolaryng Head Neck Surg*. 2000;122:11–18.

PART II

Pathology Affecting the External and Middle Ear

CHAPTER 4

Pathology of the External Ear

Jewel Greywoode and Gregory J. Artz

ANATOMY

The external auditory canal (EAC) begins at the external auditory meatus laterally and ends at the tympanic membrane (TM) medially. The canal is bordered by the floor of the middle cranial fossa superiorly, mastoid posteriorly, parotid and parapharyngeal space inferiorly, and the temporomandibular joint (TMJ) anteriorly. Derived from the first branchial cleft ectoderm, the EAC develops as a result of apoptotic recannalization in a medial to lateral direction. Failure of this recannalization results in congenital aural atresia and its associated conductive hearing loss.[1]

Lined entirely by squamous epithelium, elastic cartilage comprises the lateral one-third of the canal and a portion of the temporal bone makes up the medial two-thirds. There is no subcutaneous layer in the bony portion of the canal and the skin tightly adheres to the surface of the bone. Beneath the skin overlying the cartilage, the subcutaneous layer contains apocrine glands, sebaceous glands, and hair follicles. Termed apoliposebaceous units, these structures produce cerumen as part of the self-cleansing mechanism of the external canal.[2] Preformed pathways in the lateral cartilaginous portion of the canal, the fissures of Santorini, allow for spread of infection and/or tumor between the EAC and parotid gland. Medially, there can be an embryologic remnant defect, the foramen of Huschke, which also communicates with the parotid gland and glenoid fossa.[1]

Sensation to the canal is the result of innervation by several cranial and somatic nerves. The auriculotemporal nerve, a branch of the 3rd division of the Vth cranial nerve, supplies the anterior surface and roof of the canal. Arnold's nerve, auricular branch of the Xth cranial nerve, supplies the posterior wall and floor of the canal.[2] This contribution is responsible for the cough a patient may get during speculum examination and debridement of the external ear canal. This cough reflex appears to be more pronounced in the elderly population due to increased sensitivity of the ear canal skin. Hitselberger's sign is numbness of the conchal bowl and EAC due to decreased sensation of cranial nerve VII due to neural compression from a vestibular schwannoma.

FUNCTION

The EAC is a self-cleaning passageway responsible for the collection of sound. The shape of the EAC confers an acoustic advantage to transmit and funnel sound to the tympanic membrane and ossicular chain. The EAC in addition to the tympanic membrane provides protection for the middle ear space from foreign bodies and environmental factors. Cerumen is a common and normal finding in the ear canal. The major component of cerumen is desquamated keratin and is slight acidic in nature creating an unfavorable environment for bacteria or fungus. The self-cleaning mechanism of the EAC has been studied and is the result of lateral migration of epithelium from the TM to the external auditory meatus. Debris and cerumen produced by the apoliposebaceous units is carried toward the meatus by this migrating epithelium. Many patients will attempt self-cleaning; however, use of cotton-tipped applicators and other similar objects, particularly sharp objects, should be discouraged. There are several other methods to atraumatically remove cerumen from the external canal. Irrigation of the canal with water can be effective, but care should be taken to avoid extremes of temperature, as this may induce vertigo. Another common method for removal of cerumen is suctioning and/or curetting with a handheld otoscope or under otomicroscopic guidance.

PATHOLOGY

A wide variety of conditions affect the external auditory canal ranging from infectious and inflammatory etiologies to benign masses and tumors (Table 4–1). Otitis externa is one of the most common inflammatory/infectious conditions of the external canal. This condition usually follows trauma to the canal from instrumentation or moisture related to water exposure, hearing aids, ear plugs, music headphones, "earbuds," or excessive sweating. Traumatic temporal bone fractures can cause lacerations of the EAC. Dermatologic conditions of systemic diseases can also manifest within the ear canal, such as in psoriasis, eczema, or xerosis (dry skin). These dermatologic conditions lead to itching of the ear canal predisposing to infection from trauma and microtears and abrasions in the ear canal epithelium. Exostoses and osteomas are benign mass that are often found incidentally in the ear canal, and are rarely treated unless causing hearing loss or chronic infections. Examples of malignant neoplasms include squamous cell carcinoma, basal cell carcinoma, and adenoid cystic carcinoma from the adjacent parotid gland.[3] This chapter serves to highlight the important points in the pathophysiology, diagnosis, and

Table 4–1. Differential Diagnosis of External Auditory Canal Pathology

Infectious/Inflammatory	**Neoplasm/Mass**
Otitis externa (OE)	Benign
Acute	Papilloma
Chronic	Hemangioma
Malignant	Ceruminoma
Fungal otitis externa	Exostosis
Eczematous otitis externa	Osteoma
Dermatitis	Keratosis obturans
Atopic	External canal cholesteatoma
Contact	Fibrous dysplasia
Seborrheic	Eosinophilic granuloma
Psoriasis	Malignant
Systemic lupus erythematosus	Squamous cell carcinoma
Folliculitis/Furunculosis	Basal cell carcinoma
Bullous myringitis	Adenoid cystic carcinoma
Trauma	**Miscellaneous/Other**
Iatrogenic	External auditory canal stenosis
Foreign body	Idiopathic
Temporal bone fracture	Elderly
	"Itchy ear"
Congenital	Encephalocele
Complete aural atresia	Displaced temporomandibular joint
External auditory canal stenosis	
Branchial cleft anomaly (Type I and II)	

treatment of the most common external auditory canal pathology. Topical treatments utilized in the treatment of these external ear canal disorders are also discussed.

INFECTIOUS/INFLAMMATORY

Otitis Externa

Otitis externa (OE) is an inflammatory process of the external auditory canal that occurs as a result of irritation to the canal skin. Acute otitis externa occurs when the acidic and hydrophobic environment created by cerumen is disrupted. This can occur as a result of trauma to the thin canal skin from instrumentation by a fingernail, cotton-tipped applicator, or other foreign body. A breach in the integrity of the ear canal skin barrier allows opportunistic normal flora to cause inflammation and infection. Prolonged exposure to water (eg, swimming) or a moist environment from a tympanic membrane perforation or draining pressure equalization tube can create the perfect conditions for the proliferation of bacteria. Additional causes of moisture buildup in the ear canal that can lead to infections include hearing aids, ear plugs, "ear bud" headphones, and excessive sweating. In addition, any process that disrupts the self-cleansing mechanism of the ear canal, such as overproduction of cerumen, prominent exostoses or osteomas, or accumulation of squamous keratin debris called keratosis obturans, may result in otitis externa.[4] The clinical picture of otitis externa is a spectrum ranging from itching and mild discomfort to severe pain and life-threatening involvement of the temporal bone. Recognition of this common disease process is essential to appropriate diagnosis, treatment, and prevention of complications. When interviewing patients, they sometimes report a distinct incident of canal trauma or prolonged exposure to water; however, many patients cannot recall any inciting event related to the problem. In milder/early acute otitis externa, symptoms include itching and discomfort. On physical exam, the canal is often tender, edematous, and can partially obscure the view of the tympanic membrane. Debris may be present and can be white, yellow, and green in color. In more severe or advanced stages, there is severe pain, intense purities, and copious otorrhea. The canal will become tender and edematous, such that the tympanic membrane is usually not visible. In many cases, the patient may have decreased hearing in the affected ear from the debris and associated ear canal and tympanic membrane edema.

The most common organisms involved are *Pseudomonas* and *Staphylococcus aureus* species.[5] Management involves creating a dry environment unsuitable for the growth and proliferation of these bacteria. An antibiotic drop is commonly used and the addition of steroids (eg, dexamethasone) to the preparation has been shown to be effective in reducing inflammation. Some commonly used topical medications include combinations of ciprofloxacin with dexamethasone, tobramycin with dexamethasone, ofloxacin, and neomycin with hydrocortisone. Ofloxicin is the only one listed that is not combined with a steroid. Care must be used when prescribing tobramycin or neomycin if a tympanic perforation is present due to the risk of ototoxicity. Because of the amount of edema that can occur in the canal, an ear canal wick is often placed to facilitate the drops reaching the medial canal. Pain control with anti-inflammatory or oral narcotics is usually required.

Chronic otitis externa is a chronic thickening of the external ear canal due to a low-grade infection/inflammation of the canal skin. Signs and symptoms can be similar to acute OE, but most often, these patients complain of dry, "itchy" ears. On exam, the canal can be erythematous, but marked edema is noticeably absent. Treatment is aimed at reducing inflammation and/or infection, and includes topical corticosteroids, antibiotic drops, and regular office EAC debridement. Systemic therapy can include oral antibiotics such as ciprofloxacin or doxycycline. Surgical intervention can include canalplasty with a split-thickness skin graft; however, this may not address the underlying skin pathology.

Malignant Otitis Externa (MOE)

Malignant otitis externa is a severe, localized infection of the temporal bone and/or skull base that occurs from progression of otitis externa in diabetics and immunocompromised individuals. Pseudomonas is the most common organism involved and these patients complain of severe otalgia. Severe cases can progress to skull base osteomyelitis (SBO) and may present with VIIth cranial nerve palsy or have multiple cranial neuropathies. Other common microbes that cause otitis externa include Staphylococcus species, and gram-negative rods. Findings on physical exam include generalized edema of the ear canal skin with exudate, and in severe cases granulation tissue can be seen at the bony cartilaginous junction of the external canal. Treatment of these individuals involves conservative ear canal cleaning and debridement with the addition of long-term systemic antibiotics, preferably directed by microbiology culture results. The infection may spread along the temporal bone and become a skull base osteomyelitis. The treatment paradigm has shifted over the past few decades away from aggressive surgical debridement of the skull base to use of intravenous antibiotics with hyperbaric oxygen, except in cases of severe cranial neuropathies.[5] There is also controversy regarding the best radiologic study to follow patients with MOE and/or SBO and how to best determine response to antibiotic treatment. A pre-treatment MRI and CT scan of the temporal bone is recommended and then a follow-up MRI after completion of antibiotic therapy. A bone scan can also be helpful pre- and post-treatment to evaluate for resolution of inflammation and skull base involvement.

Fungal Otitis Externa

Fungal otitis externa (otomycosis) is a condition that usually occurs from overgrowth of fungal organisms in the ear canal. The usual mechanism involves overuse of antibiotic drops, which can kill normal bacterial flora and change the pH of the ear canal allowing for the proliferation of these fungal organisms. Diabetics and other immunocompromised individuals are at a greater risk for developing these opportunistic infections. It is also not uncommon to encounter this in patients with occlusive hearing aid molds. Signs and symptoms can be similar to nonfungal OE. Pruritis and thick otorrhea are common. Culture usually reveals *Candida* or *Aspergillus* species.[6] The spores of the *Aspergillus* species, known as conidiophores, can sometimes be seen lining the EAC. Initial management is aimed at eliminating the warm, moist environment in which these organisms thrive. The canal is carefully debrided with suction under otomicroscopic guidance and agents such as acetic acid, gentian violet, boric acid, or thimerosal are utilized to dry and acidify the canal, reducing colonization. Topical antifungal medications such as clotrimazole and itraconazole can also be effective. Avoidance of the triggering factors is important in preventing recurrence. One of the most commonly used topical agents is a clotrimazole/betamethazone combination cream. It can be applied into the ear canal through a syringe and 18-gauge angiocatheter. The ear canal is filled with the cream with 0.5–1.0 cc of medication and the patient returns in 1 week for evaluation and debridement. Patients must be counseled that they will have hearing loss in the affected ear for several days due to the application of the cream. This cream, when applied in the office, is very successful in managing otitis externa due to infectious or dermatologic causes.

Eczematous Otitis Externa

Eczematous otitis externa is a general term to describe dermatologic conditions affecting the external auditory canal.[7] Patients usually complain of dry, scaly, pruritic canals and are at risk of developing otitis externa as a result of instrumentation to relieve itching. Conditions involved include lupus erythematosus, psoriasis, dermatitis (atopic, contact, seborrheic), and xerosis (dry skin). Individuals with atopic dermatitis will usually have a family or personal history of allergies. Atopic dermatitis of the ear canal can range from mild erythema or scaling to severe crusting and exudative lesions. Topical steroids are the mainstay of treatment. Creams seem to work best for exudative lesions and ointments for thick, scaly lichenified lesions.[8] When applying a cream or ointment to the ear canal for a dermatitis, one can try to not completely occlude the ear canal and suction out the center portion of the ointment so the patient's hearing is not compromised. Contact dermatitis occurs in individuals with exposure to certain irritants. Neomycin sensitivity is one of the most well-recognized causes of contact dermatitis in the external canal. Treatment involves stopping the offending agent and treatment with corticosteroid/antibiotic drops. Seborrheic dermatitis, or dandruff, occurs most often on the scalp and forehead, but can involve the external auditory canal. Treatment is with topical corticosteroids or medicated shampoos. Lupus erythematosus and psoriasis are systemic, chronic inflammatory, autoimmune conditions that may require dermatology consultation for management. Topical corticosteroids in cream or drop form can be helpful to relieve local symptoms, such as itching, and reduce inflammation. Proper application in the ear canal is critical to effectively treat these dermatoses with topical steroid preparations. Patient often try to apply ointments and creams with cotton-tipped applicators unsuccessfully as they cover only a small area of the outer ear canal skin. The most effective treatment is repeated applications in the office using a syringe and 18-gauge angiocatheter.

Bullous Myringitis

Bullous myringitis refers to inflammation of the outer epithelial layer of the tympanic membrane. Frequently, this extends onto the medial portion of the ear canal. Patients usually experience severe otalgia, otorrhea, and hearing loss. On examination, bullae can be seen on the drum surface and a serous otitis media may be present. There is an association with upper respiratory infections, specifically those caused by *Mycoplasma*. The hearing loss is usually sensorineural and more than half of patients will regain their hearing. Treatment involves antibiotic ear drops, oral analgesics, and oral antibiotics to treat the *Mycoplasma*.[6] If there is any sensorineural hearing loss on audiogram, one may consider treating this similar to a sudden sensorineural hearing loss patient with 60 mg of prednisone for at least a week with repeat audiometry at one week. Intratympanic dexamethasone injections are an option if the sensorineural hearing loss persists despite treatment with oral medications.

NEOPLASMS/MASSES

There are several different masses that can occur in the external ear canal. Most of these are benign and are easily treated with medical therapy and/or surgical intervention. When evaluating an ear canal mass, it is important to consider not only structures within the canal, but also the structures that border the canal. For example, a defect in the tegmen, may allow herniation of cerebral contents into the middle ear cavity. This condition is not uncommon with increased intracranial pressure, such as in pseudotumor cerebri or benign intracranial hypertension. A defect in the anterior wall of the canal (rare) or trauma can displace the temporomandibular joint posteriorly into the external canal space. Prior surgery can also raise suspicion for an iatrogenic external ear canal cholesteatoma anywhere in the ear canal where the epithelium was disrupted, most commonly in the bony EAC from a prior skin incision.

Benign

Exostosis/Osteoma

Exostoses are bony growths in the external canal believed to be a reactive process to repeated cold water exposure.[4] They are multiple, broad-based hyperostotic lesions, usually bilateral in nature, and tend to occur in the medial portion of the bony canal where the ear canal skin is thinnest. Histologically, the lesions are composed of concentric layers of dense lamellar bone, resembling an "onion-skin." Typically asymptomatic, large lesions can cause obstruction of the canal causing conductive hearing loss and/or otitis externa. Additionally, the physical obstruction to cerumen clearance predisposes the individual to other processes such as keratosis obturans or external auditory canal cholesteatoma.[9] Management of exostoses involves treating the associated medical conditions that may develop such as otitis externa. Surgery is only recommended for those patients with recurring symptoms of hearing loss, pain, infection, otorrhea and keratin buildup. Surgical management can be performed transcanal or through a postauricular incision depending on the patient's anatomy and experience of the surgeon. The surgery involves raising a tympanomeatal skin flap, drilling the lesions, and completing a canalplasty. A skin graft may be needed if there is loss of skin and /or large areas of exposed bone. Recurrence of these lesions is related to continued exposure to cold water.[10]

Osteomas are unilateral, solitary, pedunculated, bony growths that usually occur at the tympanosquamous or tympanomastoid suture lines. Histologically, they are also composed of dense lamellar bone, but the orientation is irregular and there is intervening fibrovascular tissue.[11] The exact etiology of these lesions is unknown and growth of these lesions can also cause obstruction of the canal resulting in cerumen accumulation or hearing loss. Treatment involves excision of symptomatic lesions.

Keratosis Obturans/External Canal Cholesteatoma

Previously thought to be the same entity, keratosis obturans and external canal cholesteatoma are two distinct entities unique in etiology, presentation, and treatment. First described by Toynbee in 1850, keratosis obturans refers to the accumulation of keratin plugs in the external canal causing acute severe pain and conductive hearing loss.[12] Typically bilateral, they occur in younger patients and there is an observed association with bronchiectasis and sinusitis in these patients.[9] These lesions usually are not destructive and treatment involves careful mechanical removal of the epidermal plug. Treatment of any associated otitis externa is also addressed.

External auditory canal (EAC) cholesteatoma is the accumulation of epithelium that is identical to the middle ear cholesteatoma and petrous apex epidermoid, but occurs in the external canal. EAC cholesteatoma is less frequent than middle ear cholesteatama and usually caused by trauma, prior ear surgery, or persistent cerumen accumulation. These lesions are locally destructive, and in rare, advanced stages can invade nearby structures.[13] Otorrhea is a common symptom, but hearing loss is rare because there is no physical obstruction of the drum. Because of the destructive nature of external canal cholesteatoma, biopsy is important to rule out a malignancy such as squamous cell carcinoma. Naim et al[13] proposed a classification system based on the extent of involvement of the external canal. Stage I is limited to hyperplasia of the canal epithelium; stage II evolves to periosteitis; stage III includes a defective bony canal; and stage IV presents with erosion of adjacent anatomic structures. Treatment of stage I disease involves periodic cleaning of the canal to prevent progression of the disease. Stage II and III are managed surgically with excision to a clear margin of normal skin. Any underlying erosive bone is to be excised to smooth bone and repair achieved with soft tissue, cartilage, or fascia. The most destructive lesions, stage IV require a mastoidectomy to remove all infected tissue and devitalized bone. Because of the rare nature of this disease entity, long-term results are currently unavailable.

Ceruminoma

Ceruminous glands are modified apocrine sweat glands and benign tumors can occur. Termed ceruminous adenoma or pleomorphic adenoma, theses lesions are usually asymptomatic until they cause hearing loss, aural fullness, or secondary external otitis.[5] Treatment includes biopsy to rule out malignancy and local excision. A split-thickness skin graft may be needed when resection results in a large defect.

Malignant

Primary malignant neoplasms of the external ear canal or temporal bone are rare. Most often, lesions that prove to be malignant are spread of tumor from the surrounding structures such as the auricle or parotid gland. Squamous cell carcinoma is the most common malignant tumor of the canal, followed by basal cell carcinoma and adenoid cystic carcinoma.[5] Treatment usually involves surgical excision and adjuvant radiotherapy for advanced lesions.

Miscellaneous

External Auditory Canal Stenosis

Stenosis of the EAC can be primary or acquired. Primary causes include congenital atresia or stenosis from failure or incomplete recannalization of the canal. Acquired stenosis can be the result of trauma, surgery, or masses and can be very difficult to treat. These patients require wide excision with canalplasty and split thickness skin grafts. Restenosis is common and beneficial adjunctive therapies include topical steroids and kenalog injections.

A common problem in the elderly is reduced elasticity of the conchal bowl cartilage leading to a narrowing of the ear canal laterally. This is often referred to as "lateral ear canal collapse." This problem leads to a buildup of cerumen and can be troublesome when fitting patients for hearing aids. Routine ear canal debridement every 6 to 12 months usually prevents severe impactions and surgical meatoplasy is rarely indicated.

TOPICAL TREATMENTS

Various topical medications have been applied to the external canal to treat various conditions. The basic function of these ototopical agents is direct killing of the organisms involved or changing the environment of the canal. These topical medications come in various forms and usually have more than one function (Table 4–2). The addition of other agents such as a steroid or acetic acid gives them added anti-inflammatory and acidification properties, respectively. In the presence of a tympanic membrane perforation, the acidic nature of many of the drops can cause pain and discomfort. Moreover, most of the drugs are ototoxic and should not be allowed to enter the middle ear space. Ophthalmic solutions are often used in the ear canal and tend to have a pH closer to neutral, thereby causing less pain and discomfort if there is a perforation.[6]

Table 4–2. Topical Treatments in the External Auditory Canal

Antibacterial	**Acidification and Drying**
Fluoroquinolone	Acetic acid (VoSol™)
Ciprofloxacin	Aluminum acetate (Domeboro™)
Ofloxacin (Floxin™)	Boric acid
Aminoglycosides	Gentian violet
Gentamicin	Thimerosal
Neomycin	**Other**
Tobramycin	Hydrogen peroxide
Other	Carbamide peroxide (Debrox™)
Chloramphenicol	Fluocinolone Acetonide (DermOtic™)
Antifungal	
Clotrimazole (Lotrimin™)	
Itraconazole (Sporanox™)	
Tolnaftate (Tinactin™)	
Methylcresyl acetate (Cresylate™)	

Antibacterial

Antimicrobials, specifically antibacterial drops, are commonly used to treat bacterial infections of the external ear, as in otitis externa. Fluoroquinolones (eg, ciprofloxacin, ofloxacin) are effective against associated microorganisms such as *Pseudomonas* and *Staphylococcus* species and are generally considered safe to use in the presence of a tympanic membrane perforation. The addition of a steroid such as dexamethasone (Ciprodex™) or hydrocortisone (Cipro HC™) gives added anti-inflammatory properties.

Aminoglycosides such as neomycin, gentamicin, and tobramycin are also effective against *Pseudomonas* and *Staphylococcus* species, but are known to be ototoxic and should not be used in the presence of a tympanic membrane perforation. Neomycin can be combined with polymyxin, and hydrocortisone (Cortisporin™), to achieve added anti-inflammatory properties, but neomycin is a common cause of allergic sensitivity and contact dermatitis. This is usually suspected if there is no improvement or worsening of the drainage after 48 to 72 hours of treatment. Tobramycin (Tobradex™) a common prescribed topical ophthalmic preparation with dexamethasone, can be used for chronic otitis externa and otitis media in patients with multiple drug allergies, however the potential for ototoxicity must be clearly stated to the patient. Chloramphenicol, now rarely used, except in refractory cases, is effective against bacterial and fungal organisms.

Antifungal

Fungal colonization of the external canal is usually treated by drying and acidification of the ear, but antifungal agents can also be effective in eradicating organisms. An over-the-counter preparation such as clotrimazole (Lotrimin™) is effective. *Aspergillus* infections may be resistant and itraconazole is a good alternative. The only antifungal considered safe for use with a tympanic membrane perforation is tolnaftate (Tinactin™), which can be made into a powder form for easier application to the EAC skin. Topical m-cresyl acetate (Cresylate™) has been shown to be very effective and also has antibacterial properties.[14]

Acidification and Drying

Acetic acid (VoSol™, Acetasol™) has long been used in the preparation of topical ear drops. The most common use is to acidify the ear with otitis externa and to reduce fungal colonization. When combined with alcohol, there is a drying effect as well. In the presence of a perforation, this can cause severe discomfort and should be avoided. Related preparations include acetic acid with hydrocortisone (VoSol HC™), which has minimal antibacterial properties, but is effective at acidifying the ear canal and reducing associated itching and swelling in otitis externa. Aluminum acetate, available as a powder, is a topical astringent that is water soluble and can be added to the acetic acid solution (Domeboro™) achieve acidification and anti-inflammatory effects.[14] One must be aware that many of these acidifying agents can be painful and uncomfortable for patients during the first few days, particularly with severe infections where there is excoriation of the ear canal skin and ulcerations. These medications are not recommended when there is a tympanic membrane perforation due to the risk of ototoxicity and pain.

The most common drying agents include boric acid and gentian violet. Boric acid is a commercially available hydrophilic powder that is frequently combined with other agents (eg, dexamethasone, clotrimazole, ethanol) to treat mastoid cavities. Gentian violet is not only considered a drying agent, but an antifungal as well, particularly effective against *Candida* species. Commonly used as a drying agent and to reduce fungal colonization of the canal, its use should be avoided with a tympanic membrane perforation.

Cerumen Management/Pruritis

Hydrogen peroxide can be used with an intact eardrum to soften cerumen and facilitate atraumatic removal. Caution should be used with a tympanic membrane perforation or patent tympanostomy tube as it usually causes discomfort and pain if it enters the middle ear. Debrox™ is a useful over-the-counter wax-softening agent with carbamide peroxide and glycerin. It is very effective in managing cerumen buildup. Dermotic™, a combination of fluocinolone and mineral oil is very successful in helping patients with troublesome ear canal pruritis. Other agents that help with pruritis are topical steroid creams (eg, Elocon™, Cordran, Hydrocortisone) and ointments that can be applied with a cotton-tipped applicator.

REFERENCES

1. Kelly KE, Mohs DC. The external auditory canal: anatomy and physiology. *Otolaryngol Clin North Am.* 1996;29:725–739.
2. Couch ME, Blaugrund J, Kunar D. History, physical examination, and the preoperative evaluation. In: Cummings CW, ed. *Otolaryngology: Head and Neck Surgery.* 4th ed. St. Louis, MO: Mosby, Inc; 2005:8–9.
3. Marsh M, Jenkins H. Temporal bone neoplasms and lateral cranial base surgery. In: Cummings CW, ed. *Otolaryngology: Head and Neck Surgery.* 4th ed. St. Louis, MO: Mosby, Inc; 2005:3717–3720.
4. Kroon DF, Lawson ML, Derkay CS, Hoffman K, McCook J. Surfer's ear: external auditory exostoses are more prevalent in cold water surfers. *Otolaryngol Head Neck Surg.* 2002;126:499–504.
5. Bojrab DI, Bruderly T, Abdulrazzak Y. Otitis externa. *Otolaryngol Clin North Am.* 1996;29:761–782.
6. Ruckenstein MJ. Infections of the external ear. In: Cummings CW, ed. *Otolaryngology: Head and Neck Surgery.* 4th ed. St. Louis, MO: Mosby, Inc; 2005:2979–2986.
7. Shea CR. Dermatologic diseases of the external auditory canal. *Otolaryngol Clin North Am.* 1996;29:783–794.
8. Ball SS, Pillsbury HC III. Allergic disease and the external ear. In: Krouse JH, ed. *Allergy and Immunology: An Otolaryngologic Approach.* Baltimore, MO: Lippincott William & Wilkins; 2001:185–191.
9. Tran LP, Grundfast KM, Selesnick SH. Benign lesions of the external auditory canal. *Otolaryngol Clin North Am.* 1996;29:807–825.

10. Whitaker SR, Cordier A, Kosjakov S, Charbonneau R. Treatment of external auditory canal exostoses. *Laryngoscope.* 1998;108:195–199.
11. Sheehy JL. Osteoma of the external auditory canal. *Laryngoscope.* 1958;68:1667–1673.
12. Piepergerdes JC. Keratosis obturans and external auditory canal cholesteatoma. *Laryngoscope.* 1980;90:383–391.
13. Naim R, Linthicum Jr F, Shen T, Bran G, Hormann K. Classification of the external auditory canal cholesteatoma. *Laryngoscope.* 2005;115:455–460.
14. Sander R. Otitis externa: a practical guide to treatment and prevention. *Am Fam Physician.* 2001;63:927–936.

CHAPTER 5

Tympanic Membrane Perforation and Tympanoplasty

Patrick Antonelli

INTRODUCTION

Tympanoplasty is by far the most common procedure performed by most otologists and general otolaryngologists who perform ear surgery. Although certain techniques may be used in the majority of cases, excellent outcomes may be achieved with many different techniques. The techniques described in this chapter should be viewed as representative of those that are currently most commonly used. Awareness of the range of options for middle ear reconstruction may be helpful in specific circumstances.

DEFINITION

Tympanoplasty is defined as any modification or repair of the middle ear and tympanic membrane (TM). The term should not be used interchangeably with myringoplasty, in which the procedure is limited to the tympanic membrane and the middle ear space is not altered. The term tympanoplasty includes ossicular chain reconstruction and stapedectomy, but these terms are commonly considered separately. Similarly, mastoidectomy may be included under the umbrella of tympanoplasty. This chapter focuses on reconstruction of the tympanic membrane and will include only superficial attention to mastoidectomy and ossicular chain reconstruction. The other topics are covered in separate chapters.

INDICATIONS AND GOALS

There are three general reasons to perform a tympanoplasty: to eradicate disease, to improve hearing, and to improve quality of life. Chronic suppurative otitis media (CSOM), with or without cholesteatoma, is the most common middle ear pathology that is treated with tympanoplasty. Middle ear tumors, such as glomus tympanicum, are far less common. Conductive hearing loss due to TM perforation and ossicular chain discontinuity or fixation is typically found in association with these middle ear diseases, but may also occur in isolation. Finally, many ears with chronic, stable TM perforations may have no associated infection, cholesteatoma, or significant conductive hearing loss. These ears may require reconstruction to allow for other lifestyle choices, such as swimming or wearing hearing aids, which may lead to middle ear infection in the presence of a TM perforation.

When the primary indication for tympanoplasty is eradication of disease, the primary goal is obtaining a safe, healthy ear and a secondary goal is hearing improvement. Patients should be reminded of this, as the primary and secondary goals may be at odds, at least in the short term.

PATHOGENESIS OF CHRONIC SUPPURATIVE OTITIS MEDIA AND CHOLESTEATOMA

The state of the middle ear may impact treatment outcomes. Some of the factors that lead to the development of CSOM and cholesteatoma are not corrected by tympanoplasty. It is critical that both the surgeon and the patient remain mindful of the pathogenesis of these disorders, because they are likely to become issues postoperatively.

Eustachian tube dysfunction (ETD) is thought to be central to the pathogenesis of all forms of otitis media. ETD initially leads to resorption of oxygen and carbon dioxide from the middle ear space and the development of negative middle ear pressure.[1,2] The negative pressure may lead to relatively sterile chronic otitis media with effusion, aka "hydrops ex vacuuo."[3] ETD and negative middle ear pressure also predispose to infection with acute respiratory pathogens, such as *Streptococcus pneumoniae*.[4] These respiratory tract pathogens may promote the middle ear inflammatory process, which perpetuates the ETD, and increases middle ear susceptibility to chronic middle ear pathogens, such as *Pseudomonas aeruginosa*.[5–7] Middle ear bacteria may elaborate inflammatory proteases that can weaken the TM.[8] Persistent ETD, chronic negative middle ear pressure, and high levels of protease activity lead to progressive atelectasis, perforation, and cholesteatoma.[9–12]

Debris from a cholesteatoma creates a nidus for CSOM, elevated activity levels of proteolytic enzymes, and activation of osteoclasts. A perforation will allow both reflux of nasopharyngeal secretions and contamination from the ear canal. Nonhealing of wounds such as a perforation may result from high levels of microbes in the tissue. In recent years, these high counts of microbes in tissue have been ascribed to biofilms, a phenotype that renders the microbes resistant to both host defenses and conventional antimicrobial agents. Nonhealing of the tympanic membrane may also result from infolding of the squamous epithelium into the middle ear space.[13] Thus, there may be some overlap between persistent TM perforations and cholesteatoma.

MIDDLE EAR WOUND HEALING

Understanding middle ear repair is predicated on a broader understanding of the processes involved in middle ear wound healing. Healing of middle ear mucosa is similar to that of other tissues. The initial tissue injury involves activation of the clotting cascade, degranulation and aggregation of platelets, and formation of a thrombus. Inflammatory mediators and growth factors released from the damaged tissue and platelets lead to the recruitment of neutrophils, followed by macrophages, and the release of elastase and collagenase. Damaged cells and stroma are broken down. Macrophages produce additional cytokines and growth factors, which promote the ingrowth of fibroblasts and epithelial cells, and angiogenesis. The initial fibrin matrix is converted to glycosaminoglycans and proteoglycans, and ultimately collagen and elastin.

Healing of the TM follows the same initial steps, but cell proliferation is led by the squamous epithelium and followed by the fibroblast ingrowth.[14–16] This activity is unsupported by deeper tissues, over the middle space, which is vulnerable to pressure changes and infection. When TM healing occurs adjacent to mucosal injury, such as often occurs with removal of disease from the middle ear cleft, the healing process may become confluent, with scar bands or obliteration of the middle ear cleft. Loss of epithelium lateral to the reconstructed TM (eg, with concomitant bony canalplasty) may similarly lead to proliferation of the healing process laterally. This is most commonly encountered with "anterior blunting" with the lateral graft technique. The converse may also occur: excessive levels of collagenase and elastase activity resulting from overexpression of these enzymes by either the host or resident flora or insufficient levels of protease inhibitors may lead to loss of tissue grafts and recurrent TM perforation.

ERADICATION OF DISEASE

The first step in tympanoplasty is treatment of the involved disease. This may be a very limited step in the case of an isolated perforation (eg, removal of the perforation margin). With cholesteatoma and middle ear tumors, this can constitute the bulk of the procedure. Preoperative planning must take into account the likely and possible extent of disease, which will dictate approach and reconstructive options. Inadequate exposure and disease eradication may lead to failed reconstruction. Eradication of disease commonly requires bony canalplasty, atticotomy, or mastoidectomy for sufficient exposure. Cholesteatoma, tumor, and mucosal disease are often intimately adherent to adjacent TM, mucosa, ossicles, and the chorda tympani. Inexperienced surgeons may be reluctant to "sacrifice" these structures, but this is often necessary to achieve the first goal of surgery: a safe, healthy ear. Surgeons must also be vigilant for occult pathology that may compromise outcomes, such as infected foreign bodies (eg, welding slag in the eustachian tube or intruded tympanostomy tubes).

Clearance of reversible disease, such as otorrhea, by medical management is advocated by some otologists prior to tympanoplasty. However, clinical outcomes with "wet" ears may be equivalent to dry ears.[17] Furthermore, clearing a chronic suppurative process may only be possible through surgical treatment.

RECONSTRUCTION

Myriad strategies may be used to reconstruct the tympanic membrane. The optimal choice depends on the status of the middle ear once all disease has been eradicated.

Nonoperative

In chronic, stable TM perforations without associated disease or ossicular pathology, minimally invasive, office-based procedures may be employed. The classic, conservative approach is the "paper patch." This involves removal of the epithelial margin of the perforation and application of a thin paper across the perforation. The former incites the healing response and the latter provides a scaffold to support regeneration of the TM. Roughly 30 to 60% of small perforations will close when treated with a paper patch.[18–20] Techniques using other scaffolding have been reported with good rates of hearing improvement and/or TM healing.[18,21,22] TM cauterization (eg, with trichloroacetic acid) has also yielded excellent rates. While hearing loss has been reported with this technique, it is exceedingly rare.[23] TM cauterization is an excellent means of salvaging early failures with other tympanoplasty techniques. Growth factors have received a great deal of attention as a means of treating chronic TM perforations, but evidence of efficacy has been lacking.[24–28]

Myringoplasty

With small to medium size perforations (ie, less than 50% of the TM surface area), and the absence of other middle ear pathology or ossicular pathology, reconstruction limited to the TM, "myringoplasty," may be performed. These procedures may be performed in the office or the ambulatory surgical suite with appropriately selected patients. The quickest and easiest to perform is the fat-plug myringoplasty.[29] After removing the epithelium from the perforation margin, fibro-fatty tissue is placed through the perforation as seen in Figure 5–1. With larger perforations, placement of gelatin sponge medially and laterally may help to secure the fat graft. These grafts may take many months to take on a relatively normal thickness and appearance. Successful closure is obtained in 70 to 80% of treated ears.

An elegant and more efficacious alternative is the cartilage-inlay technique.[30] Cartilage from the conchal bowl or tragus is shaped to be 2 to 3 mm larger than the perforation, and then the lateral margin is incised to create flanges analogous to those on a tympanostomy tube. After freshening the perforation margin, the cartilage is inserted into the TM, just like a tympanostomy tube (Figure 5–2). Gelatin sponge may be placed lateral to the cartilage to promote healing. Success rates on the order of 95% can be expected.

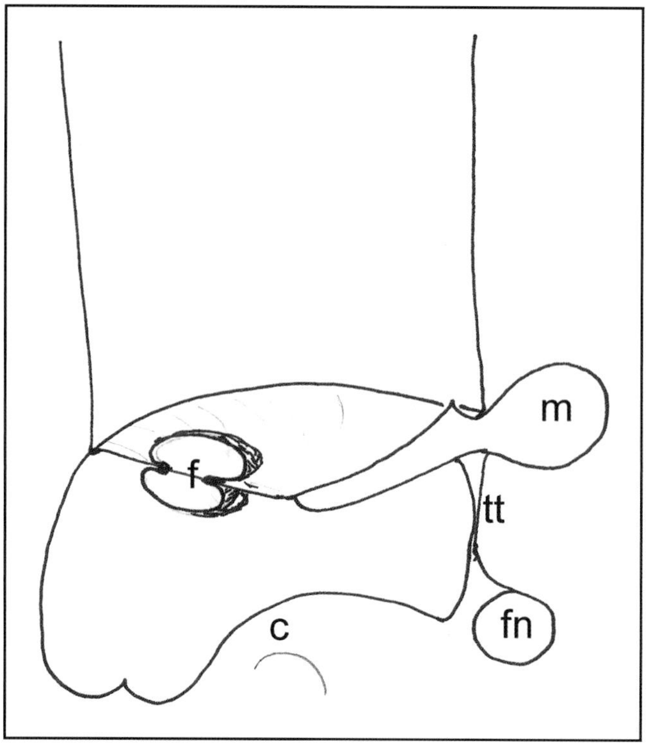

Figure 5–1. The fat plug myringoplasty is illustrated in a coronal cross-section of a left ear with a perforation just caudal to the malleus (m). The fat graft (f) forms a dumbbell shape with the waist at the perforation. Gelatin sponge may be placed between the cochlear promontory (c) to support larger grafts. The tensor tympani (tt) and facial nerve (fn) are also shown.

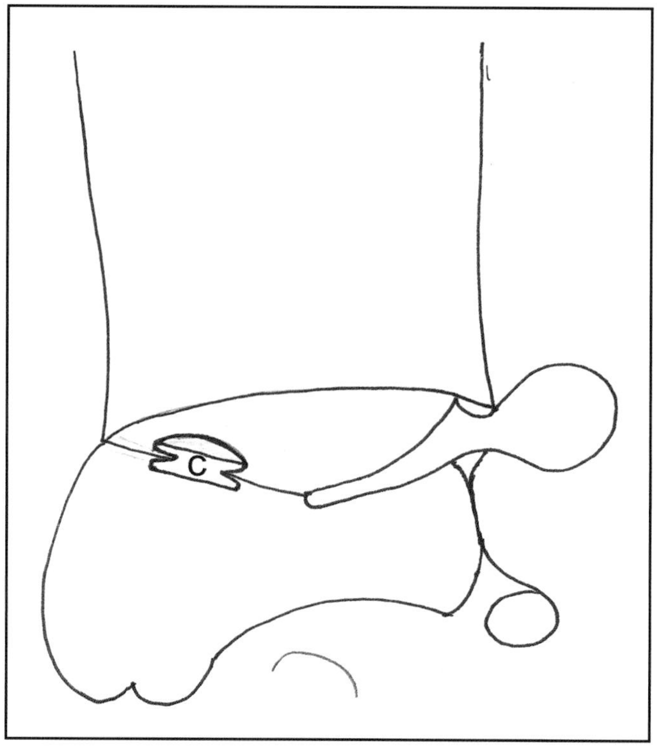

Figure 5–2. The cartilage inlay myringoplasty is shown in a coronal cross-section. The cartilage graft (c) has been cut along its edge to form a bivalve with flanges that engage the tympanic membrane both medially and laterally.

A less known option is the Plester tympanoplasty.[31] This involves sandwiching a fascia graft lateral to the residual lamina propria and deep to the skin. Skin elevation may be limited to the TM, but more commonly includes an adjacent margin of the canal. Gelatin sponge is placed in the middle ear for support, the tissue graft is applied, the skin is returned to its native position, and gelatin sponge is placed over the skin. Success rates over 90% are seen.

Tympanoplasty

Larger perforations, concomitant disease, or the presence of ossicular pathology, require formal evaluation and reconstruction of the middle ear. The medial or underlay technique is the most popular for repair of larger perforations.[32,33] Canal incisions are made and a tympanomeatal flap (eardrum and adjoining ear canal skin) are raised (Figure 5–3). Fibrous tissue, typically fascia, or perichondrium, is placed medial the TM and secured with gelatin sponge (Figure 5–4). The TM and graft are returned to the appropriate position and the lateral aspect of the TM is covered with gelatin sponge (Figure 5–5). If ossicular chain reconstruction is performed, the prosthesis or transposed ossicle is placed after packing the anterior portion of the mesotympanum. The posterior mesotympanum is packed and the prosthesis is covered with autologous cartilage before returning the fascia and drum remnant to the native position. This technique yields closure of the TM in roughly 90% of cases.

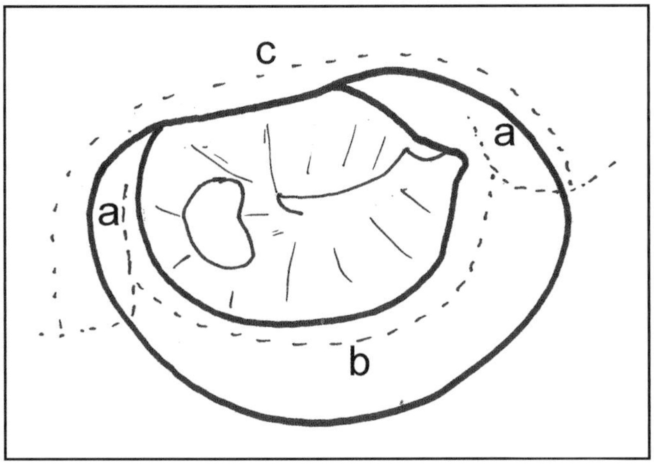

Figure 5–3. External view of external auditory canal incisions used for both medial and lateral graft tympanoplasty techniques. Cuts are made parallel to the axis of the canal, roughly at 6 and 12 o'clock (a). A third cut (b) connects these incisions, allowing entry into the middle ear and exposure of the eardrum after reflection of the pinna. The lateral graft technique typically involves removal of the skin from the anterior canal wall and remaining tympanic membrane. A fourth incision just medial to the anterior bony-cartilaginous junction (c) allows anterior skin elevation.

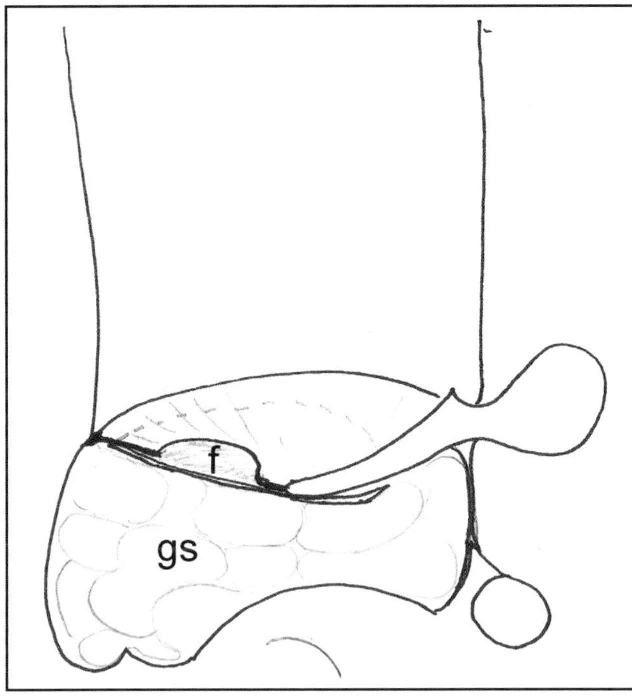

Figure 5–4. The medial technique tympanoplasty is shown in a coronal cross-section. The fascia graft (f) is held against the tympanic membrane remnant with gelatin sponge (gs).

If the perforation is quite large or anterior and a medial technique is to be used, small clips may be used to secure the graft to the anterior drum remnant or tympanic ring.[34] Clips can be made by coiling 30 gauge wire around a small caliber otologic suction tip then cutting the coil along its axis. The clips are easily applied with a microcups forceps (Figure 5–6).

The largest and most anterior perforations can most reliably be closed with a lateral technique.[33,35] As the name implies, this involves placing a fibrous tissue graft lateral to at least a portion of the TM remnant. Before the fibrous tissue graft is placed, skin must be elevated off the TM remnant. Failure to remove the squamous epithelium may lead to the development of cholesteatoma medial to the fibrous tissue graft. With a postauricular approach, the posterior canal skin is elevated as a "vascular strip" in continuity with the meatus and pinna. The anterior canal skin is removed and saved for later replacement as a free skin graft. The anterior canal skin can also be elevated from medial to lateral, leaving it attached to the tragus. The bony canalplasty is performed, particularly anteriorly. This facilitates visualization for graft placement and postoperative care. It also increases the angle between the canal and the

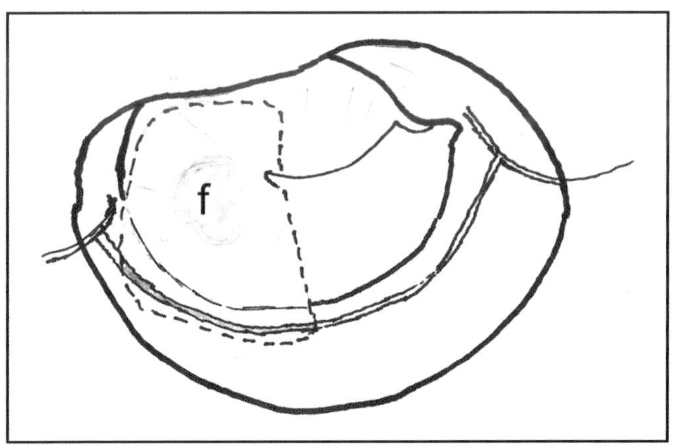

Figure 5–5. External view of the tympanic membrane after replacement of the flaps used in the medial graft tympanoplasty technique. The fascia graft (f) is seen through the perforation with the dotted lines illustrating conventional margins of the graft.

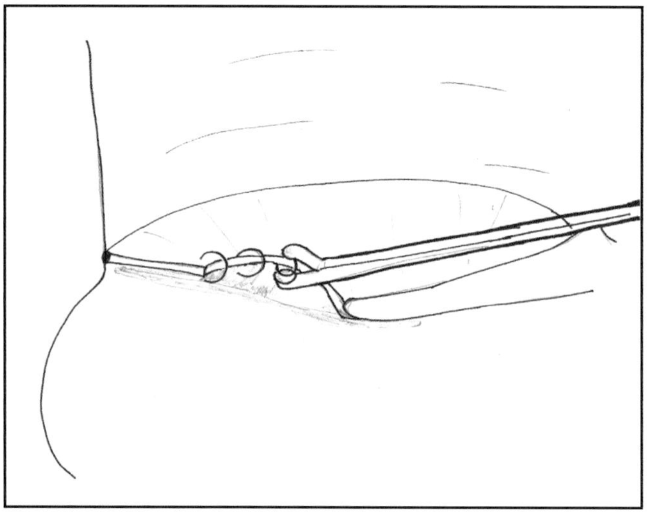

Figure 5–6. Coronal cross-section of a medial technique tympanoplasty with application of microclips to secure the graft to the perforation margin.

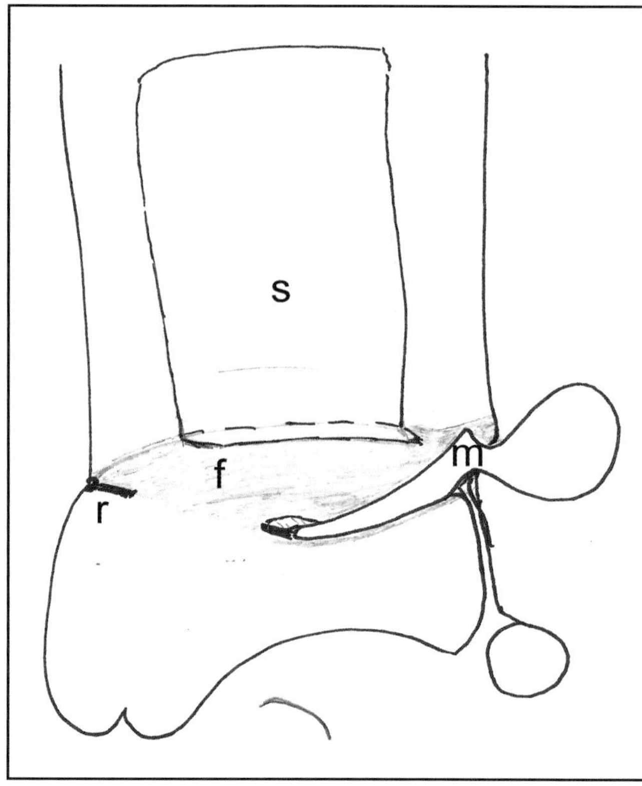

Figure 5–7. The lateral technique tympanoplasty is shown in a coronal cross-section. The fascia graft (f) abuts the anterior tympanic ring, just lateral to the tympanic membrane remnant (r) after passing under the long process of the malleus (m). The anterior canal skin (s) has been replaced over the anterior sulcus.

anterior drum, thereby reducing the risk for anterior blunting (ie, accumulation of scar in the angle between the anterior tympanic ring and the tympanic membrane). After removing any remaining epithelium and any atrophic TM or problem areas of tympanosclerosis, a fibrous tissue graft is placed medial to the malleus and lateral to the TM remnant (Figure 5–7). An ossicular chain reconstruction prosthesis or transposed incus can be placed, secured with gelatin sponge, and covered with cartilage. Gelatin sponge need not be placed in the middle ear to support the TM. Canal skin is replaced as seen in Figures 5–7 through 5–9, with some of the epithelium extending onto the anterior TM and fascia graft to reduce the risk of anterior blunting. Many surgeons also place gelatin film into the anterior sulcus to prevent blunting. Success rates on the order of 95% are reported with this technique.

The lateral graft technique is most readily performed in ears with an intact malleus and anterior annulus. Loss of the malleus renders the graft vulnerable to lateralization. Both situations may be addressed by more securely fixing the fibrous tissue graft anteriorly. This may be accomplished in a number of ways. The fibrous graft may be placed between the anterior tympanic ring and the protympanic mucosa (if robust). More reliably, a 0.5 to 1.0-mm groove can be drilled into or through the tympanic ring at the anterior bony sulcus. The graft can be tucked into the groove. Wire microclips can also be used to secure the fibrous graft anteriorly.

Another alternative to an anterior perforation is the over-under tympanoplasty technique. This involves delicate dissection of the tympanic membrane so that it may be detached from the malleus. The laser aids in this dissection, especially when separating these structures at the umbo. Care must be taken with this approach so that vibratory trauma is not transmitted along an intact ossicular chain. This approach allows wide exposure to the anterior aspect of the middle ear, tympanic membrane, and even the eustachian tube. This approach can be very

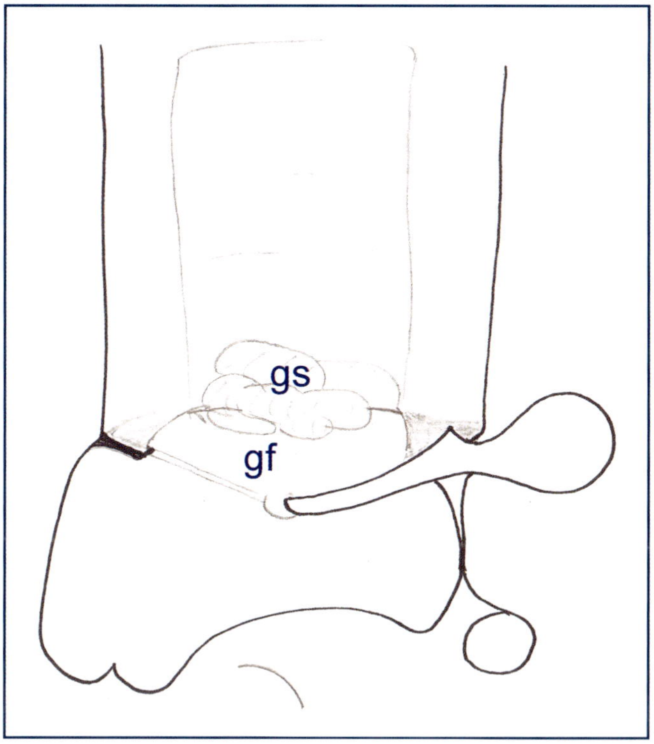

Figure 5–8. The lateral technique tympanoplasty is shown in a coronal cross-section after placement of gelatin film (gf) into the anterior sulcus and gelatin sponge (gs) lateral to the film.

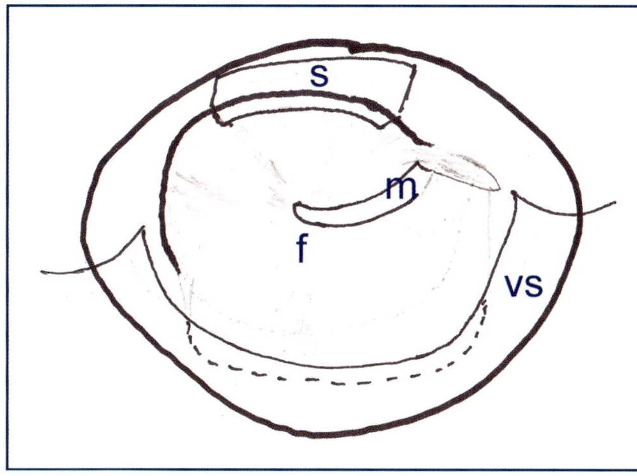

Figure 5–9. External view of the tympanic membrane after replacement of the flaps used in the lateral graft tympanoplasty technique. The fascia graft (f) is seen under the long process and over the neck of the malleus (m) with coverage by the skin graft (s) anteriorly and the vascular strip (vs) posteriorly.

effective and reduces the risk of blunting from the lateral technique.

Another alternative for reconstruction of a middle ear with a large perforation and an absent malleus is a homograft tympanoplasty. This requires procurement of a cadaveric TM from a tissue bank. Such specimens typically include a cuff of soft tissue from the adjacent canal and the malleus. Specimen preparation takes a few hours to remove the fixative prior to placement. A magnetic stir-plate and sterile magnet are used to agitate the rinse solution around the homograft and ensure removal of fixative. Placement is remarkably easy. Exposure and canalplasty are performed as described above for a lateral technique tympanoplasty. The cuff of soft tissue around the homograft TM can be divided in a number of areas from laterally to adjacent to the annulus to allow the graft to better fit in the reconstructed canal. Gelatin sponge is placed over the mesotympanum. A transposed homograft incus or ossicular chain prosthesis (usually with a cartilage graft) is placed, and then the homograft TM is set on top of the prosthesis or transposed ossicle. The homograft TM can be rotated to allow for optimal alignment of the homograft malleus with the prosthesis or transposed ossicle. The skin is brought down over the cuff and the canal is filled with gelatin sponge.

OVERCLOSURE OF THE EAR CANAL

Patients with deaf ears or those that prove refractory to standard tympanoplasty techniques may be considered for overclosure of the ear canal. Briefly, all squamous epithelium is removed from the bony external canal and middle ear. Laterally based skin flaps are developed both posteriorly and anteriorly. These are everted and their deep surfaces approximated with slowly absorbing suture. This yields a safe, dry ear in nearly all cases. Satisfactory auditory rehabilitation may be accomplished with bone-anchored hearing devices.

TISSUE GRAFTS

A fibrous tissue graft is used in the majority of tympanoplasties. Autologous fascia is usually readily available from the temporalis muscle, except in cases of multiple revisions. Fascia is naturally thin, strong, and easy to manipulate. Although some shrinkage may occur, it usually maintains its cut shape reasonably well. Many surgeons favor drying the fascia to facilitate graft shaping and placement.

"Fool's fascia" is the areolar tissue overlying the true temporalis fascia. In many individuals, this is fairly thick. It is often adequate for TM grafting, but its loose nature makes it much more difficult to shape and place, as it becomes rather amorphous when wet.

Perichondrium, especially from the tragus, is an excellent alternative to fascia. It is even stronger and easier to manipulate, particularly without drying. This requires another incision, with the added potential for additional pain, and the amount available is more limited. This is an excellent choice when cartilage will also be used.

Cartilage may be used in lieu of a fibrous tissue graft. Use of cartilage as an interposition graft reduces the rate of prosthesis extrusion through the TM. The cranial aspect of the conchal bowl is easily harvested through a postauricular incision. Though curved in situ, this relaxes tremendously after removal and stripping of the perichondrium. Its thickness often does not require thinning. Removal from the upper aspect of the conchal bowl preserves the more caudal perichondrium, which can help to maintain a wider meatoplasty upon closure of a postauricular incision. If a meatoplasty is to be performed, the excised conchal cartilage can be used. Its shape and thickness require some preparation to achieve an appropriate TM graft. Tragal cartilage may be used with attached perichondrium. Although preservation of the cartilage-perichondrial integrity may offer additional stability with the reconstruction, it may be easier to shape and place the cartilage and fibrous tissue grafts independently. Appropriate shaping of the cartilage graft depends on the indication (eg, covering a prosthesis vs filling an atticotomy defect), technique (eg, inlay vs underlay vs palisade), and location (eg, central portion of the TM without associated malleus vs abutting the malleus). Shaping is readily accomplished with a scalpel (#15 blade), but special cutting devices may be used to thin the cartilage more reliably.

Any fibrous material, such as scar from an old incision, devoid of skin, of course, can be shaped for use in tympanoplasty. Even a narrow, thick piece of scar can be bivalved, crushed with a clamp, then flattened with a fascia press to achieve an adequate graft. Such grafts are often a little thicker than fascia, which may be desirable for individuals with significant eustachian tube dysfunction.

In addition to TM homografts, homologous fascia, dermis, and other fibrous materials may be used in tympanoplasty. Such "off-the-shelf" products may be attractive as timesavers and ready sources of grafting material after multiple revision procedures. Host-responses are more favorable with current tissue processing technologies, but tissue healing with such materials may be less predictable than with autologous materials. Also, the cost of these materials must be factored.

Synthetic materials have also been considered as TM grafting material. These have not been widely adopted. Use of collagen sheeting for middle ear reconstruction has been reported to result in cholesteatoma formation in an animal model.[36]

PACKING MATERIALS

Tissue grafts and prostheses often need support during the acute healing process. This is provided by the use of packing material. Bleeding may also be attenuated by the use of these materials. By far, the most commonly used middle ear packing material is gelatin sponge. This is relatively inexpensive and widely available. High success rates are achieved with tympanoplasty using gelatin sponge. However, gelatin sponge may promote excessive scarring, which could compromise long-term hearing results.[37,38] Gelatin film has been promoted as an adjunct to gelatin sponge to minimize the extent of scarring.[39] Less scarring has been observed with other packing materials, such as hyaluronic acid foam and collagen,[40–42] but this has not been borne out as improved outcomes with tympanoplasty.[43]

Fibrin glue may be used in place of packing material. This has been shown to be safe in animal studies and highly effective in human trials. [44,45]

The ear canal may be packed with a variety of materials, including those used in the middle ear. Additionally, ribbon gauze, wick sponges, Silastic, and various ointments have been used successfully.[46] In some cases, no canal packing may be necessary.[47]

APPROACH

There are three basic approaches to perform tympanoplasty surgery: transcanal, endaural, or postauricular. The transcanal approach involves performing the procedure through the ear canal, typically using a speculum. Small perforations or limited ossicular chain repair can be done in this fashion. The endaural approach involves making a cut from the medial bony canal at approximately 12 o'clock, out through the incisura. This allows access to temporalis fascia, tragal cartilage, the conchal bowl, and the mastoid. Most tympanoplasties can be done with this approach, but it is more dependent on surgeon experience. The postauricular approach begins with incisions in the ear canal as shown previously in Figure 5–3, typically at 12 o'clock and either at the tympanomastoid suture or as low as 6 o'clock. These are connected with a "transverse" incision lateral to the posterior TM. An incision is made in or behind the postauricular crease and carried down to the level of the temporalis fascia and mastoid periosteum. The latter is divided and the anterior extent elevated forward along the mastoid, down into the tympanic ring, until the posterior canal skin is elevated in continuity with the pinna. This yields the best and most flexible view of the mastoid and the middle ear. Failure is likely to result if tympanoplasty is attempted with inadequate exposure; thus, the postauricular approach is the workhorse for middle ear reconstruction.

PERIOPERATIVE MANAGEMENT

Tympanoplasty candidates require little special preoperative care beyond that of any presurgical patient. Use of anticoagulants should be avoided if possible, but these are not absolute contraindications for middle ear reconstruction.

Many, if not most, cases can be done using the surgeon and patient's choice of anesthetic. Local anesthesia with intravenous sedation can be extremely efficient and effective. If disease is extensive, the patient is relatively anxious, or the surgeon is inexperienced, general anesthesia is preferred. Infiltration of local anesthetic combined with epinephrine around the pinna (ie, a ring block) and throughout the ear canal will reduce the need amount of general anesthesia needed and will facilitate the procedure through vasoconstriction. Inhalational anesthetics have traditionally been avoided in ear surgery, as these agents tend to accumulate in the middle ear. With proper surgical technique, inhalational agents should not pose any serious issues or compromise tympanoplasty success. Administration of dexamethasone on induction has been shown to significantly reduce postoperative nausea and vomiting with tympanoplasty.

Prophylactic antibiotics are commonly used, but their use is controversial, at best. Older cephalosporins and penicillin derivatives have not demonstrated benefit.[48] Cefuroxime has been shown to reduce postoperative infection with tympanoplasty in the presence of infection, but this agent does not have adequate coverage of all pathogens that are known to be present with a non-intact TM (eg, *Pseudomonas aeruginosa*).[49] Tympanoplasties performed in the presence of overt infection are associated with postoperative cellulitis, perichondritis, or abscess in roughly 5% of cases. These benefit from packing removal and administration of both systemic and topical antibiotics directed at *P. aeruginosa* and *S. aureus*.

Pressure dressings are commonly applied to the ear postoperatively. They may prevent hematoma and pain from accidental contact with the wound. They have not, however, been shown to significantly improve outcomes.

Postoperative pain control is usually achieved with oral non-opioids and narcotics. Post-tympanoplasty pain seems to result from involved musculature. Nonsteroidal anti-inflammatory agents (eg, ibuprofen) can be even more effective than narcotics postoperatively. They may be used as the first line of analgesia, with narcotics reserved for break-through pain. Pain is usually the most severe over the first 24 hours, gradually decreasing thereafter. Pain that is intractable immediately after surgery should raise concerns for a hematoma or overly tight pressure dressing (eg, forehead ischemia). Pain that worsens after the first couple of days should be suspect for wound infection.

Ototopical drops are commonly administered postoperatively. These can help to reduce microbial growth and soften the packing to facilitate removal.

Packing can be removed at any time postoperatively. Practices range widely, with initial debridement occurring between 1 and 6 weeks postoperatively.

Hearing assessment may be performed at any time following the procedure. However, if this is done before middle ear packing has had time to be cleared and eustachian tube function has normalized, it may be of limited value. Most surgeons wait at least 3 months to perform the first postoperative audiometry.

REFERENCES

1. Elner A. Quantitative studies of gas absorption from the normal middle ear. *Acta Otolaryngol (Stockh)*. 1977;83:25–28.
2. Doyle WJ, Seroky JT. Middle ear gas exchange in rhesus monkeys. *Ann Otol Rhinol Laryngol*. 1994;103:636–645.
3. Casselbrandt ML, Cantekin EI, Dirkmaat DC, Doyle WJ, Bluestone CD. Experimental paralysis of tensor veli palatini muscle. *Acta Otolaryngol (Stockh)*. 1988;106:178–185.
4. Meyerhoff WL, Giebink, GS, Shea D. Pneumococcal otitis media following middle ear deflation. *Ann Otol Rhinol Laryngol*. 1981;92:72–76.
5. Post JC, Preston RA, Aul JJ, et al. Molecular analysis of bacterial pathogens in otitis media with effusion. *JAMA*. 1995;273:1598–1604.
6. Antonelli PJ, Juhn SK, Goycoolea MV, Giebink GS. Pseudomonas otitis media after eustachian tube obstruction. *Otolaryngol Head Neck Surg*. 1992;107:511–515.
7. Antonelli PJ, Juhn SK, Goycoolea MV, Giebink GS. Middle ear susceptibility to pseudomonas infection during acute otitis media. *Ann Otol Rhinol Laryngol*. 1993;102:531–536.
8. Antonelli PJ, Schultz GS, Kim KM, et al. Alpha 1-antitrypsin and Ilomastat inhibit inflammatory proteases present in human middle ear effusions. *Laryngoscope*. 2003;113: 1347–1351.
9. Bluestone CD, Klein JO. Otitis media, atelectasis, and eustachian tube dysfunction. In: Bluestone CD, Stool SE, Kenna MA, eds. *Pediatric Otolaryngology*, Vol 1. Philadelphia, PA:WB Saunders Co; 1996:388–582.
10. Sade J, Berco E. Atelectasis and secretory otitis media. *Ann Otol Rhinol Laryngol*. 1976;85(suppl 25 pt 2):66–72.
11. Wells MD, Michaels L. Role of retraction pockets in cholesteatoma formation. *Clin Otolaryngol*. 1983;8:39–45.
12. Wolfman DE, Chole RA. Experimental retraction pocket cholesteatoma. *Ann Otol Rhinol Laryngol*. 1986;95:639–644.
13. Amoils CP, Jackler RK, Milczuk H, Kelly KE, Cao K. An animal model of chronic tympanic membrane perforation. *Otolaryngol Head Neck Surg*. 1992;106:47–55.
14. Gladstone HB, Jackler RK, Varav K. Tympanic membrane wound healing. An overview. *Otolaryngol Clin North Am*. 1995;28:913–932.
15. Makino K, Amatsu M, Kinishi M, Mohri M. Epithelial migration in the healing process of tympanic membrane perforations. *Eur Arch Otorhinolaryngol*. 1990;247:352–355.
16. Stenfors LE, Carlsoo B, Salen B, Winblad B. Repair of experimental tympanic membrane perforations. *Acta Otolaryngol*. 1980;90:332–341.
17. Vartiainen E, Kansanen M. Tympanomastoidectomy for chronic otitis media without cholesteatoma. *Otolaryngol Head Neck Surg*. 1992;106:230–234.
18. Laurent C, Söderberg O, Anniko M, Hartwig S. Repair of chronic tympanic membrane perforations using applications of hyaluronan or rice paper prostheses. *ORL J Otorhinolaryngol Relat Spec*. 1991;53:37–40.
19. Dursun E, Dogru S, Gungor A, Cincik H, Poyrazoglu E, Ozdemir T. Comparison of paper-patch, fat, and perichondrium myringoplasty in repair of small tympanic membrane perforations. *Otolaryngol Head Neck Surg*. 2008;138:353–356.
20. Golz A, Goldenberg D, Netzer A, et al. Paper patching for chronic tympanic membrane perforations. *Otolaryngol Head Neck Surg*. 2003;128:565–570.
21. Kartush JM. Tympanic membrane patcher: a new device to close tympanic membrane perforations in an office setting. *Am J Otol*. 2000;21:615–620.
22. Kakehata S, Hirose Y, Kitani R, Futai K, Maruya S, Ishii K, Shinkawa H. Autologous serum eardrops therapy with a chitin membrane for closing tympanic membrane perforations. *Otol Neurotol*. 2008;29:791–795.
23. Taylor PH. Sudden deafness following chromic acid application to a perforation of the tympanic membrane. *J Laryngol Otol*. 1975;89:1075–1078.
24. O'Daniel TG, Petitjean M, Jones SC, et al. Epidermal growth factor binding and action on tympanic membranes. *Ann Otol Rhinol Laryngol*. 1990;99:80–84.
25. Amoils CP, Jackler RK, Lustig LR. Repair of chronic tympanic membrane perforations using epidermal growth factor. *Otolaryngol Head Neck Surg*. 1992;107:669–683.
26. Vrabec JT, Schwaber MK, Davidson JM, Clymer MA. Evaluation of basic fibroblast growth factor in tympanic membrane repair. *Laryngoscope*. 1994;104:1059–1064.
27. Soumekh B, Hom DB, Levine S, Juhn SK, Antonelli PJ. Treatment of chronic tympanic-membrane perforations

with a platelet-derived releasate. *Am J Otol.* 1996;17:506–511.

28. Ramsay HA, Heikkonen EJ, Laurila PK. Effect of epidermal growth factor on tympanic membranes with chronic perforations: a clinical trial. *Otolaryngol Head Neck Surg.* 1995;113:375–379.
29. Gross CW, Bassila M, Lazar RH, Long TE, Stagner S. Adipose plug myringoplasty: an alternative to formal myringoplasty techniques in children. *Otolaryngol Head Neck Surg.* 1989;101:617–620.
30. Eavey RD. Inlay tympanoplasty: cartilage butterfly technique. *Laryngoscope.* 1998;108:657–661.
31. Singleton GT. Symposium: methods of reconstruction in tympanoplasty. V. Prevention of blunting the anterior canal drum head contour—Plester technique. *Laryngoscope.* 1976;86:193–195.
32. Austin DF, Shea JJ Jr. A new system of tympanoplasty using vein graft. *Laryngoscope.* 1961;71:596–611.
33. Rizer FM. Overlay versus underlay tympanoplasty. Part I: historical review of the literature. *Laryngoscope.* 1997;107:1–25.
34. Weider DJ. Tympanoplasty: medial grafting using Williams' microclips. *Arch Otolaryngol.* 1977;103:468–472.
35. Sheehy JL, Glasscock ME 3rd. Tympanic membrane grafting with temporalis fascia. *Arch Otolaryngol.* 1967;86:391–402.
36. Hueb MM, Goycoolea MV, Muchow D, Duvall AJ, Paparella MM, Sheridan C. In search of missing links in otology. III. Development of a new animal model for cholesteatoma. *Laryngoscope.* 1993;103:774–784.
37. Hellstrom S, Salen B, Stenfors LE. Absorbable gelatin sponge (Gelfoam) in otosurgery: one cause of undesirable postoperative results? *Acta Otolaryngol.* 1983;96:269–275.
38. Liening DA, Lundy L, Silberberg B, Finstuen K. A comparison of the biocompatibility of three absorbable hemostatic agents in the rat middle ear. *Otolaryngol Head Neck Surg.* 1997;116:454–457.
39. McGhee MA, Dornhoffer JL. The effect of gelfilm in the prevention of fibrosis in the middle ear of the animal model. *Am J Otol.* 1999;20:712–716.
40. Li G, Feghali JG, Dinces E, McElveen J, van de Water TR. Evaluation of esterified hyaluronic acid as middle ear-packing material. *Arch Otolaryngol Head Neck Surg.* 2001;127:534–539.
41. Krupala JL, Gianoli GJ, Smith RA. The efficacy of hyaluronic acid foam as a middle ear packing agent in experimental tympanoplasty. *Am J Otol.* 1998;19:546–550.
42. Laurent C, Hellstrom S, Stenfors LE. Hyaluronic acid reduces connective tissue formation in middle ears filled with absorbable gelatin sponge: an experimental study. *Am J Otolaryngol.* 1986;7:181–186.
43. Bagger-Sjoback D, Holmquist J, Mendel L, Mercke U. Hyaluronic acid in middle ear surgery. *Am J Otol.* 1993;14:501–506.
44. Epstein GH, Weisman RA, Zwillenberg S, Schreiber AD. A new autologous fibrinogen-based adhesive for otologic surgery. *Ann Otol Rhinol Laryngol.* 1986;95:40–45.
45. Sakagami M, Yuasa R, Yuasa Y. Simple underlay myringoplasty. *J Laryngol Otol.* 2007;121:840–844.
46. Zeitoun H, Sandhu GS, Kuo M, Macnamara M. A randomized prospective trial to compare four different ear packs following permeatal middle ear surgery. *J Laryngol Otol.* 1998;112:140–144.
47. Borgstein J, de Zwart G, Bruce IA. Ear packing after ear surgery: is it really necessary? *J Laryngol Otol.* 2008;122:253–254.
48. Jackson CG. Antimicrobial prophylaxis in ear surgery. *Laryngoscope.* 1988;98:1116–1123.
49. Govaerts PJ, Raemaekers J, Verlinden A, Kalai M, Somers T, Offeciers FE. Use of antibiotic prophylaxis in ear surgery. *Laryngoscope.* 1998;108:107–110.

CHAPTER 6

Cholesteatoma

Robert Standring, Brian Duff, and Seilesh Babu

INTRODUCTION

Cholesteatoma is a benign disease, which may behave like a malignancy with erosion of normal structures and high likelihood of recurrence. It occurs when keratinizing stratified squamous epithelium accumulates in the temporal bone resulting in a destructive process that can erode important surrounding structures. This can lead to serious complications, such as conductive hearing loss, dizziness, meningitis and brain abscess. Cholesteatoma may remain clinically silent for a significant period of time until the disease has become quite extensive. Common symptoms include hearing loss, otorrhea, and otalgia. Surgical therapy is the mainstay of management. The primary surgical objective is eradication of all diseased tissue with establishment of a dry, safe ear. Maintenance or restoration of hearing is a secondary goal.

HISTORY

In 1858, Muller described cholesteatoma as a fatty tumor with cholesterol, and thus named it such.[1] Schuknecht termed the name "keratoma" to more appropriately describe this lesion, as it does not contain cholesterol.[1] Management of these lesions was traditionally accomplished with a radical mastoidectomy to allow visualization and exteriorization of the disease. Current treatment has evolved to become tailored to the amount of disease found in the middle ear and mastoid cavity, resulting in possible canal wall-up or canal wall-down mastoidectomy procedures, as is further discussed.

ANATOMIC CONSIDERATIONS

A basic knowledge of the anatomy of middle ear and mastoid cavity will allow sound treatment of cholesteatoma from a surgical standpoint. The tympanic cavity develops from the endoderm of the first branchial pouch. Numerous pathways form from the mucosal folds of this pouch, which allow for the spread of cholesteatoma throughout the tympanic cavity and mastoid antrum.

Cholesteatoma usually develops from a retraction pocket in the epitympanum, especially in an area described as Prussak's space.[2] This space is bounded by the neck of the malleus medially, par flaccida laterally, lateral process of the malleus and its associated horizontal folds inferiorly, and the lateral malleal fold superiorly. Cholesteatoma may extend from here to other areas through paths of least resistance along the incus and into the posterior mesotympanum. The scutum, or lateral wall of the epitympanum, can be eroded and may serve as a radiologic sign of an aggressive process in the mesotympanum.

Several structures are important to recognize in the posterior mesotympanum: the facial recess and sinus tympani. The facial recess is bounded by the facial nerve posteromedially, fossa incudis superiorly, and chorda tympani nerve laterally. The sinus tympani is located medial to the fallopian canal between the canal and medial wall of the posterior mesotympanum, bordered superiorly by the ponticulum and inferiorly by the subiculum.[3] This area is difficult to visualize directly during surgery, and therefore becomes a common location that cholesteatoma may recur. Opening the facial recess through the mastoid may be helpful in visualizing residual cholesteatoma within the sinus tympani. Classically, a mirror was used to view this area in search of residual disease. Novel techniques including the use of 30- and 70-degree endoscopes may also prove useful to evaluate the sinus tympani.

Cholesteatoma can also spread to the anterior epitympanum, where it may involve the facial nerve or extend into the supratubal recess. If the facial nerve is involved, a canal wall-down mastoidectomy is usually indicated, as discussed later, due to the facial nerve being the medial border of the canal wall in this space.

PATHOGENESIS OF CHOLESTEATOMA

A possible etiology of accumulation of squamous and keratin debris from a retraction pocket or a tympanic membrane perforation may be due to the migration of epithelium of the tympanic membrane and the external auditory canal. The source of posterior mesotympanic retraction pockets stem from eustachian tube dysfunction (ETD), whereas the source of epitympanic retraction pockets is less defined. Poor tubal function most likely plays a role in recurrent disease as it leads to persistent negative middle ear pressure, effusion, and tympanic membrane retraction.

Several theories attempt to explain the cause of cholesteatoma formation.[2] (1) Implantation of squamous epithelium into middle ear space from trauma (i.e. myringotomy with tubes); (2) Invasion of squamous epithelium into the middle ear via a persistent tympanic membrane perforation; (3) Invagination of a retraction pocket until it becomes so deep that it leads to cholesteatoma; (4) Metaplasia of normal middle ear mucosa; and (5) Congenital rest of trapped epithelium.

CLASSIFICATION OF CHOLESTEATOMA

Cholesteatoma can be classified as congenital or acquired. Acquired cholesteatoma may be further subdivided into primary or secondary.

Congenital Cholesteatoma

Congenital cholesteatoma arises from trapped squamous epithelium that is abnormally located in the temporal bone during development. By definition, a child diagnosed with congenital cholesteatoma does not have a history of recurrent suppurative ear disease, previous otologic surgery, trauma, or tympanic membrane perforation. The diagnosis is usually made in children of preschool age with an intact tympanic membrane.[4] Cholesteatoma usually presents as an incidental white mass in the anterior-superior quadrant of the middle ear (Figure 6–1). Patients are usually asymptomatic unless the ossicular chain is involved. The cholesteatoma is usually diagnosed by the pediatrician during routine examination and the visualized lesion usually represents the "tip of the iceberg."

Acquired Cholesteatoma

Acquired cholesteatoma is usually diagnosed in older children and adults and associated with a previous history of middle ear disease. The cholesteatoma is most often found in the posterosuperior quadrant of the tympanic membrane with the associated presence of tympanic membrane retraction and/or perforation (Figure 6–2). Patients usually present with hearing loss, otorrhea, and otalgia.

Primary Acquired Cholesteatoma

Accumulation of squamous debris in a retraction pocket may result in a primary acquired cholesteatoma. The pars flaccida is weaker and negative pressure has a larger force on this portion of the tympanic membrane. A retraction pocket ensues and the lateral wall of the epitympanum (scutum) is eroded. The

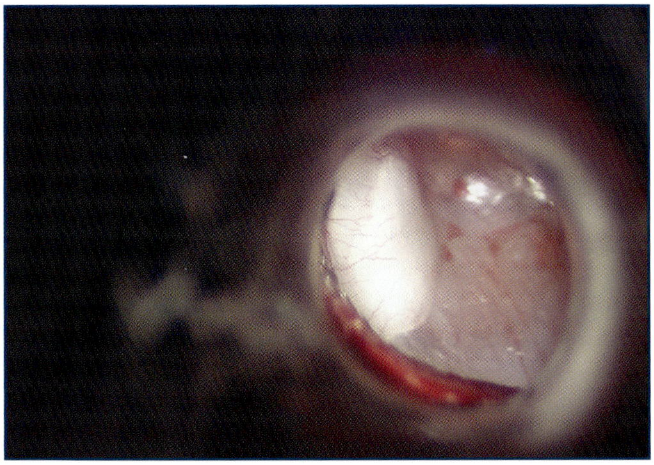

Figure 6–1. Right tympanic membrane with central and anterior-superior white mass noted consistent with congenital cholesteatoma.

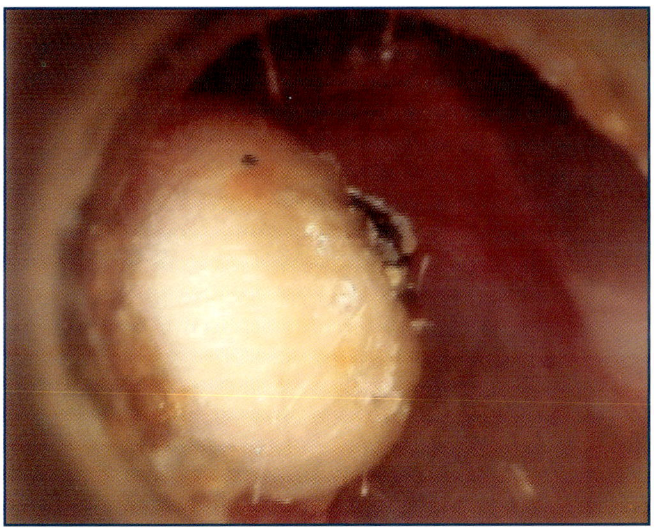

Figure 6–2. Right ear canal with cholesteatoma extending through posterior-superior tympanic membrane into the canal itself.

epitympanum containing the head of the malleus and short process of the incus may become involved. The thin bone between the epitympanum and the cranial cavity (tegmen tympani) may become eroded and result in epidural abscess, meningitis, or brain abscess. Bony erosion occurs by 2 principal mechanisms. First, pressure effects produce bony remodeling, as occurs normally throughout the entire skeleton when pressure is applied consistently over time. Second, enzymatic activity at the margin of the cholesteatoma enhances osteoclastic activity, which greatly increases the speed of bone resorption. The level of these osteolytic enzymes appears to increase when a cholesteatoma becomes infected.

Secondary Acquired Cholesteatoma

Secondary acquired cholesteatoma is usually accompanied by trauma to the tympanic membrane with subsequent migration of squamous epithelium into the middle ear. This may be from implantation of squamous epithelium through placement of tympanostomy tubes or from a perforation of the tympanic membrane.

Despite the classification system for cholesteatomas, their mode of presentation and their treatment are quite similar.

CLINICAL PRESENTATION

Patients may not present until the cholesteatoma has become infected or symptomatic due to mass effect or erosion. They may be asymptomatic or not seek medical attention until symptoms become troublesome. Patients with cholesteatoma present with persistent, foul-smelling otorrhea. Hearing loss is also common as ossicular damage is frequently present and can result in a conductive loss. Dizziness is a relatively uncommon symptom, unless erosion has occurred along the stapes footplate or from a labyrinthine fistula. Symptoms such as vertigo, as well as headache and facial nerve weakness, may indicate impending intratemporal or intracranial complications and should prompt immediate assessment and treatment.

Physical Examination

The physical examination consists of a thorough head and neck examination with particular attention to the otologic exam. A general overall assessment of the patient is necessary to diagnose fever, changes in mental status, or other findings that might afford clues to the development of a potential complication.

Otomicroscopy aids in the evaluation and diagnosis of cholesteatoma. Thorough aural suctioning is performed in order to remove otorrhea, debris, or crusting which may hinder adequate visualization. With extensive cholesteatoma only a large polyp or mucopurulence may be seen in the ear canal. Care and caution should be taken prior to office removal of ear canal polyps. The polyp may be connected to underlying vital structures, such as the facial nerve or stapes. Imaging may be warranted to check the integrity of the tegmen to rule out dural herniation prior to removal of this tissue.

The tympanic membrane is examined for evidence and location of any retraction pockets or perforations. The retraction pocket is usually located in the posterior-superior quadrant with accumulated squamous and keratin debris. Evaluation of the middle ear mucosa is performed through the perforation. Weber and Rinne tests with 512-Hz tuning fork are most likely to indicate a conductive hearing loss and should be compared with subsequent audiometric findings. Failure to observe appropriate correlation with the expected results may prompt further investigation, such as imaging studies. Facial nerve function should be carefully checked and documented to rule out a chronic facial palsy. Typically, acute facial paralysis is an obvious finding based on history and physical.

Audiologic Testing

Pure tone audiometry with air and bone conduction, speech reception thresholds, and word recognition usually establish a conductive hearing loss. The degree of conductive loss will vary depending on the extent of disease. In fact, some patients will have significant disease along with ossicular erosion but suffer from minimal hearing loss. The cholesteatoma in this situation provides mass effect that is able to conduct the sound relatively well. Tympanometry findings will vary as well and may suggest decreased compliance or tympanic membrane perforation. A sensorineural component of hearing loss may raise suspicion for erosion into the horizontal canal or of the stapes footplate or associated with chronic serous labyrinthitis.

Imaging

Most patients presenting with cholesteatoma do not require preoperative imaging. In cases of recurrent disease, unusual presentation, or a suspected complication, a CT of the temporal bone may be helpful. The CT may show erosion of the scutum, labyrinthine fistula, tegmen defects, ossicular erosion, and abnormalities of the fallopian canal. If an intracranial complication is suspected, MRI scanning may be indicated as well. Cholesteatoma will be hypointense on T1 imaging, hyperintense on T2 imaging, and may enhance after administration of gadolinium on T1-weighted sequences. Diffusion-weighted imaging shows restricted diffusion. It is possible that recurrent cholesteatoma may be able to be identified on MRI scan.[5]

MANAGEMENT OF CHOLESTEATOMA

Cholesteatoma is a surgical disease, but, depending on the clinical circumstances, non-surgical management options may be appropriate for some patients. Elderly or poor surgical candidates may be carefully monitored in the clinic setting with nonsurgical treatments, such as routine aural toilet. Despite numerous medical treatments to reduce infection and dry the ear, success of eradicating cholesteatoma may be limited. Topical and systemic antibiotics are usually not helpful as there is little absorption into the cholesteatoma sac itself.

The goal of cholesteatoma treatment is eradication of the disease to create a safe, dry ear that reduces the risk of complications occurring. Improvement of hearing is a secondary goal.

Office-Based Treatment

Certain cholesteatomas may be managed in the office with otomicroscopy and aggressive aural toilet. Thorough cleaning at routine intervals with removal of all accessible squamous debris may be adequate to prevent extension of the disease process and development of infection and other complications. This regimen is particularly useful in those patients in whom disease is limited to an attic or posterosuperior retraction pocket that allows adequate visualization and access. A reliable and cooperative patient is essential. This may provide a dry ear prior to surgery; however, this is not always possible. Regular cleaning can help control infection and may slow growth, but it does not stop further expansion and does not eliminate risk.

Topical therapy with antibiotic and steroid medications may be useful as well. Irrigations with vinegar or acetic acid may reduce the burden of squamous debris.

Surgical Management

Surgery is the mainstay for management of cholesteatoma. The goal is to completely remove the disease and prevent recurrence. Table 6–1 shows the goals of cholesteatoma surgical treatment. Several surgical options/philosophies exist in regard to this manner, but no consensus exists as to the most efficacious procedure.

Atticotomy

Atticotomy is performed by removing the scutum to allow for access to limited attic disease. The scutal defect is subsequently reconstructed, usually with autologous cartilage, to reduce the possibility of retraction pocket formation and development of recurrent cholesteatoma.

Table 6–1. Goals of Surgical Management of Cholesteatoma

To make the ear safe by eliminating the cholesteatoma and infection
To make the ear problem-free for all the usual activities of daily living, including swimming
To conserve residual hearing and improve hearing if possible
To provide an acceptable cosmetic appearance
To reconstruct the ear in a manner that reduces the chances of recurrence

Radical Mastoidectomy

Radical mastoidectomy is performed by creating one large cavity that allows visualization through an enlarged meatus. The tympanic membrane and ossicles are removed and the eustachian tube is plugged. This allows complete exteriorization of the disease. No ossicular chain reconstruction is performed.

Modified Radical Mastoidectomy

This is similar to the radical procedure, except that the tympanic membrane and ossicles are left in place without any ossicular chain reconstruction. Also referred to as the Bondy procedure, this technique more specifically describes the procedure where the middle ear space is not entered, but a common cavity is created implying that cholesteatoma did not violate the tympanic membrane. This approach is adequate for larger attic cholesteatomas located lateral to the ossicles in patients with a sclerotic mastoid.

Tympanoplasty with Mastoidectomy

This procedure describes the actual type of mastoidectomy that is routinely performed with middle ear reconstruction. This allows eradication of disease in the middle ear and mastoid, reconstruction of the ossicular chain, and repair of the tympanic membrane. This procedure can be characterized further as canal wall-up or canal wall-down, both implying that work was performed on the middle ear.

Risks of Surgery

As with any surgical procedure, careful preoperative patient counseling is mandatory. The risks, complications, and benefits of the surgery must be completely explained. Postoperative care and need for routine follow-up care must also be discussed.

A variety of complications exist in surgical treatment of cholesteatoma. They include bleeding, infection, hearing loss, taste disturbance, vertigo and dizziness, tinnitus, facial nerve injury, CSF leak, meningitis, and possible recurrence requiring further surgery, as well as the risks of general anesthesia. The most feared complication is facial nerve paralysis. In the hands of experienced surgeons, the rate of permanent facial nerve injury following cholesteatoma surgery is around 1%. In a large retrospective study from an experienced neurotologist looking at over 1,400 surgeries for cholesteatoma over a 30-year period, there was a 1.2% rate of facial nerve paralysis and greater than a 30% chance of dehiscence.[6] Facial nerve monitoring may reduce this risk, although controversy exists regarding this. The chorda tympani nerve may be involved with cholesteatoma requiring section. This may result in alteration of taste for several weeks to months after surgery. The risk of complete sensorineural hearing loss or severe dizziness is 1%, usually as a result of damage from the cholesteatoma itself.

Numbness of the external ear is a natural consequence of an incision behind the ear. Some sensation returns several months later but return is usually incomplete. Most patients do not find this troublesome. Shortly after surgery the ear may protrude slightly. The ear almost always returns to normal as the wound behind the ear heals.

Treatment of Retraction Pocket

The cause of the retraction pocket seems to stem from ETD. The importance of ET function in the successful management of cholesteatoma and other chronic middle ear diseases cannot be overstated.[6] Treatment is limited for this problem, but potential exists for evaluation and treatment in the future with eustachian tube surgery. Tympanostomy tube insertion with middle ear aeration may be beneficial in alleviating this. If the pathologic process can be arrested before irreversible changes have occurred, then development of a cholesteatoma may be averted. Many cases are noted to have continued retraction of the tympanic membrane despite tympanostomy tube placement.

Congenital Cholesteatoma Management

Congenital cholesteatoma limited to the mesotympanum may be accessed and treated with a transcanal approach and elevation of a tympanomeatal flap. Careful dissection from surrounding ossicles and the tympanic membrane allows removal. Occasionally, a portion of the tympanic membrane must be delicately elevated from the malleus to allow access to the anterior mesotympanum. Careful postoperative observation must be followed due to recurrence in these patients.

Tympanomastoidectomy: Canal Wall-Up Surgical Technique

To access the middle ear and mastoid, post-auricular and ear canal incisions are commonly employed. Endaural incisions are occasionally performed based on experience in this approach. Incisions are made in the ear canal. Several types of incisions have been described, but the H-flap incision works well. Twelve o'clock and 6 o'clock incisions are made laterally from the annulus. An incision is made 4mm lateral from the annulus in a parallel fashion connecting the 12 and 6 o'clock incisions. Gelfoam soaked in adrenaline is then placed in the ear canal while the mastoid work is done.

The surface landmarks are identified, including the spine of Henle and the linea temporalis or temporal line. The mastoidectomy is then performed using appropriately sized drill bits and suction-irrigation. A large cutting bur (usually a size 6) is initially used to saucerize the edges of the mastoid bone starting along the temporal line, which usually demarcates the level of the tegmen. As one uses the larger burs for dissection, there is less of a chance to damage critical structures. The boundaries of the exposure is the sigmoid sinus posteriorly, the ear canal anteriorly, the tegmen superiorly, and mastoid tip/digastric ridge inferiorly. The ear canal needs to be thinned to allow adequate exposure into the aditus ad antrum and the ear canal angle is what guides one to the antrum. The tegmen or dural plate should be left intact and can be identified by small amounts of bleeding that occurs as well as change in the drill noise as it becomes higher pitched when near the thin bone. The air cells are completely removed and Koerner's septum is identified. This thick bone is removed and the aditus ad antrum is seen (Figure 6–3). In sclerotic cases, the dural plate and the sinodural angle need to be followed to avoid inadvertent injury to the incus, facial nerve, or horizontal canal. Dissection continues anteriorly into

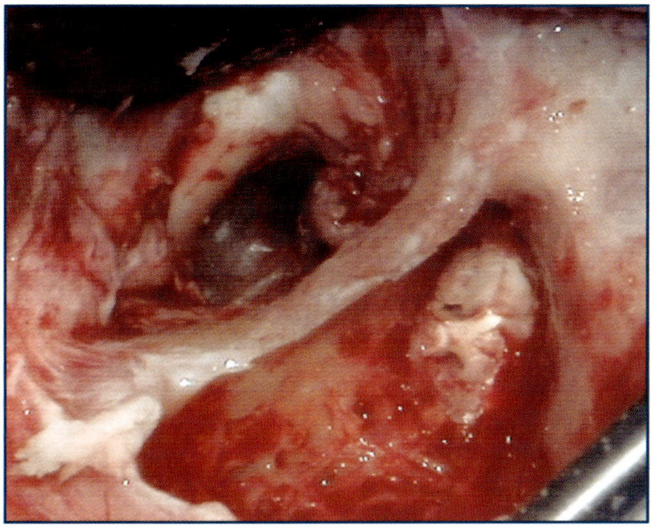

Figure 6–3. Intraoperative view of left intact canal wall mastoidectomy with cholesteatoma noted filling the antrum and bulging in the posterior-superior quadrant of the tympanic membrane.

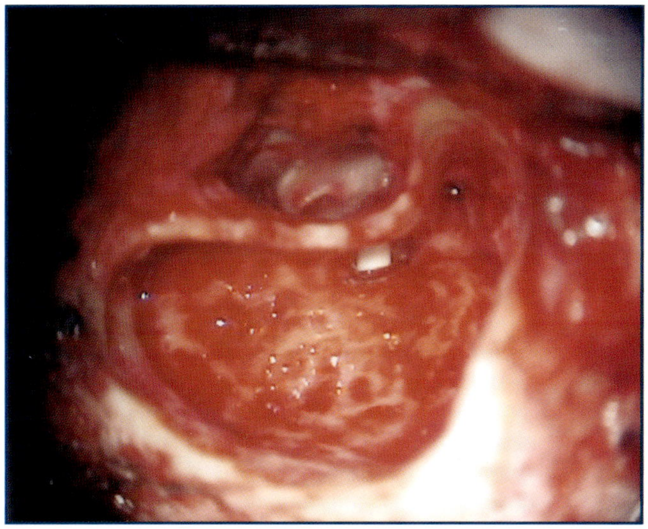

Figure 6–4. Intraoperative view of left intact canal wall mastoidectomy with facial recess opened. Cholesteatoma has been removed and ossicular chain reconstruction has been performed as noted by white mass visible through the facial recess.

the zygomatic root with enough exposure superior to the ear canal that the horizontal canal is seen. The reflection of the incus can be seen in the water from the irrigation. Care must be taken when drilling near the incus, especially if the ossicular chain continuity is not known.

The facial recess (bounded by the fossa incudis, the facial nerve, and the chorda tympani nerve) may be opened to allow access to the posterior aspect of the mesotympanum. The short process of the incus points to the facial recess and this can be thinned with a smaller diamond (usually a size 2) bur until it is eggshell thin. Drilling should be done under constant irrigation to prevent heat injury to the facial nerve and in a direction parallel to the nerve. Drill speed can be reduced to allow better control in this critical area as well. Once thin enough, the triangular opening can be widened with sharp instruments and usually has a 1.5-mm opening (Figure 6–4).

The tympanomeatal flap is elevated and the middle ear space is entered. The chorda tympani nerve is identified and preserved. Cholesteatoma is identified and carefully dissected from surrounding ossicles and tissue. Stimulating instruments with nerve monitoring makes identification of the facial nerve and dissection of cholesteatoma off it safer. The ossicular chain is inspected and palpated. If involved with disease, ossicles need to be excised to prevent recurrence. The decision to reconstruct the ossicular chain may be challenging and can be performed at the initial resection or as a planned second procedure. The tympanic membrane may be reconstructed with fascia or cartilage graft if necessary. Cartilage grafting may prevent further retraction pocket formation, as well as limit extrusion of the reconstructive prosthesis.

Intact canal wall mastoidectomy is suitable in cases with a cholesteatoma in the attic, antrum, and possibly the posterior mesotympanum with an adequately aerated middle ear and mastoid. A staged procedure is often necessary with a scheduled second look at 6 to 9 months for removal of residual cholesteatoma and ossicular chain reconstruction. Staging becomes important in the presence of extensive abnormalities of middle ear mucosa, residual cholesteatoma, and ossicular erosion.

Tympanomastoidectomy: Canal Wall-Down (CWD)

The goal of mastoid surgery is to eliminate and prevent recurrent disease and sometimes this can only be accomplished with removal of the posterior canal wall. Often, the decision to remove the canal wall is made intraoperatively, although sometimes this can be determined prior to the surgery. Preoperative or Intraoperative findings that may suggest that removal of the canal wall is indicated include: patient with history of poor compliance with unreliable follow-up, extensive sinus tympani involvement (although visualization is not significantly improved with this approach), significant erosion of the canal wall, or identification of a labyrinthine fistula. Finding cholesteatoma in an only hearing ear may be an indication for a CWD procedure in an attempt to prevent further complications with subsequent hearing loss. Also, previous failed surgical attempts at controlling the disease may be reason enough to perform the CWD exteriorization procedure.

The surgical technique is similar to the canal wall-up procedure. The canal wall itself is removed and taken down to the level of the facial nerve from the zygomatic root to the digastric ridge. Removal of all air cells, including those within the retrofacial, retrolabyrinthine, and subarcuate air cell tracts is performed. The facial ridge is lowered until the fallopian canal is barely visible. Facial nerve monitoring and stimulation allows complete removal of the facial ridge as low as possible. The mastoid tip may need to be addressed so that debris cannot collect there in the future. It may be amputated from attached muscles. A large meatoplasty is created by removing conchal cartilage to allow adequate air circulation into the cavity.

Mastoid obliteration provides a means of decreasing the size of the mastoid cavity to avoid bowl complications such as accumulation of debris with subsequent infection as well as caloric effects of an open mastoid cavity. Obliteration may have benefit initially, but has variable efficacy over time. Various flaps and materials have been advocated for this purpose, including temporoparietal fascial flaps, periosteal-pericranial flaps, bone chips, bone pate, and bone cement.

Postoperative Care

Regular office visits are necessary following surgery. Packing material is removed and healing is carefully followed. Mastoid incisions are monitored for possible infections. Open mastoid cavities heal slowly and may require 6 months to fully epithelialize.

Frequently, granulation tissue forms in the open cavity as it heals. Granulation tissue may be helpful because it can contract the size of the cavity. Steroid creams, steroid-containing drops, and regular applications of gentian violet can be used to help control the development and extent of granulation tissue. Silver nitrate cautery effectively eliminates or reduces granulation tissue, but care must be taken near the facial nerve.

Both aminoglycoside and fluoroquinolone topical preparations provide appropriate antibacterial coverage for healing wounds. The complete absence of potential ototoxicity among the fluoroquinolones makes them more appealing. If a nonsteroidal otic preparation is desired, either ciprofloxacin (Ciloxan) or ofloxacin (Floxin otic) are excellent choices. If granulation tissue is present, steroid-containing drops may be preferred. In such cases, ciprofloxacin/dexamethasone (Ciprodex) is an excellent choice.

Long-Term Care

Patients with cholesteatoma will require routine office visits at least every 6 months for many years for evaluation of hearing and inspection for recurrent disease. Patients with an exposed mastoid cavity may require lifelong visits. Once healed, the mastoid cavity should not cause much difficulty and will need routine removal of debris. Removal of crusting and debris allows better aeration of the cavity. Use of alcohol and vinegar irrigations may allow maintenance of a healthy cavity as well. Water precaution is recommended for patients with a large open cavity.

Persistent drainage from a canal wall-down cavity can arise for a number of reasons. The most common cause of persistent drainage is either a sequestered air cell that continues to harbor infection or small areas of osteitis. Granulation tissue in the mastoid bowl is potentially the result of infection or underlying inflammation and should be removed or further investigated. If the area of osteitis is large and postoperative otorrhea has persisted for months or years, skin grafting is a consideration for treatment. Skin grafts are especially useful in cavities that have developed mucosal epithelial linings.

Occasionally, use of topical steroidal, antibacterial, antifungal, and antifibroblastic (Mitomycin C) preparations may reduce the granulation tissue as well.[7] Reoperation may be necessary in some patients to maintain the cavity.

Hearing rehabilitation after surgical resection for cholesteatoma includes staged ossicular chain reconstruction, hearing aid amplification, and implantable hearing solutions such as the bone-anchored hearing aid.

Results of Therapy

Due to the nature of the cholesteatoma disease process, randomized, prospective clinical studies are difficult to implement. It is often difficult to assess whether disease found after surgery is due to residual disease or recurrent cholesteatoma. Therefore, many reports use the term recidivism to encompass both residual and recurrent disease.

Although there has been no consensus as to the most appropriate surgical approach for the optimal surgical management of cholesteatoma, most studies demonstrate a higher degree of recidivistic disease in cases treated with an intact canal wall approach. Nevertheless, strong proponents of both intact canal wall and canal wall-down continue to debate.

A retrospective study reviewed their cases of 66 pediatric patients with cholesteatoma followed for an average of 3 years. Recidivistic disease was noted in 41% of the patients having intact canal wall mastoidectomy compared with 12% recidivism in those having a canal wall-down procedure.[8] Hearing results were comparable for the two procedures with a postoperative speech reception threshold of less than 30 dB in 75% of cases with intact canal wall and 72% of cases with canal wall-down. Another study found similar results, with surgeon experience also being a consideration in the success of intact call wall mastoidectomy.[9]

Another study for pediatric patients found that surgeons preferred the canal wall-down approach. These authors showed rates of recidivistic disease were 11% for tympanoplasty, 19% for intact canal wall mastoidectomy, 5% for modified radical mastoidectomy, and 0% for radical mastoidectomy.[10] Others have reported a need for fewer revisions with canal wall-down surgery and similar hearing results with this approach.[11]

Controversy in Cholesteatoma Treatment

The principal controversy surrounds intact canal wall versus canal wall-down mastoidectomy for removal of disease. The approach to each case is based on many factors, including those relating to the ear itself, patient issues, as well as the experience of the surgeon. Management needs to be tailored specifically for each patient separately.

In certain circumstances, the surgeon can make the decision to use a canal wall-down technique preoperatively. If the patient has had several episodes of recurrence of the cholesteatoma and wishes to avoid future operations, or they are not interested in a possible second-look procedure, then the canal wall-down technique is most applicable and safer. Sometimes, this decision is not possible until the operation has begun and a clear understanding of the extent of disease has been obtained. Canal wall-down operations have the highest probability of permanently ridding the patient of the cholesteatoma.

Canal wall-up procedures have the advantage of maintaining a normal appearance, but they have a higher risk of persistent or recurrent cholesteatomas. This risk of recurrence is high enough that most surgeons recommend a second-look procedure 6–9 months later to confirm lack of disease and allow easier removal of recurrent cholesteatoma.

Treatment results are variable in terms of eradication of disease and hearing between the intact canal and CWD procedures. Advantages and disadvantages for each approach are summarized in Tables 6–2 and 6–3. Whatever the chosen approach, complete eradication of disease should remain at the forefront of the surgical decision-making process.

Another area of controversy is the use of facial nerve monitoring. The debate surrounds whether facial nerve monitoring is the standard of care. Many experienced otologists use it frequently even though they know the anatomy extremely well. In fact, this extra piece of knowledge may be more beneficial to them than to an inexperienced operator. On the other hand, predicting the cases in which the facial nerve is at risk is not possible and one could argue

Table 6–2. Advantages and Disadvantages of Intact Canal Wall Mastoidectomy

Advantages	Disadvantages
Rapid healing	Mastoid not accessible without 2nd look
Minimal post-op care	Residual disease more likely
No water precautions	Retraction pocket formation more likely
Easier hearing aid fit	May require further surgical procedures to eradicate disease

Table 6–3. Advantages and Disadvantages of Canal Wall-Down Mastoidectomy

Advantages	Disadvantages
Easy detection of residual disease	Longer healing time with special care of cavity possible
Usually single procedure to eradicate disease	Routine cleaning required as debris accumulates
	Water precautions necessary
	More difficult hearing aid fit

that monitoring should be performed in every case. Facial nerve monitoring can be utilized as a precaution, much like pulse oximetry, that may be potentially useful in any given case. The senior author (SB) routinely uses facial nerve monitoring for all cases involving cholesteatoma.

COMPLICATIONS

Complications can occur from the disease process itself but the surgeon must take great care to avoid iatrogenic ones.

Conductive hearing loss is a common complication of cholesteatoma, resulting from ossicular erosion or mass effect. Usually the poor blood supply at the incudostapedial joint leads to a common site of erosion, especially the lenticular process of the incus. The degree of conductive hearing loss varies considerably depending on the amount of cholesteatoma and erosion present. A maximal conductive loss may be evident with erosion the lenticular process of the incus and the stapes superstructure.

Labyrinthine fistula, most commonly of the lateral semicircular canal, should be suspected in patients with sensorineural hearing loss or vestibular symptoms at presentation. Sometimes, a labyrinthine fistula is suggested based on the preoperative CT scan images; other times, a fistula is a complete surprise. If the fistula appears superficial, gently remove the matrix at the end of the case and cover the defect with fascia.[12] However, if the fistula is large and it appears that the cholesteatoma matrix is attached firmly to the membranous labyrinth itself, consider leaving the matrix in position due to the potential risk of hearing loss and permanent balance disorder. If this is the case, it is reasonable to perform a canal wall-down mastoidectomy. Regardless, both broad-spectrum intravenous antibiotics and steroids should be administered immediately to reduce the risk of bacterial labyrinthitis.

It is the goal of the surgeon to prevent iatrogenic facial nerve injuries with proper pre-operative planning and meticulous surgical technique. The most dreaded complication in cholesteatoma surgery is facial nerve injury. Weakness of the facial nerve may be a presenting symptom and would prompt immediate surgical intervention. Disease-related facial nerve injury may also be noted only at the time of surgery and should be addressed during the procedure. It is the goal of the surgeon to prevent iatrogenic facial nerve injuries with proper pre-operative planning and meticulous surgical technique. The tympanic segment of the facial nerve is a common site of iatrogenic injury both during mastoidectomy and removal of cholesteatoma from the middle ear.[6]

If intraoperative damage has occurred, most medical-legal experts recommend obtaining a second opinion for management decisions. Treatment may require facial nerve decompression proximal and distal to the injury. The severity of the injury needs to be assessed. If more than 50% of the diameter of the nerve is deemed nonviable because it has been cut, crushed, or stretched, then this segment of nerve needs to be resected and repaired primarily or with an interposition nerve graft.

More commonly, patients wake up in the recovery room with facial nerve weakness. If complete paralysis is present, the surgeon will have significant stress and may find it difficult to remember the events of the surgery that may have lead to any problems. If the surgeon is not absolutely sure that the facial nerve is anatomically intact, then the patient should be taken back to surgery immediately and any injury should be repaired. One should also wait several hours to make sure that this is not a consequence of the local anesthetic, if the facial nerve was not at risk. If facial paralysis persists 3 to 4 hours beyond recovery from anesthesia, remove the packing, although it is unlikely that pressure from a dressing is causing the problem.

If the facial nerve was clearly visualized at the time of surgery and the operating surgeon is absolutely certain that the nerve is anatomically intact, treat the injury like any other posttraumatic nerve paralysis. Begin electroneuronography (ENOG) testing approximately 72 hours postoperatively. If, within the first 2 to 3 weeks, the compound action potential on the affected side drops to less than 10% of the compound action potential on the normal side, the surgeon may consider re-exploration.

Encephalocele may occur as a result of iatrogenic dural exposure and disruption in the area of the tegmen tympani or mastoideum. Leakage of cerebrospinal fluid may or may not be evident. When recognized at the initial procedure, the dural defect should be repaired with temporalis fascia or similar material. Cartilage may be necessary to provide support for larger defects. Leakage of CSF may necessitate placement of a lumbar drain for management.

Intratemporal or intracranial complications of cholesteatoma are serious and may be life-threatening. Expeditious evaluation and management are mandatory.[13]

SUMMARY

Cholesteatoma occurs due to the presence of keratinizing stratified squamous epithelium in the middle ear and mastoid. Eradication of disease is the primary surgical goal, followed by maintenance or restoration of hearing. The surgical treatment must be tailored to the individual patient and disease process, but it must be accepted that cholesteatoma is a chronic disease with a high rate of recidivism and requires diligent long-term follow-up. Canal wall-down tympanomastoidectomy offers a very low rate of recurrence or persistence of a cholesteatoma. This compares quite favorably to the 20 to 40% recurrence rates associated with closed-cavity techniques. Hearing results and care of the cavity afterward must play a role in decision making as well. Complications from cholesteatoma can be life-threatening and must be quickly diagnosed.

REFERENCES

1. Strunk CL. Cholesteatoma. In: Bailey BJ. *Head and Neck Surgery-Otolaryngology*. 2nd ed. Philadelphia, PA: JB Lippincott; 1998;2:2041–2051.
2. Kemppainen HO, Puhakka HJ, Laippala PJ, et al. Epidemiology and aetiology of middle ear cholesteatoma. *Acta Otolaryngol*. 1999;119(5):568–572.
3. Pickett BP, Cail WS, Lambert PR. Sinus tympani: anatomic considerations, computed tomography, and a discussion of the retrofacial approach for removal of disease. *Am J Otol*. 1995;16:741–750.
4. Weber PC, Adkins WY. Congenital cholesteatomas in the tympanic membrane. *Laryngoscope*. 1997;107:1181–1184.
5. Jeunen G, Desloovere C, Hermans R, Vandecaveye V. The value of magnetic resonance imaging in the diagnosis of residual or recurrent acquired cholesteatoma after canal wall-up tympanoplasty. *Otol Neurotol*. 2008;29(1):16–18.
6. Quaranta N, Cassano M, Quaranta A. Facial paralysis associated with cholesteatoma: a review of 13 cases. *Otol Neurotol*. 2007;28(3):405–407.
7. Babu SC, Kartush JM, Patni A. Otologic effects of topical mitomycin C: phase I. evaluation of ototoxicity. *Otol Neurotol*. 2005;26(2):140–144.
8. Dodson EE, Hashisaki GT, Hobgood TC, Lambert PR. Intact canal wall mastoidectomy with tympanoplasty for cholesteatoma in children. *Laryngoscope*. 1998;108:977–983.
9. Graham MD, Delap TG, Goldsmith MM. Closed tympanomastoidectomy. *Otolaryngol Clin North Am*. 1999;32(3):547–554.
10. Hirsch BE, Kamerer DB, Doshi S. Single-stage management of cholesteatoma. *Otolaryngol Head Neck Surg*. 1992;106:351–354.
11. Roland PS, Meyerhoff WL. Open-cavity tympanomastoidectomy. *Otolaryngol Clin North Am*. 1999;32(3):525–546.

12. Busaba NY. Clinical presentation and management of labyrinthine fistula caused by chronic otitis media. *Ann Otol Rhinol Laryngol*. 1999;108(5):435–439.

13. Schwaber MK, Pensak ML, Bartels LJ. The early signs and symptoms of neurotologic complications of chronic suppurative otitis media. *Laryngoscope*. 1989;99:373–375.

CHAPTER 7

Complications of Cholesteatoma and Otitis Media

Nouha Alammar and Seilesh Babu

INTRODUCTION

Otitis media (OM) is one of the most common pediatric diagnoses made in the United States today. The advent of antibiotics in the 1940s revolutionized the clinical picture and treatment of otitis media. In addition, modern radiographic imaging have allowed for earlier diagnosis and treatment. Despite the widespread use of antibiotics and improved imaging, the complications of OM still occur and cause significant morbidity and mortality. Early diagnosis and prompt treatment of these complications are essential for a good prognosis.

Complications from OM can be classified as intratemporal and intracranial. Intratemporal complications include: mastoiditis, facial paralysis, petrositis, and labyrinthitis from labyrinthine fistula. The intracranial complications of OM include: meningitis, sigmoid sinus thrombosis, otitic hydrocephalus brain abscess, subdural empyema, and extradural abscess[1] (Table 7–1). These infections may arise from acute otitis media (AOM) or chronic otitis media (COM). The pathophysiology, clinical presentation, diagnosis, and management of the individual complications of OM are presented.

Table 7–1. Complications of Otitis Media

Intratemporal Complications	Intracranial Complications
Mastoiditis	Meningitis
Petrous apicitis	Sigmoid sinus thrombosis
Labyrinthitis with labyrinthine fistula	Otitic hydrocephalus
Facial nerve paralysis	Epidural abscess
	Subdural empyema
	Brain abscess

INTRATEMPORAL COMPLICATIONS OF OTITIS MEDIA

Coalescent Mastoiditis

Mastoiditis is a disease entity that lies along a spectrum ranging from asymptomatic effusion, to coalescent disease, and finally to abscess formation. Mastoiditis develops when acute or chronic otitis media fails to resolve and leads to mucosal thickening and mastoid effusion with corresponding changes in the bone and mastoid air cell system. As the disease progresses, edema of the mucoperiosteal lining disrupts aeration leading to an osteoclastic process in the inflamed periosteum. This causes coalescence of small air cells into a large cavity with loss of trabecular bone.

Coalescent mastoiditis is a progressive disease usually seen in young children. It is classically described in patients with well-pneumatized mastoids and rarely develops in those with history of chronic ear disease. Clinical presentation includes symptoms of postauricular pain, purulent otorrhea, fever, and toxicity. The physical findings include mastoid tenderness to palpation, postauricular erythema, edema, and displacement of the auricle anteriorly. Evaluation of the patient consists of a complete hematologic workup and a computed tomography (CT) scan. The CT scan will demonstrate the loss of mastoid air cell trabeculation and opacification of the pneumatized spaces and is the hallmark of mastoiditis.

Coalescent mastoiditis is a serious complication requiring prompt treatment. Initial treatment includes intravenous antibiotic therapy and usually requires decompression of the mastoid. This may temporarily be accomplished with a myringotomy and pressure equalizing tube (PET), but usually a complete mastoidectomy with precise eradication of devitalized and necrotic bone is necessary. Another approach is placement of a ventilating tube in conjunction with 3 to 6 weeks of antibiotics therapy as an alternative.[2]

Petrous Apicitis

The petrous apex constitutes the anterior superior portion of the temporal bone. It can either be characterized as sclerotic, underdeveloped, or pneumatized. Air cell tracts are found between the mastoid system and the petrous apex, which allows for extension of mastoid infection into the apex leading to petrous apicitis. The pathology of this infection mimics that which is seen in mastoiditis. It ranges from an effusion, to the destruction of the bony partitions, and formation of an abscess. Because of the anatomic proximity to the middle and posterior cranial fossa, this infection can lead to serious intracranial infections.

The symptomalogy of petrous apicitis is a reflection of increased pressure within the petrous apex, which contains the trigeminal ganglion in Meckel's cave and the sixth cranial nerve (CN VI) as it travels through Dorello's canal. This results in referred deep retro-orbital pain from irritation of the trigeminal ganglion and sixth nerve palsy. Along with otorrhea, this triad is collectively known as *Gradenigo's syndrome*.[3] When this disease is suspected, a CT scan is obtained to document the septae of air cells and contour of the petrous apex. A magnetic resonance imaging (MRI) scan may aid in differentiating marrow from CSF and evaluating for intracranial complications. Serial C-reactive protein (CRP) levels and erythrocyte sedimentation rate (ESR) may be used to follow progression and response to therapy.[4]

The management of petrous apicitis is dependent on the duration, severity, and presence of complications. With the widespread use of antibiotics, the prevalence of apicitis markedly has decreased, and IV antibiotics have become the initial treatment of petrous apicitis. However, in the presence of necrotic bone, abscess, or persistent disease, surgical intervention is a necessity. The petrous apex lies in close proximity to the otic capsule and carotid artery making surgical access complex. The surgical approach is dictated by the air cell tracts that are found on imaging. In a hearing ear, the possible approaches include: infracochlear, infralabyrinthine, retrolabyrinthine, subarcuate, and the middle fossa. In a nonhearing ear, surgical access can be gained via the translabyrinthine or transcochlear approaches.[5]

Labyrinthine Fistula

Labyrinthine fistula and labyrinthitis represent complications of chronic otitis media with cholesteatoma. Labyrinthitis, which is more common, may occur from spread of the infection and inflammation near the semicircular canals. A fistula results from loss of protective endochondral bone covering the labyrinth without involving the perilymph. This erosion of the bone involving the otic capsule allows mass-induced motion of endolymphatic system leading to vestibular and auditory symptoms. Because of its proximity to the antrum, 90% of these fistulas involve the lateral semicircular canal (SCC). There are reported cases involving the superior SCC, posterior SCC, or the cochlea as well and may present with similar symptoms so thorough evaluation of the CT scan is essential.[6] The mechanism of erosion of the bone is thought to be due to inflammatory mediators in absence of cholesteatoma, or activated mediators in the presence of cholesteatoma. This can lead to demineralization and loss of substance covering the labyrinth.

Patients present with vestibular symptoms consisting of brief episodes of vertigo, disequilibrium, or imbalance which can be provoked by loud sounds (Tullio's phenomenon). On physical examination, a positive fistula test can be elicited by occluding the external auditory canal with the pneumatic otoscope and assessing for eye motion deviating away from the side of compression. The fistula test is shown to be present in 32 to 50% of patients with a fistula during ear exploration.[6] Still, the absence of the above symptoms does not confirm the presence of an intact bony labyrinth. Therefore, the definitive diagnosis of a fistula can only be made intraoperatively. The use of preoperative CT imaging may be helpful in surgical planning as well.

The management of labyrinthine fistulas is surgical. A mastoidectomy is essential for the treatment of cholesteatoma and diagnosis of the labyrinthine fistula. The most appropriate surgical approach depends on the size, extent, and location of the fistula. Some reports indicate that treatment of a small fistula involving the labyrinth can be performed in a single-stage operation.[6] On the other hand, a large fistula can be approached by removing the cholesteatoma matrix and then repairing the defect with bone pate and fascia. Identification of the fistula may be difficult until the cholesteatoma and inflammatory tissue is removed and the fistula exposed. One must think about the possibility of a fistula prior to removal of this matrix in order to prevent damage to the endolymph and reduce hearing and vestibular loss. A canal wall-down mastoidectomy may be necessary in this instance as some cholesteatoma matrix will be left in place. Furthermore, to minimize the risk of hearing loss, corticosteroids can be used during removal of cholesteatoma from the fistula.

Facial Paralysis

Facial nerve paralysis may result from otogenic causes such as acute OM or chronic suppurative OM with or without cholesteatoma. Facial paralysis with OM is presumed to be secondary to the release of bacterial toxic metabolites that affect the fallopian canal.[7] This usually occurs in the setting of a congenital nerve dehiscence within the facial canal, or via vascular channels that communicate between the fallopian canal and the mastoid air cells. As a result, neuropraxia can develop either from edema, ischemia, or nerve compression.

The development of facial paralysis with chronic suppurative OM or cholesteatoma is a result of direct invasion of the fallopian canal and bony erosion. The destruction by cholesteatoma occurs mostly at the tympanic and mastoid segments which lead to nerve compression.[7]

Children with facial paralysis or paresis, in the setting of acute otitis media, will usually present 7 to 10 days after the onset of the ear infection. The facial nerve weakness presents abruptly, with an incomplete paresis that is short-lived. The lacrimal function is rarely affected. In the case of paralysis secondary to COM or cholesteatoma, the course is one of gradual weakness and carries a worse prognosis.

The diagnosis of otogenic facial paralysis is based on a complete history and physical, with clinical differentiation between acute or chronic otitis media. The Schirmer test allows assessment of lacrimal function and helps in delineating the location of the lesion. It is also important to perform a detailed examination of the individual facial nerve branches to assess for Neumann's sign. This occurs when a single nerve branch weakness progresses to affect the function of others, and has been known to be suggestive of a cholesteatoma.[8]

In the setting of complete facial paralysis, electrophysiologic testing of the nerve should be obtained to assess the nerve degeneration that will help determine the prognosis. These tests are described in Chapter 12. Furthermore, CT imaging of the temporal bones can be useful in surgical planning where an intracranial process is presumed. On the other hand, in the setting of incomplete paralysis with AOM, spontaneous recovery is expected and the role of electrophysiologic testing is not necessary.

Incomplete facial paralysis with AOM can be treated conservatively with intravenous antibiotics and myringotomy with tympanostomy tube. Broad-spectrum coverage is needed for *H. influenzae, Streptococcus, M. catarralis*, and *Staphylococcus* species.

The treatment for complete facial paralysis from acute mastoiditis, chronic suppurative otitis media, or cholesteatoma requires surgical intervention. In the case of chronic suppurative OM without cholesteatoma, the surgeon should perform an intact canal wall mastoidectomy with facial nerve exploration from the geniculate ganglion to the stylomastoid foramen. If granulation tissue or cholesteatoma is encountered containing the facial nerve, a diamond bur is used to thin the fallopian canal. The nerve sheath is then exposed proximal and distal to the diseased segment. The surgeon should avoid opening the nerve sheath, which can serve as a barrier to direct infection, and also decreases the risk of further nerve injury.[8]

INTRACRANIAL COMPLICATIONS OF OTITIS MEDIA

Meningitis

Despite advancing treatments of OM in the post-antibiotic era, meningitis remains the most common intracranial complication of acute and chronic OM. However, in children, meningitis more commonly follows acute OM. This usually occurs as a result of direct bacterial migration, or hematogenous seeding of the meninges and the subarachnoid space. Meningitis associated with COM is thought to arise secondary to direct spread of middle ear or mastoid disease. The route of extension can follow several different paths which include the preformed channels known as Hyrtl's fissures, the labyrinth, the petrous apex cells, or paths caused by bony erosion.

Patients with meningitis caused by acute OM present with a rapid downward course. Initially, they present with a headache associated with nuchal rigidity. This is followed by persistent fevers, chills, irritability, and vomiting. Finally, photophobia and decreased neurological status ensues.

The diagnosis of meningitis relies on obtaining CSF cultures, followed by antibiotic therapy tailored to the results. The most common organisms include: *S. pneumoniae, Group A Streptococcus,* and *H. influenzae type B*. Prior to performing a lumbar puncture, a CT scan is obtained to rule out coexisting pathology such as a Mondini malformation, a fistula, or any osseous defects. This may also prevent any intracranial complications from the lumbar puncture.

Sigmoid Sinus Thrombosis

Sigmoid sinus thrombosis or lateral sinus thrombosis compromises 17 to 19% of otogenic intracranial complications. It usually occurs by way of bony destruction secondary to chronic OM, or cholesteatoma. There is a direct extension caused by the infection and inflammation moving from the middle ear and temporal bone to the dura adjacent to the sigmoid sinus. Thrombosis begins with platelet aggregation and the development of an intramural thrombus. The mural thrombus can propagate retrograde to the transverse sinus, or antegrade to involve the internal jugular vein or cavernous sinus. Embolization of the infected thrombus at this point increases the risk of distant lung emboli and septicemia.[5]

The clinical presentation of sigmoid sinus thrombosis includes high spiking ("picket fence") fevers, headache, ear pain, neck stiffness, and lethargy. In addition, increased intracranial pressure can lead to papilledema and visual deficits. Also, mastoid emissary vein thrombosis can present with Griesinger's sign, which is characterized by tenderness and edema over the posterior mastoid. Diagnostic imaging studies include CT scan and MRI which shows the characteristic "delta" sign of sinus thrombosis.[8] Furthermore, MRA can depict lack of flow and determine the thrombosis and is considered the gold standard for diagnosing dural sinus thrombosis.

The first-line treatment of sigmoid sinus thrombosis is IV antibiotics with blood brain barrier penetration for six weeks. This may be followed by surgical intervention in the presence of COM or cholesteatoma. The surgical procedure consists of performing a mastoidectomy, with exposure of the sigmoid sinus, dural venous sinus, and surrounding granulation tissue. In the past, some advocated aspiration of the sinus and a thrombectomy. Currently, outcomes have not been affected by thrombectomy and mastoidectomy and IV antibiotics are sufficient treatment.[4] Internal jugular vein ligation is recommended when evidence of septicemia and distant pulmonary emboli exists. Anticoagulation may be necessary when the thrombus extends into the transverse sinus, cavernous, or internal jugular vein.

Otitic Hydrocephalus

Otitic hydrocephalus represents a condition that is a misnomer. It was originally described as increased intracranial pressure with normal CSF findings on a lumbar puncture. In 1931, Symonds defined this condition as an infection of the transverse sinus with retrograde extension into the superior sagittal sinus.[7] This thrombophlebitis can prevent CSF absorption which leads to increased intracranial pressure. Otitic hydrocephalus is a complication that can be secondary to AOM, COM, or otologic surgery. It has been shown to carry a favorable prognosis when diagnosed promptly.

The symptoms and signs of otitic hydrocephalus are the result of the increased intracranial pressure and they include headache, visual changes, lethargy, nausea, and vomiting. On ophthalmic examination, papilledema, diplopia, and sixth nerve palsy may be present. In addition, an MRI and MRV can be performed to assess for thrombosis of the dural sinus or ventricular dilation. Still, the diagnosis is one of exclusion and can be based entirely on clinical symptoms.

Treatment of otitic hydrocephalus requires decreasing the intracranial pressure and eradicating any underlying otogenic process. The goal is to prevent optic nerve atrophy. In the case of COM with sinus thrombosis, a mastoidectomy with exposure of the dural venous sinus is indicated. Medical management is aimed at decreasing intracranial pressure. Some of the medications used include mannitol, acetazolamide, fluid restriction, and corticosteroids. If such treatments are unsuccessful, serial lumbar drainage and lumboperitoneal shunting may be required to normalize the intracranial pressure.

Epidural Abscess

Epidural abscesses occur when purulent material and granulation tissue is located superficial to the dura. These abscesses present as early intracranial complications. They result from bony destruction caused by chronic OM with cholesteatoma or a coalescent mastoiditis. They are usually found incidentally during surgery and can occur at the following sites: (1) between the tegmen and the middle fossa dura, (2) along the sigmoid sinus, and (3) along the posterior fossa dura. These abscesses can cause other intracranial complications such as brain abscess, sigmoid sinus thrombosis, and otitic hydrocephalus.

The clinical presentation of epidural abscess is mainly silent. Occasionally, the patient will complain of increased otalgia or headache which is similar to a chronic OM presentation. The diagnosis is usually made intraoperatively, but a CT scan or MRI is warranted if suspicion for an intracranial pathology is present.

The management of an epidural abscess is centered on the treatment of the underlying cause. A mastoidectomy is performed and the bone overlying the sigmoid sinus, posterior fossa dura, and middle fossa dura is removed until healthy dura can be appreciated. Postoperative treatment consists of continuous IV antibiotics until signs of the disease have resolved.

Subdural Empyema

Subdural empyema is defined as an infection located between the dura and arachnoid layers of the brain. It is the least common complication of otitis media. Subdural empyema is found to be more common in children with chronic OM rather than acute OM. Granulation tissue or cholesteatoma will move through the bone and dura at the location of the tegmen tympani. Another possible route is via the venous system characterized by a retrograde spread of the infection. The final route of spread is secondary to abscess rupture into the subdural space.

The clinical signs and symptoms can include headache, nausea, and vomiting. After several days, the disease progresses and symptoms of seizures and neurological deficits develop. Imaging with CT scan or MRI makes the diagnosis. These images will show an area of low-density cerebral convexity with rim enhancement of the brain matter. Surgical debridement is necessary with neurosurgical consultation and a mastoidectomy is usually performed simultaneously.

Brain Abscess

Brain abscess is described as a collection of purulent infection surrounded by encephalitis mostly affecting the temporal lobe and cerebellum. It is the second most common intracranial complication after meningitis and may be caused by chronic OM. These abscesses can develop from venous thrombophlebitis, and normally will reveal sterile cultures. However, evidence of a positive culture will usually contain multiple organisms with *Proteus* as the predominant species.

Brain abscesses occur in four pathologic stages. The first stage is known as the encephalitic stage. It is the result of thrombophlebitis with the infection propagating to the white matter of the brain. This stage is followed by necrosis and liquefaction of brain matter. The third stage occurs within 10 days and marks the formation of an abscess with capsule formation. The final stage represents the abscess expansion that may eventually lead to rupture.

The clinical presentation occurs in correlation with the pathologic stages. In the first stage symptoms include fever, nausea, vomiting, and headache. This is followed by a clinically silent period. After several weeks, fever, lethargy, mental status change, seizures, and papilledema can occur. The presence of these symptoms indicates an intracranial involvement and a CT scan or MRI should be performed while initiating broad-spectrum antibiotics. Failure to recognize this would result in progression of the disease to its final stages. The patient in stage four becomes hemodynamically unstable and the disease is fatal.

The treatment of a brain abscess usually will require surgical intervention. The patient should be started on IV steroids and anticonvulsants prior to neurosurgical drainage. This is usually performed within 24 hours of presentation. However, in the case of acute OM, a myringotomy with culture of fluid is sufficient initially. In the setting of chronic OM with or without cholesteatoma, a mastoidectomy is performed at the time of the abscess drainage. It has been advocated that parenteral antibiotics should be given for several weeks followed by CT scan to check for disease resolution.

CONCLUSION

Despite appropriate antibiotic therapy and access to physicians, serious intracranial and intratemporal complications of OM still occur. Early recognition of the signs and symptoms suggestive of otogenic complications will prevent many neurological problems. Physicians should maintain a high index of suspicion when faced with OM, especially when complications exist. Antibiotics should be started when the diagnosis is suspected, and radiological imaging should be performed, followed by effective surgical management as dictated by the presentation.

REFERENCES

1. Leskinen K. Complications of acute otitis media in children. *Curr Allergy Asthma Reports*. 2005;5:308–312.
2. Dubey SP, Larawin V. Complications of chronic suppurative otitis media and their management. *Laryngoscope*. 2007;117:264–267.
3. Smith JA, Danner CJ. Complications of chronic otitis media and cholesteatoma. *Otolaryngol Clin N Am*. 2006; 39:1237–1255.
4. Agrawal S, Husein M, MacRae D. Complications of otitis media: an evolving state. *J Otolaryngol*. 2005;34:533–539.
5. Bento R, de Brito R, Ribas GC. Surgical management of intracranial complications of otogenic infection. *ENT Journal*. 2006;85:36–39.
6. Magliulo G, Celebrini A, Cuiuli G, Parrotto D. Surgical management of the labyrinthine fistula complicating chronic otitis media with or without cholesteatoma. *J Otolaryngol*. 2008;37:143–147.
7. Kitsko DJ, Dohar JE. Inner ear and facial nerve complications of acute otitis media, including vertigo. *Curr Allergy Asthma Reports*. 2007;7:444–450.
8. Neely JG. Facial nerve and intracranial complications of otitis media. In: Jackler et al. *Neurotology and Skull Base Surgery*. Philadelphia, PA; Elsevier Mosby; 2004:chap 52.

CHAPTER 8

Ossicular Chain Reconstruction

Travis Pfannenstiel and Dennis Bojrab

INTRODUCTION

Success in ossicular chain reconstruction (OCR) is achieved when a mobile tympanic membrane and a secure sound-conducting mechanism to the inner ear fluids are present in the absence of infection or cholesteatoma. Further criterion for success may be introduced; however, in achieving these fundamental goals one produces a healthy ear capable of receiving amplification without the risks associated with chronic otitis media and cholesteatoma. Historically, the radical mastoidectomy was the only operation for patients with chronic otomastoid disease producing a safe, dry ear, with poor function. Wullstein[1] and Zollner[2] first introduced the term tympanoplasty in 1951 to describe surgical reconstruction of the middle ear hearing mechanism.

This chapter reviews the history of ossicular chain reconstruction, the materials used for OCR, and factors predicting success in ossicular chain reconstruction. The mechanics of hearing is briefly discussed in this chapter.

ACOUSTIC MECHANICS

The middle ear functions to convey sound pressure waves from the air into the fluids of the inner ear. The difference between these media through which sound is conducted through the external auditory canal, ossicles, and the fluids of the cochlea makes the middle ear an impedance-matching system minimizing energy loss.

The acoustic transformation theory describes the middle ear transformer as a series of three lever systems: the tympanic membrane lever, the ossicular lever, and the hydraulic lever. As a result of these three lever systems, the middle ear creates a gain of approximately 27 to 34 dB.[3]

In some diseased and reconstructed ears (Types IV, V tympanoplasties), loss of the tympanic membrane and ossicular chain can cause a hearing loss that exceeds 30 dB. This is explained by sound waves having access to both the round and oval windows causing cochlear fluid wave cancellation and interference. Shielding of the round window with cartilage or fascia results in redirection of all sound energy into the oval window.[3] Acoustic coupling theory thus applied allows for closure of the air bone gap to near 20 dB.

Status of the Middle Ear

Under normal conditions the middle ear air pressure is less than the external canal air pressure, providing an environment conducive to ossicular coupling and promoting tympanic membrane displacement. If middle ear aeration is poor and the space is reduced, the pressure of the middle ear increases relative to the external canal pressure and the impedance increases. This pressure difference leads to a reduction in ossicular and tympanic membrane motion. 0.5 mL has been calculated as the minimal amount of middle ear air space required to maintain ossicular coupling within 10 dB of normal.[4]

In outlining potential risk factors for failure in ossiculoplasty various authors have found the status of the middle ear as a consistent predictor of success. The Middle Ear Risk Index (MERI) attempts standardization in reporting various perioperative factors, but it has not been widely utilized. The MERI takes into account otorrhea, perforation, cholesteatoma, ossicular status, presence of granulation tissue or effusions, prior surgery, and smoking history.[5] Although a useful tool the MERI has not been validated, and to date no validated questionnaire or staging system for ossicular chain reconstruction is available to otologists for clinical investigation.

REPORTING OSSICULOPLASTY SUCCESS

The first step in consistently reporting success in chronic ear surgery is accurate description of the type of surgical procedure performed. One widely accepted classification scheme breaks tympanoplasty into five subtypes. Type I tympanoplasty (myringoplasty) involves reconstruction of a tympanic membrane defect with a completely intact ossicular chain. Type II tympanoplasty involves reconstruction of an eardrum in the absence of a usable malleus; hence, the tympanic membrane is brought into contact with the incus and stapes assembly. Type III tympanoplasty grafts the eardrum directly to a mobile stapes superstructure, and Type IV tympanoplasty involves grafting the tympanic membrane directly to a mobile stapes footplate and shielding the round window niche from external sound. Finally, Type V tympanoplasty involves removal of a fixed stapes footplate/superstructure and replacement with a fat or vein graft combined with obstruction of the round window niche.[3]

Multiple variables affecting the operative and reported outcomes following ossiculoplasty such as surgeon experience, patient population, consistent reporting criteria, and professional conflict of interest, make comparing trials of prostheses exceptionally difficult. Unfortunately, a significant determinant of the prostheses selected by various surgeons remains individual experience and training.

IMPLANT CHARACTERISTICS

Many materials have been used for ossicular chain reconstruction. The ideal prosthesis for ossicular reconstruction should be: biocompatible, capable of maintaining its shape, rigidity, and acoustic properties, cost-effective, and simple to deploy.

AUTOGRAFTS

Autograft material, such as cartilage and bone, was one of the first materials used for ossiculoplasty.[6] Over several decades of clinical investigation into the utility of autograft prosthesis, cartilage has been shown to be an inferior substrate. Cartilage has been shown to lose rigidity and mass density through neovascularization and periods of chondritis during long term implantation in the middle ear.[7,8] Schuknecht and Shi[9] investigated the stability of osseous middle ear implants and found no evidence of bone erosion and little resorption.

Autologous incus grafts have been used for many years for middle ear reconstruction by modifying them to fit between the manubrium of the malleus and the stapes capitulum (Figure 8–1). Autograft

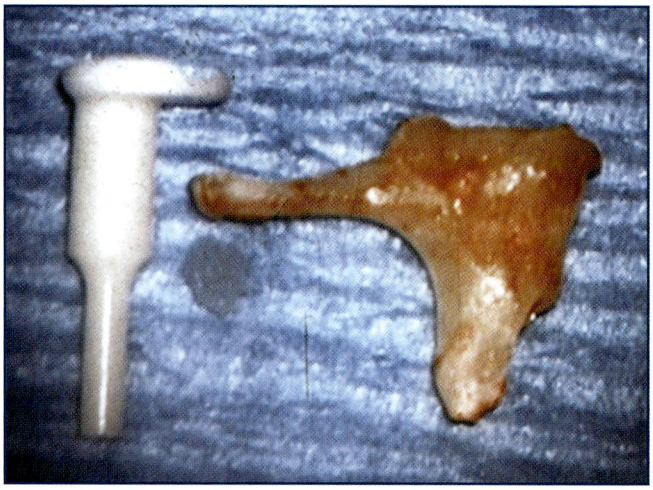

Figure 8–1. *Left:* Bojrab Universal HAPEX prosthesis (Gyrus ENT, Bartlett, TN) and *Right*: autologous incus graft.

incus has been shown to maintain contour, shape, size, and physical integrity for at least 11 years.[7] In a series of 2,200 cases, allograft and homograft prostheses yielded better hearing results than even the most biocompatible allograft prostheses.[10]

With numerous advantages, autograft bone also has several disadvantages when compared to "off-the-shelf" artificial prosthetics. Autografts are associated with prolonged operative time in obtaining and reshaping the bone, lack of availability in chronically diseased or previously operated ears, and possible resorption. Furthermore, the delicate sculpting of the autograft into a serviceable prosthesis adds an order of complexity to a highly complex surgery.

Past critics of autograft bone had proposed progressive osteitis and bone remodeling within the autografted ossicles and an increased risk of residual cholesteatoma. One recent study demonstrated a 5% incidence of residual cholesteatoma in incus and malleus specimens harvested from ears undergoing surgery for cholesteatoma. Interestingly, the incidence approached zero percent when ossicles deemed unserviceable for reconstruction were excluded.[11] These data combined with the above large case series make a strong argument for autograft prosthesis as a primary surgical option in appropriately selected patients.

HOMOGRAFTS

To overcome some of the disadvantages of autografts, irradiated homograft ossicles and cartilage were introduced in the 1960s. Homograft ossicles or cartilage are either presculpted by the processor or sculpted during surgery. Their use was common among early ossicular chain reconstructive surgeons with hearing results and biocompatibility being equivalent to autograft. The environment surrounding homograft material has changed since 1986 with wider awareness of risk toward communicable diseases (human immunodeficiency virus, Creutzfeldt-Jakob disease).[12] Furthermore, ethical and moral issues may be encountered in acquiring autograft material of any kind when the intent and consent of family and donor are uncertain and a profit incentive exists to the supplier. With the improved biocompatibility and utility of artificial materials use of homograft prosthesis has decreased dramatically in recent years.

ALLOPLASTS

Alloplastic or synthetic materials provide consistency in design and availability making them simpler to utilize with more consistent outcomes. Recently, alloplasts have become the most commonly used materials for ossicular reconstruction. Materials include: polyethylene tubing, Teflon, Silastic tubing, stainless steel, titanium, gold, high-density polyethylene sponge (HDPS), bioglasses, and bioceramics.

The earliest biocompatible materials, such as polyethylene, Teflon, and Proplast, demonstrated high rates of migration, extrusion, and reactivity causing fibrosis. Plastipore, a high-density polyethylene sponge (HDPS), was developed to closely mimic human bone in density, but its composition and interaction with the immune system were dramatically different.[13] Although a promising advancement in technology, the long-term stability of these prostheses was limited by a lack of biocompatibility. Extrusion frequently occurred if HDPS prostheses were brought into contact with the tympanic membrane or subjected to otitis media.[14] Rates of extrusion are reduced considerably when cartilage is placed between any prosthesis with limited biocompatibility and the tympanic membrane; however, even in experienced hands extrusion rates have averaged 3 to 5% in series with 5 to 10 years of follow-up.[15]

In designing more biocompatible middle ear implants, the bioceramics were introduced. Composed of calcium phosphate, this series of prosthesis closely resemble the mineral matrix of human bone allowing them to incorporate with human tissue and negating an unfavorable immune response.

Hydroxyapatite (HA) is a type of bioceramic commonly used in middle ear reconstructions. HA has many of the ideal characteristics required to be a good prosthesis. It is biocompatible, exhibits a low extrusion rate, and provides good sound transmission. Microscopic analysis of explanted HA prostheses demonstrates complete epithelialization with all cell types characteristic of the middle ear, thus producing an ideal outcome.[16] HA also forms a chemical bond with living bone that is osteoconductive with little biodegradation, allowing improved stability.[17] Placing HA prostheses directly against the tympanic membrane or fascial graft does not necessitate a cartilage cap (Figure 8–2). One pitfall is placement of an HA prosthesis near the scutum which may result in unfavorable osseointegration with subsequent conductive hearing loss. Hearing results have been consistent and extrusion rates for HA have been low (3%).[18,19]

HA is a brittle material which may fracture during intraoperative modification with otologic drills or sharp instrumentation. Technically, at the time or surgery, shaping of the HA prosthesis may be performed with a diamond drill bit. Experience is necessary in this technique to limit the possibility of fracturing.

HAPEX, a combination of HA and polyethylene, provides similar mechanical properties to HA while maintaining the excellent biocompatibility of the HA line. Microscopic analysis of HAPEX implants at revision surgery has revealed overgrown fibrous tissue without evidence of macrophages or foreign body giant cells associated with foreign body reaction. The addition of the polyethylene component allows HAPEX to be more readily modified intraoperatively with less fracture tendency. The primary limitation of HAPEX at the present time is the cost of the biomaterial itself.

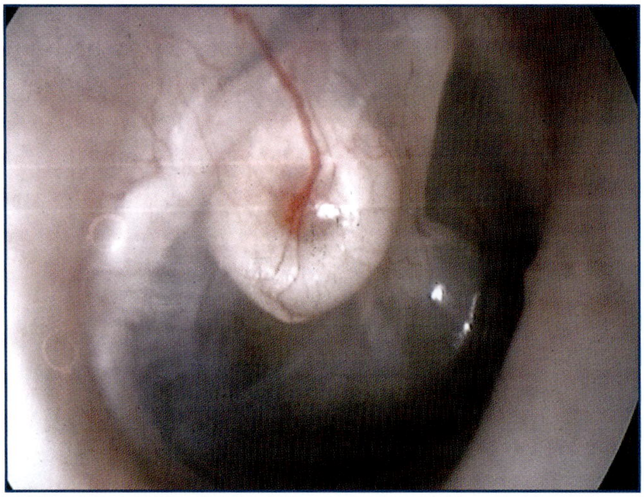

Figure 8–2. Transaural endoscopic digital photo of a biocompatible prosthesis in contact with the tympanic membrane years after implantation. Note the neovascularization of the tympanic membrane lateral to the prosthesis.

Titanium has become increasingly popular for use in middle ear implants. The physical properties of titanium make it possible to manufacture an extremely fine and light prosthesis with substantial rigidity in the shaft. Titanium forms a biostable titanium oxide layer within the middle ear.[20] Studies in rabbits have shown that within 28 days after implantation, a thin layer of epithelium forms over the inserted implant.[21]

Differential machining of titanium surfaces triggers unique tissue reactions. Rough milling a titanium implant increases available contact points and increases the strength of integration between the implant and surrounding tissues. Rough-milled surfaces are most appropriate in areas that contact cartilage grafts, stapes capitulum, or footplate. Conversely, the smoother the surface the less connective tissue reaction occurs and the epithelial covering is minimized.[22]

Pure titanium prosthesis have benefited from utilizing a cartilage cap to reduce extrusion. Controversy exists over the significance of titanium's favorable physical properties relative to the HA line. Titanium's acoustic impedance is higher than HA allowing a more efficient transfer of sound energy in addition to titanium having a lighter weight and greater versatility in prosthesis design. Some prostheses have begun to incorporate a combination of both HA and titanium components to find an ideal middle ground.

Nickel titanium (Nitinol) is a combination metal alloy of nickel and titanium in equal percentages that results in unique properties that may be useful in ossicular chain reconstruction: shape memory and superelasticity. Shape memory allows the metal to be deformed and then revert back to it original shape after heating to designated temperature. Superelasticity is a property that is not dependent on temperature and allows the material to exhibit enormous elasticity when being deformed but maintaining its original form. This material is becoming popular for stapes pistons/prosthesis and ossicular chain prostheses. Consideration must be made for reactivity to the nickel portion of the prosthesis in susceptible patients. Questions should be asked regarding nickel allergies to all patients where a prosthesis may be used.

SUCCESS IN OSSICULOPLASTY

Nothing fails like success because we don't learn from it. We learn only from failure.

Kenneth Boulding

To achieve success in ossiculoplasty, one must relentlessly analyze the failures. Poor outcomes in ossiculoplasty result from movement at the lateral attachment of the prosthesis, movement at the medial attachment, extrusion of the prosthesis, or from poor Eustachian tube function. In an attempt to minimize these complications, many implant designs have been developed with myriad materials, shapes, sizes, and weights. With some variation the success rates remain comparable.

Two broad categories of ossicular prostheses exist: Total Ossicular Replacement Prostheses (TORPs) and Partial Ossicular Replacement Prostheses (PORPs). TORP and PORP are trademarked names of early ossicular replacement prostheses from Smith Nephew Richards, Memphis, TN. Their design and approach to hearing restoration earned them the distinction of becoming part of the vernacular within the otologic community. The name TORP implies the prosthesis is being placed directly to the footplate of the stapes without involving the stapes superstructure. PORP denotes a prosthesis placed onto the capitulum of the stapes utilizing the superstructure to affect vibrational motion of the inner ear fluids.

TORPs are utilized in Type I tympanoplasties where there is absence or abnormality of the stapes superstructure. The TORP is placed between the malleus and footplate or directly to the tympanic membrane and footplate. PORPs are utilized in Type I tympanoplasties where a stapes superstructure is present. The PORP is placed between the stapes superstructure and malleus or tympanic membrane. Due to the presence or absence of a malleus for ossicular reconstruction being a significant predictor of hearing restoration other classification systems have been proposed which better describe the prereconstructive status of the middle ear and positioning of the prosthesis. Of note, tympanoplasty types II, III, IV, and V imply ossicular reconstruction was not attempted, but rather the tympanic membrane is allowed to adhere to the remnant of the ossicular conducting system.

Multiple variables present intraoperatively which complicate the optimal positioning of an ossicular reconstructive prosthesis including: the stapes to malleus offset (angle and distance), presence of a usable malleus, volume of the middle ear space, and angle of the stapes superstructure. Prosthesis have been modified and refined to address some of these variables. For securing the prosthesis to the malleus some prostheses have been designed with hooks or cradles. Other prostheses more commonly used in connecting directly to the tympanic membrane have included rough milled titanium surfaces and barbs to secure the prosthesis to a cartilage cap. On the medial side of the prosthesis several advancements have occurred to secure the prosthesis from slipping. Some surgeons utilize cartilage blocks, fascia, or a footplate shoe to stabilize the prosthesis from movement laterally, and for placing the prosthesis on to the stapes superstructure various receiving ends have been designed to grab the capitulum (Figures 8–3 and 8–4).

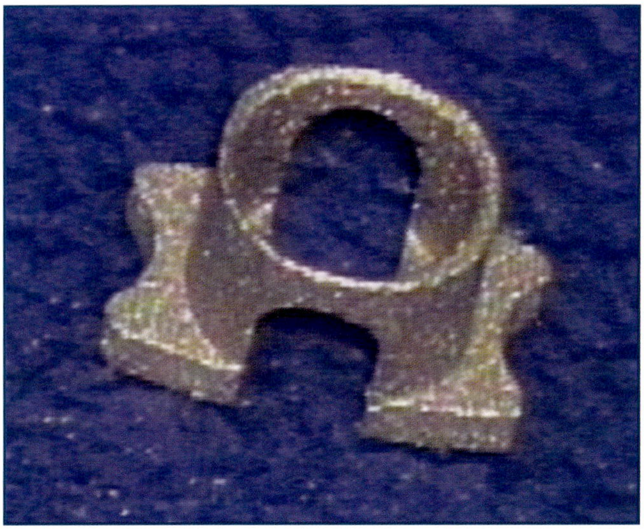

Figure 8–3. Bojrab footplate shoe (Grace Medical, Memphis, TN).

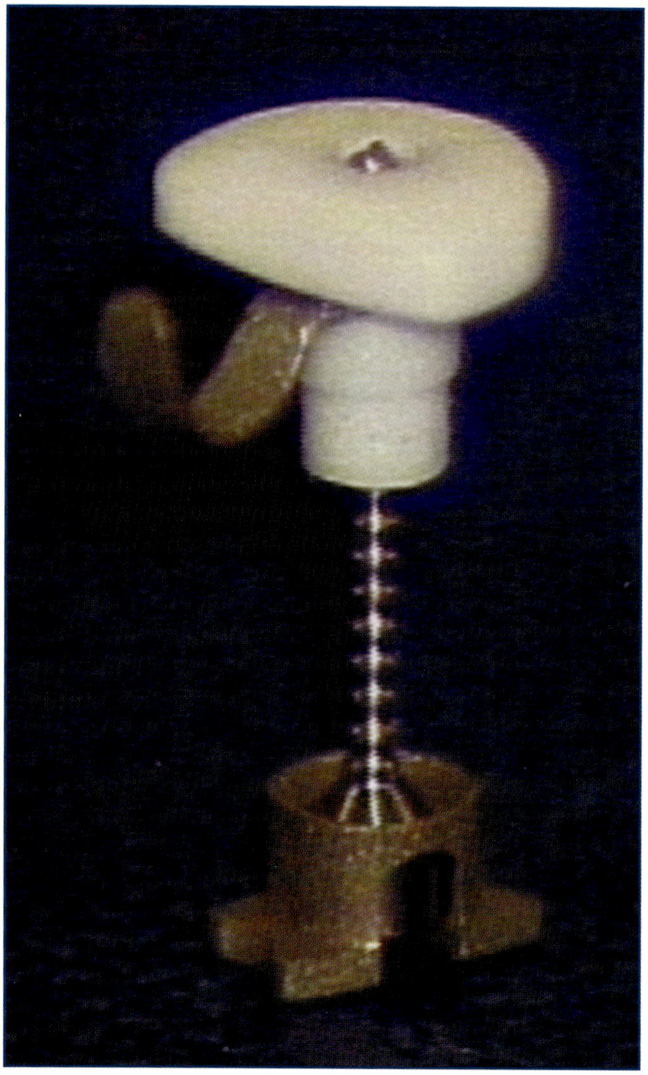

Figure 8–4. Bojrab Grace Alto Total Ossicular Replacement Prosthesis with titanium clip for grasping the malleus (Grace Medical, Memphis, TN) balanced in a Bojrab footplate shoe (Grace Medical, Memphis, TN) providing medial stabilization.

Improvements in bioavailability, reducing the load on the footplate, reduced operative complexity, and a greater understanding of how and when to deploy specific implants have advanced ossiculoplasty to a new era of elevated expectations. Newer prosthesis designs and materials may blend the knowledge of middle ear mechanics and biomedical engineering to create the "ideal" prosthesis.

PROSTHESES COMMONLY USED AT MICHIGAN EAR INSTITUTE

Grace Alto Bojrab Titanium + HA (Grace Medical, Memphis TN)

This prosthesis is a lightweight adjustable length titanium implant available in both a total and partial configuration with a HA head and titanium extension to fit under the malleus, if present (Figure 8–5). The shaft is shortened utilizing a simple tool provided in the peel pack (Figure 8–6). The ability to quickly customize the length of the prosthesis intraoperatively reduces the likelihood of overloading the annular ligament and limiting the motion of the stapes superstructure. If the malleus to stapes anatomy is unfavorable the head of the prosthesis may be covered with a cartilage cap to increase stability with the tympanic membrane and further reduce extrusion. When utilizing the total version of the Grace Alto the authors have found benefit to stabilizing the medial aspect of the prosthesis at the footplate with a titanium footplate shoe, as shown in Figure 8–4.

Gyrus Bojrab HAPEX Universal (Gyrus ENT, Bartlett, TN)

The Universal prosthesis has the benefit of composite design, with easy intraoperative modification to be utilized as a partial or total ossicular replacement prosthesis. The Universal prosthesis was designed with a hydroxyapatite head to minimize extrusion when directly in contact with the tympanic membrane. The HA head contains a groove designed to fit under the malleus providing stability to the lateral aspect of the prosthesis. The HAPEX (hydroxyapatite-polyethylene composite) shaft can be easily modified. HAPEX, unlike conventional HA, can be cut with a knife without fracturing. The distal shaft is narrow allowing it to function as a total prosthesis by oscillating the footplate. To utilize an intact stapes superstructure the distal shaft is trimmed revealing a wider hollow shaft for use as a partial prosthesis, fitting over the capitulum of the stapes. In patients

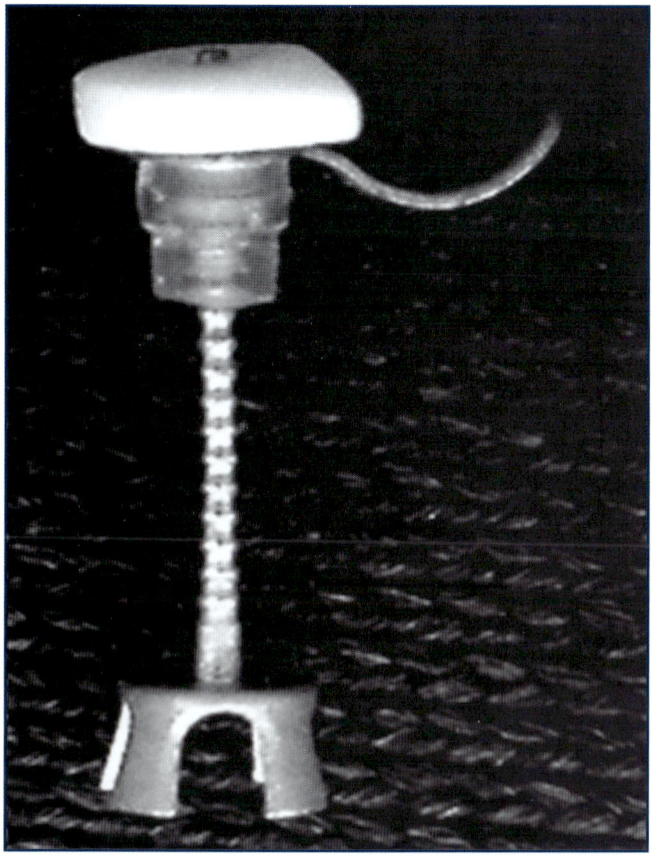

A

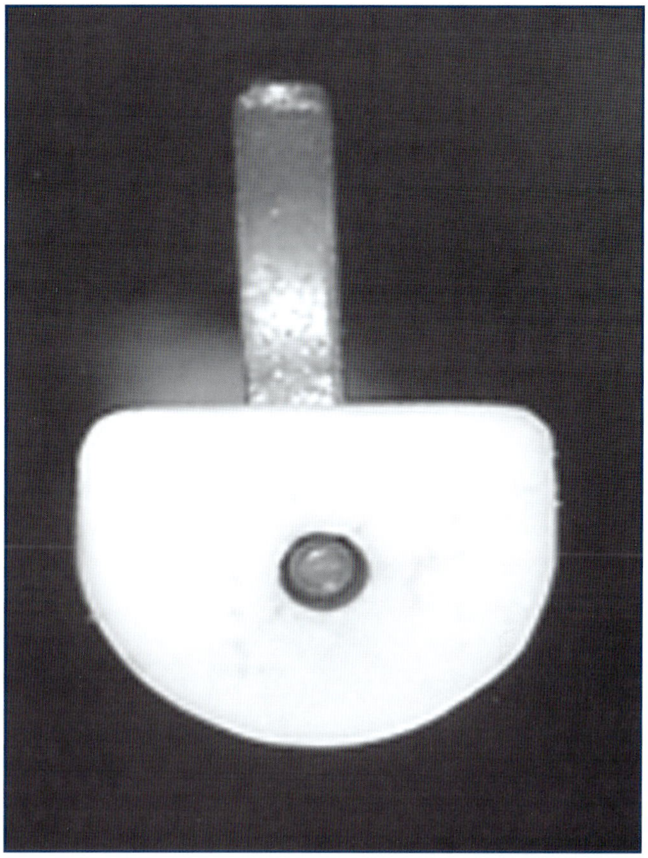

B

Figure 8–5. A. Bojrab Grace Alto Partial Ossicular Replacement Prosthesis (Grace Medical, Memphis, TN) with medial stabilization cage for securing onto the stapes capitulum. **B.** Bojrab Grace Alto Partial Ossicular Replacement Prosthesis (Grace Medical, Memphis, TN) demonstrating the hydroxyapatite head and titanium clip.

with an intact stapes superstructure and favorable malleus orientation, the head and distal shaft are removed creating a hollow strut graft. From a hospital system standpoint the Universal prosthesis can be utilized in a wide variety of reconstructive situations drastically reducing the number of prosthesis needing to be stocked and reducing confusion and cost within the operative theater.

Kartush Incus Strut

Composed of hydroxyapatite the Kartush Incus Strut (Smith Nephew Richards, Memphis, TN) allows for direct connection of the malleus to stapes capitulum. The strut design eliminates the top-heavy cap of many earlier prostheses minimizing the weight of the prosthesis; furthermore, the rigidity and composition of the prosthesis closely mimics an incus interposition graft without the necessary intraoperative sculpting. A malleus to stapes offset angle of less than 60 degrees is required with the preferred offset less than 45 degrees. Extrusion rates are low as the prosthesis is hidden medial to the malleus and the hydroxyapatite composition of the strut allows for mucosalization. As previously discussed, hydroxyapatite when in contact with the tympanic membrane will have the lowest extrusion rate of biomaterials presently available due to its similarity to native ossicular bone (Figure 8–7).

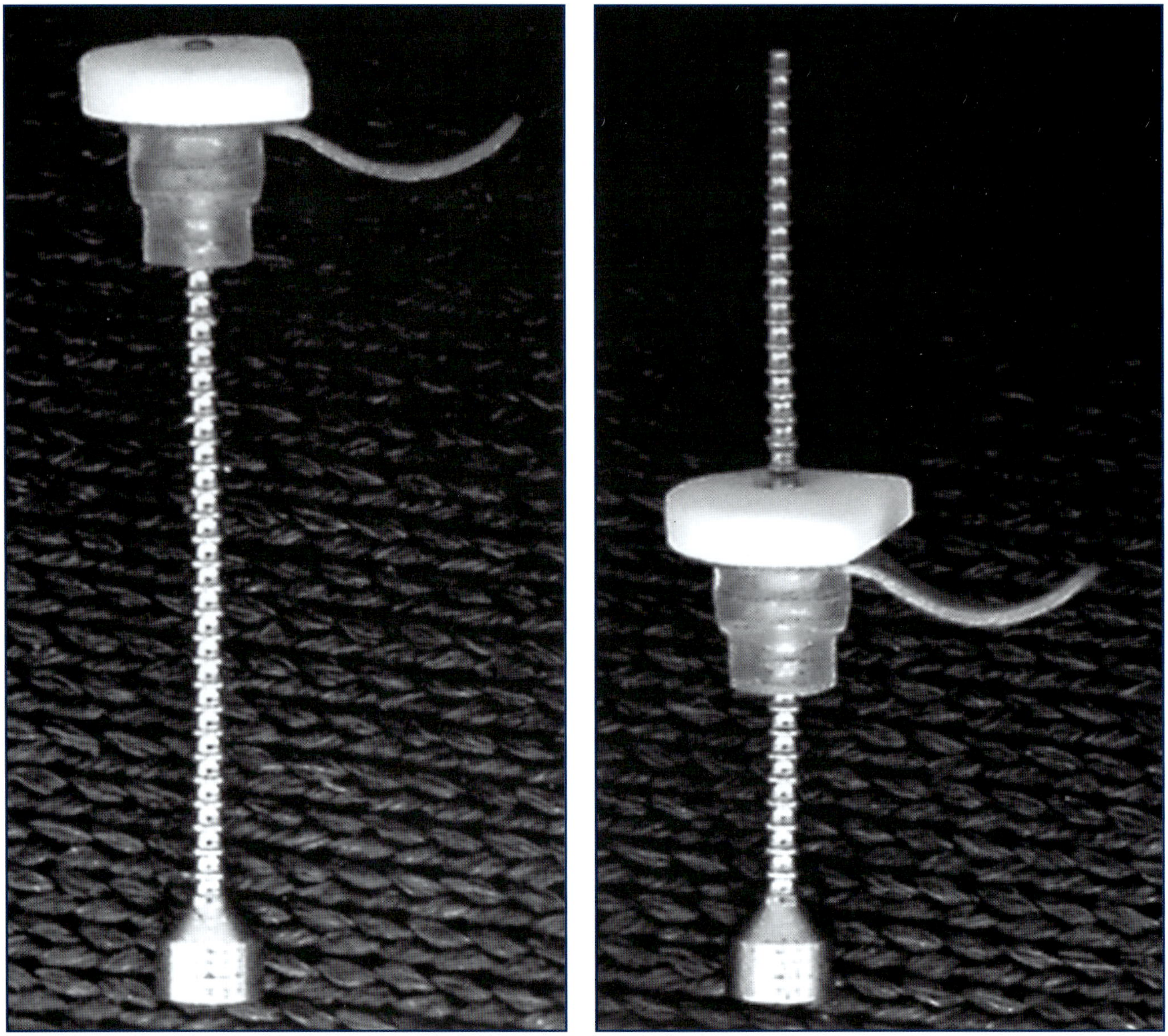

A

B

Figure 8–6. A. Fully extended Bojrab Grace Alto Total Ossicular Replacement Prosthesis (Grace Medical, Memphis, TN). **B.** Shortened Bojrab Grace Alto Total Ossicular Replacement Prosthesis (Grace Medical, Memphis, TN) for accommodating a contracted middle ear space.

OTHER PROSTHESES USED

There are several companies that manufacture prosthesis utilizing various materials and designs to accomplish successful reconstruction of the ossicular chain. Companies such as Olympus (which purchased Gyrus ENT), Grace Medical, Medtronic, and Kurz produce commonly used prostheses. Various head designs, materials, and coupling techniques are developed by each company and can be found on their appropriate websites. Kurz has developed

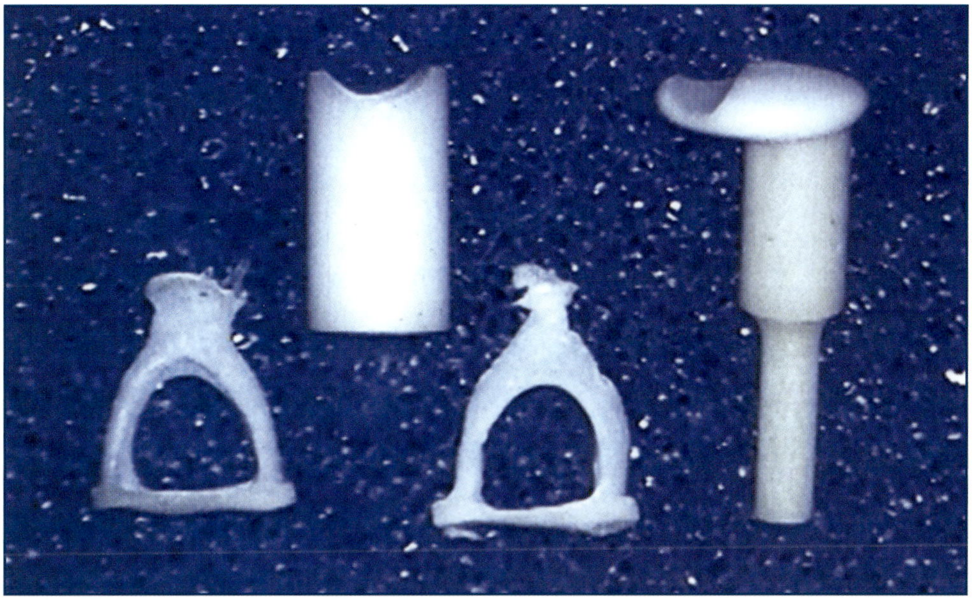

Figure 8–7. Size comparison image of two human stapes bones in relation to *left* Kartush Incus Strut (Smith Nephew Richards, Memphis, TN) and *right* Bojrab Universal Prosthesis—Total configuration (Gyrus ENT, Bartlett, TN).

some unique titanium prosthesis for partial, total, and stapes reconstruction that are commonly used in Europe. In choosing appropriate types of prosthesis to stock, the surgeon must rely on past experience with successful outcomes in training or practice, as well as the experience and innovative ideas/design of each company.

COMPLICATIONS

Immediate, intraoperative complications can occur from using an oversized prosthesis or being too aggressive in manipulating the ossicular chain. These maneuvers can result in fracture of the stapes superstructure, dislocation of the stapes or stapes footplate, tear of the annular ligament with a perilymphatic fistula, and possibly severe or total sensorineural hearing loss. Controlled microsurgical techniques and extensive practice in temporal bone laboratories and under the supervision of experienced surgeons will limit the occurrence of the above. In the event of an annular ligament tear or crack in the footplate, a tissue seal of fat or fascia is recommended combined with discontinuing the operative procedure and returning at a later date.

Immediate postoperative complications include vertigo and sensorineural hearing loss. Vertigo can be related to an unrecognized perilymphatic fistula or oversized prosthesis. If a complete vestibular evaluation fails to elucidate other causes middle ear exploration and revision ossicular chain reconstruction may be necessary. Sensorineural hearing loss is an uncommon complication potentially related to perilymphatic fistula, serous labyrinthitis, excessive manipulation of the ossicular chain, or idiopathic causes. Treatment with corticosteroids either oral or transtympanic is recommended and consideration should be given to middle ear exploration if the response is suboptimal.

Delayed postoperative complications include erosion or extrusion of the prosthesis and recurrent conductive hearing loss. The cause of either may be recurrent middle ear cholesteatoma, poor healing, graft failure, dislocation of the prosthesis, ossicular fixation or erosion, or severe retraction of the tympanic membrane. In the presence of this complication the patient's candidacy for ossicular reconstruction should be re-evaluated. Patients with severe eustachian tube dysfunction, extensive cholesteatoma, or persistent chronic otitis media may benefit from a Type III, IV, or V tympanoplasty without the introduction of foreign material into the middle ear space.

CONCLUSION

Ossicular chain problems are frequently encountered in otologic surgery and are amenable to reconstruction. Because various materials are used for ossiculoplasty, it is important to determine which type of prosthesis is appropriate. This decision is based on the status of the diseased ear and the surgeon's preference. Considerations must be made for the presence of absence of the malleus, the anatomic relationship of malleus to stapes, the severity of eustachian tube dysfunction, and tympanic membrane status. As newer materials are developed for use in the middle ear and implant design continues to be modified, the hearing results for patients will continue to improve.

REFERENCES

1. Wullstein H. The restoration of the function of the middle ear in chronic otitis media. *Ann Otol Rhinol Laryngol.* 1971;80:210–217.
2. Zollner F. The principles of plastic surgery of the sound conducting apparatus. *J Laryngol Otol.* 1955;69:637–652.
3. Merchant SN, Ravicz ME, Puria S, et al. Analysis of middle ear mechanics and application to diseased and reconstructed ears. *Am J Otol.* 1997;18:139–154.
4. Gan RZ, Dyer RK, Wood MW, Dormer KJ. Mass loading on the ossicles and middle ear function. *Ann Otol Rhinol Laryngol.* 2001;110:478–485.
5. Becvarovski Z, Kartush JM. Smoking and tympanoplasty: implications for prognosis and the Middle Ear Risk Index (MERI). *Laryngoscope.* 2001;111:1806–1811.
6. Hall A, Rytzner CI. Stapedectomy and autotransplantation of ossicles. *Acta Otolaryngol.* 1957;47:318–324.
7. Smyth G. Long term results of middle ear reconstructive surgery. *J Laryngol Otol.* 1971;85:1227–1230.
8. Merchant SN, Nadol JB Jr. Histopathology of ossicular implant. *Otolaryngol Clin North Am.* 1994;27:813–833.
9. Schuknect HF, Shi SR. Surgical pathology of middle ear implants. *Laryngoscope.* 1985;95:249–258.
10. Portmann M. Results of middle ear reconstruction surgery. *Ann Acad Med Singapore.* 1991;20:610–613.
11. Ng SK, Yip WWL, Suen M, et al. Autograft ossiculoplasty in cholesteatoma surgery: is it feasible? *Laryngoscopy.* 2003;113:843–847.
12. Glasscock ME III, Jackson CG, Knox GW. Can Acquired immunodeficiency syndrome and Creutzfeldt-Jakob disease be transmitted via otologic homografts? *Arc Otolaryngol Head Neck Surg.* 1988;114:1252–1255.
13. Bayazit Y, Goksu N, Beder L. Functional results of Plastipore prostheses for middle ear ossicular chain reconstruction. *Laryngoscope.* 1999;109:709–711.
14. Shinohara T, Gyo K, Saiki T, Yanagihara N. Ossiculoplasty using hydroxyapatite prosthesis: long-term results. *Clin Otolaryngol.* 2000;25:287–292.
15. Sheehy JL. TORPs and PORPs: causes of failure—a report on 446 operations. *Otolaryngol Head Neck Surg.* 1984;92:583–587.
16. Horman K, Donath K. Is hydroxyapatite ceramic an adequate biomaterial in ossicular reconstruction? *Am J Otol.* 1987;8:402–409
17. Grote JJ. Reconstruction of the middle ear with hydroxyapatite implants: long-term results. *Ann Otol Rhinol Laryngol.* 1990;99(suppl 144):12–16.
18. Goldberg RA. Hydroxyapatite ossicular replacement prostheses: results in 157 consecutive cases. *Laryngoscope.* 1992;102:1091–1096.
19. Meijer AG, Verheul J, Albers FW, Segenhout HM. Cartilage interposition in ossiculoplasty with hydroxyapatite prosthesis: a histopathologic study in the guinea pig. *Ann Otol Rhinol Laryngol.* 2002;111:364–369.
20. Dalchow CV, Grun D, Stupp HF. Reconstruction of the ossicular chainwith titanium implants. *Otolaryngol Head Neck Surg.* 2001;125:628–630.
21. Schwager K. Titanium as a biomaterial for ossicular replacement: results after implantation in the middle ear of the rabbit. *Eur Arch Otorhinolaryngol.* 1998;255:396–401.
22. Bojrab DI. Alternatives in biocompatible ossicular implants. *Insights Otolaryngol.* 1992;7:1–7.

CHAPTER 9

Otosclerosis and Stapes Surgery

Yoav Hahn and Jack Kartush

DEFINITION

Otosclerosis is a disease limited to the temporal bone that primarily affects the otic capsule. This process may cause a conductive hearing loss, a mixed conductive-sensorineural hearing loss, or more rarely a sensorineural hearing loss. Suggested etiologies of otosclerosis include hereditary, endocrine, biochemical, metabolic, infectious, traumatic, vascular, and autoimmune.

HISTORY

Ankylosis of the stapes was first described by Valsalva in 1704.[1] During dissection of the temporal bone of a cadaver, he noted the immobility of the stapes bone in the footplate. Toynbee first described hearing loss caused by fixation of the stapes.[2] In 1894, Politzer first published the histologic characteristics of otosclerosis and established it as a primary disorder of the otic capsule.[3] Bezold further described the clinical findings associated with otosclerosis in 1908, when he discussed the historical, audiometric, and physical findings.

Successful surgery for hearing restoration began with Lempert's fenestration operation described in 1938.[4] Rosen,[5] a student of Lempert, discovered that footplate mobilization improved hearing immediately in a patient with otosclerosis. He continued to improve on this technique until Shea, his student, opened the era of stapedectomy. Stapedectomy has been performed for otosclerosis since first introduced by Shea in 1956. In 1969, Schuknecht and Applebaum[6] introduced the technique of stapedotomy in which the stapes superstructure is resected but the footplate preserved. The adaptation of the laser to microsurgery has been a more recent innovation.[7–9]

PATHOLOGY

The embryologic formation of the temporal bone likely plays a role in the development of otosclerosis. The otic capsule arises from mesenchyme surrounding the otic vesicle at 4 weeks of development. In the 8th week of embryologic development, the cartilaginous framework is begun. In the 16th week, endochondral bone replacement occurs. However, in some individuals, complete bony replacement does not occur and some of the cartilage framework persists. The fissula ante fenestrum, located just anterior to the footplate, is the last area of the otic capsule to have endochondral bony replacement and is affected in 80 to 90% of patients with otosclerosis.[10] In addition, the other areas of predilection for otosclerotic lesions include the border of the round window niche, the apical medial wall of the cochlea, the area posterior to the cochlear aqueduct, the region adjacent to the semicircular canals, and the stapes footplate itself.

The sequential changes in the morphologic features of otosclerosis begin with resorption of endochondral bone that is probably caused by the action of lysosomal hydrolases and osteoclasts.[11] Osteoid is then laid down within the collagen matrix and produces islands of immature basophilic bone called blue mantles. New mature laminated bone leads to the highly mineralized mosaic patterns typical of the disease.

CLINICAL FINDINGS

Conductive hearing loss is the principal finding associated with otosclerosis. This hearing loss typically occurs in early or mid-adult life, but may present earlier. Conductive hearing loss in children is not covered in this chapter but may be treated similarly to adults, but with a more cautious plan due to the increased risk of hearing loss with surgical treatments and congenital deformities of the ossicular chain and inner ear. A positive family history is found among approximately 50% of patients.[12] Hearing impairment is usually progressive, often reaching a plateau in the patient's mid-forties. The degree of eventual sensorineural involvement is unpredictable. Otosclerosis is estimated to be unilateral in approximately 15% of cases.[13–15] Tinnitus may also be associated with otosclerosis and varies in intensity and character.

A progressive pattern is seen on audiometry in patients with otosclerosis. Initially, a low frequency conductive loss is seen secondary to the stiffening of the stapediovestibular joint.[16] The air-bone gap widens and affects more frequencies as the stapedial footplate becomes fixed. The disease advances more rapidly at times, depending on environmental factors such as pregnancy. Cochlear involvement may produce a high frequency sensorineural hearing loss and also a drop in speech discrimination score. In other audiometric testing, impedance plethysmography often is normal or can show reduced tympanic membrane compliance. Stapedial reflexes classically are abnormal; however, they may be within normal limits depending on the degree of stapes fixation and can make differentiation between causes of conductive hearing loss difficult in certain instances.

Carhart Notch

An apparent loss in bone conduction occurs around 2000 Hz on audiometry in patients with otosclerosis. This was first described by Carhart in 1950.[17] This is secondary to loss of the middle ear contribution to bone conduction. Upon vibration of the mastoid bone, the ossicular chain vibrates slightly out of phase, causing a relative movement of the stapes footplate to the cochlea. In otosclerosis, this does not occur. Carhart found that otosclerosis reduces bone conduction thresholds by 5 dB at 500 Hz, 10 dB at 1000 Hz, 25 dB at 2000 Hz, and 15 dB at 4000 Hz.

DIFFERENTIAL DIAGNOSIS

The diagnosis of otosclerosis is made based on clinical and audiometric findings. Progressive conductive hearing loss, normal otoscopic exam with an intact and mobile tympanic membrane, no evidence of eustachian tube dysfunction, a negative Rinne test result, and absent stapedial reflex are typically found with otosclerosis. Other processes should be considered in patients with conductive hearing loss. Ossicular discontinuity, middle ear effusion or disease, tympanosclerosis, Paget's disease, osteogenesis imperfecta, and degenerative arthritis may all cause conductive deafness. In addition, causes of ossicular fixation should be considered including lateral ossicular fixation and incus-annulus fusion. Another consideration is superior semicircular canal dehiscence. The stapedial reflex can help differentiate this condition from otosclerosis as the reflex should be intact with superior semicircular canal dehiscence, although variability may exist in early otosclerosis, where the reflux may still be intact. VEMP testing and CT scan of the temporal bone may be used to rule out superior semicircular canal dehiscence but not necessary in the typical case of conductive hearing loss.

MANAGEMENT OF OTOSCLEROSIS

Amplification

Patients with conductive hearing loss caused by otosclerosis may use hearing aids as an alternative to surgery. Surgery for otosclerosis is an elective procedure and patients should be counseled about other options, including no treatment and use of hearing aids. Patients are advised that a hearing aid, although a very low risk, will do nothing to stop the otosclerotic process. The disadvantage of using hearing aids for a long period is that it may reduce the success rate and increase the complication rate of surgery years later if the disease is very advanced. If the patient has a significant sensorineural component to their hearing loss, a hearing aid may still be required after successful stapes surgery. However, with successful surgery, the patient may require a less powerful, more effective hearing aid.

Medical Management:

The value of medical therapy for otosclerosis is controversial. Medical therapy may be considered for patients that cannot or choose not to undergo surgery or for patients with a predominant sensorineural hearing loss or vestibular symptoms thought to be secondary to otosclerosis.

Shambaugh first predicted stabilization of otosclerotic lesions with the use of sodium fluoride.[18] Fluoride ions replace the usual hydroxyl ion, forming a fluorapatite complex instead of hydroxyapatite crystal. The fluorapatite complex is more stable and theoretically resists osteoclastic action. The mechanism of otospongiotic disease leading to otosclerosis is the reversal of the enzymatic equilibrium. Cochlear otosclerosis occurs when the normal balance of enzymatic activity is disrupted in favor of tryptic activity, resulting in the sensorineural hearing loss. Sodium fluoride medical treatment can act directly on trypsin and other enzymes that are considered to be causative for cochlear otosclerosis.[19] It is thought to slow down or halt the progression of otosclerotic hearing loss by neutralizing and inactivating the hydrolytic and proteolytic enzymes of otospongiotic lesions.[20] Sodium fluoride promotes maturation of active otospongiosis by reducing its vascularity and its bone resorption activity and by increasing new bone formation to eventually produce inactive otosclerosis.

Several double-blind, placebo-controlled studies have been reported on small groups of patients that have verified the positive value of sodium fluoride in reducing progression of sensorineural hearing deterioration in stapedectomized patients.[21] A prospective clinical, double-blind, placebo-controlled study to evaluate the effect of sodium fluoride treatment on otospongiosis was performed in 142 patients with otospongiosis and no history of surgical treatment.[22] Treatment consisted of 20 mg of sodium fluoride as enteric-coated tablets twice a day, containing 500 mg of calcium gluconate, and 400 units of vitamin D and placebo consisted of similar tablets without sodium fluoride but containing the same dose of calcium gluconate and vitamin D. In this study, the authors showed a statistically significant worse deterioration of the hearing loss in the placebo group than in the active treated (40 mg sodium fluoride daily) group, supporting the view that sodium fluoride can change otospongiotic, active lesions to more dense, inactive otosclerotic lesions.

In patients that have cochlear symptoms in an ear that would also benefit from stapedectomy, fluoride therapy may be considered for several months to reduce the otospongiotic foci and harmful enzymatic activity. This may potentially decrease the likelihood of intraoperative sensorineural hearing loss. Patients with early otosclerosis may be considered for fluoride therapy for 6 months followed by repeat hearing test to assess if progression of hearing loss can be slowed or halted.

Side effects of fluoride (Florical and Monocal are the two preparations available over the counter) include occasional stomach upset, allergic itching, and increased joint pains. Fluorosis, the most severe side effect in the treatment of osteoporosis, has not been noted with the lower doses of fluoride therapy. If an increase in arthritis symptoms occurs, the fluoride is stopped and the joints return to their previous state in a few weeks. Women of childbearing age should be informed that fluoride medication can be teratogenic in the first 6 weeks of fetal development. In addition, patients with gallstones, kidney stones, or GI disturbance are at higher risk if started on fluoride therapy.

Monocal is a preparation that is absorbed in the intestine rather than in the stomach and may cause fewer side effects. Although some authors recommend doses of 2 tablets three times a day (Florical) and 1 to 2 tablets three times a day (Monocal), we typically advise lower doses such as 1 to 2 tablets per day to minimize side effects, knowing that the benefits may not be as great. With this low dose, we have had no patients in the last 25 years with fluorosis, teratogenic effects, or serious adverse events.

Surgical Management

Stapedectomy is typically considered for patients with an air-bone gap of at least 15 dB and reversal of Rinne testing with a 512-Hz tuning fork, speech discrimination scores of 60% or better, and no contraindication to surgery. The worst hearing ear should be addressed first. Stapedectomy was described by Shea with a polyethylene strut prosthesis over a vein graft to seal the oval window defect.[23] Early procedures entailed removal of the entire stapedial footplate with placement of grafted tissue over the oval window followed by the piston. With the advent of the microdrill and laser technology, stapedotomy has more commonly become the procedure of choice, wherein the stapes superstructure is removed and an opening created in the otosclerotic footplate. Results of several studies have implied lower risk for immediate and late cochlear loss with stapedotomy and better hearing results compared with traditional techniques.[24–26]

Stapedectomy Prostheses

Many different prostheses have been developed for stapedectomy over the past 30 years. Some of the designs that have proved most effective and are still in use today include the McGee piston, Robinson bucket handle prostheses, and the Smart piston. Many different materials have been used. The metallic properties of middle ear prostheses need to be considered with the advancements in MRI technology and potential for complication if the prosthesis moves or generates heat in the magnetic field.

Metallic Properties of Pistons

Stainless steel has been widely used in the design of middle ear prostheses for decades but there are a variety of types some of which have greater or lesser ferromagnetic qualities than others. A recent study showed that some "nonmagnetic" stainless steel prostheses may move in the presence of high magnetic fields.[27] In this study, the authors demonstrated that the "nonmagnetic" stainless steel pistons were deflected when subjected to 4.7 tesla magnetic field interactions. Platinum based prostheses were also studied and they showed no motion when subjected to the same magnetic field. As MRI magnetic fields become increasingly stronger, prostheses with even minimal ferromagnetic properties are at risk for movement and may cause hearing loss, tinnitus, or dizziness.

An additional study evaluating different types of middle ear implants in an MRI scanner showed displacement of only a single lot of McGee platinum-stainless steel pistons.[28] The authors concluded that MRI could pose a hazard to patients who have had stapedectomy using certain platinum-stainless steel piston prostheses. Subsequent to this, the manufacturer (Gyrus ENT) recommended that patients implanted with specific production lots of these pistons not undergo MRI secondary to the risk of prosthesis motion. In a later study, titanium middle ear prostheses were examined for magnetic field interactions at 3.0 tesla.[29] No deflection or heating of these titanium prostheses was noted.

Fortunately, recent studies have shown that most stapes prostheses, even stainless steel types, appear to have a very low risk of movement under magnetic fields. Nonetheless, unless totally non-ferromagnetic materials are used, there will remain some risk to these patients if they undergo MRI scanning.

Many poststapedectomy patients have been able to forego MRI imaging with CT scanning instead. However, when that alternative is not acceptable, and when the implanted prosthesis is of stainless steel composition or when the prosthesis type is unknown, patients may need to consider having their old prostheses replaced with newer nonferromagnetic material.

Stapes Prostheses

The initial prosthesis used was the Shea Teflon prosthesis, a shaved piece of polyethylene tubing (Figure 9–1). This prosthesis, like some of the newer prostheses, was popular because crimping was not necessary. The eye of the piston is expanded to a C-shape of sufficient size, placed over the incus, and the loop closes itself around the incus. While

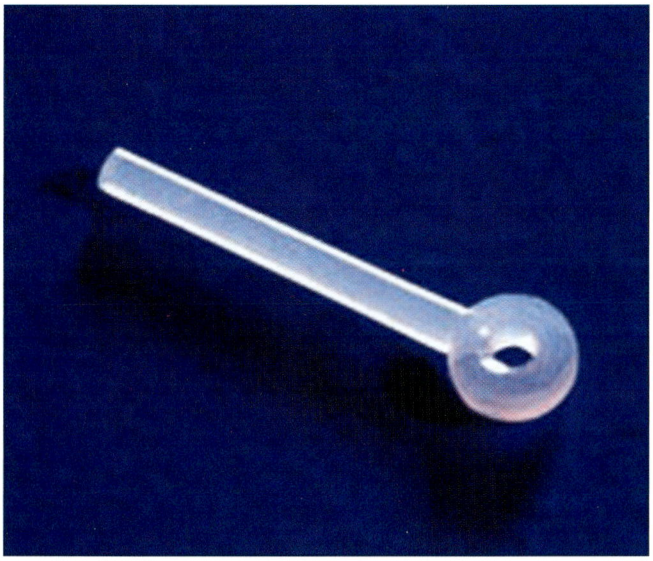

Figure 9–1. Shea Stapes piston: The eye of the prosthesis is spread open and the loop is placed over the incus. The loop self crimps around the incus.

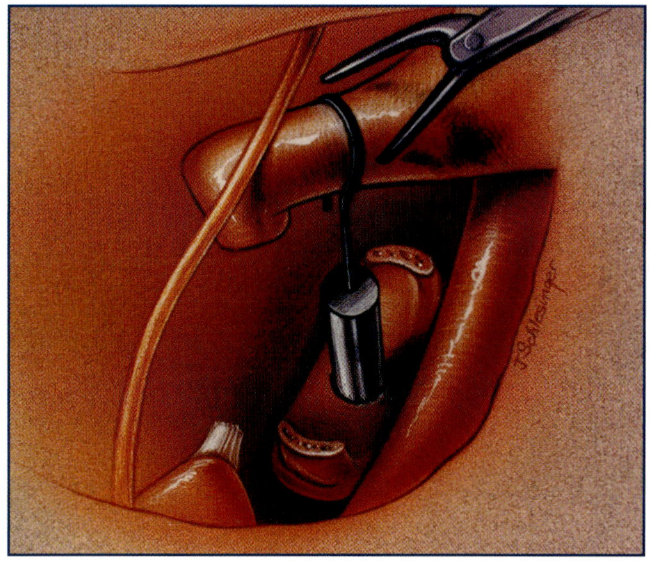

Figure 9–2. The McGee piston: A classic example of piston design. (Copyright Jack M. Kartush, MD, 1987)

it was effective in many patients, in some it led to inner ear complications and consequently many different materials and designs have been tried. The Schuknecht fat wire stapedectomy prosthesis was used quite commonly years ago. Due to loosening of the wire, erosion of the lenticular process of the incus, and perilymph fistulas due to atrophy of the fat graft, this design is rarely used today. Each prosthesis has its unique pros and cons: none are perfect and new designs will no doubt continue to evolve. A few of the commonly used prostheses are discussed.

McGee Piston. The McGee piston (Gyrus, Bartlett, TN) is a classic example of piston design, and many pistons have subsequently followed this design utilizing a ribbon that crimps around the lenticular process of the incus (Figure 9–2). The original prosthesis was made entirely of stainless steel but was later enhanced to use a platinum ribbon to improve crimping and reduce lenticular necrosis. Many studies have shown excellent results utilizing these pistons. Although there has been great success, use of this piston does require crimping of the ribbon onto the lenticular process, which some surgeons find difficult and anxiety provoking. The thin loop is difficult to grasp and crimp on the incus while the thin shaft crumples easily during insertion. Because the wire is very thin on these pistons, they may have sub-optimal conformity to the lenticular process occasionally leading to overcrimping, and a higher incidence of incus necrosis. Furthermore, as noted above, a certain lot of McGee pistons were mistakenly manufactured with a ferromagnetic alloy in the 1980s, making them incompatible with MRI. These factors led us to modify the classic McGee design.

Big Easy Piston. To deal with these potential difficulties and complications, the Big Easy piston (Medtronic, Jacksonville, FL) was developed (Figure 9–3). The Big Easy piston is made entirely of non-ferromagnetic titanium and platinum, ensuring MRI compatibility. This piston addresses some of the problems associated with prior iterations. The soft platinum piston loop is three times wider, affording easier and more precise crimping (Figure 9–4). When placing the loop over the incus, there is improved conformity to the contour of the lenticular process with less movement and rocking prior to crimping. The stronger shaft is twice the width of previous pistons, reducing inadvertent bending upon insertion.

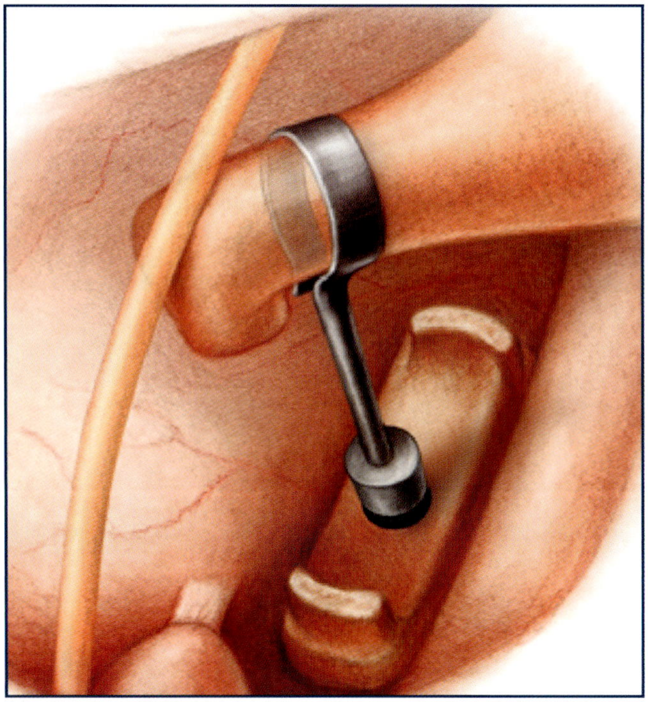

Figure 9–3. The Big Easy piston: This piston is 3 times as wide and has twice the strength of a conventional piston. (Copyright Jack M. Kartush, MD, 1987)

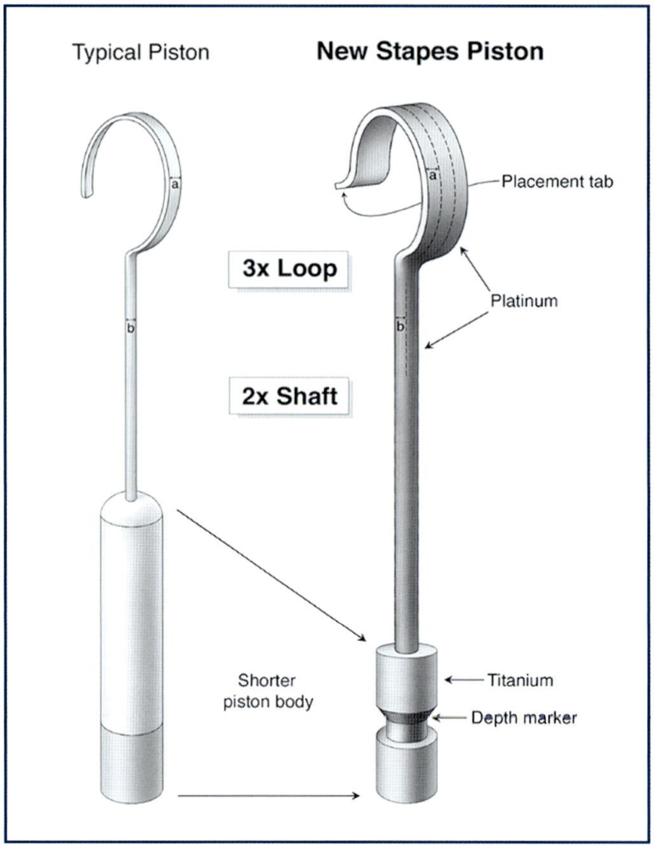

Figure 9–4. A comparison of the conventional McGee piston and the Big Easy piston. The Big Easy wire loop is three times wider and the shaft is twice the width of previous pistons.

The short piston body and longer platinum shaft improves visualization during placement. In addition, there is a depth marker at 0.5 mm that identifies optimal depth within the fenestra.

Robinson Bucket Handle Prosthesis. The Robinson bucket handle prosthesis (Gyrus, Bartlett, TN), a stainless steel prosthesis, has been very popular through the years because it avoids the need to crimp (Figure 9–5). Due to concerns of MRI compatibility, new titanium versions have become available. This prosthesis has a "bucket handle" to place over the incus but its use does not appear to be a necessity for stabilization if there is an adequate soft tissue graft beneath it, typically vein. In experienced hands, it is extremely safe and effective. However, some inexperienced or occasional surgeons gravitate toward prostheses such as this to avoid crimping. Although crimping is avoided, it is replaced by another delicate microsurgical maneuver: it requires the surgeon to lift up the incus with one hand while the other hand pushes the piston under the incus onto the vein graft.

Too great an elevation of the incus may cause subluxation. Too little incus elevation may cause intrusion of the prosthesis into the vestibule.

The greatest numbers of poststapedectomy profound sensorineural hearing loss cases that have been referred to our Institute have come from occasional surgeons using the Robinson prostheses wherein the prosthesis has been implanted too deep within the vestibule. Grafted tissue must be placed over the oval window to prevent intrusion of the prosthesis into the vestibule. This requisite tissue, however, obscures the new fenestra, which may then lead to malpositioning the piston along the edge of the fenestra. This is in contrast to pistons that are first placed into the fenestra and the fascia placed

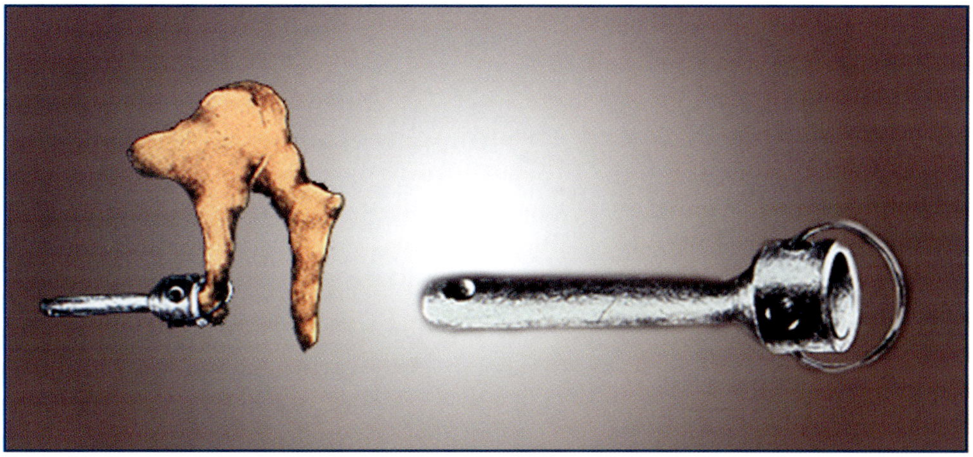

Figure 9–5. The Robinson Bucket Handle prosthesis. ®Registered mark of Mendell Robinson, MD.

subsequently. Surgeons that feel they do not have the experience or technical ability to crimp a ribbon over the incus should also consider their abilities relative to safely placing a bucket handle prosthesis.

Smart Piston. The Smart piston (Gyrus, Bartlett, TN), a Nitinol/Fluoroplastic prosthesis, has recently become popular because of its Nitinol technology that also avoids crimping[30] (Figure 9–6). The self-crimping mechanism works with application of heat to the ribbon using bipolar cautery or laser. Unlike the bucket handle prosthesis, there is no need to neither elevate the incus nor place a vein graft first. However, one needs to be cautious with the application of thermal energy to avoid injury to the chorda tympani or acceleration of ischemic necrosis of the distal incus due to devascularization of its tenuous blood supply.

The material is called Nitinol because of the nickel and titanium components. Reaction to nickel is the most common metal allergy in humans.[31] Many otologists are unaware of the nickel content of these pistons and should check with the manufacturer regarding implantation in nickel sensitive patients or consider preoperative skin testing.

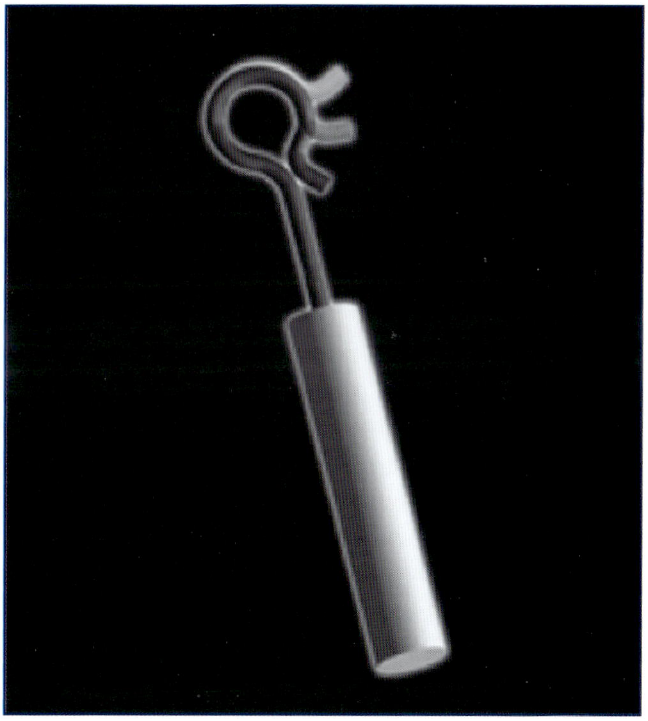

Figure 9–6. Smart piston with Nitinol loop. This prosthesis has a heat-activated loop for crimping. (From Gyrus ENT product brochure)

There is also some concern that the heat-induced crimp of the Smart piston around the incus may loosen over time. In a recent study assessing short term (6 weeks to 1 year) and intermediate term (greater than 1 year) results after stapedotomy utilizing the Smart Piston, the air-bone gap was <10 dB in 88% of the short-term group but worsened to 79% of the intermediate group.[32] The decrease in number of patients with closure of the air-bone gap over time may be secondary to the loosening crimp around the incus. Such loosening has been noted in clinical practice in patients implanted with the Smart piston. In a single otologic practice, eight patients have been noted to have loosening of the crimp around the incus during revision surgery (W.H. Lippy, Personal communication, November 12, 2008). Longer term studies are required with this relatively new prosthesis.

Lasers in Stapedotomy

Several different types of lasers have been adapted for stapedotomy. Laser technology allows precise and mechanically atraumatic cutting as well as hemostasis.[33] Complex revision stapes surgery that traditionally has been of high risk and low success is now performed much more effectively with laser. The laser-tissue interaction must be fully understood to safely and optimally utilize this technology.

Tissue characteristics of laser energy should ideally permit the vaporization of the stapes footplate or oval window soft tissue with minimal thermal effect to the vestibule and without passing through the perilymph to damage the delicate structures of the inner ear.

Argon and KTP Laser

Argon and KTP lasers have similar wavelengths and properties. The wavelength of the argon laser is 488 nm while the KTP laser wavelength is 532 nm. The visible wavelength of these two lasers provides excellent target accuracy, as the aiming beam and surgical beam are the same. Both fiberoptic handheld probes and micromanipulators can be used with these lasers. The use of argon laser in otologic surgery was first reported in 1980, and KTP use followed thereafter. [8,34]

Argon and KTP laser radiation is poorly absorbed in bone and perilymph, thus increasing the potential risk to the saccule and utricle during use. Lesinski and others have performed extensive study of the penetration of the argon and KTP laser beam through the perilymph. Delivery of the laser beam with the microscope-mounted micromanipulator delivery system projects the laser beam with a small convergence angle. With the fiberoptic delivery system, the beam of laser spreads out with a more broad angle of divergence, thus the power density rapidly decreases with increasing distance from the tip.[35] Recommendations have been made to use a lower wattage to vaporize the footplate and to pause for several seconds between laser bursts to decrease the incidence of postoperative symptoms.[34]

Due to inadequate power, the KTP and Argon lasers cannot create a 0.7-mm fenestra in a single application. Therefore, a "rosette" technique is used in which multiple 0.2-mm laser applications are used to create a 0.7-mm fenestra through which the prosthesis will pass. Once the fenestra has been created, extreme caution should be exercised because direct application of visible laser energy to the open vestibule can produce dramatic temperature rises, up to 175 degrees C, in the vestibule at the level of the utricle and saccule.[36]

CO_2 Laser

Many experimental studies and clinical trials have demonstrated the safety and effectiveness of the CO_2 laser in stapes surgery.[37,38] The wavelength of the invisible CO_2 laser is 10,600 nm. CO_2 lasers are absorbed in bone and perilymph, ideal characteristics for performing stapedotomy safely. Studies have shown that use of the CO_2 laser on the open vestibule caused a rise in the perilymph temperature of only 0.3 C.[37] One of the advantages of the CO_2 laser for stapedotomy is its high absorption of radiation in the perilymph with a resultant low penetration depth of only 0.01 mm.

As the CO_2 laser beam is invisible, a second aiming beam (HeNe 612 nm) is required: calibration of these two lasers must be ensured. Until recently, the CO_2 laser has only been available for use with a micromanipulator (Lumenis, Santa Clara, CA). Fiberoptic delivery of the CO_2 laser has been recently introduced allowing direct application of the laser energy with handheld, precise control, although the expense of the fiber may need to be considered.

Although the CO_2 laser is also extremely effective in creating a fenestra using a rosette technique using 0.2-mm diameter applications, a "Single-shot" fenestra is possible utilizing newer technology (Figures 9–7A and 9–7B). The CO_2 laser may be applied with microprocessor-controlled rotating mirrors, known as scanner systems (Lumenis, Santa Clara, CA) to perform stapedotomy. Within a fraction of a second, a spiral figure is traced, enabling the CO_2 laser to achieve high power density with minimal side effects.[39] The field of laser irradiation can be set, typically to 0.6 or 0.7 mm, suitable for stapedotomy. A single-shot footplate perforation of preselected diameter is thus created. The ability to achieve a circular footplate perforation with a single application of laser irradiation without appreciable thermal damage to the surrounding area is a significant advantage of this technology because it prevents the need to have overlapping rosette applications that could enter the vestibule.

Erbium Laser

With its wavelength of 2940 nm, erbium laser energy is totally absorbed by water or water-containing tissue. Thus, ablation of bone is characterized by high

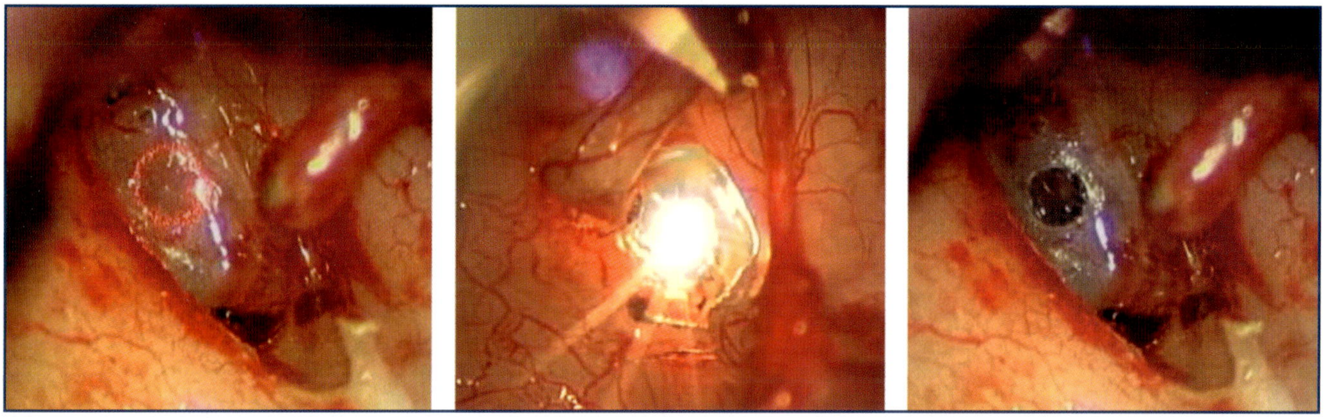

A

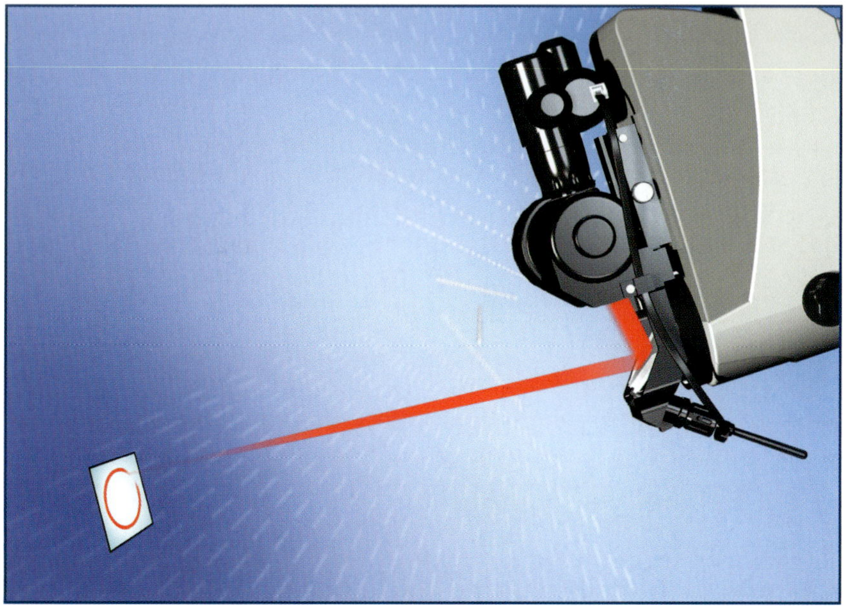

B

Figure 9–7. A. "Single-shot" fenestra using Lumenis CO_2 Surgi-Touch Scanner attachment. Note the aiming beam and subsequent circular footplate perforation. (Copyright Jack M. Kartush, MD, 2001). **B.** Scanner technology robotically creates a precise spiral in a fraction of a second.

precision and a very restricted thermal effect. This tissue ablation in erbium laser is achieved through explosive, rather than thermal, effects. The pressure wave that is generated, though, may lead to acoustic trauma. One study showed that the peak sound pressure level associated with the erbium laser was 132 dBA.[40] Concerns about possible high-frequency hearing loss after erbium laser stapedotomy have been published, noting a 10- to 30-dB hearing loss between 1 kHz and 10 kHz in guinea pigs.[41]

When compared to microdrill stapedotomy and CO_2 laser with scanning technology, the Erbium laser showed significantly higher degrees of hearing loss. Recently, however, several clinical studies have been published showing erbium laser technology to be a useful and safe tool for laser stapedotomy.[42,43]

Although the erbium laser offers advantages in bone ablation, as soon as bleeding occurs, the oligothermic Erbium laser radiation is completely absorbed by blood and no longer reaches the target area. Thus, as opposed to CO_2, argon, and KTP lasers, it has no hemostatic properties. Because of this and the concern for acoustic trauma, this technology is rarely today used for stapedotomy in the United States.

Fenestration and Postfenestration Stapedectomy

The fenestration procedure was introduced by Lempert in 1938 and, although not performed today, should be understood as the otolaryngologist may need to care for a patient that has undergone this procedure in the late 1950s.[4] Endaural canal wall down mastoidectomy is performed to expose the dome of the horizontal semicircular canal. The canal wall skin is preserved and the incus and head of the malleus are removed. The bone over the dome of the horizontal semicircular canal is gradually thinned down with a diamond bur without injuring the membranous labyrinth. The tympanomeatal flap is positioned so that its thinnest portion covers the new fenestra and allows sound to enter the cochlea by way of the horizontal canal.

Although there are relatively few patients still alive that have undergone this procedure, the otolaryngologist needs to understand the procedure and use caution in mastoid debridement at the horizontal semicircular canal in such a patient. Furthermore, if a patient has a persistent or recurrent conductive hearing loss after fenestration surgery, revision surgery may be considered. In addition to avoiding trauma to the fenestrated horizontal semicircular canal, the otolaryngologist must be aware that there will be no incus present, as it would have been removed during the fenestration procedure. Consequently, the prosthesis must be placed between the manubrium of the malleus and the oval window. The option of amplification with hearing aid should be considered in these patients. In the patient with persistent conductive hearing loss who is unable to wear a conventional hearing aid, a bone-anchored hearing implant (BAHA) is also an option.

Stapedotomy Procedure

Intravenous sedation is preferred for adults as this allows the surgeon to test hearing results at the conclusion of the case and to detect vertigo from manipulations at the oval window. General anesthesia is used in children, in anxious adults, and for those in whom the airway may be compromised during heavy sedation. A "whisper test" is performed at the conclusion of the surgery to assess hearing improvement. In addition, intraoperative audiometry has been described utilizing 500 Hz and 1000 Hz tones to ensure desired improvement in hearing results.[44]

Preparation for the procedure and attention to details is of utmost importance before the procedure even begins. The correct ear should be marked in the preoperative area by the surgeon after confirming the side with the patient.

The laser should be assessed to ensure proper function and the chosen prosthesis should be available. In addition, the surgeon should ensure that the speculum holder is on the table and correctly positioned. Preoperative antibiotics and, often, steroids are given preoperatively.

A small amount of postauricular hair is shaved in preparation for the infrequent case where the external auditory canal is narrow or tortuous, requiring a postauricular approach. Using 1% lidocaine with 1:100,000 epinephrine, the postauricular and meatal areas are anesthetized prior to antiseptic prep and surgical draping, to allow time for the anesthetic and hemostatic effects to take place. The use of "custom" local anesthetic solutions with high epinephrine concentrations should be avoided to reduce the risk of cardiac arrhythmia and inadvertent injection of mistakenly high concentrations.

After sterile prep and draping, a moist sponge is placed over the patient's eyes. Further infiltration of local anesthetic is now performed using the microscope to allow deeper injection. This should be performed slowly and deliberately, observing blanching of the ear canal skin to ensure adequate anesthesia and hemostasis. Infiltration should be monitored closely for blebs in the canal skin as this weakens the epithelium and may lead to tearing of the canal skin during elevation and further complication. If a bleb does occur during local anesthetic infiltration, immediately aspirate back on the syringe to decompress the bleb.

Next, a small piece of subcutaneous fascia or fat is harvested from a postauricular incision and saved for later use. Always harvest enough fascia for tympanoplasty, should it become necessary. Press the fascia and let dry naturally on a Teflon block. Some of this will be cut up and moistened for use as tissue seal in oval window.

The speculum should then be secured into the speculum holder. The largest speculum that can comfortably fit into the ear canal should be used for greatest exposure.

The operating microscope with an attached CO_2 laser with micromanipulator is used (Lumenis, Santa Clara, CA). An 8-mm tympanomeatal flap is created. The chorda tympani nerve is preserved and the middle ear entered. After the tympanomeatal flap is elevated and prior to drilling, a small piece of Gelfoam with 1:1000 topical epinephrine is placed on the promontory for both hemostasis and to collect bone dust while drilling.

Adequate exposure is attained using a microdrill and curette on the osseous annulus until the stapedial tendon and inferior portion of the tympanic facial nerve are well seen (Figure 9–8). The chorda tympani nerve is exposed with a small curette *after* the canal is drilled to intentionally leave bone as a natural protector. A canalplasty may be necessary in some patients through either a transcanal or postauricular approach. A foil "protector" can be created using a portion of suture package to protect the tympanomeatal flap during drilling of the annulus or external ear canal (Figure 9–9). Malleus and incus mobility are ensured and stapes fixation is confirmed.

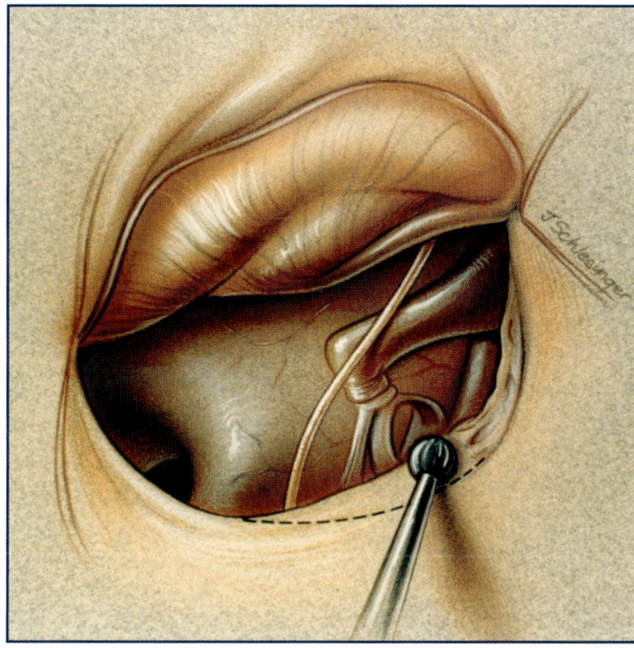

Figure 9–8. Drilling of the scutal area using a small cutting bur to achieve exposure. (Copyright Jack M. Kartush, MD, 1987)

The CO_2 laser is initially used in conventional single pulse mode: 0.3 watt, 0.1 sec, 0.2-mm spot size through the micromanipulator for hemostatic cutting. The microscope is set to a working distance of approximately 300 mm to coincide with a 300-mm focal length on the laser-preset parameters. Although the laser parameters may be altered, we have found that a distance of 300 mm optimizes working distance. The spot size may be increased for coagulation without cutting. Although coagulation may be accomplished by lowering the power on the laser unit, it is most readily performed by the surgeon simply de-focusing the micromanipulator rather than repeatedly asking the nurse to make changes in the power setting.

The incudostapedial joint is lasered prior to separating it with a joint knife (Figure 9–10). This prevents bleeding from the tiny artery that is always present and makes separation of the joint easier. To allow better stability of the stapes superstructure,

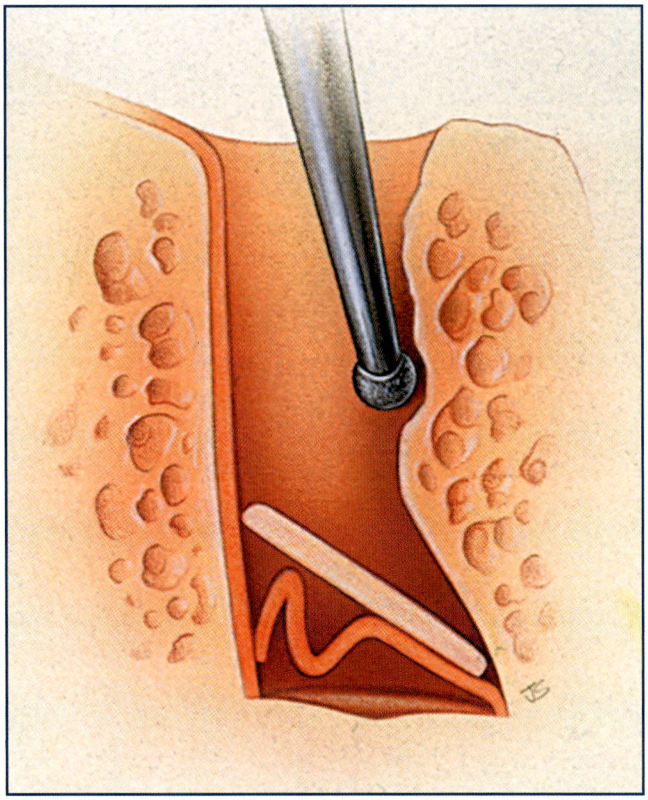

Figure 9–9. Placement of a flap protector when canalplasty is required can minimize injury to external auditory canal skin and tympanic membrane. (Copyright Jack M. Kartush, MD, 1987)

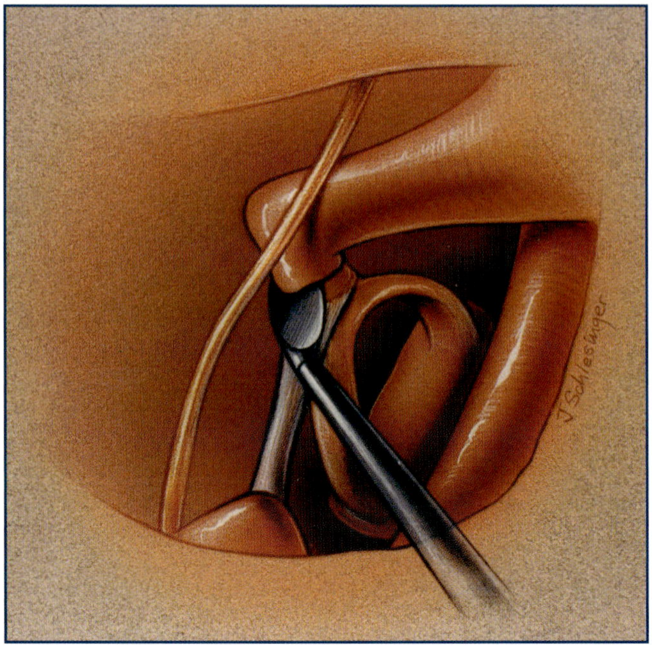

Figure 9–10. Separation of the incudostapedial joint prior to division of the stapedius tendon. Note the clear visualization of the facial nerve, origin of stapedius tendon at the pyramidal eminence, and posterior crus of stapes superstructure. (Copyright Jack M. Kartush, MD, 1987)

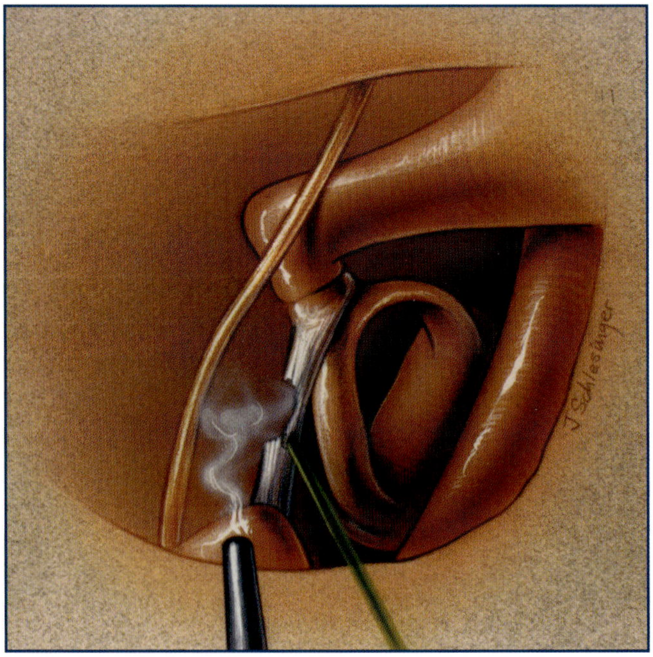

Figure 9–11. Division of the stapedius tendon using laser. (Copyright Jack M. Kartush, MD, 1987)

the stapes tendon is lasered *after* separating the joint (Figure 9–11). The posterior crus of the stapes is then lasered as close to the footplate as possible to prevent the stump of the crus from later interfering with placement of the piston (Figure 9–12). If the anterior crus is visible, it can also be lasered. The superstructure is then briskly down-fractured away from the facial nerve and removed.

Small fenestra laser stapedotomy can be performed using the conventional single pulse mode parameters that are used for the initial middle ear work: 0.3 W, 0.1 sec, and 0.2-mm spot size. A rosette technique is used wherein multiple laser applications with the 0.2-mm spot size are used to gradually create a 0.7-mm fenestra (Figure 9–13). Although the CO_2 wavelength will minimize the risk to the inner ear, care must still be taken not to allow the laser to pass through adjacent previously created holes in

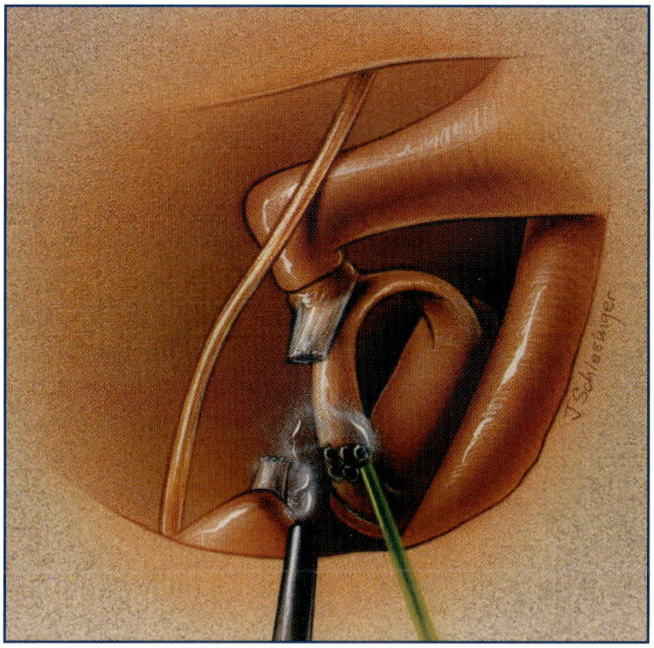

Figure 9–12. Removal of the posterior crus as close to the footplate as possible. (Copyright Jack M. Kartush, MD, 1987)

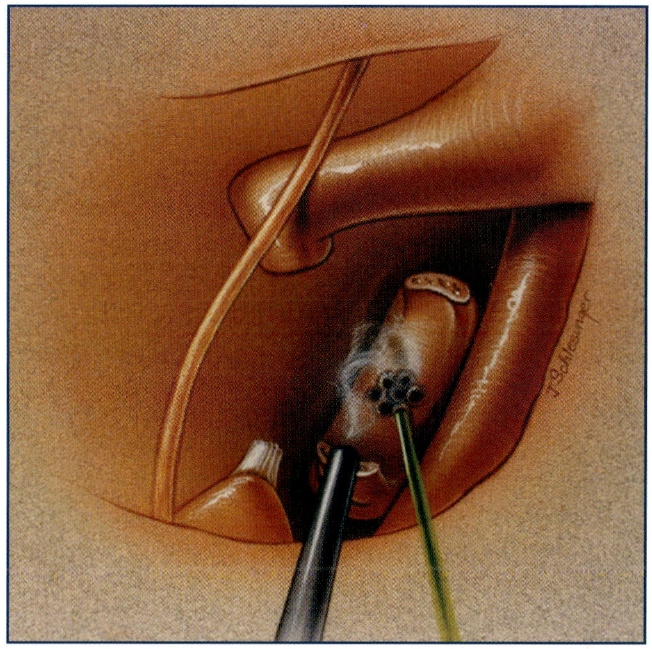

Figure 9–13. Small fenestra laser stapedotomy utilizing CO_2 laser with micromanipulator. (Copyright Jack M. Kartush, MD, 1987)

order to prevent injury to the inner ear, especially if perilymph has leaked out to cause a dry fenestra. Absence of perilymph takes away the natural protection of the vestibular end organs. For those who choose to use visible spectrum lasers (KTP or Argon) instead of the invisible wavelength CO_2 laser, even greater care must be taken because visible lasers can pass through perilymph, potentially causing injury to the inner ear.

In contrast to the classic rosette technique, our preferred approach today is to create a "Single Shot" fenestra using the Surgi-Touch Scanner attachment. This eliminates the need to repeatedly laser the footplate and thus prevents the possibility of individual laser hits inadvertently passing through the previous laser holes, as may occur with the rosette technique. The Surgi-Touch Scanner parameters are ensured and then a "Single-shot" fenestra is created in a tenth of a second. Parameters used are 28 W, 0.7-mm spot size with a focal length of 300 mm (to match the microscope working distance). With extremely thick footplates (obliterative otosclerosis), a 0.5-mm diamond drill is used to thin the bone and then the laser is used to open the thinned footplate.

One of the benefits of hemostatic lasers and use of epinephrine-soaked Gelfoam early in the procedure is that typically there will be little or no bleeding once the fenestra is opened. This is an extremely important point because if blood pools over the fenestra, the surgeon is placed in a predicament. If the blood is suctioned away, visibility will be improved but perilymph may also inadvertently be aspirated, which can cause vertigo and a dry vestibule. In contrast, if the surgeon does not wish to risk suctioning at the fenestra, there is the risk that the piston may not be appropriately placed through the fenestra due to lack of visibility.

The stapes piston is then inserted into the fenestra with a small alligator forceps (Figure 9–14). In our current practice, a Medtronic "Big Easy" Stapes Piston is inserted, 4.25 mm in length, 0.5 mm in diameter. Due to the challenges associated with working in a narrow external auditory canal and middle ear under binocular microscopy, parallax effects and coaxial instrumentation make accurate measurement of the distance from the oval window to the lenticular process difficult in determining prosthesis length.

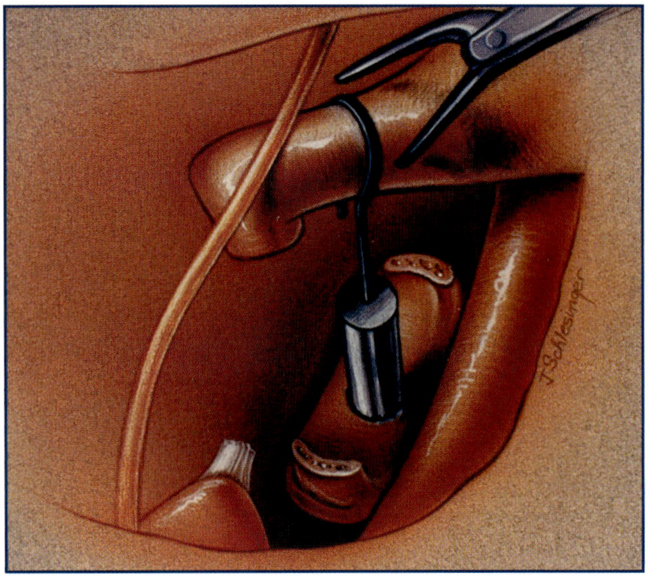

Figure 9–14. The stapes piston is carefully placed over the lenticular process of the incus and crimped gently. (Copyright Jack M. Kartush, MD, 1987)

Thus, in our experience with thousands of stapes procedures, we have found that a prosthesis length of 4.25 mm for the McGee and Big Easy pistons is optimal in 95% of adults. Unless the middle ear appears to be grossly shallow or deep, the best measuring device is to start with a 4.25-mm prosthesis. If the prosthesis is too short, it should be obvious to the surgeon by looking at the depth notch on the piston and by doing a tap test: the base of the piston is tapped and if it is too short, it will swing out of the fenestra. In contrast, a piston that is too long will be detected by the depth notch being too deep and virtually invisible beneath the fenestra. In addition, in a sedated patient, they may immediately experience vertigo. The ability to detect intraoperative vertigo secondary to a deep piston is another benefit of intravenous sedation.

Once the piston position is confirmed, the MRI-safe piston is crimped onto the incus and then its position at both the incus and the footplate are confirmed under high power magnification. The prior harvested fascia is cut into 3-mm pieces, which are moistened and packed around the piston at the fenestra. A critical maneuver before closure is to now move the malleus and look for movement of both incus and piston. If the piston does not move well, the fenestra may need to be widened. The tympanomeatal flap is then replaced. A whisper test confirms improved hearing and several pieces of saline-soaked Gelfoam are placed over the tympanomeatal flap and tympanic membrane. A non-ototoxic antibiotic ointment, such as Bacitracin, is then instilled in the external auditory canal. Most patients may be discharged the same day if they live within an hour or two of the hospital.

STAPEDECTOMY PEARLS

Approach

- The patient's head is turned 30 degrees away from the operative surgeon and is taped gently to the bed. If agitation occurs intraoperatively, movement of the head will be minimized.
- The ipsilateral shoulder should be gently pulled inferiorly and strapped for safety and to prevent elevation into the surgical field.
- When harvesting fascia, always obtain enough not only to cover the fenestra but also to ensure that there is sufficient surplus in the event a tympanoplasty is required.
- The speculum holder is placed consistently with adjustment controls at the right hand position for ease of adjustment. Align speculum itself with wide end oriented vertically.
- When making tympanomeatal incisions, make the superior cut high so that it is well above the pars flaccida. Use sickle knife for both superior and inferior horizontal incisions.
- The thicker vascular strip skin is more difficult to cut with sickle knife; therefore, Bellucci scissors are routinely used to complete the incision.
- Use a 7200 Beaver blade to connect superior and inferior incisions; rock the blade from side to side to ensure that the canal skin is not torn.

- Ensure that the elevated tympanomeatal flap can be folded easily over the tympanic membrane for complete visualization of the middle ear. If this cannot be achieved, it means the flap incisions are not complete.
- Just before elevating the annulus, place 1:1000 epinephrine-soaked Gelfoam for a few moments to assure hemostasis of the ear canal.
- Elevate annulus at the easiest spot where it can be visualized without a lip of overhanging bone.
- When elevating the annulus, scrape back and forth with a curved needle instrument. This sharp curved instrument will ensure elevation *beneath* the fibrous annulus. If you do not appropriately elevate under the fibrous annulus and instead are lateral to it, the tympanic membrane will be thinned and there will be increased risk of perforation.
- Place topical 1:1000 epinephrine-soaked Gelfoam in the middle ear before drilling to absorb bone dust and to ensure hemostasis.
- Use a 2.4 mm-cutting bur initially to drill scutal area and then switch to a small diamond burr.
- Start drill with bur off bone to prevent skipping. Do not expose chorda tympani yet. Leave a shell of bone over this to maintain protection while drilling, which is initiated posterior and superior to chorda tympani. Have the nurse drip in saline as needed. Remove the last segment of bone over the chorda with small bone curette/hook.
- Goal when removing posterior canal bone is to visualize: (1) posteriorly, the posterior crus and stapedius tendon, and, if possible, the pyramidal eminence; and (2) superiorly, the inferior aspect of the facial nerve and enough of the lenticular process of the incus to allow for ease of piston placement and crimping.
- Use care to prevent too great a scutal defect that could allow a retraction pocket to develop postoperatively.

Middle Ear Work

- When performing stapedotomy on a sedated patient, the patient may be moving their head slightly with every breath. Fine surgical work should be performed after patient exhales as this affords surgeon greatest time period to proceed. This will minimize errant lasering and decrease risk of injury.
- The incudostapedial joint can be located by gentle lateral traction on the incus. This will demonstrate the articulation between the incus and stapes.
- Use suction to evacuate smoke to allow cooling between laser hits if using rosette technique. Do not suction perilymph: use only small suction tips, for example, 24 French, once the fenestra is opened.
- 0.3-mm oval window rasp (McGee-Farrior/Storz) or additional lasering may be utilized to enlarge the fenestra.
- Especially for the inexperienced surgeon, placing a saline-soaked Gelfoam in the hypotympanum prior to placing the prosthesis will prevent wasted time and effort searching for piston if it falls during insertion.
- When crimping piston, use index finger on crimping instrument to open and close the instrument. It may be intuitive to control the instrument by moving the thumb, but the index finger should perform the motion so that the instrument does not move during crimping (Figure 9–15).
- When crimping, use one hand to stabilize and one hand to guide the piston into place with slow, deliberate, and gentle motion.
- Shift the microscope such that your line of site is inferior to the crimper so you can observe the crimper without losing depth of field.
- If the crimper is inadequate due to a thin long process, use an alligator turned backward to crimp the piston loop.
- A "tap test" should be performed: a slight tap with a curved needle at the base of the piston is used to observe whether it slides

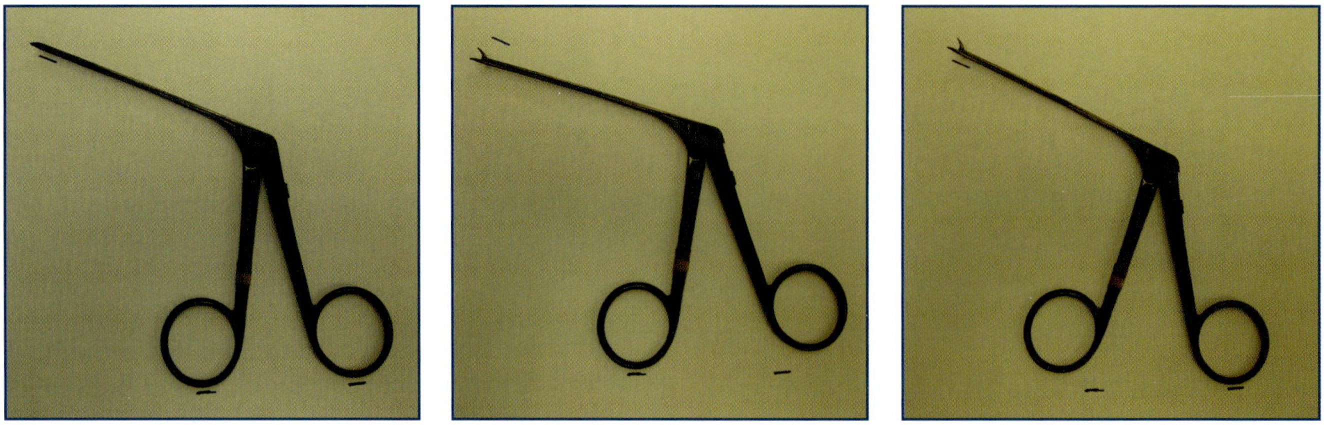

A B C

Figure 9–15. **A**. Crimping instrument. Notice the markings indicating location of instrument. **B**. Using the thumb to open the device, there is considerable movement of the instrument, approximately 1 cm at the distal aspect. This can be appreciated by noting relationship to markings. **C**. Using the index finger when crimping keeps the device stable and leads to greater success.

out of the fenestra, indicating that it is too short or is poorly placed.

- A final critical check is to then move the malleus and confirm movement of both incus and piston.
- A piston that is clearly in the fenestra but does not move well alerts the surgeon that they must recheck for either too tight of a fenestra or undetected ossicular head fixation.
- When replacing flap at end of procedure, suction the air out of the middle ear to hold the flap down and to improve hearing.
- Place moist Gelfoam over the tympanic membrane and tympanomeatal flap before filling the outer meatus with Bacitracin to stabilize flap and prevent ointment from getting injected underneath the flap.

INTRAOPERATIVE ISSUES

Narrow Oval Window Fenestra

A difficult scenario in stapes surgery is dealing with a narrow oval window niche. This limits the surgeon's ability to create an appropriately sized fenestra and makes it difficult to know if the fenestra created may in fact be too narrow, which will restrict movement of the piston.

A narrow niche often can be markedly improved by using the laser to vaporize approximately 1 mm of promontory bone just below the stapes. This is especially helpful if there is a low, dehiscent facial nerve. In our cochlear microdissections, we found that there is nearly always 2 mm of bone that can be lasered away in this area before exposure of the cochlear periosteum occurs. Thus, with care, improved exposure can be attained safely with the laser.

Stapes surgery requires that the fenestra be sealed to prevent a perilymph fistula. How the fenestra is sealed can also affect how well the piston fits within the fenestra. There are two main techniques for sealing the oval window: (1) place the piston in the fenestra and then pack tissue around it; and (2) cover the fenestra with tissue and then place the piston over it. Although the latter technique is required for the Robinson and Lippy Bucket handle designs, it is optional for McGee-type pistons. We prefer the former approach. If the fenestra is narrow and the surgeon places tissue over it, it may be difficult to know with certainty if the piston is truly within the fenestra or caught on the edge. Furthermore, the surgeon must account for the fact that the graft will take up some of the fenestra space; thus, always assure there is sufficient space for both piston and graft. Confirm appropriate fit by moving the malleus and assuring unrestricted movement of the piston.

Incus Erosion/Subluxation

Erosion of the incus is a common finding at revision stapedectomy (Figures 9–16 and 9–17). No prosthesis will ever be completely free of delayed incus necrosis because the tenuous blood supply of the lenticular process comes from the head of the incus medially and from the stapes capitulum laterally. Thus, the simple act of disarticulating the incudostapedial joint will always cause some degree of devascularization of the lenticular process.

In dealing with incus erosion, the surgeon must assess whether reconstruction is possible with the remaining incus or whether reconstruction to the malleus or drum is necessary. Alternative prostheses such as the Big Easy Offset piston or the Lippy Modified-Robinson prostheses can be effective if the incus erosion is mild to moderate (Figure 9–18) If incus erosion is severe, a malleus to oval window prosthesis may be utilized (Figure 9–19).

Revision surgery for incus lenticular necrosis requires removal of a greater amount of scutum to fully visualize the entire remaining lenticular process. If this is not performed, crimping of the piston will be difficult or impossible. Due to the necrotic incus, we typically use a slightly longer Big Easy Offset piston: usually 4.5 mm. There are separate right and left offsets so the correct piston must be selected depending upon which ear is being operated on.

When incus necrosis is severe, neither the Big Easy Offset nor Lippy piston may suffice, and thus reconstruction to the malleus (or drum) is necessitated. Although it is possible to use a TORP directly to the tympanic membrane, there is a concern for retraction of the TORP into the fenestra due to Eustachian tube dysfunction. If a TORP is used, a graft of adequate thickness must be placed underneath the prosthesis rather than around it.

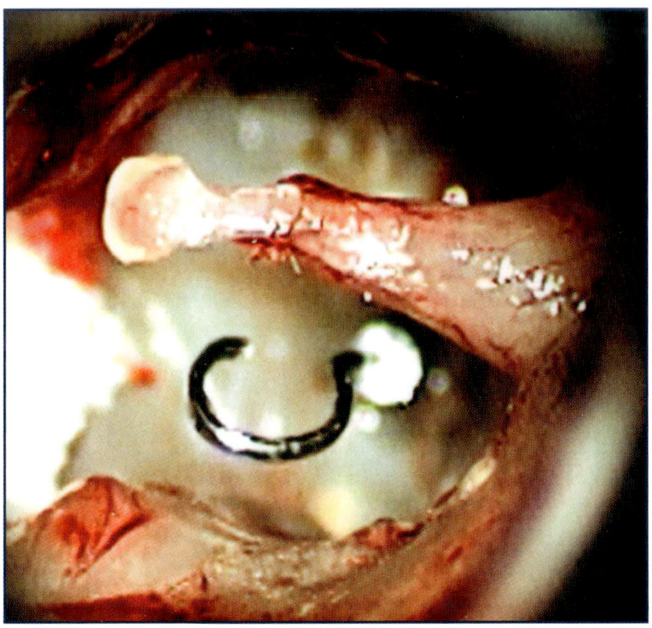

Figure 9–16. Incus erosion secondary to prior piston placement.

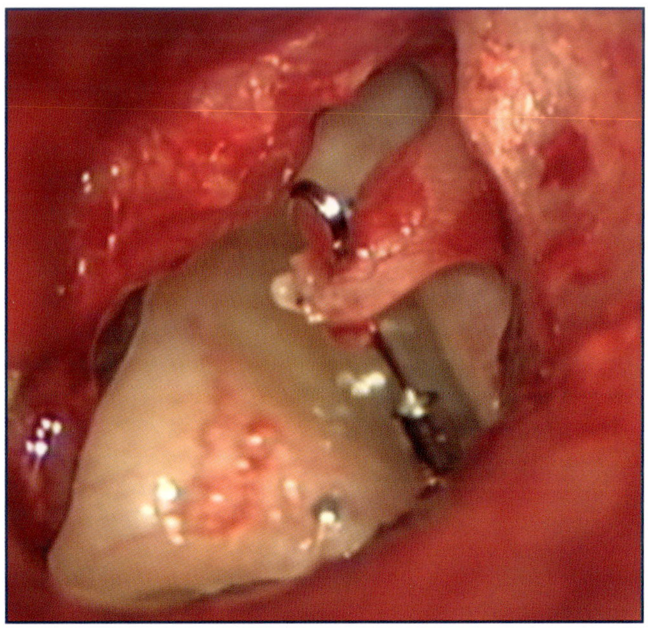

Figure 9–17. Severe erosion of distal aspect of the lenticular process of the incus.

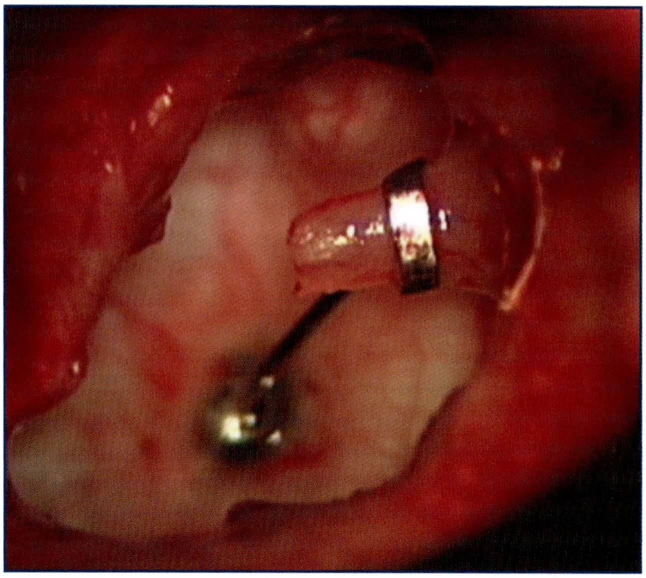

Figure 9–18. Placement of an offset piston to the more proximal aspect of the incus. Note the difficult angle that is addressed with an offset piston.

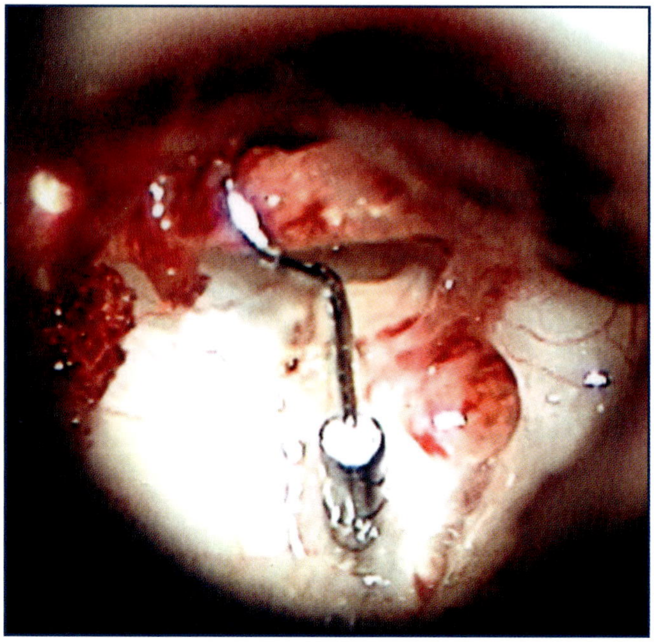

Figure 9–19. Malleus to oval window piston.

In order to perform a malleus to oval window reconstruction, the drum must be separated from the malleus. Although this can be readily accomplished along the superior manubrium, the transition of tympanic membrane to periosteum at the umbo makes separation of the drum from the umbo difficult without creating a perforation. Although it is possible to leave the drum attached to the umbo, this makes crimping the prosthesis extremely difficult.

Therefore, we have found that completely elevating the drum from the malleus and anticipating the potential of a tiny perforation at the umbo can be readily treated with an over-under tympanoplasty, wherein fascia is placed medial to the drum and lateral to both the manubrium and the ribbon of the prosthesis (Figure 9–20). This allows excellent exposure of the malleus for crimping.

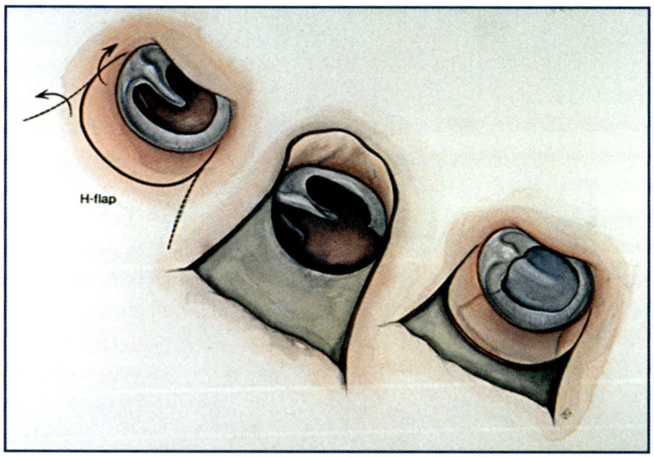

Figure 9–20. Over-under tympanoplasty. The fascia graft is placed under the tympanic membrane and over the malleus. (Copyright Jack M. Kartush, MD, 1987)

The distance between the malleus and the oval window is much more variable than from the incus to the oval window. This distance can vary from 3.75 mm to over 5 mm. Also, the location along the shaft of the malleus varies in distance to the oval window as the manubrium is always slanted medially toward the promontory at the umbo. Thus, it is critical in this situation that the surgeon measure the distance from the malleus to the oval window as best as can be done given the anatomic and visual constraints.

Placement of the piston over the malleus can be made easier by loading the prosthesis onto the alligator at a more obtuse angle. This is accomplished by angling the alligator more perpendicular and less in line to the shaft of the prosthesis. Use of the crimper with the greatest curve allows easier crimping over the malleus. Following crimping, the piston shaft will tend to rest on the anterior ledge of the stapes fenestra, as the malleus is more anterior than the oval window. To correct this, take a hook in one hand and suction or strut guide in the other hand and gently rotate the prosthesis posteriorly until it no longer rests on the promontory or anterior fenestral ledge.

Intraoperative Complications Pearls

- If a tympanic membrane tear occurs, previously harvested fascia should be utilized to repair the defect.
- If the chorda tympani is inadvertently (or rarely intentionally) sectioned during exposure, it can sometimes be successfully repaired by re-approximating edges of the nerve over a bed of Gelfoam followed by fascia. The tympanic membrane is then gently replaced.
- If a floating footplate occurs when downfracturing the stapes superstructure, use the laser to complete the stapedotomy in order to avoid mechanical manipulation of a floating footplate which risks medial displacement of footplate fragments and resultant vestibular injury.
- When the anterior crus is difficult to downfracture, attempt to fracture in an inferior and anterior direction. Also, lasering the anterior crus sometimes becomes possible after the posterior crus has been lasered away.
- Although we prefer the single-shot technique for stapedotomy, the rosette technique should be considered if there is a dehiscent or prolapsed facial nerve, or if the patient is restless under sedation with frequent and unpredictable movements. Under these scenarios, the risk of unintentionally lasering adjacent tissue is increased. Therefore, the rosette technique is selected because the amount of laser energy used during each application is substantially less than the energy delivered during the single-shot technique. In addition, a tiny pledget of moist Gelfoam can be placed over a dehiscent facial nerve.
- If the facial nerve is significantly prolapsed to the area over the oval window, and adequate exposure cannot be obtained by lasering or drilling the bone inferior to the oval window, avoid use of the laser along the nerve. Place aluminum foil over nerve to protect it and use a diamond microdrill to perform the stapedotomy. Ensure foil is removed prior to conclusion of the case.
- If severe facial nerve prolapse is present over the oval window, the case should be abandoned and hearing aid or BAHA considered.
- A persistent stapedial artery may course between the stapes crura. This small artery is nearly always readily controlled with the laser. With an extraordinarily large stapedial artery, the procedure may be terminated and hearing aid or BAHA considered.
- During revision stapes surgery, the laser makes removal of scar around the prior stapedotomy site significantly safer than conventional mechanical techniques. Under these circumstances, use single pulse settings at low laser energy at the neomembrane of the oval window unless residual or new bone is encountered.

POSTOPERATIVE COMPLICATIONS

In the postoperative patient with significant dizziness, tinnitus, and/or hearing loss, one must consider the most likely differential diagnosis. Etiologies include serous labyrinthitis, perilymphatic fistula, a deep piston, or reparative granuloma. These patients should be monitored closely with timing and severity of symptoms as well as physical exam as the key factors in determining likely cause and treatment.

Serous Labyrinthitis

The most common cause of postoperative inner ear symptoms after routine stapedotomy is thought to be "serous labyrinthitis." This is often seen after completely routine procedures wherein "everything goes right." This complication may be associated with individual variations in inner ear sensitivity. Most of these patients appear to benefit from a short course of oral steroids. If rapid improvement is not noted, the packing should be removed even at an early stage postoperatively, the ear examined, and the hearing assessed. Reparative granuloma, perilymph fistula or a deep/long piston should be excluded.

Oval Window Fistula

Oval window fistula was relatively common in the past when Gelfoam and blood were used in the fenestra instead of tissue seals. In addition, prior to the McGee type of piston, a "fat-wire" piston was commonly employed in which a piece of fat was placed on the end of a wire loop fashioned at the time of the surgery. These cases had a not insignificant incidence of late complications because the fat would occasionally atrophy, resulting in fistula and lateralization of the wire from the fenestra.

Oval window fistula after stapedectomy may occur in the early postoperative period or years later. Our routine immediate postoperative instructions include avoiding strenuous activity and hard nose blowing. Fluctuating or progressive hearing loss is noted with tinnitus, with or without vertigo. Trauma or barometric pressure change may precede symptoms. Clinical exam may include positive fistula testing, typically performed simply with digital pressure or pneumotoscopy eliciting dizziness. Audiometric findings include sensorineural hearing loss, although hearing loss is not always present on audiogram. The diagnosis is rarely seen when a tissue seal of fascia or vein has been used. Middle ear exploration with grafting of the oval window using tissue is indicated if a fistula is thought to be present.

Deep Piston

The incidence of deep insertion of the piston within the vestibule is low in experienced hands. Most commonly, this complication occurs when the chosen piston length is greater than the standard of 4.25 mm. The diagnosis is strongly considered when either a longer prosthesis has been used or if the patient experienced dizziness during placement of the piston through the fenestra intraoperatively. As in perilymph fistula, digital pressure or pneumotoscopy often elicits dizziness; however, the onset of symptoms is usually immediately after surgery, in contrast to fistulas which may occur quite late. CT imaging after stapedectomy has not been shown to be reliable in determining depth of piston insertion within the vestibule.[45] Thus, imaging after stapedectomy has limited value in identifying the piston that is too deep within the vestibule.

Other etiologies of vertigo should be considered including benign paroxysmal positional vertigo (BPPV), a depressed footplate fragment, or reparative granuloma. BPPV may be seen in the postoperative period secondary to surgical injury to the utricle or due to free flowing particles from the fenestra. This condition typically is self-limiting and often benefits from canalith repositioning maneuvers.

Reparative Granuloma

The hallmark of reparative granuloma is progressive sensorineural hearing loss after earlier postoperative hearing improvement. This may be associated with vertigo, aural fullness, or tinnitus. Often, the audiogram reveals a mixed hearing loss most severe in the high frequencies. If this diagnosis is considered, the packing in the external auditory canal should be removed and the ear examined. The tympanic membrane typically appears thickened and bright red tissue is visualized along the tympanomeatal flap and lenticular process of the incus.

Use of Gelfoam as an oval window sealant is believed to have contributed to this complication in the past. Most surgeons now use a tissue seal, making this complication much less common. Talcum powder was also considered a cause of reparative granuloma. However, surgical gloves are now virtually always talc free. The current cause of this rare complication is unknown. As noted previously, there has been a case of reparative granuloma in our institution associated with Smart piston using Nitinol in a patient with a nickel allergy.

Prompt surgical exploration is indicated if this complication is suspected. Significant granulation tissue around the oval window and prosthesis is noted on exploration. Multinucleated giant cells are noted histologically, signifying foreign body reaction.

If reparative granuloma is encountered on re-exploration, the granuloma should be lasered away, the prosthesis removed and a tissue seal placed over the oval window. We typically do not reconstruct with a new prosthesis at re-exploration because many patients will have a significant sensorineural hearing loss. Therefore, we wait approximately 6 months to determine if there is sufficient cochlear reserve to consider revision surgery. Alternatively, a hearing aid or BAHA may be considered.

Persistent Postoperative Conductive Hearing Loss

In the case that postoperative audiogram shows no improvement in hearing, one must consider malleus fixation, too tight of a fenestra, piston displacement, or superior canal dehiscence. After superior canal dehiscence is ruled out, the patient may be re-explored, ideally with IV sedation. If malleus head fixation is found, mobilization may be considered, which is ideally done after the incudostapedial joint (or piston) has been separated to minimize labyrinthine trauma. Re-fixation of the malleus after mobilization, however, is not uncommon. Thus, alternatively, an atticotomy may be performed to remove the malleus head and the incus with subsequent ossicular reconstruction performed between the malleus and oval window.

Postoperative Otitis Media

Acute otitis media in the postoperative period is a rare complication. This is an especially concerning condition as bacteria may enter the labyrinth and could rarely lead to meningitis. Antibiotic therapy should be instituted, myringotomy considered, and the patient's condition monitored closely.

RESULTS OF STAPES SURGERY

Approximately 90% of patients undergoing primary stapes surgery have a conductive deficit of 10 dB or less when measured 6 to 12 months after stapedectomy. In these studies, about 5% of patients have an unsatisfactory result estimated at 15 dB or higher average air-bone gap.[46–48] The air-bone gap closure typically remains stable through time.[49] A long-term sensorineural hearing loss affecting the high frequencies may occur with time that may be a consequence of presbycusis or cochlear otosclerosis.

The experience of the surgeon is clearly a predictor in stapes surgery outcomes.[50] Experienced surgeons in this study more accurately placed the stapes prosthesis and caused less cochlear trauma than novice surgeons. There has been a significant decline in the number of resident stapedectomies performed in training programs over the past several decades, and more recent graduates have become progressively more reluctant to perform stapes surgery.[51] Consequently, although an otologic fellowship is not a prerequisite for stapes surgery, otolaryngologists should honestly evaluate their training, experience and microsurgical skills before opting to perform stapes surgery.

Revision stapes surgery is significantly more complicated and is associated with greater risk and poorer results. In a large study of revision stapedectomy over 25 years ago at a time that fat-wire prostheses were common, displacement of the prosthesis to the inferior edge of the fenestra was the most common cause of failure with an incidence of 41%.[52] Incus necrosis (17%) and fistula (16%) followed in frequency. After revision, less than 50% of patients had a 10 dB air-bone gap and 7% of patients had a sensorineural hearing loss, half of them a total loss. Now, with more modern prostheses and use of tissue seals, incus necrosis and slippage of the prosthesis are the most common findings. Revision stapes surgery brings with it heightened risk to any remaining hearing and, in our opinion, should be performed by an experienced otologic surgeon using laser technology.

SUMMARY

Otosclerosis is a common cause of conductive hearing loss for which surgical treatment is highly successful with a low incidence of complications in experienced hands. Nonsurgical treatment of otosclerosis includes fluoride therapy and amplification. Laser stapedotomy is the definitive treatment for hearing restoration.

Generous exposure of the middle ear, use of laser technology, and compulsive attention to detail before, during, and after stapedectomy are critical elements to achieve optimal results and minimize complications.

REFERENCES

1. Canalis RF. Valsalva's contribution to otology. *Am J Otolaryngol.* 1990;11(6):420–427.
2. Toynbee J. *Diseases of the Ear*. Philadelphia, PA: Blanchard and Lea; 1860.
3. Politzer A. Veber primare Erkankung der Knochernen Labyrinth Kapsel. *Ohrenheilkd.* 1894;25:309–312.
4. Lempert J. Improvement of hearing in cases of otosclerosis: a new, one stage surgical technic. *Arch Otolaryngol.* 1938;28:42–97.
5. Rosen S. Restoration of hearing in otosclerosis by mobilization of the fixed stapedial footplate; an analysis of results. *Laryngoscope.* 955;65(4):224–269.
6. Schuknecht HF, Applebaum EL. Surgery for hearing loss. *N Engl J Med.* 1969;280(21):1154–1160.
7. Perkins RC. Laser stepedotomy for otosclerosis. *Laryngoscope.* 1980;90(2):228–240.
8. DiBartolomeo JR, Ellis M. The argon laser in otology. *Laryngoscope.* 1980;90(11 pt 1):1786–1796.
9. McGee TM. The argon laser in surgery for chronic ear disease and otosclerosis. *Laryngoscope.* 1983;93(9):1177–1182.
10. Schuknecht HF, Barber W. Histologic variants in otosclerosis. *Laryngoscope.* 1985;95(11):1307–1317.
11. Schuknecht H. *Pathology of the Ear*. Cambridge, MA: Harvard University Press; 1974.
12. Donnell GN, Alfi OS. Medical genetics for the otorhinolaryngologist. *Laryngoscope.* 1980;90(1):40–46.
13. Soifer N, Weaver K, Endahl GL, Holdsworth CE Jr. Otosclerosis: a review. *Acta Otolaryngol Suppl.* 1970;269:1–25.
14. Levin G, Fabian P, Stahle J. Incidence of otosclerosis. *Am J Otol.* 1988;9(4):299–301.
15. Cawthorne T. Otosclerosis. *J Laryngol Otol.* 1955;69(7):437–456.
16. Goodhill V, Moncur JP. The low-frequency air-bone gap. *Laryngoscope.* 1963;73:850–867.
17. Carhart R. The clinical application of bone conduction audiometry. *Trans Am Acad Ophthalmol Otolaryngol.* 1950;54:699–707.
18. Shambaugh GE Jr. Clinical diagnosis of cochlear (labyrinthine) otosclerosis. *Laryngoscope.* 1965;75(10):1558–1562.
19. Causse JR, Uriel J, Berges J, Shambaugh GE Jr, Bretlau P, Causse JB. The enzymatic mechanism of the otospongiotic disease and NaF action on the enzymatic balance. *Am J Otol.* 1982;3(4):297–314.
20. Parahy C, Linthicum FH Jr. Otosclerosis: relationship of spiral ligament hyalinization to sensorineural hearing loss. *Laryngoscope.* 1983;93(6):717–720.
21. Bretlau P, Salomon G, Johnsen NJ. Otospongiosis and sodium fluoride. A clinical double-blind, placebo-controlled study on sodium fluoride treatment in otospongiosis. *Am J Otol.* 1989;10(1):20–22.
22. Bretlau P, Causse J, Causse JB, Hansen HJ, Johnsen NJ, Salomon G. Otospongiosis and sodium fluoride. A blind experimental and clinical evaluation of the effect of sodium fluoride treatment in patients with otospongiosis. *Ann Otol Rhinol Laryngol.* 1985;94(2 pt 1):103–107.
23. Shea JJ Jr. Fenestration of the oval window. *Ann Otol Rhinol Laryngol.* 1958;67(4):932–951.
24. Smyth GD, Hassard TH. Eighteen years experience in stapedectomy. The case for the small fenestra operation. *Ann Otol Rhinol Laryngol Suppl.* 1978;87(3 pt 2 suppl 49):3–36.
25. Fisch U. [Surgical results of stapedectomy or stapedotomy (author's transl)]. *HNO.* 1979;27(11):361–367.
26. McGee TM. Comparison of small fenestra and total stapedectomy. *Ann Otol Rhinol Laryngol.* 1981;90(6 pt 1):633–636.
27. Williams MD, Antonelli PJ, Williams LS, Moorhead JE. Middle ear prosthesis displacement in high-strength magnetic fields. *Otol Neurotol.* 2001;22(2):158–161.
28. Applebaum EL, Valvassori GE. Further studies on the effects of magnetic resonance imaging fields on middle ear implants. *Ann Otol Rhinol Laryngol.* 1990;99(10 pt 1):801–804.
29. Martin AD, Driscoll CL, Wood CP, Felmlee JP. Safety evaluation of titanium middle ear prostheses at 3.0 tesla. *Otolaryngol Head Neck Surg.* 2005;132(4):537–542.
30. Rajan GP, Atlas MD, Subramaniam K, Eikelboom RH. Eliminating the limitations of manual crimping in stapes surgery? A preliminary trial with the shape memory Nitinol stapes piston. *Laryngoscope.* 2005;115(2):366–369.
31. Christensen OB. Nickel dermatitis. An update. *Dermatol Clin.* 1990;8(1):37–40.
32. Sorom AJ, Driscoll CL, Beatty CW, Lundy L. Retrospective analysis of outcomes after stapedotomy with implantation of a self-crimping Nitinol stapes prosthesis. *Otolaryngol Head Neck Surg.* 2007;137(1):65–69.

33. Lesinski SG, Palmer A. CO_2 laser for otosclerosis: safe energy parameters. *Laryngoscope.* 1989;99(6 pt 2 suppl 46): 9–12.
34. Silverstein H, Rosenberg S, Jones R. Small fenestra stapedotomies with and without KTP laser: a comparison. *Laryngoscope.* 1989;99(5):485–488.
35. Gherini S, Horn KL, Causse JB, McArthur GR. Fiberoptic argon laser stapedotomy: is it safe? *Am J Otol.* 1993;14(3): 283–289.
36. Vollrath M, Schreiner C. The effects of the argon laser on temperature within the cochlea. *Acta Otolaryngol.* 1982; 93(5-6):341–348.
37. Lesinski SG. Lasers for otosclerosis—which one if any and why. *Lasers Surg Med.* 1990;10(5):448–457.
38. Lesinski SG, Stein JA. CO_2 laser stapedotomy. *Laryngoscope.* 1989;99(6 pt 2 suppl 46):20–24.
39. Jovanovic S, Schonfeld U, Scherer H. CO_2 laser stapedotomy with the "one-shot" technique—clinical results. *Otolaryngol Head Neck Surg.* 2004;131(5):750–757.
40. Michaelides EM, Kartush JM. Implications of sound levels generated by otologic devices. *Otolaryngol Head Neck Surg.* 2001;125(4):361–363.
41. Kiefer J, Tillein J, Ye Q, Klinke R, Gstoettner W. Application of carbon dioxide and erbium:yttrium-aluminum-garnet lasers in inner ear surgery: an experimental study. *Otol Neurotol.* 2004;25(3):400–409.
42. Parrilla C, Galli J, Fetoni AR, Rigante M, Paludetti G. Erbium: yttrium-aluminum-garnet laser stapedotomy—a safe technique. *Otolaryngol Head Neck Surg.* 2008;138(4): 507–512.
43. Keck T, Burner H, Rettinger G. Prospective clinical study on cochlear function after erbium:yttrium-aluminum-garnet laser stapedotomy. *Laryngoscope.* 2005;115(9):1627–1631.
44. Lippy WH, Schuring AG, Rizer FM. Intraoperative audiometry. *Laryngoscope.* 1995;105(2):214–216.
45. Hahn Y, Diaz, R, Hartmann, J, Bobinski, M, Brodie, H. Assessing stapes piston position using computed tomography: a cadaveric study. *Otol Neurotol.* In press.
46. Sheehy JL. Stapedectomy wire prosthesis for use with tissue grafts. *Trans Sect Otolaryngol Am Acad Ophthalmol Otolaryngol.* 1976;82(1):108–109.
47. Sheehy JL, Nelson RA, House HP. Stapes surgery at the Otologic Medical Group. *Am J Otol.* 1979;1(1):22–26.
48. Ginsberg IA, Hoffman SR, Stinziano GD, White TP. Stapedectomy—in depth analysis of 2405 cases. *Laryngoscope.* 1978;88(12):1999–2016.
49. Shea JJ. Thirty years of stapes surgery. *J Laryngol Otol.* 1988;102(1):14–19.
50. Rothbaum DL, Roy J, Hager GD, et al. Task performance in stapedotomy: comparison between surgeons of different experience levels. *Otolaryngol Head Neck Surg.* 2003; 128(1):71–77.
51. Caughey RJ, Pitzer GB, Kesser BW. Stapedectomy: demographics in 2006. *Otol Neurotol.* 2006;27(6):769–775.
52. Sheehy JL, Nelson RA, House HP. Revision stapedectomy: a review of 258 cases. *Laryngoscope.* 1981;91(1):43–51.

CHAPTER 10

Paragangliomas of the Temporal Bone

Matthew Kircher and Aftab Patni

HISTORY

Paragangliomas of the head and neck are tumors that are uniquely derived from paraganglionic or glomus tissue. Van Haller, in 1743, is credited with describing the carotid body, but its function was unknown.[1] Guild, in 1941,[2] identified vascular tissue on the promontory of the middle ear and convexity of the jugular bulb. He documented the histologic appearance and anatomic locations of glomus formations along the tympanic branch of the glossopharyngeal nerve, along the auricular branch of the vagus nerve and in the adventitia of the jugular bulb. He pointed out that the innervation of these glomerula is from nonmyelinated fibers of the adjacent nerve. Rosenwasser, in 1945,[3] was the first to recognize the relationship between the unusual vascular tumors of the temporal bone and the normally occurring glomus formations in the temporal bone as described by Guild.

Paragangliomas are reported with differing nomenclature. Within the temporal bone, they are most commonly referred to as glomus (glomus jugulare and glomus tympanicum) tumors, although chemodectomas, nonchromaffin tumors, resectomas, and tympanic body tumors are terms that have been used in the past. The preferred terminology refers to these tumors as jugulotympanic paragangliomasis.

PHYSIOLOGY, PATHOLOGY, AND PATHOPHYSIOLOGY

The paraganglionic system is considered important in fetal development as a source of catecholamines. Later, the developed adrenal gland takes over this secretory function. Paraganglia continue to serve a chemoreceptive role in central regulation of respiration. The carotid body signals changes in arterial pH, pCO_2, and pO_2 to the brainstem via the glossopharyngeal nerve.

Paraganglia contain two types of cells: chief and sustentacular cells. Type I or chief cells contain dense-core granules seen on electron microscopy. These granules contain catecholamines. Chief cells have traditionally been classified as part of the amine precursor uptake decarboxylase (APUD) system and more recently as a member of the diffuse neuroendocrine system. Chief cells are of paraganglionic origin and originate from neural crest cells. In contrast, type II or sustenacular cells are supporting cells and do not contain secretory granules. Paraganglia, in addition, possess an abundant microvasculature.[4]

Paraganglia are associated with the autonomic nervous system and its ganglions. Because of this association, paragangliomas in the temporal bone may be found in the region of the jugular fossa in the adventitia of the jugular bulb. Paraganglia or glomus bodies can be found in the tympanic canaliculus, cochlear promontory, retrofacial air cell tract, and the area of the geniculate ganglion within the temporal bone. Paraganglia follow the course of Jacobson's nerve (tympanic branch of glossopharyngeal nerve) and Arnold's nerve (auricular branch of vagus nerve) within the temporal bone. Within the remainder of the head and neck, these cells may be found at the bifurcation of the common carotid artery (carotid body), in the orbit in relation to the ciliary nerve (orbital body), at the ganglion nodosum (vagal body), and in the larynx along the superior and inferior laryngeal nerves.[5]

Paragangliomas are abnormal proliferations of paraganglia tissue. The most common location of paragangliomas in the head and neck is the carotid body (carotid body tumor), followed by the jugulotympanic region (glomus jugulare and glomus tympanicum). Paragangliomas of the vagus nerve (glomus vagale) are less prevalent. Temporal bone paragangliomas receive their vascular supply primarily from the inferior tympanic branch of the ascending pharyngeal artery, a branch of the external carotid artery.

Pathologically, paragangliomas have a characteristic histologic appearance with three common features: chief cells, sustentacular cells, and numerous capillaries. Chief cell predominate and are arranged in an organoid-nested pattern, known as zellballen. These clusters of cells are separated by a fibrovascular stroma with abundant small blood vessels and unmyelinated nerve fibers[6,7] (Figure 10–1). With electron microscopy, secretory granules are identified within the chief cells. Using immunohistochemistry, chief cells stain positively with neuron-specific enolase, chromogranin A, synaptophysin, and serotonin. Sustentacular cells stain positively with S-100 and glial fibrillary acidic protein[8] (Figure 10–2). Preoperative biopsies and fine needle aspirations of paragangliomas are difficult both due to their location within the temporal bone and their risk of profuse bleeding. Hence, definitive pathologic diagnosis is typically made post-tumor excision.

Paragangliomas can exhibit malignant potential in 10% of cases, though the incidence of malignant temporal bone paragangliomas is likely closer to 4%.[4] Histologically, it is difficult to differentiate between malignant tumors and their benign counterpart. Divisions based on degree of mitosis and invasiveness is unreliable. The only reliable indicator is identification of tumor in sites not known to contain paraganglia. The regional lymph nodes, bony skeleton, lung, and liver are common sites when metastasis is truly present. The aggressive

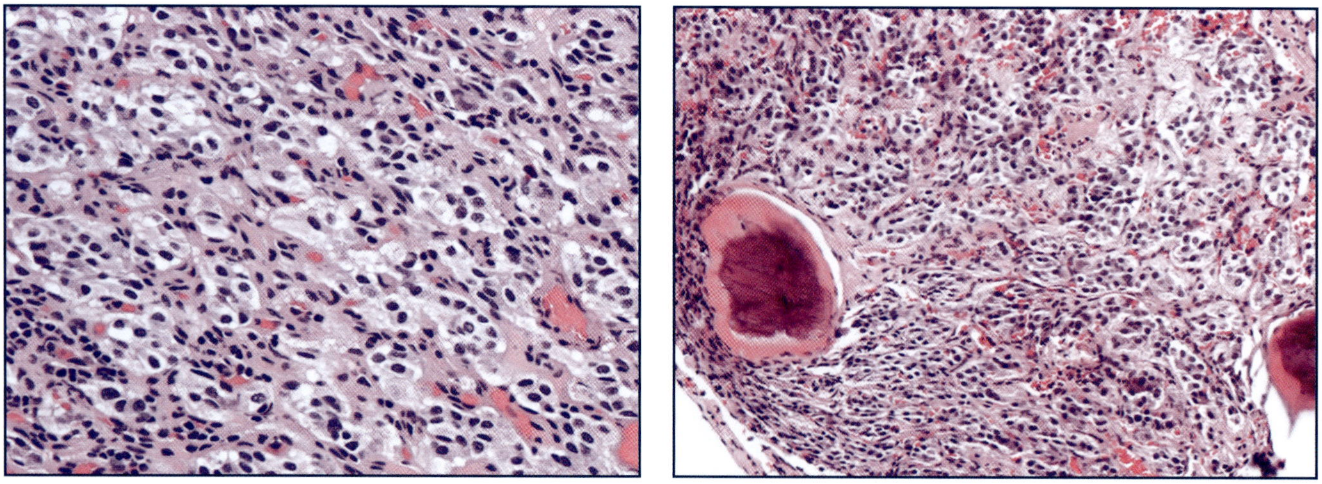

A B

Figure 10–1. A. H&E (hematoxylin and eosin) stain showing the polygonal to oval tumor cells arranged in the distinctive cell balls, called *zellballen* (200×). These cells are separated by fibrovascular stroma and surrounded by sustentacular cells. **B.** H&E stain demonstrates bone invasion (100×).

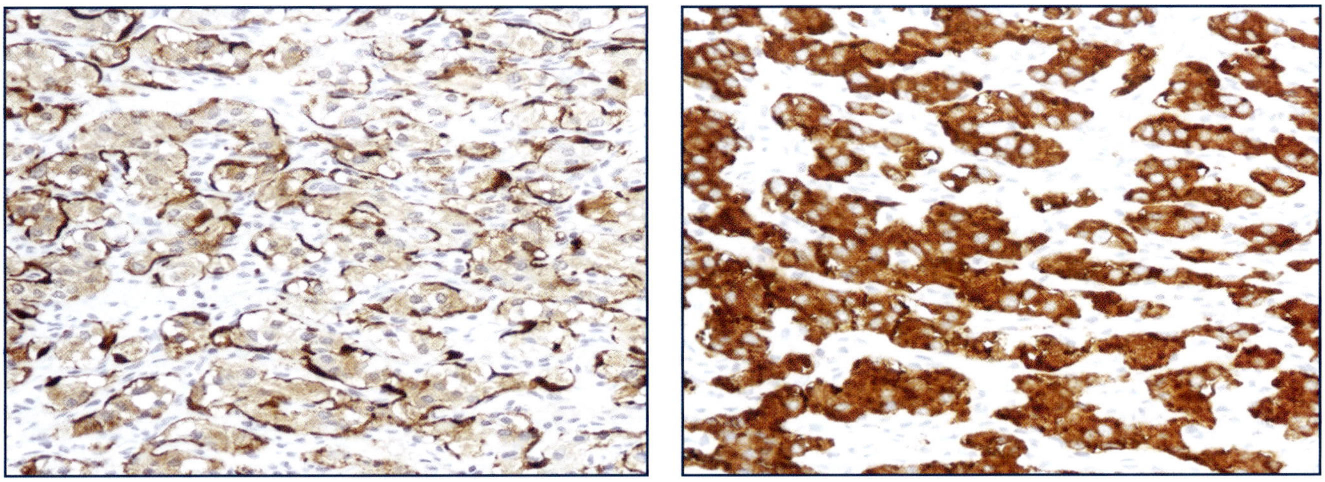

A B

Figure 10–2. A. S-100 stain: stains the sustentacular cells (brown) surrounding the tumor cells (200×). **B**. Synaptophysin stain: stains the tumor cell cytoplasm brown (200×).

local behavior of these tumors does not imply malignancy as these lesions have a propensity to erode the skull base, involve the carotid artery, and spread intracranially. In addition, 10% of paragangliomas can be multicentric.

The carotid body is extremely sensitive to changes in oxygen tension. A higher incidence of carotid body tumors is found in humans inhabiting higher altitudes and in patients with cardiopulmonary diseases, such as COPD and congenital cyanotic heart disease.[9,10] It is unclear whether these factors contribute to the formation of temporal bone paragangliomas.

The ability to synthesize catecholamines in paragangliomas does not imply a functional tumor, as is more frequently seen in pheochromocytomas. Approximately 2% of tumors are functional and produce symptoms, though essentially all glomus tumors have the potential to secrete catecholamines.[11] Experimentally, it takes a five-fold increase in norepinephrine to produce symptoms. Symptoms related to catecholamine excess are headache, sweating, palpitations, and hypertension. A functional tumor should prompt a search for catecholamines and their metabolites, metanephrines and vanillymandelic acid. Head and neck paraganglia do not contain the enzyme that converts norepinephrine to epinephrine. Hence, the presence of excess epinephrine should alert the physician to search for a concurrent adrenal pheochromocytoma. Glomus tumors can have endocrine activity with the secretion of hormones including serotonin, kallikrein, and histamine. When present, the clinical presentation may include diarrhea, hyperglycemia, abdominal pain, and bronchoconstriction.

Somatostatin receptors are found in high density within paragangliomas and other neuroendocrine and neural tumors. This information can help detect primary, multiple, and metastatic paragangliomas via octreotride scintigraphy.[12] In addition, ^{111} indium octreotide, a somatostatin analog, may have adjunctive use as a tumor growth inhibitor.

Similarly, meta-iodobenzylguanidine (MIBG) is selectively taken up by paragangliomas and can be used both diagnostically and therapeutically as radiolabeled ^{131} I-MIBG.[13] A dopamine analog, 18-fluorodopamine, can also be used in diagnosing multicentric disease.[14]

EPIDEMIOLOGY

Paragangliomas are usually benign lesions. They represent the most common benign tumor of the temporal bone, behind acoustic neuromas. Generally, paragangliomas occur in the fifth decade of life, though they can occur at any age and tend to demonstrate considerable biologic variability in their clinical behavior and growth patterns.

Most paragangliomas are solitary. Multiple or asynchronous tumors can occur in 4 to 10% of patients. The most common reported combination is a glomus tympanicum with a carotid body tumor.[15] Multiple paragangliomas and pheochromocytomas can be seen in familial syndromes. The proportion of patients with a positive family history is variably estimated at 10% in the United States and up to 50% in the Netherlands. These patients with a positive family history have a 30% incidence of multiple glomus tumors.[16] Syndrome of familial paragangliomas, multiple endocrine neoplasia types IIA and IIB, neurofibromatosis I, and von Hippel-Lindau disease have all been described.

Syndrome of familial paragangliomas is a hereditary form of the disease where head and neck paragangliomas can be inherited without other tumors. It is associated with germline mutations in the mitochondrial complex II subunits encoded by genes SDHB, SDHC, and SDHD. A mutation in the SDHD gene appears to be responsible for a chronic hypoxia signal within the chief cell leading to cellular proliferation and paraganglioma formation through an unknown mechanism. These mutations are found in the majority of familial paragangliomas, but also in 11% of nonfamilial head and neck paragangliomas.[17,18] Interestingly, the disease phenotype is transmitted via paternal genetic imprinting, where it is passed only through the fathers, whereas mothers do not transmit the disease.[19] An affected father will pass on the disease to 50% of his offspring. Identification of these genes has important clinical implications for diagnosis and genetic counseling.

MEN IIA syndromes present as a triad of medullary thyroid carcinoma, pheochromocytoma, and parathyroid hyperplasia, whereas MENIIB also includes mucosal neuromas without parathyroid hyperplasia. Von Hippel-Lindau syndrome presents with retinal angiomas, and cerebellar hemoangioblastomas.[20] Carney[21] described a triad of gastric leiomyosarcoma, pulmonary chondroma, and extraadrenal functional paragangliomas as Carney's complex.

GROWTH PATTERNS

Most temporal bone paragangliomas follow an indolent and protracted course of slow growth. They can cause marked local bony erosion and local invasion. They migrate through naturally occurring tissue planes via naturally occurring fissures, foramina, and air cell tracts following a path of least resistance. In the hypotympanum, glomus jugulare tumors have access to the hypoglossal canal, jugular foramen, and carotid canal. They can extend to involve the posterior fossa and then expand intracranially. Glomus tumors can follow the internal carotid artery to the cavernous sinus and the middle cranial fossa. They may involve the facial nerve by extension into the facial recess and retrofacial air cells. In addition, tumors can tract along the peritubal air cells to the petrous apex. Extensive middle ear involvement can lead to ossicular chain impairment, erosion of the tympanic membrane, external canal involvement, and otic capsule invasion via the round window. Rarely, glomus tumors may exhibit rapid, aggressive growth characteristics, resulting in short-term survival.[5] Paragangliomas that spread hematogenously are given a diagnosis of malignancy as long as metastasis are documented in sites known to not contain paraganglia, hence ruling out synchronous lesions.

NATURAL HISTORY

Paragangliomas of the temporal bone, though slow to grow, can cause a significant amount of morbidity and morbidity. Tumor growth is the rule over the lifetime of the individual. Intracranial extension occurs in 15 to 36%. Based on the pathway of extension, cranial nerve abnormalities and deficits may be seen in up to 37 to 46% of patients.[22–24] The associated mortality is typically low and these patients can live many years, even with advanced disease. The reported mortality from temporal bone paragangliomas regardless of the type of treatment received is about 6%, thus the majority of patients will have a normal life expectancy.[25,26] Despite the low mortality, paragangliomas can cause progressive local destruction which results in significant functional compromise with debilitating symptoms.

SYMPTOMS AND SIGNS

The most common presenting symptom of jugulotympanic paragangliomas is pulsatile tinnitus followed by conductive hearing loss. The increased vascularity of the mass results in a pulsatile tinnitus that is synchronous with the heartbeat and is present in up to 98% of patients. Occasionally, these pulsations may be objectively documented by using an impedance audiometer, the waves increase in magnitude with jugular vein compression and decrease in magnitude with carotid artery compression. Involvement of the middle ear causes a conductive hearing loss in approximately 60% of patients via compression of the ossicles, adherence to the tympanic membrane, or invasion of the tympanic membrane. Sensorineural hearing loss occurs in 13% of patients with tumor invasion into the cochlea or labyrinth or with intracranial extension with cochlear nerve involvement. Vertigo may be present if the growth compresses the footplate of the stapes or invades the labyrinth.[5,22–24]

The most common finding is a red, vascular, pulsatile middle ear mass in the hypotympanum or promontory (Figure 10–3). In the later stages, a paragangliomas may extend through the tympanic membrane and present as a bleeding aural polyp (Figure 10–4). Brown's sign is present when positive pressure applied with a pneumatic otoscope produces a distinct blanching of the tympanic membrane or the mass behind it. It is highly suggestive of a vascular tumor. Tuning forks will likely reveal a conductive hearing loss, though a sensorineural hearing loss may be present and suggests cochlear invasion or retrocochlear compression (Figure 10–5). Vestibular testing may show unilateral caloric weakness

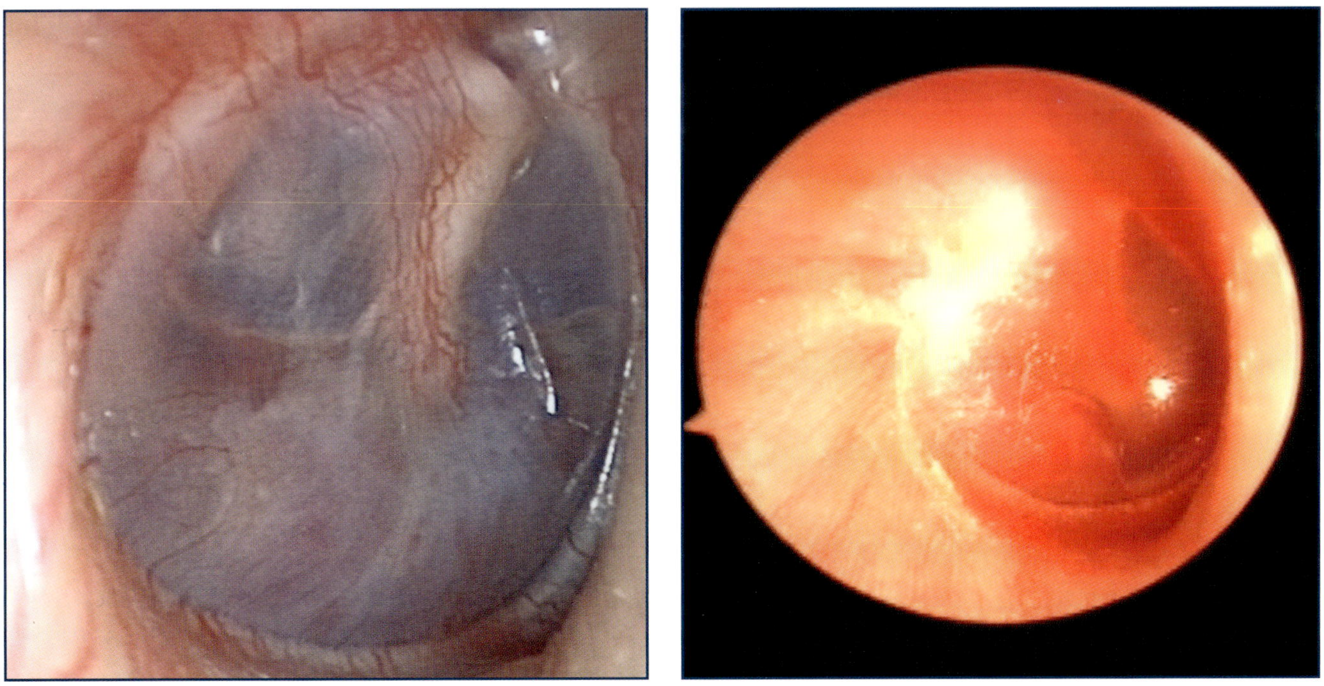

A B

Figure 10–3. A. Right glomus tumor seen through tympanic membrane filling inferior half of middle ear space. **B.** Glomus tumor seen through tympanic membrane.

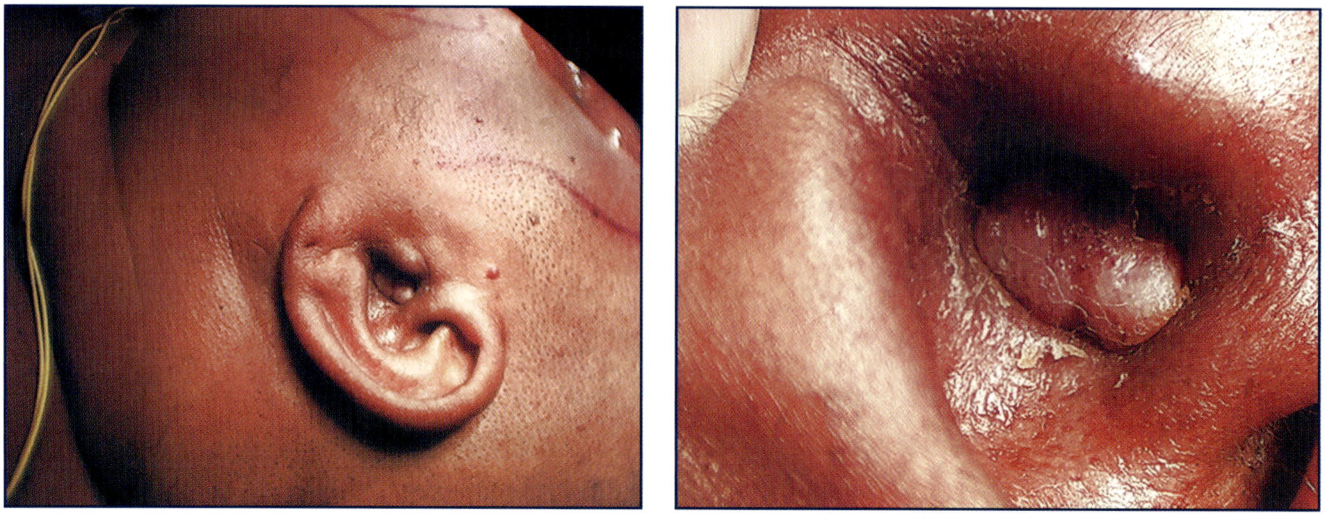

A B

Figure 10–4. **A**. Patient has a large firm ear canal polyp with bloody otorrhea. Interestingly, pressure application would cause acute vertigo with nystagmus secondary to underlying labyrinthine fistula. **B**. Close-up view of polyp of EAC.

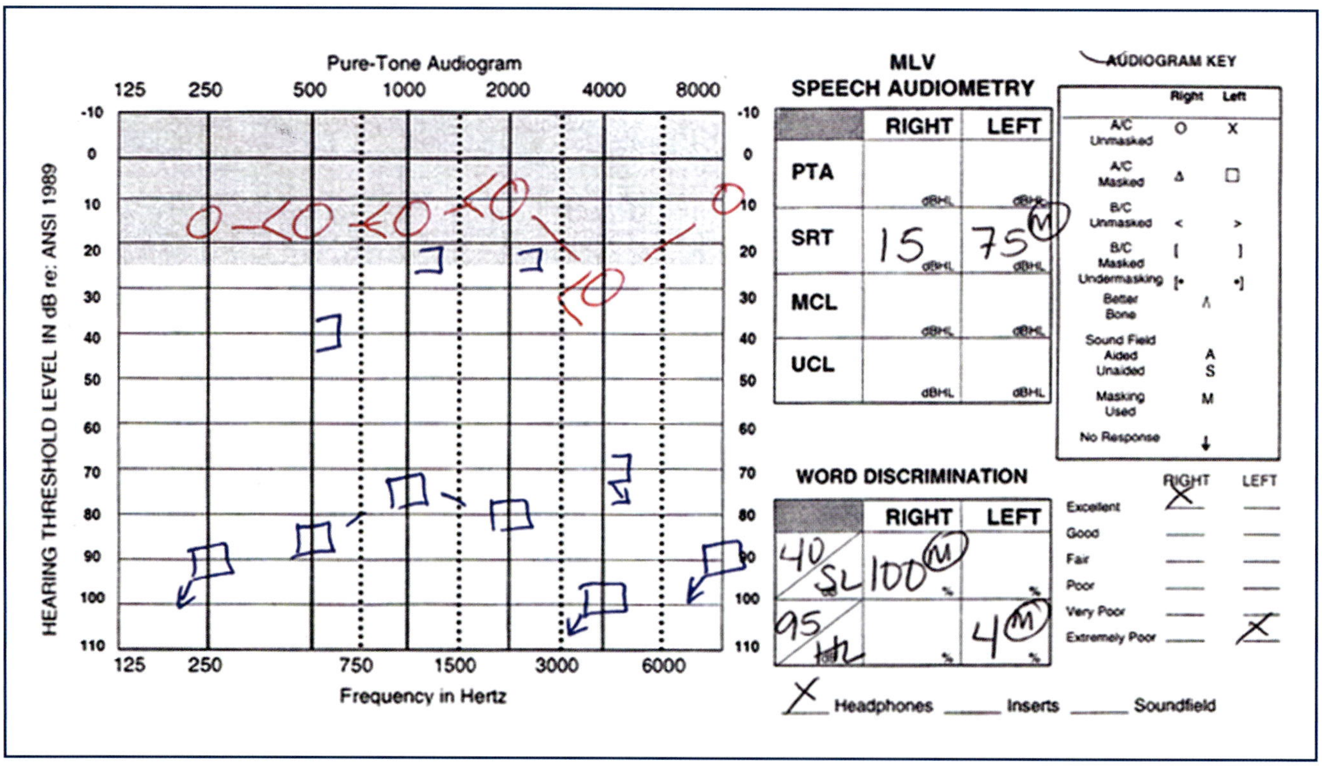

Figure 10–5. This patient's glomus tumor caused extensive erosion of the ossicles and labyrinthine invasion, hence the mixed hearing loss with poor discrimination score.

and office head-shake testing may confirm a nystagmus with the fast phase of nystagmus toward the opposite ear in advanced disease.

Tumors extending into the jugular foramen can produce a range of symptoms and signs. Because of the generous space of the jugular foramen and the relative compressibility of the jugular bulb and vein, tumors may grow to a sizeable lesion prior to causing lower cranial nerve palsies. Encroachment of the carotid artery by tumor can lead to Horner's syndrome secondary to sympathetic plexus involvement. The patient may have facial paresis or paralysis in 18 to 66% of cases, which results from either a compression neuropathy or direct neurolysis by the tumor anywhere along the fallopian canal. Hoarseness, dysphagia, and aspiration are by far the most common symptoms of lower cranial nerve involvement.[22–24] Vagus nerve invasion causes a vocal cord paresis or paralysis in approximately 30% of patients. Decreased gag reflex, shoulder, and tongue weakness are found in 21%, 17%, and 25% of patients, respectively. The overall incidence of any cranial nerve involvement by tumor is 37 to 46% and that of intracranial extension 15 to 36%.[22–24] The presence of preoperative cranial nerve deficit is associated with a higher incidence of intracranial extension.

Involvement of the posterior fossa may be entirely asymptomatic. With mass effect, symptoms of cerebellar compression, ataxia, dysdiadochokinesia, nystagmus with diplopia, and occipital headache can occur.[5] Posterior fossa extension was discovered in 50% of patients with jugular foramen syndrome and in 75% of patients with CN XII palsy.[22] Middle fossa involvement may be associated with diplopia, sensory changes in the distribution of any branches of CN V, and retro-orbital headache. Middle fossa extension was discovered in 50% of patients with Horner's syndrome (ptosis, miosis, and anhydrosis).[5]

Catecholamine secreting tumors may cause headache, sweating, palpitations, hypertension, tremor, anxiety, syncope, or weight loss. In addition, they can produce endocrine symptoms of diarrhea, hyperglycemia, abdominal pain, and bronchoconstriction. Frequently these symptoms occur in paroxysms lasting minutes to hours, with symptom-free periods between attacks.

DIFFERENTIAL DIAGNOSIS

Other middle ear vascular lesions, vascular anomalies, and tumors can mimic a paraganglioma. The high riding or dehiscent jugular bulb is the most common vascular variant of the middle ear. It is seen as a blue mass extending above the tympanic annulus and can be present in up to 6% of patients. An aberrant internal carotid artery or an internal carotid artery aneurysm can be seen as a red mass behind the tympanic membrane. Office binocular microscopy in conjunction with imaging will help in differentiating these variants and avoid biopsies that can result in massive hemorrhage.[27,28] Middle ear cholesterol granulomas, a hemotympanum, and Schwartze's sign of otosclerosis can mimic a glomus mass. Benign and malignant tumors of the middle ear, including hemangiomas, neuromas, meningiomas, adenomas and adenocarcinomas can occur. Patients who present with a mass of the jugular foramen can have a schwannoma of the IX, X, XI, and XII cranial nerves. Jugular foramen meningiomas and metastatic lesions are also seen.

METABOLIC EVALUATION

Though a catecholamine secreting tumor is uncommon, their presence must be determined pre-treatment. All tumors should be screened for secretion of dopamine, epinephrine, and norepinephrine and their metabolites: normetanephrine, metanephrine, and vanillylmandelic acid. This should be done with both blood plasma levels and 24-hour urine collection samples. Plasma catecholamines, normetanephrines, and metanephrines levels have a sensitivity of 97%, while 24-hour urine collection to examine for catecholamines, vanillymandelic acid, normetanephrine and metanephrines has a sensitivity range of 50 to 74%.[29] Unlike pheochromocytomas, head and neck paragangliomas cannot convert norepinephrine into epinephrine because they lack the enzyme, phenylethanolamine-N-methyltransferase. Hence, high levels of epinephrine should prompt a search for a concomitant pheochromocytoma.

Catecholamines act on the heart and blood vessels through alpha and beta adrenoceptors. The overall cardiovascular response is increased cardiac output and increased peripheral vascular resistance, which results in an elevation in arterial blood pressure. Secreting tumors can cause significant intraoperative hemodynamic changes, thus perioperative invasive pulse and blood pressure monitoring and management is important. The cardiovascular actions of catecholamines can be blocked by treatment with an alpha- and beta-receptor blocker.

IMAGING STUDIES

Imaging studies are essential in defining the lesion, determining the extent of tumor, and planning surgery or radiotherapy. Before CT and MRI scans, plain films and angiography were the prime methods used for diagnosis. Now CT scanning, CT angiogram, MR imaging, MR angiogram and venogram, ultrasonography, and nuclear scintigraphy are noninvasive diagnostic options.

Thin section CT scanning is very useful for paragangliomas of the temporal bone. It demonstrates the bony detail of the middle ear, mastoid, and jugular foramen. It allows assessment of tumor size and disease extent. It is particularly helpful in identifying key surgical landmarks, such as the carotid canal, the fallopian canal, the labyrinth, the ossicular chain, and the hypotympanum. In addition, soft tissue algorithms will define intracranial, infratemporal fossa, and parapharyngeal space extension. A CT scan can also help differentiate glomus tumors from other vascular anomalies.

On a CT scan, glomus tympanicum tumors will present as a mass on the cochlear promontory (Figure 10–6). Ossicular chain involvement, extension into the mastoid air cells, erosion of the labyrinth and eustachian tube are easily visible on CT (Figure 10–7). An intravenous bolus of contrast will clearly reveal the hypervascular mass with intense enhancement. Glomus jugulare tumors will show a "moth-eaten" pattern of bony destruction and enlargement of the jugular fossa (Figure 10–8). Erosion of the jugulocarotid spine, the bony septum separating the carotid canal from the jugular foramen, is classically seen. These lesions may compress or invade the jugular vein and compress or invade the carotid artery. CT angiography and venography can further evaluate the intracranial arterial and venous pathology present and may obviate need for angiogram unless preoperative embolization is planned.

MR imaging also plays a valuable role in the diagnosis and evaluation of patients. The tumor, adjacent soft tissue and vascular structures are well demonstrated. T1-weighted images identify bone marrow and fat. T2-weighted images will identify intra-axial disease and CSF.[30] A variety of MR protocols are used and complex lesions should be reviewed with a neuroradiologist.

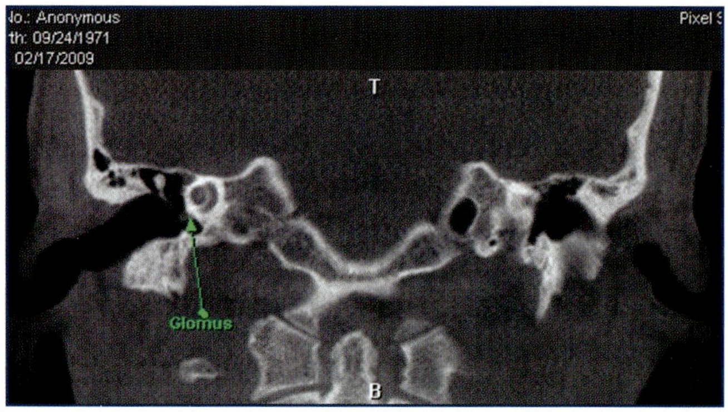

A

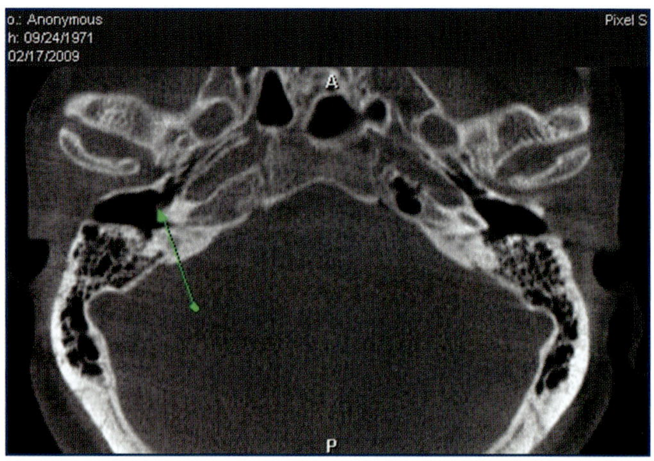

B

Figure 10–6. Coronal (**A**) and axial CT (**B**) of the temporal bone showing a small glomus tympanicum, right.

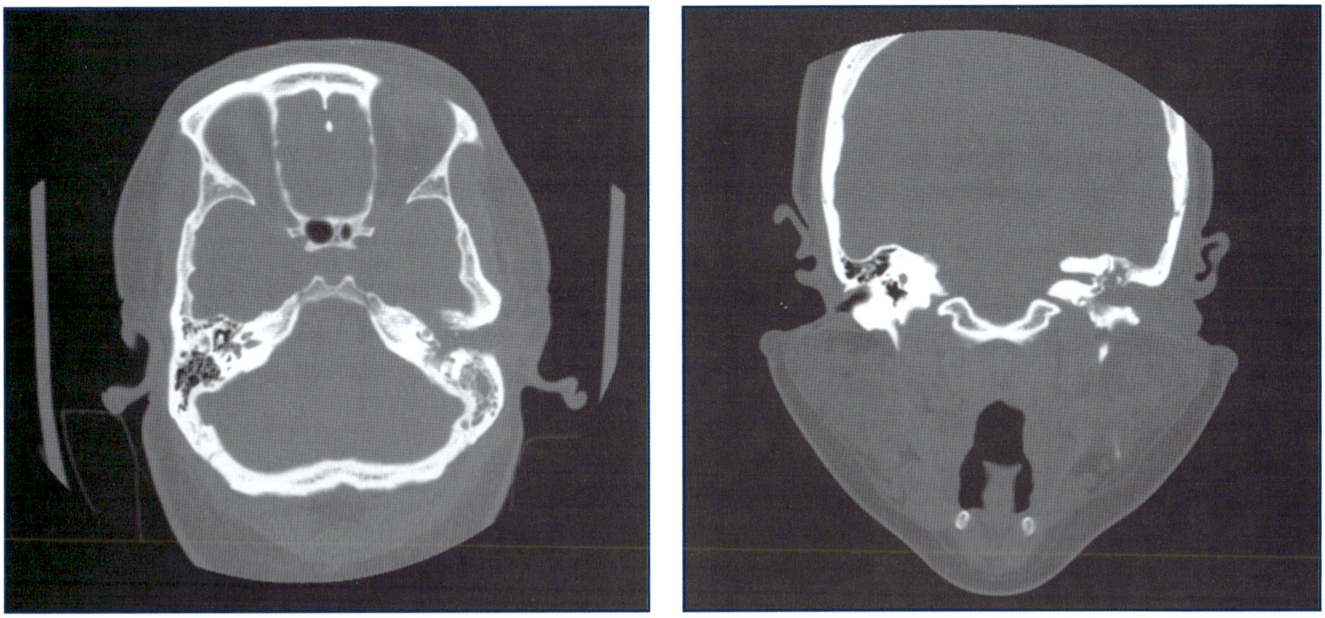

A B

Figure 10–7. CT temporal bone: **A.** axial view shows a large glomus tympanicum with erosion into the geniculate ganglion, eustachian tube, carotid canal, and round window. **B.** Coronal view shows ossicular erosion and a lateral semicircular canal fistula.

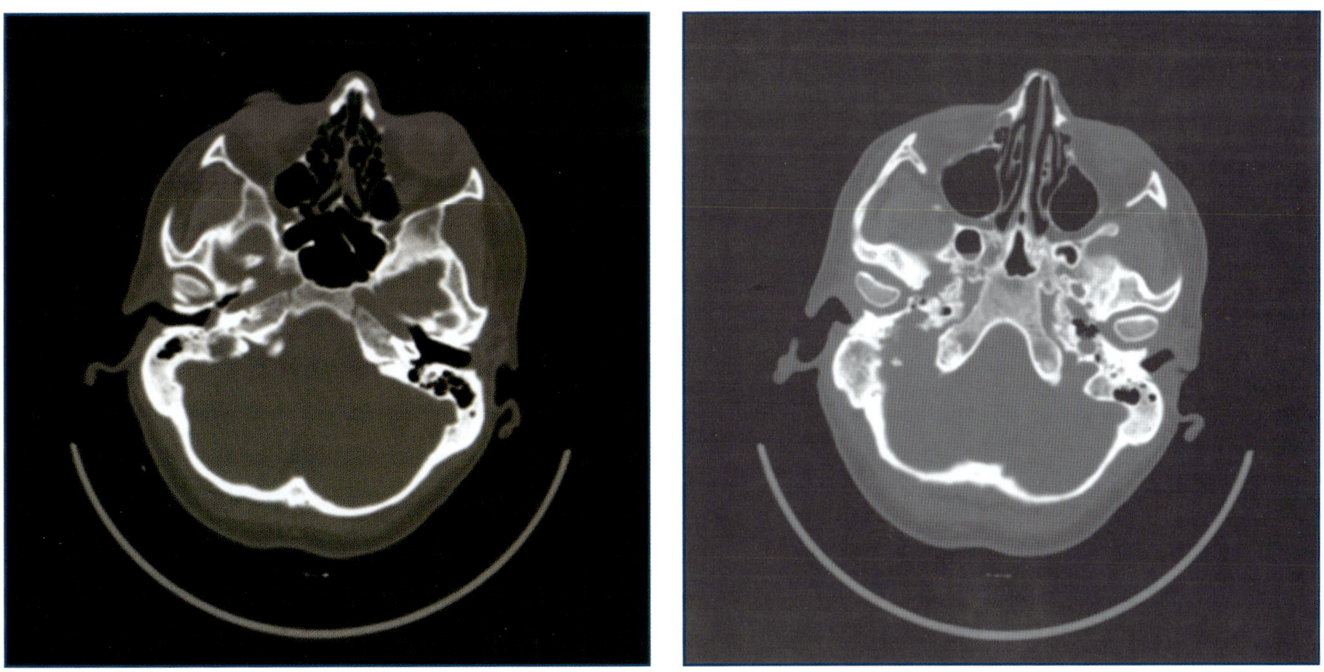

A B

Figure 10–8. CT of temporal bones: axial view. Right jugular foramen mass with destruction of the fossa. Erosion of the jugulocarotid spine and skull base is evident.

Paragangliomas have common MR imaging characteristics. A well-defined hypointense mass with areas of signal void is typically seen on T1-weighted images. A classic salt and pepper appearance is best seen on T2-weighted images but may be apparent on T1-weighted images also.[31] This bright and dark appearance represents the high vascularity within the mass with associated areas of hemorrhage, slow-flowing blood, and tumor cells. Gadolinium contrast enhancement aids in the assessment (Figures 10–9, 10–10, and 10–11). Small areas of dural and intradural extension and neural foramina involvement are readily apparent. Schwannomas and meningiomas lack such findings. Schwannomas become more dumbbell-shaped as they enlarge, extending superiorly into the basal cistern and inferiorly into the parapharyngeal space. They cause smooth enlargement of the jugular foramen without bony destruction and enhance evenly. Meningiomas have a high density on precontrast CT scans and adjacent hyperostosis may be present.

MR angiography and venography allow delineation of arterial and venous structures, obviating the need for a four-vessel angiogram until prior to the surgery in conjunction with embolization. MRA is a noninvasive technique that does not require contrast agents. The vascular images are displayed in a 3-D format. Tumor vascular supply, vessel displacement, and evidence of venous thrombosis may all be determined preoperatively[30] (Figure 10–12). MR angiograms also allow detection of synchronous ipsilateral and contralateral paragangliomas and metastatic lesions.[32] Despite the high sensitivity and specificity of MRA, the four-vessel angiogram remains the gold standard secondary to superior vascular resolution[33] (Figure 10–13).

Paragangliomas have a high density of somatostatin receptors on their cell surface and this characteristic can be used in nuclear imaging. Multiple radioactive agents have been used to provide information regarding tumor location, multicentricity, and tumor recurrence, as well as screening protocols in familial paragangliomas. Octreotide scintigraphy uses radiolabeled ^{111}indium octreotide, a somastatin analog. In addition, ^{123}I-MIBG or radioactive methyliodobenzylguanidine, ^{111}indium pentetreotide (a somastatin analog), and 18-fluorodopamine can also be used as markers.

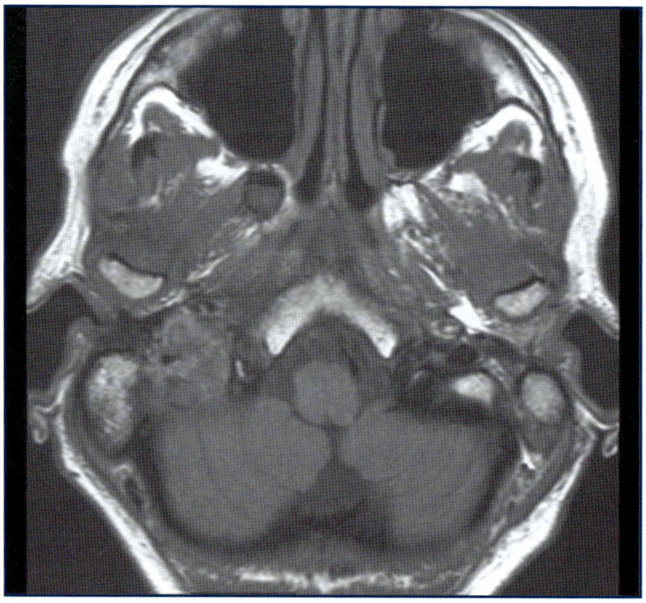

A

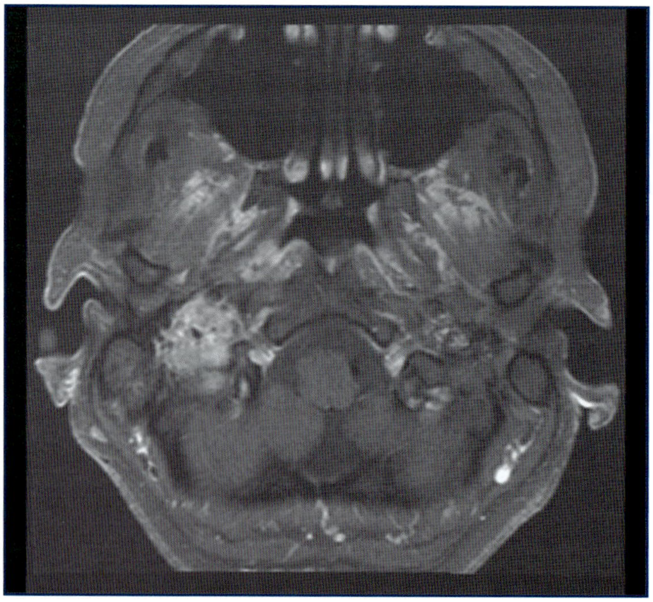

B

Figure 10–9. A. MRI T1 axial image with a right jugular foramen mass. **B.** MRI T1 SE axial image (fat suppression) with gadolinium clearly demonstrates the tumor mass.

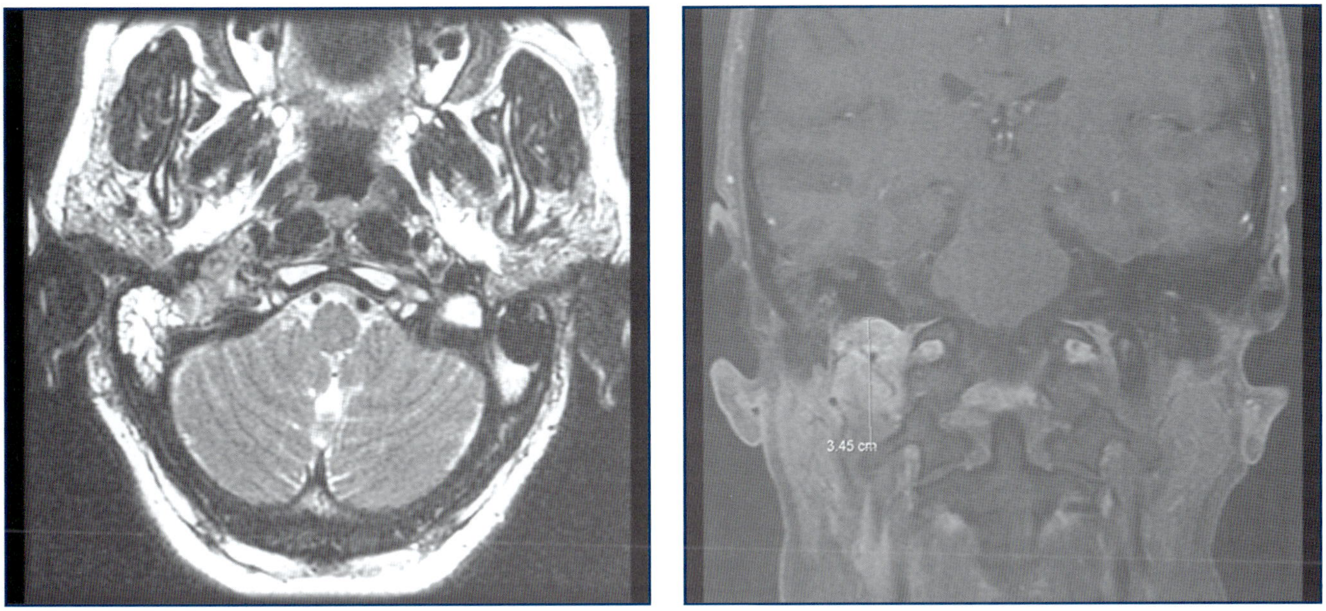

A B

Figure 10–10. **A**. MRI T2-weighted axial image demonstrates both obstructive bright fluid within the mastoid and the isotense tumor mass with salt and pepper appearance. **B**. MRI T1-weighted with gadolinium enhancement identifies inferior extension of the tumor into the parapharyngeal space.

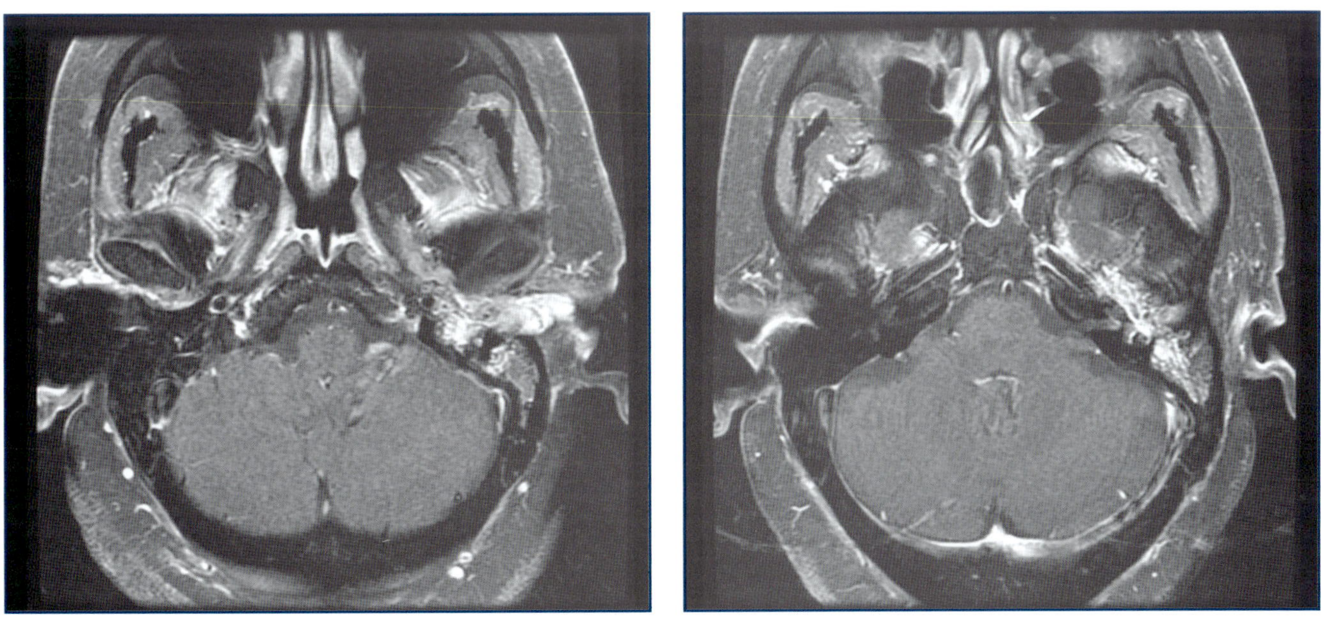

A B

Figure 10–11. MRI T1 SE with gadolinium. (**A**) Shows a massive ear canal polyp. (**B**) Tumor extends to involve the geniculate ganglion and tympanic and mastoid segments of the facial nerve. This patient had a complete facial paralysis.

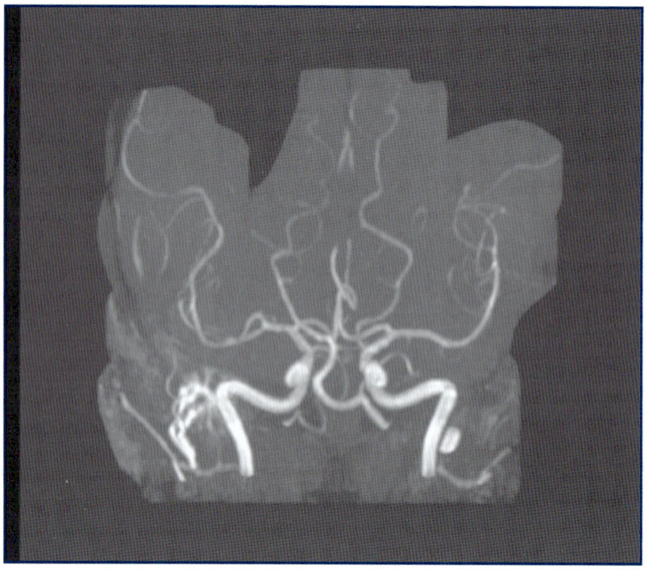

A

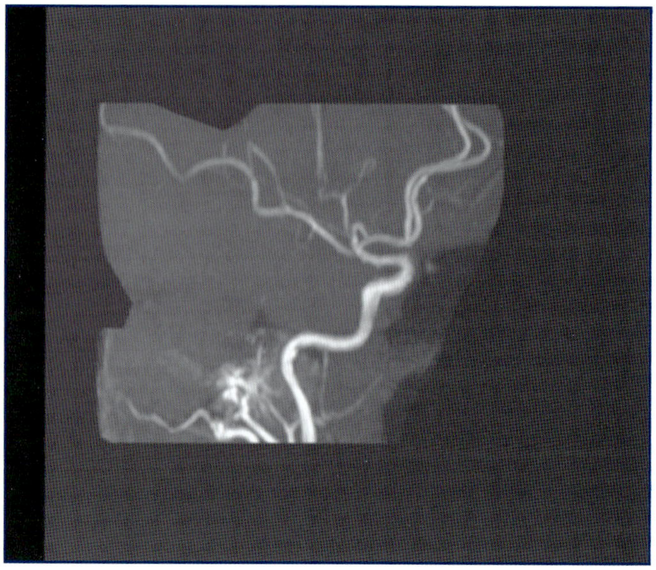

B

Figure 10–12. MRA (**A**) AP and (**B**) lateral views. Right glomus jugulare is apparent. A dilated and enlarged ascending pharyngeal artery is noted feeding the vascular tumor.

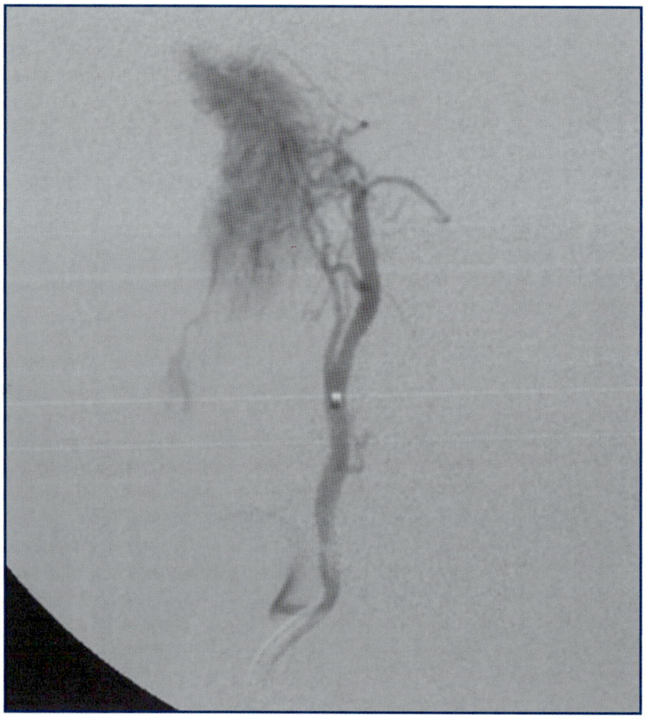

Figure 10–13. Four-vessel angiogram. This is an AP view showing tumor blush after injection of contrast into the ascending pharyngeal artery, which was the dominant vessel to the tumor.

Duplex ultrasonography is more useful in demonstrating a hypervascular mass within the confines of the neck, such as carotid body tumors. It is rarely useful for paragangliomas of the temporal bone secondary to the bony confines of the skull base. Transcranial doppler studies can provide information regarding collateral blood flow and the direction of flow within the cerebral circulation when carotid artery compromise is suspected or ligation is anticipated.

ANGIOGRAPHY AND EMBOLIZATION

Although imaging evaluation beyond MRI and high-resolution CT scan is rarely required for glomus tympanicum, angiography is obtained for most glomus jugulare preoperatively. Paragangliomas have near pathognomonic appearance on arteriography and can confirm the presurgical diagnosis. The typical appearance is of a hypervascular mass with enlarged feeding vessels. There is an intense tumor blush and an early venous phase. A standard four-vessel arteriogram assessing the carotid and vertebral arteries and the sigmoid-jugular venous system is performed. It demonstrates the primary arterial supply, collateral vessels, and vascular encroachment. The relationship of the tumor to the internal carotid artery and jugular vein is clearly shown, including degree of vascular encasement and thrombosis. The contralateral sigmoid sinus and jugular vein must be patent if surgical excision of glomus jugulare is planned to prevent intracranial hypertension.

The angiogram and MRI contribute valuable information regarding the need for vessel sacrifice. If it is likely that the internal carotid artery will be resected, then preoperative patient tolerance must be determined. The ideal preoperative method to assess tolerance to either ICA reconstruction or resection is controversial. Temporary balloon occlusion of the carotid artery assesses the adequacy of the collateral circulation of the circle of Willis. Alternatively, xenon perfusion brain scans may be employed.

Typically, glomus jugulare receive their blood supply from more than one vascular pedicle and are considered multicompartmental. This fact is crucial when these tumors are embolized because each vascular pedicle must be embolized for adequate devascularization of the entire lesion to occur. The vascular supply to these lesions is based on the normal vascular anatomy of the temporal bone. The ascending pharyngeal artery, a branch of the external carotid artery, typically is the dominant vascular pedicle for most jugulotympanic paragangliomas. The most significant branch from the ascending pharyngeal artery is the inferior tympanic artery. Other vascular sources include internal maxillary artery, occipital artery, ascending cervical artery, posterior auricular artery, and facial artery. In larger tumors, it is not uncommon to have additional vascular supply from branches of the internal carotid arteries and vertebral arteries, including the caroticotympanic branches of the intrapetrous carotid and posterior inferior cerebellar artery, respectively. Last, arteriography may identity small multicentric paragangliomas not noted on other imaging studies.

Retrograde jugular venography can demonstrate invasion or compression of the jugular bulb and collateral venous channels. Currently, it is rarely needed because MRV is a superior noninvasive method for this purpose.

Intravascular embolization entails the use of microcatheters to gain access to feeding vessels. Once the specific vessels are identified, a microparticulate embolic agent, such as polyvinyl alcohol (PVA) foam, is employed. PVA deeply penetrates the tissue and leads to thrombosis of precapillaries, capillaries, and postcapillary venules (Figures 10–14 and 10–15). The usefulness of preoperative embolization is well established but must be individualized. Benefits of embolization include reduced intraoperative time, reduced blood loss, and decreased operative risks.[34,35] Risks of intravascular embolization include stroke, blindness, cranial nerve deficits, soft tissue and skin necrosis, poor wound healing after surgical treatment, and complications at the access site. Stroke results from passage of emboli to the internal carotid circulation, whereas cranial nerve deficits result from loss of blood supply to the particular cranial nerve or from neural compression from edema and necrosis. Embolization itself is not a treatment modality and should be performed 24 to 48 hours prior to the surgery. A longer delay between surgery and embolization allows for revascularization and actually increases edema and inflammation.

CLASSIFICATION

Though no uniform classification scheme exists, three classification systems are useful for temporal bone paragangliomas. All three classifications are based on tumor location and extent of disease.

The Glasscock-Jackson classification[36] is divided based on tumor type as follows:

Glomus Tympanicum

Type I: Small mass limited to the promontory

Type II: Tumor completely filling the middle ear space

Type III: Tumor filling middle ear, extending into the mastoid process

Type IV: Tumor filling the middle ear, extending into mastoid or through tympanic membrane to fill external auditory canal; may extend anterior to internal carotid artery.

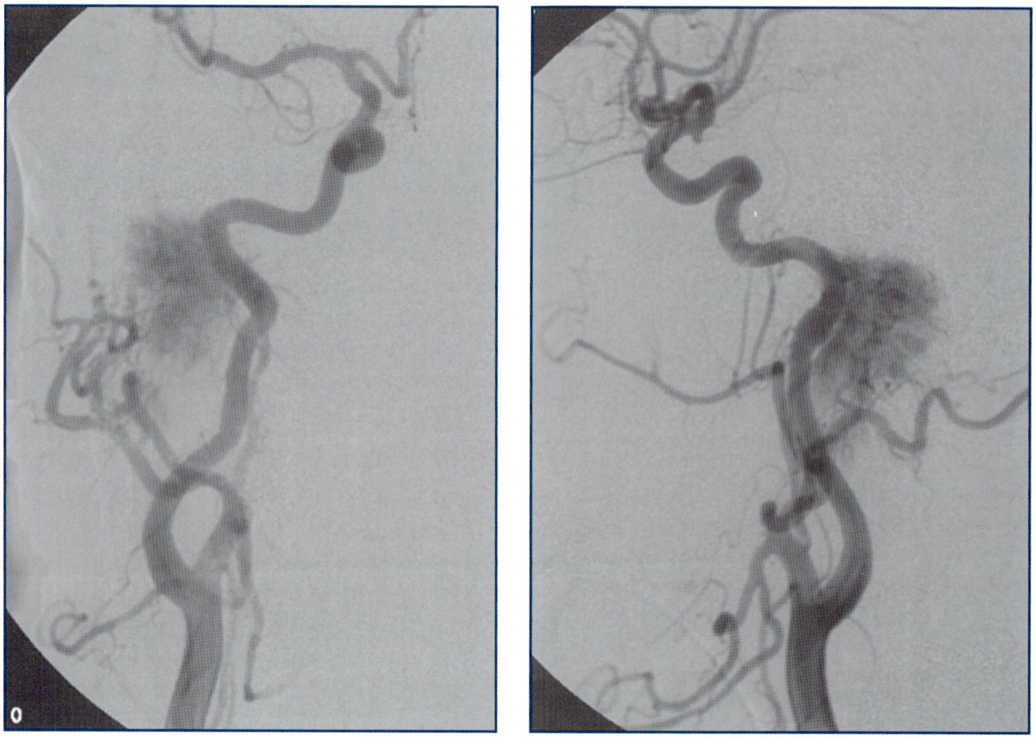

A B

Figure 10–14. Angiogram: Right common carotid artery injection with AP (**A**) and lateral (**B**) views. The enlarged ascending pharyngeal artery on the AP view is the dominant arterial supply to the tumor mass.

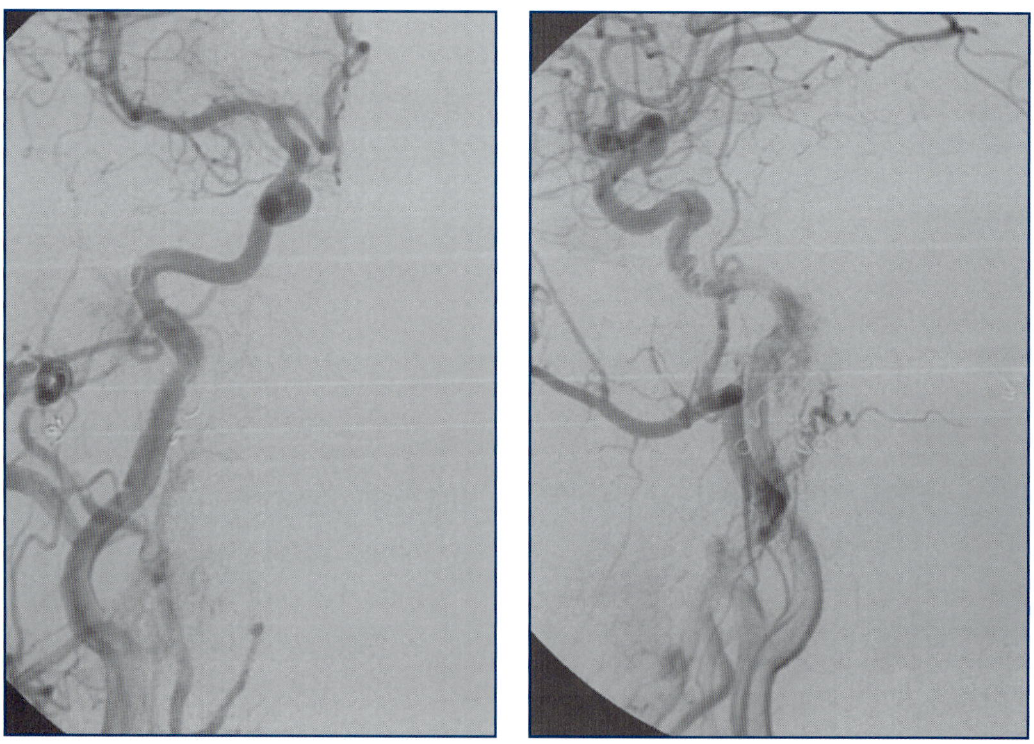

A B

Figure 10–15. Right common carotid artery injection with AP (**A**) and lateral (**B**) views. Embolization of the ascending pharyngeal artery results in loss of tumor vascularity and tumor blush.

Glomus Jugulare

Type I: Small tumor involving jugular bulb, middle ear, and mastoid process

Type II: Tumor extending under internal auditory canal; may have intracranial extension

Type III: Tumor extending into petrous apex; may have intracranial extension

Type IV: Tumor extending beyond petrous apex into clivus or infratemporal fossa; may have intracranial extension.

Fisch and Mattox[37] proposed a refined Fisch A, B, C, D classification as follows:

Type A: Tumors limited to the middle ear cleft

Type B: Tumors limited to the tympanomastoid area with no infralabyrinthine compartment involvement. Jugular bulb is intact

Type C_{1-4}: Tumors involving the infralabyrinthine compartment of the temporal bone and extending into the petrous apex. Jugular bulb is always eroded with variable carotid artery involvement (subtypes 1–4). Type C_1 may erode the carotid foramen, but does not invade the carotid artery. Type C_2 extends to involve the vertical carotid artery. Type C_3 invades both the vertical and horizontal carotid canal. Type C_4 tumors extend further to involve the entire intrapetrous carotid artery up to the cavernous sinus.

Type D_1: Tumors with an intracranial extension less than 2 cm in diameter

Type D_2: Tumors with an intracranial extension greater than 2 cm in diameter

De la Cruz[4] proposed a classification system with an associated surgical approach as follows:

1. Tympanic: Transcanal
2. Tympanomastoid: Mastoid-extended facial recess
3. Jugular bulb: Mastoid-neck (possible limited facial nerve rerouting)
4. Carotid artery: Infratemporal fossa ± subtemporal
5. Transdural: Infratemporal fossa/intracranial
6. Craniocervical: Transcondylar
7. Vagal: Cervical

TREATMENT

Management decisions regarding jugulotympanic paragangliomas are best made after a complete workup reveals the degree of clinical disability and anatomic extent of the mass. The treatment options for paragangliomas of the jugular fossa may consist of observation, radiation therapy, surgical intervention, or a combination of the above. Traditionally, surgery is considered the primary treatment for jugulotympanic paragangliomas. However, today stereotactic radiosurgery and stereotactic radiation therapy are also commonly employed as primary options. Chemotherapy at present has a limited role in aggressive locoregional disease, but may play an adjunctive role in metastatic paragangliomas.[38]

Management of Glomus Tympanicum

When small, the origin of a paragangliomas can be readily characterized as either a tympanicum or jugulare. If the jugular bulb and carotid canal are intact, then the small and intermediate sized glomus tympanicum is the least controversial management decision. This lesion can be definitively treated by surgical removal either through a transcanal or transmastoid approach. Radiation treatment may be considered for a symptomatic moribund patient.

A small tumor localized to the mesotympanum, which can be visualized in entirety through the tympanic membrane, can be approached by the transcanal approach. These tumors are typically classified as Fisch Type A, Glasscock-Jackson tympanicum Type I, or de la Cruz tympanic. A tympanomeatal flap is elevated with the inferior incision extended further anteriorly. The tumor is exposed circumferentially prior to resection to avoid blood in the operative field. The integrity of the ossicular chain is confirmed and the incudostapedial joint is disarticulated as needed. It is important to avoid mechanical trauma to the ossicular chain as this may lead to a significant sensorineural hearing loss. A KTP laser or CO_2 laser is a very useful adjunct to control bleeding. The tumor mass is typically supplied by the tympanic branch of the ascending pharyngeal artery. The tumor is removed in total if possible or piecemeal as necessary. The middle ear is packed as needed for hemostasis and the tympanomeatal flap returned with subsequent packing of the ear canal.

If the entire lesion is not visible through the eardrum, then one must determine the degree of inferior and posterior extension of the tumor. If the tumor has hypotympanic extension without erosion of the dome of the jugular bulb, then a hypotympanotomy is performed. These tumors typically are classified as Fisch Type B, and Glasscock-Jackson tympanicum Type II. After a postauricular incision, a modified tympanomeatal flap, which fully exposes the inferior bony annulus, is elevated (Figure 10–16). The inferior tympanic ring is drilled away until access to the inferior edge of the tumor is noted. The vertical facial nerve travels lateral to the bony annulus inferior to the iter of the chorda tympani nerve, therefore facial nerve stimulation and monitoring is recommended to prevent inadvertent injury. During the drilling, the facial nerve can be easily damaged if care is not taken. After tumor removal, the middle ear is packed as needed for hemostasis and cartilage may be used to reconstruct a large tympanic ring defect. The elevated tympanomeatal flap is replaced followed by packing of the ear canal (Figure 10–17).

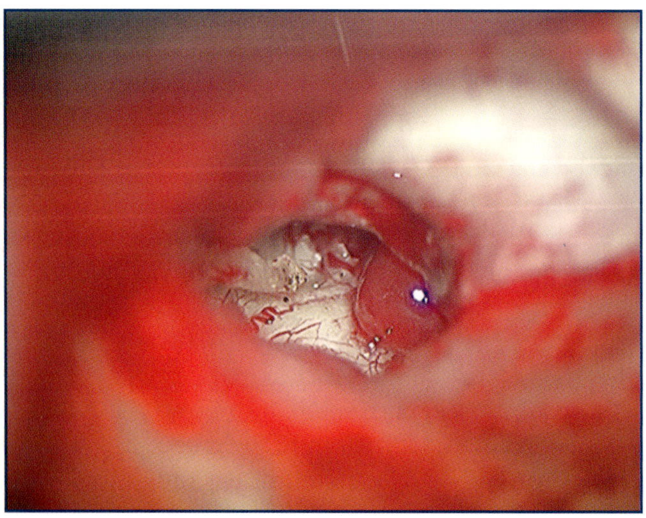

Figure 10–16. Postauricular transcanal approach. A modified tympanomeatal flap is elevated to allow for anterior exposure. Tumor extends out of view into the hypotympanum.

With extensive middle ear lesions or lesions that extend into the mastoid, an extended facial recess approach is used. Tumor extension into the mastoid can occur through the epitympanum and mastoid antrum, facial recess, or retrofacial air cells. However, in using the extended facial recess approach, the dome of the jugular bulb must be intact. These tumors typically are classified as Fisch type B, Glasscock-Jackson tympanicum Type III, or de la Cruz tympanomastoid. A modified tympanomeatal flap is elevated and a standard mastoidectomy is performed. The facial recess is opened and extended, if needed, to expose the hypotympanum by sacrificing the chorda tympani nerve. The retrofacial air tract can be drilled medial to the facial nerve and inferior to the semicircular canals as necessary. A tympanoplasty and ossicular chain reconstruction can be performed as necessary. If the tympanic membrane and posterior canal wall are extensively involved, then a canal wall mastoidectomy can easily be done to allow for complete tumor removal.

Management of Glomus Jugulare

The ideal treatment of these challenging lesions would be total tumor removal with minimal morbidity and zero mortality. Unfortunately, the complex anatomy of the jugular foramen and temporal bone makes these benign but destructive lesions difficult to treat. All glomus jugulare patients must be fully assessed to determine their symptoms, any cranial neuropathies, overall health and cardiovascular and pulmonary status, and social circumstances. Paragangliomas have been treated with radiation, surgery, or a combination of both modalities.

The presence of a paragangliomas does not necessitate surgery or radiotherapy. As paraganglio-

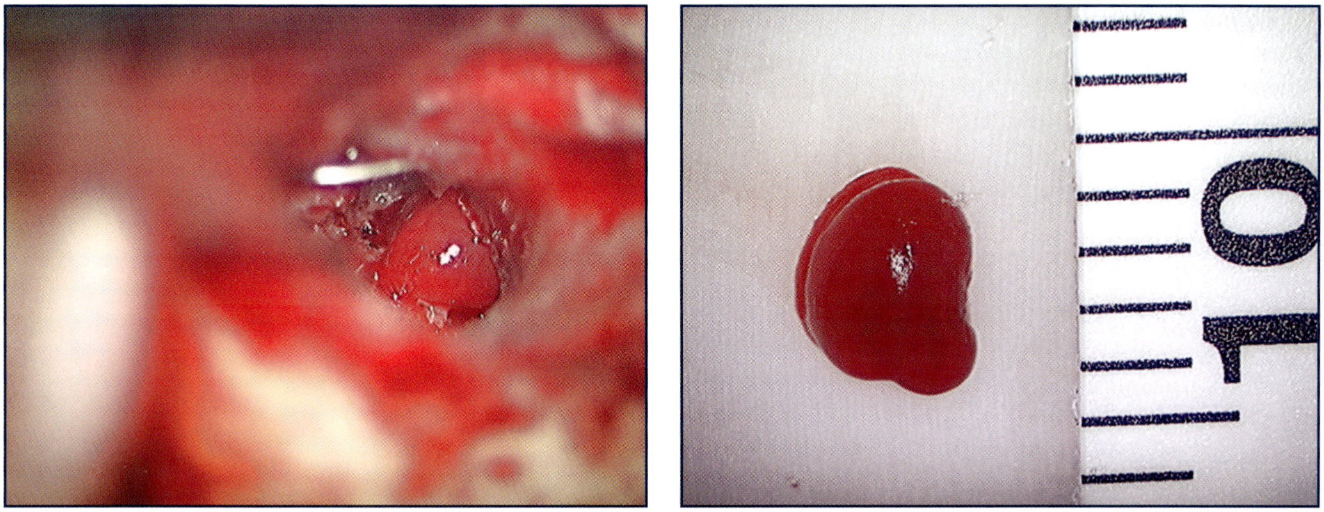

A B

Figure 10–17. A. Hypotympanotomy with inferior bony annulus drilled away exposing the inferior border of the tumor. **B.** The tumor is excised in total if possible. Piecemeal excision is also acceptable.

mas are typically slow growing, medical and radiographic observation is a treatment option. This is an appropriate choice in the elderly or infirm patient in whom the natural history of the paraganglioma is unlikely to cause significant morbidity or mortality. The paraganglioma is assessed annually with imaging studies to evaluate tumor characteristics and growth. Untreated jugulotympanic paragangliomas were found to increase in volume by 20% or more in 55% of patients over a median follow-up of 3.83 years.[39] If an aggressive tumor is thus identified, then radiation therapy is recommended to those who cannot tolerate surgical extirpation.

The role of radiation therapy as primary therapy is evolving and remains controversial. The goal of radiotherapy is cessation of paraganglioma growth or partial regression without evidence of progression on long-term follow-up. The goal is not tumor eradication or cure as it is in surgical excision. The main effect of radiation is damage to the vascular and stromal components of the glomus tumor leading to obliterative endarteritis with little effect on the tumor (chief) cells themselves. In fact, the tumor cells of irradiated patients remain viable on histological analysis.[40] Current radiation treatment options include either stereotactic radiosurgery or stereotactic radiotherapy.

Stereotactic fractionated radiotherapy entails the use of megavoltage radiation, either a ^{60}Co unit or with a linear accelerator of 4 to 15 MeV. Current studies have shown tumor control rates in the 79% to 100% range with radiation as primary, adjunctive or salvage treatment.[41–43] It appears that about 4% of patients experience a significant complication from radiotherapy, while about 7% experience minor complications.[44] Powell et al[45] reported on 59 patients treated with radiotherapy as primary or combination treatment with an actuarial rate of local control of 90% at 10 years and 73% at 25 years. Facial nerve palsy was noted in 4% of their patients. Osteoradionecrosis of the temporal bone, radiation encephalopathy, brain abscess, chronic otitis externa, stenosis of the ear canal, chronic otitis media, and lower cranial nerve palsies have all been reported. Malignant transformation after radiotherapy is a long-term concern and has been shown.[46]

Surgical Management of Glomus Jugulare

The surgical approaches used are based on tumor size, the degree of cranial nerve and neurovascular involvement, and intracranial extension. The path of the mastoid facial nerve, just lateral to the jugular bulb, puts it directly in the path of surgical dissection. The amount of carotid artery involvement varies based on tumor characteristics. Although proximal control of the carotid artery is easily achieved in the neck, distal control of the intratemporal internal carotid artery is dependent on tumor growth patterns.

Mastoid and Neck Approach

The combined mastoid and neck approach with limited facial nerve rerouting is useful for small jugulare tumors that do not involve the carotid artery and do not involve the posterior cranial fossa. In addition, this approach may be used for the large glomus tympanicum tumor with extension up to the posterior aspect of the carotid artery and extensive hypotympanic involvement with or without erosion of the jugular bulb. These tumors are typically classified as Glasscock-Jackson tympanicum type IV, Glasscock-Jackson jugulare type I, or de la Cruz jugular bulb. Any involvement of the petrous carotid artery would require an intratemporal fossa approach. Intraoperative assessment of the facial nerve is routine with continuous monitoring. In addition, it is advisable to monitor CN IX, X, XI, and XII.

The mastoid neck approach begins with a postauricular incision that extends into the neck. A complete mastoidectomy with an extended facial recess approach is performed. The sigmoid sinus is skeletonized from the sinodural angle to the level of the jugular bulb. The mastoid tip, digastric ridge, and sternocleidomastoid muscle (SCM) are released. The common (and internal, and external branches) carotid artery and the internal jugular vein are identified and dissected for control if needed. The lower cranial nerves are identified and traced superiorly. The main trunk of the facial nerve and pes anserinus is also identified and mobilization performed. The internal jugular vein is isolated, ligated and elevated superiorly to the jugular foramen. Exposure of the inferior sigmoid sinus and jugular bulb is obtained. The extent of facial nerve re-routing is based on the exposure needed. Limited anterior re-routing of the vertical mastoid segment facial nerve to the second genu can be performed for most tumors and results in excellent postoperative facial function.[47] The fascia and muscle around the stylomastoid foramen are elevated with the facial nerve to preserve its blood supply. The superior portion of the sigmoid sinus is then occluded by packing the sinus extraluminally. After both proximal and distal venous control have been obtained, the sigmoid sinus is opened just inferior to the packing. Brisk bleeding may occur from the inferior petrosal sinus which drains into the jugular bulb on its medial surface. Hemostasis is obtained by packing the jugular bulb intraluminally. While packing, caution should be used as overzealous packing can injure the glossopharyngeal nerve (CN IX) in the pars nervosa within the medial compartment of the jugular foramen. The tumor should now be fully visible and it is removed with blunt dissection and bipolar cautery for hemostasis. Identification of the lower cranial nerves by stimulating current is helpful during the dissection in difficult cases. After tumor resection is completed, the surgical field is checked for bleeding and gentle packing employed as needed. Based on the amount of tumor extension into the middle ear cleft, a tympanoplasty or ossicular chain reconstruction may be necessary.

Infratemporal Fossa Approach

When a glomus jugulare erodes anteriorly to involve the petrous carotid artery, then exposure of the infratemporal fossa (ITF) must be obtained. Fisch originally described the infratemporal fossa approach and the exposure it affords in these challenging tumors.[48] The external auditory canal is removed and the facial nerve is re-routed from the geniculate ganglion to the stylomastoid foramen. These tumors are staged as Fisch C or D, Glasscock-Jackson jugulare type III or IV, or de la Cruz stage carotid artery or transdural.

The infratemporal fossa approach begins similar to the mastoid-neck approach. However, the ear canal is transected and overclosed and a radical mastoidectomy performed with removal of the ear canal skin, the tympanic membrane, the malleus, and the incus. A maximal conductive hearing loss is an anticipated result from this procedure. The bone of the remaining anterior and inferior tympanic ring is removed. The petrous carotid artery is thus identified and the temporomandibular joint is exposed but not entered. The sigmoid sinus, digastric ridge, mastoid tip, and the posterior belly of the digastric muscle are dealt with as described above in the mastoid-neck approach. Similarly, the internal and external carotid artery, internal jugular vein, CN IX, X, XI, and XII are identified. Facial re-routing frequently entails transposing both the tympanic and mastoid segments of the facial nerve anteriorly. The mandibular condyle and ramus must be retracted anteriorly to obtain sufficient carotid artery exposure. Occasionally, a mandibular condylectomy is required. The bone over the petrous carotid artery and jugular bulb is now fully removed. The internal jugular vein, the external carotid artery, and its branches are all doubly ligated.

At this stage, the tumor extension determines the next steps. If there is no extradural tumor extension, then the superior portion of the sigmoid sinus is packed extraluminally. The sigmoid sinus is opened just inferior to the packing. Brisk bleeding from the inferior petrosal sinus is controlled with intraluminal packing. Once again, avoid overpacking as this may damage the lower cranial nerves, especially CN IX. The jugular vein, jugular bulb, and tumor are dissected with the aid of bipolar, CO_2 or KTP laser. A careful, slow dissection will help preserve lower cranial nerve function. If the tumor is not easily dissected from the carotid artery, then this may be left until the end. Small openings in the carotid can be repaired primarily and these usually occur at the caroticotympanic branches of the petrous carotid artery. The facial nerve is replaced within the fallopian canal prior to closing the defect. In an effort to reduce trauma to the facial nerve during transposition, the fallopian bridge technique can be used. In this technique, the facial nerve is left in its canal with an eggshell layer of bone. Tumor dissection proceeds by working around the facial nerve.[49]

Glomus tumors that extend intracranially may be addressed in one stage if the posterior fossa intracranial component is small. If the intracranial tumor extent is large or if there has been excessive blood loss (over 3000 mL), then a two-stage operation must be considered. Single-stage resection in large intracranial tumors is difficult because of the large defect and need to reconstruct the dural defects.

Intracranial extension of the paragangliomas modifies the surgical approach. The proximal sigmoid sinus is doubly ligated with an aneurysm suture passer after the posterior fossa dura is opened. The intracranial tumor component may be vascularized with branches from the basilar or internal carotid arteries, and these are best cauterized early in the dissection. To prevent CSF leak, the mucosa of the eustachian tube is abraded and packed with a muscle plug.

The infratemporal fossa approach can be modified to allow access to the cavernous sinus and anterior clivus if needed with a transcochlear approach. The infratemporal fossa approach can be combined with a standard retrosigmoid approach as well in patients with good cochlear function. Additional approaches for intracranial extension include the transjugular craniotomy with resection of the jugular bulb and sigmoid in a single stage without the need for ear canal closure or facial nerve mobilization.[50]

Wound closure and reconstruction are dependent on the size of the dural and bony defects. If the dural defect is large, then temporalis fascia or dural grafts can be used to prevent a CSF leak. A vascularized temporaloparietal fascia flap supplied by the superficial temporal artery or a temporalis muscle flap is useful in obliterating the large skull base defect. An abdominal fat graft may also be used to support the flap reconstruction. Very large defects or previously irradiated fields may require microvascular free-flap reconstruction. A lumbar drain is sometimes used as an adjunct postoperatively to reduce CSF pressures.

SURGICAL RESULTS

Glomus Tympanicum

Glomus tympanicum is readily amenable to surgical resection with minimal morbidity. Forest et al examined 80 patients treated surgically from 1972 to 1998.[51] Twenty-seven (34%) patients were stage I, 42 (52%) were stage II, 2 (3%) were stage III, and 9 (11%) were stage IV according to the Glasscock-Jackson classification. There were 4 subtotal resections and two tumor recurrences for a total tumor control rate of 92.5% with an average follow-up of 55 months (range 1–244 months). Long-term follow-up was recommended as one recurrence occurred 14 years after surgery. Most postoperative complications were few and minor including one wound infection, four tympanic membrane perforations, one external canal stenosis, and one cholesteatoma. One patient had an immediate facial paralysis requiring decompression with a good end result. One patient had a cerebrovascular accident with hemiplegia secondary to violation of the ICA during tumor removal. O'Leary et al[52] reviewed 73 patients with glomus tympanicum. The recurrence rate was less than 5% and usually associated with subtotal resections. There were four minor complications with 3 perforations of the tympanic membrane and 1 cholesteatoma. One patient developed a facial paralysis requiring facial nerve decompression with a favorable result.

Glomus Jugulare

Jugulotympanic paragangliomas have an intimate anatomic association with the lower cranial nerves IX to XII, the sympathetic chain, the internal carotid artery, and internal jugular vein and bulb. Hence, the surgical treatment of these vascular and infiltrative tumors can lead to unintentional damage to all of the above structures. The surgeon, in addition, must decide which anatomic structures need to be sacrificed in order to achieve total tumor removal and which structures require immediate rehabilitation to restore function.

Prior to modern microsurgical techniques, extensive jugulotympanic paragangliomas were considered unresectable. These tumors were dealt with through either subtotal resection with radiation therapy or radiotherapy alone. The morbidity and mortality in these cases were high. Rosenwasser's review[53] of his experience in 1968 showed an 80% recurrence rate and a 50% mortality rate. Today's refined skull base surgery techniques, reconstructive advancements, cranial nerve monitoring, and anesthesia have extended the limits of skull base tumor resection. Smaller lesions can often be easily separated from the medial pars nervosa with minimal risks to the lower cranial nerves. Larger lesions frequently involve the medial pars nervosa and lead to preoperative cranial nerve deficits and therefore place the lower cranial nerves at much greater surgical risk for injury or resection. Formidable lesions may be resected with well-defined intratemporal fossa approaches, which have reduced the overall morbidity and mortality.

Jackson et al[23] examined 177 patients with skull base paragangliomas with an average follow-up of 54 months. Twenty-one percent of patients were class I, 20% were class II, 35% were class III, and 23% were class IV, based on the Glasscock-Jackson scale. Subtotal resections were performed in 10% of patients, which were planned to preserve cranial nerve function. Five percent of patients developed recurrences with a median time to recurrence of 5.8 years. Surgical tumor control was achieved in 85% of all patients and 95% of patients with complete resections. Preoperative cranial nerve deficits were present in 46% of patients: CN VII in 18%, CN VIII in 13%, CN IX in 21%, CN X in 30%, CN XI in 17%, and CN XII in 24%. One or more new cranial nerve deficits occurred in 59% of all patients: CN VII in 4.4%, CN IX in 39%, CN X in 25%, CN XI in 26%, and CN XII in 21%. CSF leaks occurred in 28% of patients prior to the use of vascularized flaps and in 4.5% of patients with the use of vascularized flaps for dural reconstruction. The mortality rate was 2.7% and resulted from either internal carotid artery resection or pulmonary embolus.

Green et al[54] reviewed 52 previously untreated glomus jugulare patients. Complete surgical resection was possible in 85% of patients with no mortalities. Long-term facial function was H-B grade I or II in 95% of patients. Approximately 19% of patients required vocal fold augmentation, 4% required enteric feeding secondary to aspiration, 6% developed a wound infection, and 4% developed meningitis and CSF leak. Briner et al[55] and Moe et al[56] had a total resection in 83% of cases with the remaining having subtotal resection for extensive intracranial disease. The mortality rate was 0.7%. Dysphagia was the major complaint of patients surveyed. Seventy-five percent of patients subjectively required 1 to 2 years to recover their preoperative quality of life and 25% never reached this status.

Sanna et al[57] reviewed 53 patients with Fisch class C and D jugulotympanic paragangliomas.

They used a second-stage craniotomy for tumors with greater than 2 cm of intracranial extension. Total tumor removal was possible in 49 of these 53 patients. Local control with mean follow-up of 15 years was 83%. Postoperatively, HB I or II facial function was seen in 65.8%, although only 87.3% of these patients had good facial function preoperatively. Their incidence of new lower cranial nerve palsies was 25%.

Planned partial or subtotal removal has been recommended to help reduce the surgical morbidity of these benign slow growing lesions. Indications for this approach are unclear, and patient selection must be individualized. It must be remembered that the infiltrative nature of the tumor may allow the remnant to continue to spread to areas that are more difficult to manage surgically. This further increases the surgical risks or makes the tumor unresectable. Recently, Miller et al[58] recommended a second stage Gamma knife radiosurgery after a tailored first stage surgical resection. They removed only the middle ear and mastoid component of the tumor and treated the jugular bulb component with radiosurgery in 5 patients. Their preliminary results have shown stable or reduced tumor volumes and improved pulsatile tinnitus.

Kunzel and colleagues reported on their results with primary function-preserving surgery with or without adjuvant radiotherapy, primary stereotactic radiotherapy and observation in the treatment of jugulotympanic paragangliomas.[59] In this study, 64% of patients received primary surgery with or without adjuvant radiation, 27% underwent primary radiotherapy and 9% were observed. With a mean follow-up of 46.8 months, tumor control rate was reported at 97.2%. The authors conclude that function-preserving therapy appears to offer the greatest benefit for patients.

After surgical resection, tumor recurrence may not occur for many years. Some recurrent lesions can be difficult to identify on postoperative imaging until they have reached a considerable size. The most obvious reason for recurrent growth is incomplete resection. Additional factors that may promote recurrence despite complete resection include extensive bony infiltration, incomplete removal from the carotid artery or lower cranial nerves, unrealized dural involvement, and excessive bleeding obscuring the surgical field. Revision surgery carries increased risks because prior landmarks have been altered, facial and lower cranial nerve injury is more likely, and prior radiation may make the carotid wall more fragile.

CONCLUSION

The diagnosis and management of jugulotympanic paragangliomas has changed significantly over the last two decades. Advances in noninvasive imaging techniques have improved diagnostic certainty. Surgical resection with newer skull base techniques has reduced the surgical morbidity and mortality. In addition, stereotactic radiotherapy is being offered as a primary option for the treatment of all glomus jugulare tumor patients, not just the infirm or elderly patient.

REFERENCES

1. Marshall RB, Horn RC. Nonchromaffin paraganglioma. *Cancer*. 1961;14:779–787.
2. Guild SR. The glomus jugulare, a nonchromaffin paraganglion, in man. *Ann Otol Rhinol Laryngol*. 1953;62: 1045–1071.
3. Rossenwasser H. Carotid body tumor of the middle ear and mastoid. *Arch Otolaryngol*. 1945;41:64–67.
4. Friedman RA, Brackmann DE. Jugulotympanic paragangliomas. In: Jackler RK, Driscoll CLW, eds. *Tumors of the Ear and Temporal Bone*. Philadelphia, PA: Lippincott Williams & Wilkins; 2000:343–360.
5. Bojrab DI, Glasscock III ME, Roland PS, et al. *Glomus tumors of the temporal bone*. SIPac 88100 American Academy of Otololaryngology-Head and Neck Surgery Foundation; 1988:1–70.
6. Alford BR, Guilford FR. A comprehensive study of tumors of the glomus jugulare. *Laryngoscope*. 1962;72:765–785.
7. Wenig BM. Neoplasms of the ear. In: Wenig BM, ed. *Atlas of Head and Neck Pathology*. Philadelphia, PA: WB Saunders; 1993:368.
8. Wasserman PG, Savargaonkar P. Paragangliomas: classification, pathology and differential diagnosis. *Otol Clin North Am*. 2001;34:845–862.
9. Rodriguez-Cuevas S, Lopez-Garza J, Labastida-Almendaro S. Carotid body tumors in inhabitants of altitudes higher

than 2000 meters above sea level. *Head Neck.* 1998;20:374–378.
10. Nissenblatt MJ. Cyanotic heart disease: "low altitude" risk for carotid body tumor? *Johns Hopkins Med J.* 1978;142:18–22.
11. Farr HW. Carotid body tumors. A thirty-year experience at Memorial Hospital. *Am J Surg.* 1967;114:614–619.
12. Telischi FF, Bustillo A, Whiteman ML, et al. Octreotide scintigraphy for the detection of paragangliomas. *Otolargyngol Head Neck Surg.* 2000;122:358–362.
13. Kaltsas GA, Mukherjee JJ, Britton KE, et al. Treatment of metastatic pheochromcytoma and paraganglioma with ^{131}I-meta-iodobenzylguanidine (MIBG). *Endocrinologist.* 2003;13:321–333.
14. Hoegerle S, Ghanem N, Altehoefer C, et al. 18F-DOPA positron emission tomography for the detection of glomus tumors. *Eur J Nucl Med Mol Imaging.* 2003;30:689–694.
15. Spector GJ, Giralsky R, Maisel RH, et al. Multipe glomus tumors in the head and neck. *Laryngoscope.* 1975;85:1066.
16. Parkin JL. Familial multiple glomus tumors and paragangliomas. *Ann Otol.* 1981;90:60.
17. Baysal BE. Hereditary paraganglioma targets diverse paraganglia. *J Med Genet.* 2002;39:617–622.
18. Baysal BE. Clinical and molecular progress in hereditary paraganglioma. *J Med Genet.* 2008;45(11):689–694.
19. van der Mey Ag, Maaswinkel-Mooy PD, Cornelisse CJ, et al. Genomic imprinting in hereditary glomus tumors: evidence for new genetic theory. *Lancet.* 1989;2:1291–1294.
20. Callender GG, Rich TA, Perrier ND. Multiple endocrine neoplasia syndromes. *Surg Clin North Am.* 2008;88(4):863–895.
21. Carney JA. Gastric stromal sarcoma, pulmonary chondroma, and extra-adrenal paragangliomas (Carney triad): natural history, adrenocortical component, and possible familial occurrence. *Mayo Clin Proc.* 1999;76(6):543–552.
22. Spector GJ, Gado M, Ciralsky R, et al. Neurologic implications of glomus tumors in the head and neck. *Laryngoscope.* 1975;85:1387.
23. Jackson CG, McGrew BM, Forest JA, et al. Lateral skull base surgery for glomus tumors: long-term control. *Otol Neurotol.* 2001;22:377–382.
24. Brown LA. Glomus jugulare tumor of the middle ear: clinical aspects. *Laryngoscope.* 1953;63:281–292.
25. Carrasco V, Rosenman J. Radiation therapy of glomus jugulare tumors. *Laryngoscope.* 1993;103(suppl):23–27.
26. van der Mey AG, Frijins JH, Cornelisse CJ, et al. Does intervention improve the natural course of glomus tumors? A study of 108 patients seen in a 32-year period. *Ann Otol Rhinol Laryngol.* 1992;101:635–642.
27. Glasscock ME, Dickins JE, Jackson CG, et al. Vascular anomalies of the middle ear. *Laryngoscope.* 1980;90:77.
28. McElveen JT, Lo WM, El Gabri TH, et al. Aberrant internal carotid artery: classic findings on computed tomography. *Otolaryngol Head Neck Surg.* 1986;94:616.
29. Eisenhofer G, Lenders JW, Lineham WM, et al. Plasma normetanephrine and metanephrine for detecting pheochromcytoma in von-Hippel-Landau disease and multiple endocrine neoplasia type 2. *N Engl J Med.* 1999;340:1872–1879.
30. Lustrin ES, Palestro C, Vahessan K. Radiographic evaluation and assessment of paragangliomas. *Otol Clin North Am.* 2001;34:881–906.
31. Olsen WL, Dilon WP, Kelly WM, et al. MR imaging of paragangliomas. *Am J Roentgenol.* 1987;148:201–204.
32. van den Berg R. Imaging and management of head and neck paragangliomas. *Eur Radiol.* 2005;15:1310–1318.
33. van den Berg R, Schepers A, de Bruine FT, et al. The value of MR angiography techniques in the detection of head and neck paragangliomas. *Eur J Radiol.* 2004;52:240–245.
34. Tikkakoski I, Luotonen J, Leinonen S, et al. Preoperative embolization in the management of neck paragangliomas. *Laryngoscope.* 1997;107:821–826.
35. Valvanis A. Preoperative embolization of the head and neck: Indications, patient selection, goals, and precautions. *AJNR Am J Neuroradiol.* 1986;7:943–952.
36. Jackson CG, Bohrer PS. Glomus tumors. In: Thawley SE, Panje WR, eds. *Comprehensive management of Head and Neck Tumors.* Philadelphia, PA: WB Saunders; 1996.
37. Fisch U, Mattox D. *Microsurgery of the Skull Base.* Stuttgart; New York, NY: Georg Thieme-Verlag; 1988:136–353.
38. Fitoussi O, Debled M, Masson B, et al. Advanced paraganglioma: a role for chemotherapy? *Med Pediatr Oncol.* 1999;32:129–131.
39. Jansen JC, van den Berg R, Kuiper A, et al. Estimation of growth rate in patients with head and neck paragangliomas influences the treatment proposal. *Cancer.* 2000;88:2811–2816.
40. Hawthorne MR, Makek MS, Harris JP, et al. The histopathological and clinical features of irradiated and nonirradiated temporal paragangliomas. *Laryngoscope.* 1988;98:325–331.
41. Cole JM, Beiler D. Long-term results of treatment for glomus jugulare and glomus vagale tumors with radiotherapy. *Laryngoscope.* 1994;104:1461–1465.
42. Cummings BJ, Beale FA, Garrett PG, et al. The treatment of glomus tumors of the temporal bone by megavoltage radiation. *Cancer.* 1984;53:2635–2640.
43. Hinerman RW, Amdur RJ, Morris CG, et al. Definitive radiotherapy in the management of paragangliomas arising in the head and neck: a 35-year experience. *Head Neck.* 2008:1431–1438.
44. Springate SC, Weicheselbaum RR. Radiation or surgery for chemodectoma of the temporal bone: a review of local control and complications. *Head Neck.* 1990;12:303–307.
45. Powell S, Peters N, Harmer C. Chemodectoma of the head and neck: results of treatment in 84 patients. *Int J Radiat Oncol Biol Phys.* 1992;22:919–924.
46. Lalwani AK, Jackler RK, Gutin PH. Lethal fibrosarcoma complicating radiation therapy for benign glomus jugulare tumor. *Am J Otol.* 1993;14:398–401.
47. Jackson C. Glomus tympanicum and glomus jugulare tumors. *Otolaryngol Clin North Am.* 2001;34(5):941–970.

48. Fisch U. Infratemporal fossa approach for glomus tumors of the temporal bone. *Ann Otol Rhinol Laryngol.* 1982;91:474–479.
49. Pensak ML, Jackler RK. Removal of jugular foramen tumors. *Otolaryngol Head Neck Surg.* 1997;117(6):586–591.
50. Oghalai JS, Leung MK, Jackler RK, et al. Transjugular craniotomy for the management of jugular foramen tumors with intracranial extension. *Otol Neurotol.* 2004;25:570–579.
51. Forest III JA, Jackson CG, McGrew BM. Long-term control of surgically treated glomus tympanicum tumors. *Otol Neurotol.* 2001;22:232–236.
52. O'Leary MJ, Shelton C, Giddings NA, et al. Glomus tympanicum tumors: a clinical perspective. *Laryngoscope.* 1991;101:1038–1043.
53. Rosenwasser H. Glomus jugulare tumors: follow-up of cases. *Arch Otolaryngol.* 1968;88:35–40.
54. Green JD, Brackman DE, Nguyen CD, et al. Surgical management of previously untreated glomus jugulare tumors. *Laryngoscope.* 1994;104:917–926.
55. Briner HR, Linder TE, Pauw B, et al. Long-term results of surgery of temporal bone paragangliomas. *Laryngoscope.* 1999;109:577–583.
56. Moe KS, Daquing L, Linder TE, et al. An update on the surgical treatment of temporal bone paragangliomas. *Skull Base Surg.* 1999;9:185–194.
57. Sanna M, Jani Y, DeDonato G, et al. Management of jugular paragangliomas: the Gruppo Otologico experience. *Otol Neurotol.* 2004;25:797–804.
58. Miller JP, Semaan MT, Einstein D. Staged gamma knife radiosurgery after tailored surgical resection: a novel treatment paradigm for glomus jugulare tumors. *Stereotact Funct Neurogsurg.* 2009;87(1):31–36.
59. Künzel J, Iro H, Hornung J, Koch M, Brase C, Klautke G, Zenk J.Function-preserving therapy for jugulotympanic paragangliomas: a retrospective analysis from 2000 to 2010. *Laryngoscope.* 2012 Jul;122(7):1545–1551.

CHAPTER 11

CSF Leak and Encephaloceles

Chris Linstrom and Raj Murali

INTRODUCTION

Spontaneous cerebrospinal fluid (CSF) leakage in the temporal bone may occur in childhood and in adult life. In childhood, the most common cause is a congenital labyrinthine malformation within the temporal bone which allows a pathway of communication between the subarachnoid and perilymphatic spaces. The pressure gradient between these two spaces favors not only the flow of CSF between the internal auditory canal and the oval or round windows, but may also account for recurrent episodes of meningitis in infancy or childhood. With even minor head trauma, the integrity of the inner ear may be violated, allowing for CSF to flow into the middle ear cleft, thus predisposing the child to meningitis. Clinical examples of this abnormal CSF pressure gradient due to an abnormal pathway are perilymphatic gusher at the time of cochlear implantation in Mondini malformation, stapedotomy in X-linked progressive mixed deafness or other various perilymphatic pathways of spontaneous or congenital CSF fistulas (perilymph gusher), such as a widened fallopian canal, Hyrtl's fissure, or widened petromastoid canal through which the subarcuate artery passes.[1]

A second group of spontaneous CSF leaks is found in an older age group, roughly between 40 and 70 years of age. The most common site of leakage is the tegmen mastoideum or tympani, which is the plate of bone separating the temporal lobe from the mastoid cavity. Bony defects here allow the downward forces of brain pulsation and gravity to cause herniation and sometimes violation of the dura and/or brain, allowing encephaloceles of the petrous temporal bone include meningoceles (arachnoid tissue and CSF) and encephaloceles (dura and brain surrounded by CSF within the herniation sack) to form.

Various synonyms for encephaloceles appear in the medical literature: brain hernia, brain prolapse, cerebral hernia, brain fungus, endaural encephalocele, fungus cerebri, and meningoencephalocele.[2] Herniation of the brain into the temporal bone was first documented by Caboche in 1902.[3]

CSF otorrhea due to encephalocele is infrequently encountered and is commonly referred to the neurotologist from a general otolaryngologist. The typical history is that of an older or obese patient who presents with unilateral aural fullness and/or decreased hearing often without an antecedent history of a flu or other illness of the upper respiratory system. The patient may also have had prior otologic surgery, head trauma involving the temporal bone, or a history of meningitis. Additional risk factors include prior radiation therapy, chemotherapy, and infection from any source.[4]

Medical therapy including antihistamines, mucolytics, steroid nasal sprays, and/or antibiotics has usually been administered with no change in the patient's symptoms. The patient is found to have unilateral serous otitis media (SOM) by otoscopy. If a perforation is present, thin, watery fluid may discharge through it. A conductive hearing loss is diagnosed by tuning fork examination and confirmed with audiometric testing.

The otolaryngologist may next perform a myringotomy and tube insertion in the office and encounter clear fluid, pulsating through the tube, often resembling "spring water." At this time, the entity of encephalocele is strongly considered. This history is so characteristic that it often leads directly to the diagnosis with few intervening steps.

RELEVANT ANATOMY

The temporal bone is separated *superiorly* from the temporal lobe of the brain by the mastoid air cell system, the tegmen mastoideum and tegmen tympanum (Latin: tegere, to cover; tegmen, n., a cover; tectum, a roof or ceiling); *inferiorly* from the posterior cranial fossa and cerebellum by the mastoid air cell system and posterior fossa dura; *anteriorly* from the clivus, sphenoid and anterior cranial fossa contents by the petrous apex and petrous carotid artery. The temporal bone is "pierced" by various structures which either pass *into it* (CN VIII) or *through it* (CN VII, the petrous carotid artery, and the sigmoid sinus). The trigeminal nerve (CN V) has a groove for its ganglion cells in the anteromedial aspect of the temporal bone (Meckel's cave). A sleeve of dura invests the cranial nerves as they pass into the temporal bone.

The close proximity of the temporal lobe of the brain to the superior and anterior surfaces of the temporal bone as well as the "piercing" of it by cranial nerves and vascular structures predispose the air-filled spaces of the temporal bone to encephalocele formation.

PATHOPHYSIOLOGY

The pathophysiology of spontaneous leakage of CSF and herniation of brain into the mastoid and middle ear is not entirely clear. Several theories have been proposed to account for encephalocele formation within or around the temporal bone. With each heartbeat the brain pulsates, albeit with small linear displacement. The constant, pulsating forces of brain acting upon the temporal bone may exert a "water hammer" effect, thus wearing away the tegmen mastoideum or tegmen tympanum, thereby allowing a small "knuckle" of dura with or without brain to herniate into the air-filled spaces of the temporal bone, specifically the epitympanum and mastoid. Thus, normal variations of intracranial pressure and decades of CSF pulsations at a defective site over time may allow brain prolapse.[2] However, this may be too simple of an explanation. Autopsy series reveal many otherwise normal temporal bones with multiple foveolae granulares or little "pinhole" piercings on the inner surface of the skull vault near the tegmen but without encephalocele formation.[1]

Another explanation has been proposed by Gacek and others.[5–7] Arachnoid granulations, also called arachnoid villi or Pacchioni's granulations, are a main area of CSF resorption. They are composed of peduncles of arachnoid tissue invaginating into the lumen of the venous sinuses, such as the superior sagittal sinus and its branches. This theory suggests that arachnoid granulations that do not find a venous termination during embryonic development come to lie in a blind-ended sac against the inner bony surface of the skull. The central portion of an arachnoid granulation contains CSF, which is covered by arachnoid cells with loose attachment to a fibrous capsule, covered by endothelium. In patients with spontaneous CSF leaks, the arachnoid granulations are thought to become aberrantly located in close proximity to temporal bone dura and are covered only by a thin fibrous capsule. With time, the pressure of CSF from the subarachnoid space causes erosion through the fibrous covering of the arachnoid granulation. Pulsations of CSF from the subarachnoid space result in further erosion through the floor of the anterior, middle or posterior cranial fossae, thus resulting in a CSF leak.

Other obvious mechanisms for encephalocele formation include infectious/inflammatory disease, such as extensive chronic and extensive suppurative otitis media or cholesteatoma, prior otologic surgery that may have weakened the tegmen/dural interface or temporal bone fracture in which the integrity of the tegmen and/or dura has been compromised. Neoplasias, especially malignancies, adjacent to the tegmen may weaken it enough to lead to encephalocele formation. However, the inflammatory response to neoplasia is often so great that herniation is prevented.

Systemic predisposing factors appear to be those which cause an elevation in the resting intracranial pressure, especially obesity and hypertension. Patients with so-called benign intracranial hypertension and pseudotumor cerebri may be predisposed to this condition. There may be a trophic effect of hormonal homeostasis upon the dura in that the dura of postmenopausal women is thin and friable compared to that of premenopausal women.

Certainly any factor that causes an elevation in the normal resting intracranial pressure may lead to encephalocele formation if the normal architecture separating the brain from the temporal bone has been compromised. Some of these patients may present with a unilateral encephalocele and radiological studies may reveal bilateral tegmen defects. The contralateral side may or may not become symptomatic in the future but the clinician should be aware of this and discuss it with the patient prior to surgery.

CLINICAL PRESENTATION AND PHYSICAL EXAMINATION

It is vital that the examining physician attend to the nature, duration, and location of the patient's complaints. Knowledge of the anatomy of the temporal bone and its surrounding structures will focus the clinical examination toward the most likely site of pathology. The history is probably the single most important step in the investigative process, equaling the physical findings, which may be mild, or absent.

The clinical complaint depends on the location and the extent of the herniation and the presence or absence of an active CSF otorrhea. If the herniation is small, there may be few noticeable complaints. If larger, there may be aural fullness, hearing loss, tinnitus, dizziness, weakness of the facial nerve, or headache and, if the integrity of the dural sac is broken, extravasation of cerebrospinal fluid into the mastoid and middle ear spaces, with possible rhinorrhea or, if there is a defect in the eardrum, otorrhea. Headache in the temporal region or deep-seated otalgia are common complaints. Headache may be due to dural traction from the encephalocele or due to low intracranial pressure (ICP) in cases of CSF leak. Patients may also present acutely to the emergency room (ER), unconscious from florid meningitis. In such cases the underlying diagnosis of middle ear encephalocele may be completely missed by the ER physicians.

A complete otologic and head and neck examination should be done with a focus on cranial nerves II to XII. A microscopic examination of the tympanic membranes is usually performed, with care given to examine each and every part of the eardrum. Crusting on the eardrum, especially near the pars flaccida, may hide disease. If at all possible, this should be softened and removed.

Dizziness and/or vertigo are not common complaints in patients with encephaloceles. Clinical tests of balance should be performed as part of the overall neurotologic examination. Most patients with encephaloceles usually have normal findings on these clinical tests.

The diagnosis of CSF otorrhea or rhinorrhea is usually obvious, although it may be difficult to confirm when the leak is intermittent. If the patient has a history of otorrhea or rhinorrhea, it is important to attempt to replicate the complaint. The patient should be asked to describe the provocative position and this should be performed. This may be lying in the supine position with the offending ear undermost, or with the head straight down. A cotton ball or small cup should be placed in or near the external auditory meatus to try to catch some of the fluid. In cases of rhinorrhea, the "teapot sign" is diagnostic. The patient is given an empty beaker or test tube and is seated in a chair leaning forward with the head down. One looks for a drip of clear fluid coming from the nostril. The sign may not be elicited immediately. The patient is instructed to gently perform the Valsalva maneuver. It helps to wait about 15–30 minutes to allow the leakage to occur. If fluid can be collected, it should be sent for β2-transferrin assay, described below. Other traditional tests for CSF are reviewed but today are of diminishing value compared to β2-transferrin or radiographic studies.

INVESTIGATIONS

Audiometric

All patients with otologic complaints, regardless of the suspected lesion, should have an audiogram with a minimum battery of tests, performed separately for each ear, of pure tones, bone conduction (masked appropriately), word discrimination, and immittance with reflex decay, if the level of hearing permits.

Radiologic

Patients with unilateral otologic complaints such as hearing loss, tinnitus, and fullness/pressure should have a radiographic evaluation of the temporal bone with an appropriate study. Although cost is a significant factor in the evaluation of a patient, it is the opinion of many experienced clinicians that the patient is better served by testing more frequently than less frequently. The decision pathway is relatively easy if the complaint is one-sided, if fluid is seen within the middle ear cleft or flows from a patent pressure-equalizing tube, or if there is a conductive hearing loss. In this case, one would choose an examination that will yield the greatest amount of information about the interface between fluid and bone: a computed axial tomogram (CT). If, however, the tympanic membrane and middle ear cleft are normal and the complaint is strictly unilateral, one would be interested first in imaging soft tissue. In this case, a magnetic resonance imaging (MRI) of brain with attention to the internal auditory canal (IAC) and skull base would be the next step.

CT yields excellent information about bone and the soft-tissue/bone/air interface, but is far less sensitive and specific than MRI in detecting soft tissue neoplasia. Temporal bone CT imaging ordinarily is done without contrast, with thin slices at approximately one mm intervals, in the axial and direct coronal planes. Edge enhancing algorithms greatly aid diagnostic capabilities. Temporal bone CT imaging today has also become very quick. The average noncontrast temporal bone CT requires less than one minute of actual scanning time, i.e., it takes longer to do the paper work that the actual scan! Modern CT equipment and imaging programs allow each axis (x, y, z) of every pixel of the thousands per study to be identified and manipulated into any desired plane. Thus, even in a patient with limited cervical mobility or in a patient unable to lie supine, a scan in any plane may be obtained with little if any "pixilation" or image blurring due to reformatting. The images are sharp and clear. In patients who cannot otherwise have an MRI, CT imaging with contrast may allow definition of the great vessels within the skull and neck and may give information about infectious or inflammatory processes as well as neoplasia.

The typical CT findings in patients with encephaloceles are those of antecedent temporal bone "health," with subsequent pathology. The typical temporal bone in these cases is very well pneumatized (developed) with abundant air cells tracts around the otic capsule, often extending far into the zygomatic root and even as far as the lateral margins of the orbit. This abundant pneumatization indicates eustachian tube health. It is usually present bilaterally. On the ipsilateral side, the middle ear and mastoid are almost always opacified, without bony erosion of Körner's septum or the intra-mastoid septations. There may or may not be air/fluid levels present, depending upon the amount of fluid and the presence or absence of a drainage system (such as a tube). On coronal imaging, there may be a thinning or absence of the tegmen, often seen in several sequential slices. CT with contrast may show dural enhancement with a gap at the level of the tegmen defect, but it is less reliable for imaging brain herniation. If a tegmen defect is present that is large enough to allow for encephalocele formation, a bony defect ±soft tissue mass is often, but not always, seen on sequential coronal imaging. It is important to compare sequential slices from the normal to abnormal sides to determine if the tegmen thinning is also seen on the unaffected side. The normal tegmen may be very thin, especially in individuals with highly pneumatized temporal bones. The major differential to be decided on is chronic mastoiditis in which every air cell has become obliterated with hypertrophic mucosa but in which the tegmen is still intact.

Computed tomography and MRI are complementary to each other in the thorough evaluation of encephaloceles of the temporal bone, but MRI is not required in every single case. MRI without and with enhancement will yield the most precise information about soft tissue structures. Dura will enhance on MRI imaging with contrast and the temporal lobe dura may be may be followed along to the area of the suspected tegmen defect. In cases of larger encephaloceles, a mass may be seen herniating into the area of the mastoid or epitympanum from above. This will usually be in the exact same location as that found on the coronal CT images. However, in cases of small or suspicious tegmen defects on CT imaging, the MRI is often silent or may show an irregular pattern of dural enhancement along the tegmen, without a discrete herniation of brain. MRI has not been proven to be of uniform diagnostic utility because the herniated brain is not normal and does not have the same characteristics on MRI, as does normal brain. Flow-sensitive MRI has been studied as a promising technique in the evaluation of CSF leak.[8]

On either CT or MR imaging, the presence of air within the brain or ventricular system (pneumocephalus, pneumoventricle, respectively) is a definitive and potentially ominous sign that the integrity of the dura and/or tegmen has been violated. In its presence, especially if there is air in the ventricular system or any compression or shift of the brain or brainstem, a tension pneumocephalus due to a ball-valve effect must be excluded and neurosurgical intervention may become somewhat urgent.

Adjunctive Tests

Undoubtedly, one wants to be "proof positive" that there is real, treatable pathology in the patient before embarking upon a surgical endeavor that may result in a mastoidectomy or a craniotomy. It is incumbent upon the surgeon to exhaust every reasonable means available to support or refute the putative diagnosis. To this end, several other adjunctive tests have been developed.

These include simple measures such as the "double halo" or "double ring" sign obtained by watching the migration of fluid saved from the ear or nose on filter paper and testing the fluid for the presence and amount of glucose and protein.[9] These tests help to confirm the nature of the fluid but are often nonconclusive, yielding little definitive information.

Beta-2 transferrin, the tau fraction of transferrin, is a protein produced by neuraminidase activity in the brain that is unique to CSF and its derivatives, including perilymph and the aqueous humor of the globe. It is not found in blood, blood serum, or lymph. It is not found in the normal or inflamed middle ear space.[10,11] The sensitivity of detecting β2-transferrin via western blot analysis is very high. CSF dilutions of 1:100 remain positive for its presence. Most laboratories require a minimum of one ml to run the assay. Because it may be detected in nanomolar amounts, the fluid obtained may be diluted with sterile water if the original specimen is not sufficient.

Because perilymph is an ultrafiltration product of CSF, it would be logical to find β2 transferrin in defects of the temporal bone and dura and also to use it as a marker for CSF or its derivative, perilymph. Indeed, much effort has been expended to demonstrate that β2-transferrin is the long-awaited, unique marker for cerebrospinal fluid leaks. Its utility is somewhat limited in that it is of value when positive but of no value when negative. Its presence greatly enhances the diagnosis of encephalocele. Its absence in no way excludes it in the presence of other compelling evidence. Bearing this in mind, it is of value when one is not entirely sure that an encephalocele is the cause of chronic aural discharge. In the presence of clear discharge, a positive β2-transferrin assay will greatly tilt the evidence in favor of encephalocele or other dural compromise. It is one of many factors that will be used to formulate the plan of management for the patient.

More invasive measures include intrathecal injection of iodine-based dyes and radioisotopic cisternograms. These agents have been used in the identification of CSF leaking from patients after temporal bone or head trauma. They may also be used in refractive cases that have re-leaked after prior repair. The morbidity of these procedures must be weighed against the often low yield of clinical information.

The diagnosis of an encephalocele of the temporal bone is made by the preponderance of clinical and investigative evidence: the right complaint in the right patient with the right otological, audiometric, and radiographic findings leading to the correct diagnosis and ultimately to definitive repair. Above all, a high index of suspicion in a patient with all of the above findings will best help to yield the correct diagnosis.

DIFFERENTIAL DIAGNOSIS

The most common entity to be distinguished from an encephalocele is chronic mastoiditis. It, too, presents with many of the same clinical findings. The CT scan may be the only distinguishing feature in that there are often no air/fluid levels. The tegmen may be intact in all aspects. If this is the case, it is a safe bet that chronic hypertrophy of respiratory epithelium and mucous production from goblet cells is the cause of middle ear fluid rather than the recipient of infection. In chronic mastoiditis, placement of a myringotomy and tube may lead to resolution of fluid within the middle ear cleft and an improvement in the accompanying conductive hearing loss, only to recur when the tube becomes blocked or extrudes.

Other entities within the differential diagnosis would include cholesteatoma, cholesterin granuloma, chronic suppurative otitis media, meningitis, or brain abscess. These would each be expected to have a more severe infectious and inflammatory picture, especially in the latter two, but they may mimic encephalocele and be difficult to distinguish from it.

TREATMENT PARADIGMS

Several surgical techniques exist for the correction of an encephalocele involving the middle ear or mastoid. The surgeon must carefully review the nature and extent of the lesion and its relationship to the important structures. The surgeon must have several surgical approaches available simultaneously in the event that the selected approach fails to reach the pathology or adequately treat it. Many deficits of the temporal bone leading to encephalocele formation are managed in an extradural fashion by the neurotologist alone. If the lesion involves highly critical areas such as the petrous carotid artery or the clivus, it is wise to enlist one's neurosurgical colleague(s) to help in the care of the patient. Team effort is required for many of these cases.

The goals of surgical repair of the encephalocele or myringocele are as follows:

1. To resect devitalized and functionless cortical brain, especially if found in an infected, inflamed milieu within the mastoid.
2. To create a watertight seal at the site of the dural and bony defect(s) to prevent further CSF leakage.
3. To restore of the integrity of the intradural vault.
4. To prevent re-leakage by creating enough tensile strength in the repair to resist the intracranial pressure (ICP) head.[4]

The surgical approaches to the correction of an encephalocele may be classified:

Inferior approach (transmastoid)

Superior approach (middle cranial fossa approach)

Combined

Surgical approach from inferior approach.

A complete mastoidectomy is performed with cutting and diamond burs with these surgical landmarks: anteriorly, the posterior canal wall; posteriorly, the sinodural angle; inferiorly, the mastoid tip and jugular bulb; and superiorly, the tegmen mastoideum, extending toward the epitympanum and the tegmen tympani. Along this latter dissection, a defect in the bone with soft tissue extending through it should be encountered. Often, the dura in the area adjacent to the defect will be exposed. There may be frank cerebrospinal fluid (CSF) leaking through the defect. Where there is one defect, there may be several and the surgeon must be prepared to find and repair each one of them.

It is important to remember that the small bit of brain that has herniated from above into the mastoid is no longer functioning. Ordinarily it will cause no neurological deficit whatsoever to remove this small amount of herniated brain without or with surrounding glial tissue if it is not possible to reduce it or if it appears to be infected or inflamed.

The repair itself may be performed with a "sandwich" technique of temporalis fascia and/or cartilage with fibrin glue or another FDA-approved source of biologic adhesive. Adhesives alone should *not* be expected to provide a definitive repair. They are adjuncts only. The soft tissue and/or cartilage repair will need to be strong enough to prevent reherniation of brain from above into the mastoid cavity. If it is possible to achieve a snug fit from below, this is sufficient.

In selected cases, a small bone graft may be placed between the mastoid and the ossicular heads to prevent any soft tissue placed into the mastoid from creating a conductive hearing loss. Some surgeons find the use of bone cements aid in the reformation of the bony separation between the cranium and the middle ear or mastoid. In selected cases, abdominal fat may also be used to obliterate the mastoid. However, unless every single air cell has been drilled free of its lining of respiratory epithelium, mastoid obliteration by any soft tissue invites future problems especially mucocele formation.

The advantage of the transmastoid repair is that it will save the patient from the added morbidity of a middle fossa craniectomy. However, if the tegmen defect is too large or if it is obvious at the time of repair that the brain will likely re-herniate, it is better to proceed with a craniotomy to provide a more secure reconstruction.

In the rare case in which frank cholesteatoma with purulence is found adjacent to and surrounding herniated brain, the repair may have to be staged, with the exoneration of infected tissue first, followed by a second, definitive repair of dural and tegmen defects at a later stage. The presence or absence of active CSF leakage will guide surgical judgment regarding timing of the definitive repair. The advice of one's neurosurgical colleague must be sought.

Surgical Repair from Superior Approach

The decision to repair from the superior approach is multifactorial, depending upon the time course and likely cause of the problem, the age and body habitus of the patient with any attendant comorbidities such as obesity, the size and location of the defect, the familiarity of the surgeon, and other factors.

Extradural

In this approach, the soft tissues are prepared in such a way that both a mastoidectomy and middle fossa craniectomy may be performed, as necessary. The hairline should be drawn with a permanent marker before shaving any hair. For cosmetic reasons, the incision should never extend beyond this point. The standard postauricular incision is made and then continued superiorly in a straight or a slightly S-shaped pattern into the temporoparietal scalp. Many surgeons prefer a "dog-ear" posteriorly based scalp flap. The soft tissues are incised down to bone. If a mastoidectomy is planned, this should be done first and the tegmen defect and/or brain herniation identified from below. It is important to leave at least 3 or 4 mm of bone parallel to the tegmen and not to extend the drilling too far superiorly. This bar of bone will be necessary to help support the bony repair of the tegmen defect. Temporalis fascia is harvested. The temporalis muscle is incised and retracted in an anterior to posterior direction. A vascularized temporalis fascia graft or another soft tissue graft may be prepared at this time.

A small craniotomy measuring 3 cm by 4 cm (a "commemorative stamp size") will usually suffice for gentle retraction of the temporal lobe and extradural repair. A common mistake is to make the craniotomy too far *posteriorly* (toward the occiput). It will be important to look for encephalocele(s) at both the tegmen mastoideum *and* tegmen tympanum. Placing the craniotomy flap too far posteriorly will impede this latter evaluation. Therefore, it is prudent to place the middle of the craniotomy flap in the same coronal plane as the center of the external auditory canal. This will allow a sufficient examination of the dura both anteriorly and posteriorly.

Care should be taken not to damage the vein of Labbé or its entry in to the transverse sinus while creating the bone flap. This vein is named for Dr. Léon Labbé (1832–1916), a French surgeon who first described a large superficial vein extending between the lateral cerebral sulcus and the transverse sinus. Damage to this vein can lead to speech, memory, and/or other cognitive disorders from injury to the temporal lobe. For this reason we recommend drilling the inferior part of the craniotomy with a small bur drill bit rather than going across the bone with a craniotome. A malleable brain retractor or other middle fossa retractor (Urban retractor or Fisch retractor) may be used to evaluate the dura for deficiencies and/or herniations. A spinal drain may be inserted preoperatively, which may greatly reduce the need for brain retraction and the brain may settle in the craniotomy by gravity alone. It is vital to remember that where there is one encephalocele, there may be several. Once it has been determined how extensive the defect is, the repair is performed in a "sandwich" fashion using a bone graft, temporalis fascia (or occasionally tensor fascia lata in large defects) other soft tissue such as a vascularized temporalis flap, and possibly biologic adhesives such as Tisseal® or fibrin glue.[2,12]

A split-thickness calvarial graft of outer-table cortical bone has been described which will yield a plentiful amount of bone for the repair and still allow the original craniotomy flap to be replaced. This is done to avoid a depression at the site of the craniotomy.[13]

Alternatively, if not enough bone remains in the bone flap after harvest for tegmen repair, a titanium wire mesh cranioplasty can be done to repair the craniotomy defect. Also, bone cement may be used here. If a mastoidectomy has been performed, the repair may be visualized from below and should appear sealed and dry right away. The temporal lobe is allowed to re-expand, helping to ensure a secure repair.

Intradural

The main indications for intradural repair are large bony defects with correspondingly large encephaloceles or difficult to find encephaloceles which tend to be situated much more medially towards the petrous apex. In cases presenting with CSF otorrhea, if the source of the leak is not found during the initial extradural exploration it then becomes mandatory to open the dura, gently retract the temporal lobe, and look medially all the way up to the tentorial incisura. A tongue of brain exiting through the dura may be the clue to locating the source of the CSF leak. A spinal drain is a very useful adjunct in these cases. Intradural exploration is often required for dealing with large bony defects secondary to gunshot wounds, extensive previous skull base surgery, and radiation necrosis of temporal bone after cancer treatment.

Neurosurgeons are trained in this approach and may prefer it for very large defects or for revision surgery. All of the steps are the same as for the extradural repair with these modifications:

1. The craniotomy flap will usually be larger.
2. The dura is incised and the herniated brain *directly* observed. Infected cortical contents are not reduced intracranially and may be amputated from above and removed outside the dura. Viable and non-infected temporal lobe herniations are assessed intradurally, thus permitting cranialization whenever possible.
3. The dural defect is either repaired directly with sutures or patched with temporalis fascia, tensor fascia lata, or another dural source that is stabilized with sutures or other means.
4. The weight of the overlying temporal lobe is employed to bolster the repair and better resist the intracranial pressure.[4]

The repair of the bony defect is much the same as are the other parts of the operation. The main advantage of intradural repair is the added measure of certainty and control because herniated brain is identified at its source. It is a more definitive repair than its extradural counterpart and is of great value when indicated. For the majority of encephaloceles that a neurotologist will encounter, it would not routinely be required. For larger defects, it is important for both surgeons to discuss the patient's clinical presentation, the otologic findings, and, above all, the radiographs before deciding on the approach and technique of repair.

In large encephaloceles, where significant temporal lobe resection or manipulation is necessary, patients should be treated before surgery with antiseizure medications as the temporal lobe is especially epileptogenic.

Combined Surgical Approaches

In actual practice, most repairs of temporal bone encephaloceles are via a combined approach. It adds very little time for an experienced neurotologist to perform a complete mastoidectomy in order to visualize the defect from below. The combined approach may allow the site of herniation to be more thoroughly evaluated and repaired. There may be multiple sites of bony and dural incompetence, especially in the anterior tegmen tympani area.[2] A combined approach provides a "look from below" at the repair from above. It is the rare case that these authors repair solely from above or below.

CLINICAL AND RADIOGRAPHIC FOLLOW-UP

Most patients with suspected encephaloceles will be treated surgically. The average hospital stay will be approximately 3 to 4 days. Admission to an Intensive Care Unit is desired, but not absolutely required for extradural repairs. In repairing large defects, a spinal drain may be left in for a few days to reduce ICP and promote healing of the repair in a dry environment. CSF has excoriating properties and may not allow the repair to heal.

The patient's hearing is initially tested with tuning forks in the immediate postoperative period. The sound should lateralize to the operated ear and this should be followed throughout the healing period. A postoperative audiogram is usually obtained when the patient is well healed, at approximately 2 or 3 months. In most cases, the hearing will stay the same or improve as the middle ear cleft becomes dry.

For the majority of patients, this is the extent of postoperative investigations. In rare cases, the hearing may worsen or there may be additional complaints such as tinnitus and, even more rarely, dizziness. In these rare cases, in addition to an audiogram, one may wish to re-image the patient with CT to ascertain that the repair is stable and to look for soft tissue or bone impinging upon the ossicular chain. On post-op CT imaging, there should be improved aeration of the middle ear and mastoid, but it is very rare for the entire mastoid defect to be completely aerated. In most cases, there will be at least a small collapse of soft tissue into the lateral mastoid defect. The bony reconstruction plate is usually quite easy to identify, as well as other radio-opaque materials such as titanium mesh. On CT scanning, cartilage appears as a soft tissue thickening and it is difficult to know with certainty that a cartilaginous repair is intact, especially if the mastoid and middle ear are opacified. If symptoms are ongoing and if the radiograph does not give a definitive answer, the ear may need to be re-explored.

CASE ILLUSTRATIONS

Case 1

SF is a 52-year-old male with a one-year history of pressure and fullness in the right ear. He was treated with decongestants and antibiotics. His tuning fork lateralizes to the right and he has a mild conductive hearing loss on the right side on audiometry (Figure 11–1). He had a right myringotomy and pressure-equalizing (PE) tube inserted. Clear fluid was obtained and sent for β2-transferrin analysis that was negative. The patient continued to complain of fluid draining from the right ear. CT of the temporal bone was performed and showed near complete opacification of all air cells of the right mastoid air cell system and middle ear without destruction

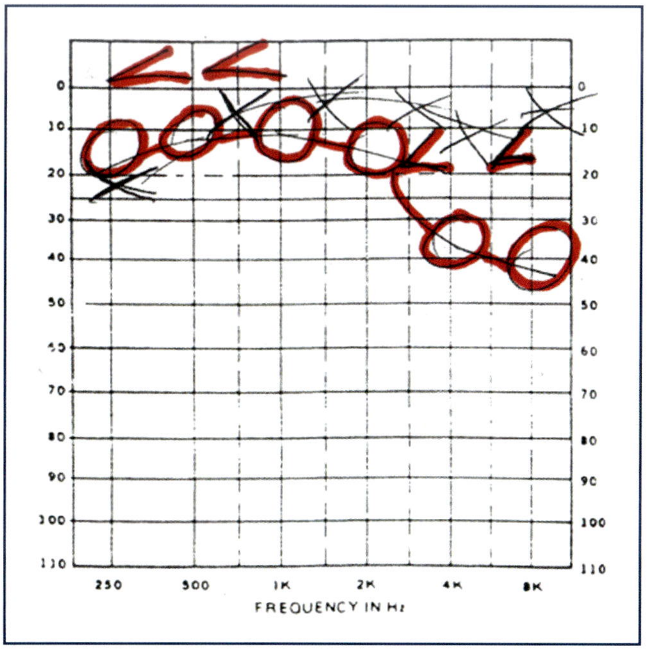

Figure 11–1. Preoperative audiogram showing mild right mixed hearing loss.

(Figure 11–2). There was soft tissue thickening around the ossicular heads, but no obvious encephalocele. A focal defect in the tegmen mastoid was seen. This was compared to the defect seen on nearly identical views on a pre-op MRI scan (Figure 11–3). Because of these findings, the patient was advised that an encephalocele was the likely cause of his leak and that surgical repair would be indicated. He agreed and this was done via a transmastoid and middle cranial fossa approach. Bone, temporalis fascia, and fibrin glue were used for the repair. He healed uneventfully, cleared the right middle ear and has had no further leak of fluid.

He has had changes of pressure in the right ear with decrease in the atmospheric barometric pressure. This was investigated with a post-operative CT. This showed that the repair was intact, with air surrounding the ossicular heads (Figure 11–4). A postoperative hearing test showed no significant change in the hearing (Figure 11–5).

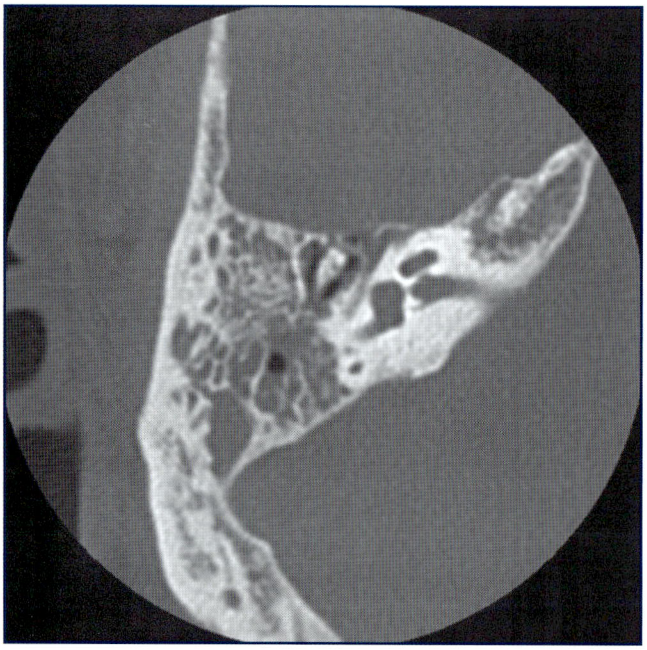
A

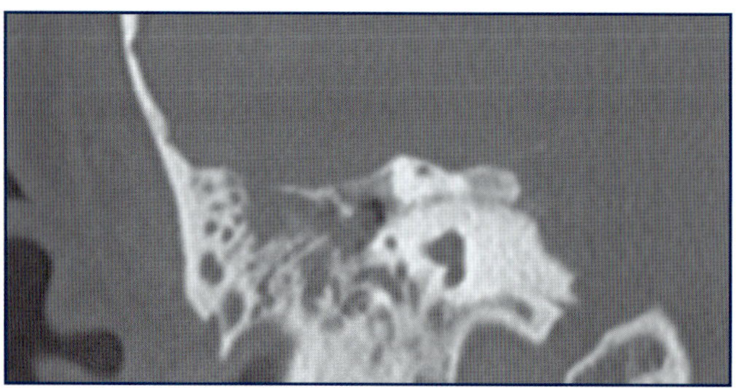
B

Figure 11–2. Pre-op CT of right temporal bones. **A.** Axial view. **B.** Coronal view. There is a defect in the right tegmen. At surgery, this was the location of the encephalocele.

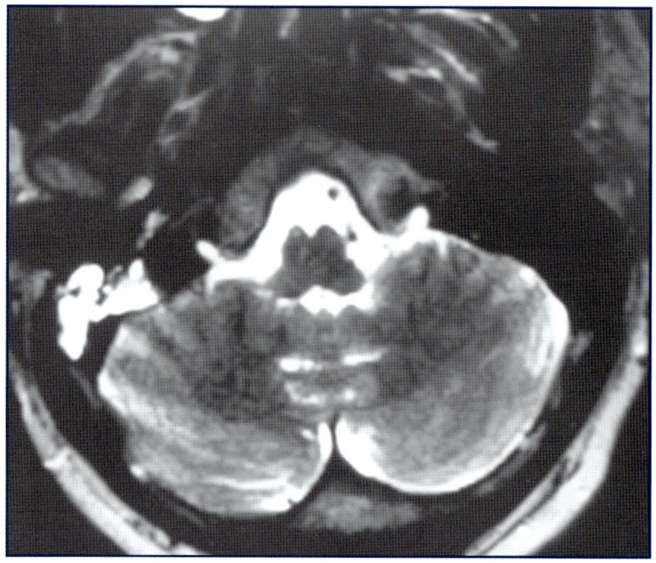
A

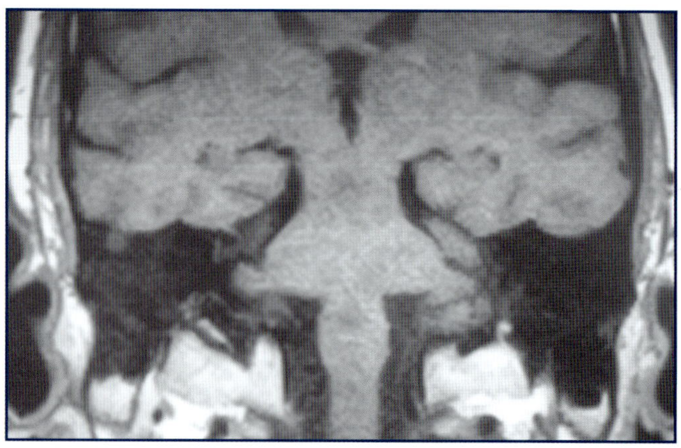
B

Figure 11–3. Pre-op MRI of temporal bones, right ear. **A.** Axial T2-weighted image. **B.** Coronal T1-weighted image. There is a defect in the right tegmen. At surgery, this was the location of the encephalocele.

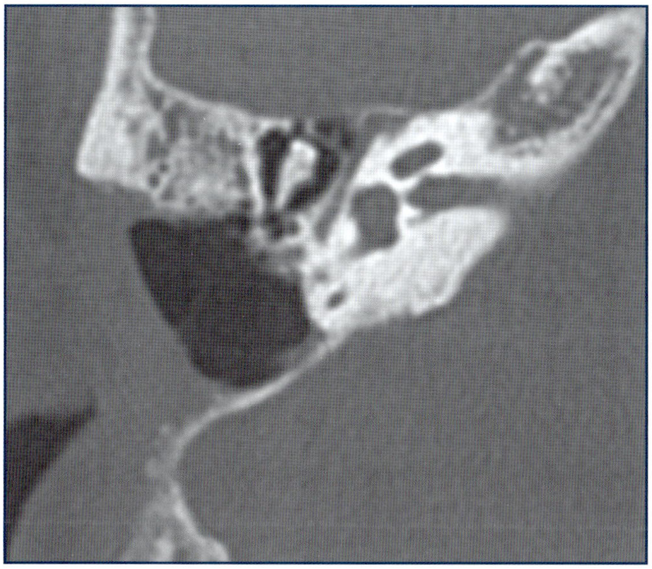

A

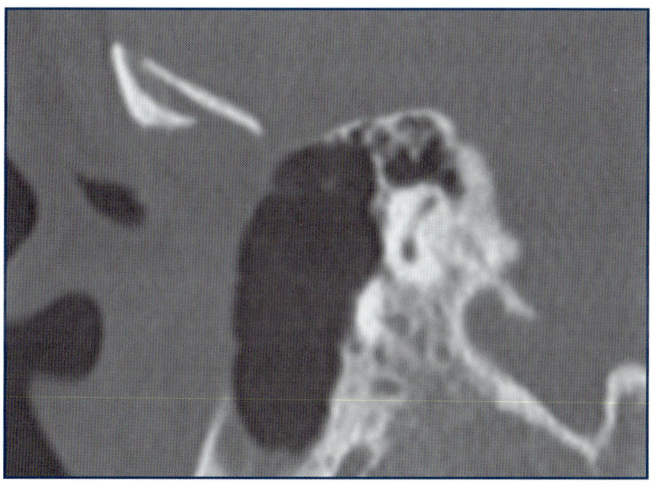

B

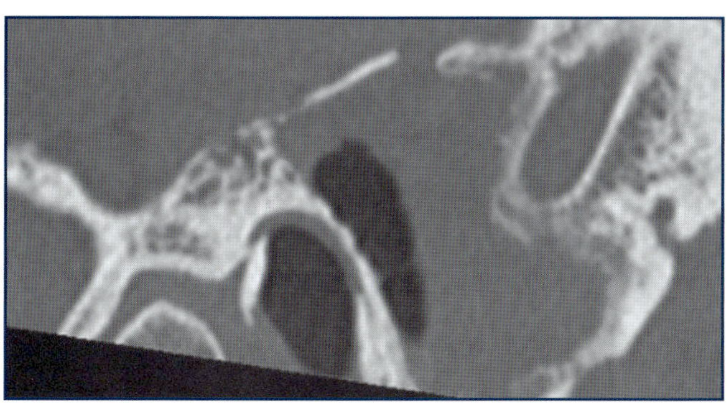

C

Figure 11–4. Post-op CT, right ear. **A.** Axial view. **B.** Coronal view. **C.** Sagittal view. The repair is intact, with air surrounding the ossicular heads.

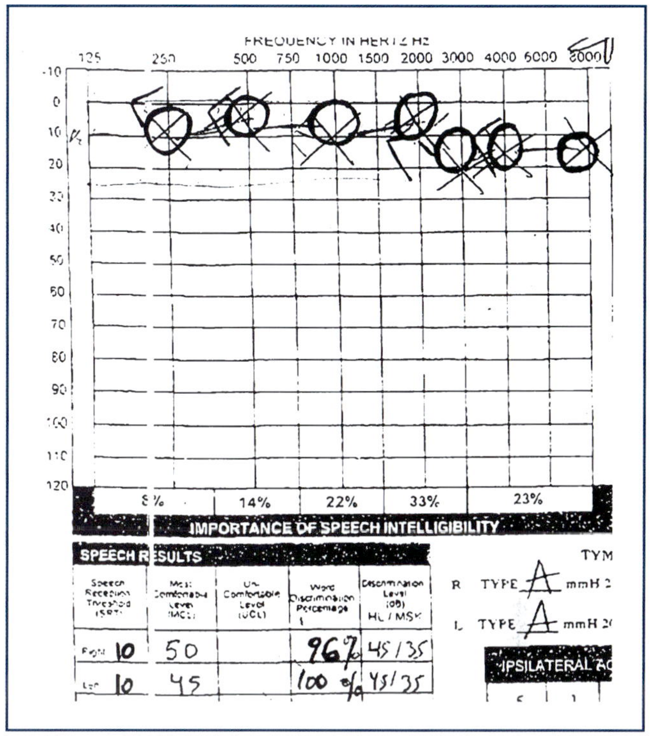

Figure 11–5. Postoperative hearing test showing little change in hearing.

Case 2

EL is a 55-year-old female with a history of hearing loss and a pulsatile tinnitus in the left ear following an influenza infection. She has some dizziness, but not vertigo. Her only significant antecedent history is that she underwent abdominal laparoscopic banding for weight reduction and over the next 5 months lost approximately 65 pounds. She has had no other contributing otologic or neurotologic history.

On otoscopic examination, all finding were normal on the right. On the left, there was retraction of the drum and fluid seen medial to the drum. She was unable to autoinsufflate the left middle ear cleft. The tuning forks at 512 and 1024 Hz were heard midline and air>bone bilaterally.

A hearing test revealed a neurosensory hearing loss on the right at 35 db/92% SDS and a mixed hearing loss on the left at 60 dB with 64% speech discrimination. There was no mass seen within the nasopharynx especially at the opening of the eustachian tube. An MRI of brain without and with gadolinium enhancement was done, revealing complete opacification of the left middle ear and mastoid air cell system. There was no obvious herniation of brain into the mastoid and no other significant findings (Figure 11–6). The overall impression was chronic serous otitis media or mastoiditis after an episode of the flu.

A repeat hearing test revealed hearing was improving bilaterally with SRT/ SDS scores 15 db/ 100% on the right and 20 dB/100% on the left with bilateral type A tympanograms and reflexes present. The patient was instructed to pop her ears and given no further treatment.

She was seen several months later still complaining of left aural fullness, pressure, and hearing loss. Otoscopy revealed fluid in the left middle ear. An audiogram done on this day revealed normal hearing on the right and a moderate to severe mixed hearing loss on the left (Figure 11–7). A myringotomy and PET insertion was performed under topical phenol anesthesia on the left. Clear, nonpulsatile fluid was obtained.

The patient then complained of nightly discharge of clear fluid from the left ear. Otoscopic examination revealed a patent grommet with a few drops of fluid. The amount did not increase with the

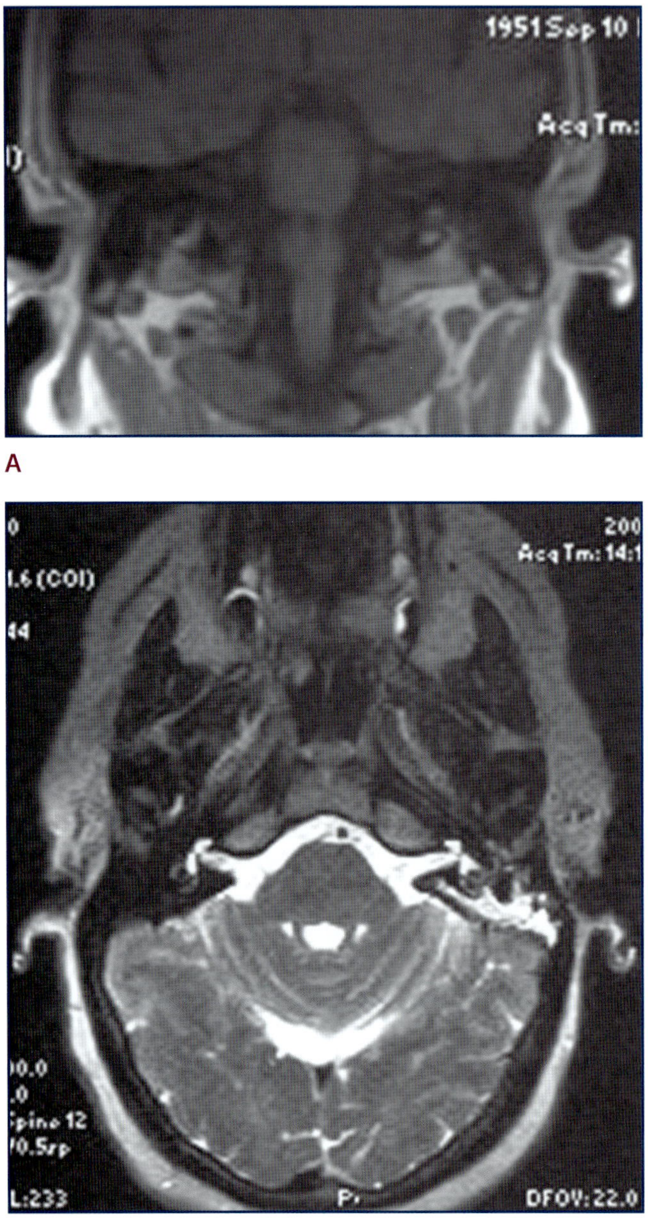

Figure 11–6. Pre-op MRI. **A.** T-1 coronal image. **B.** T-2 axial image. There is no obvious herniation of brain into the mastoid and no other significant findings.

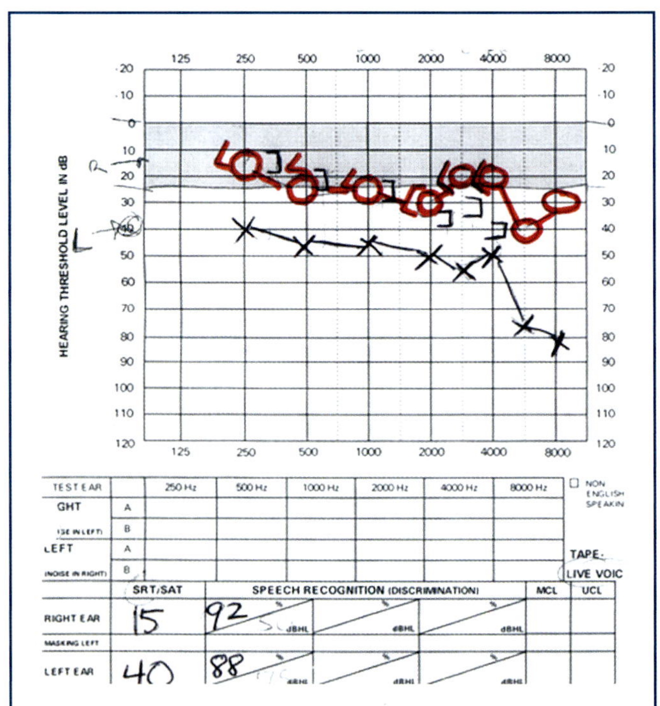

Figure 11–7. Pre-op audiogram showing normal hearing on the right and a moderate to severe mixed hearing loss on the left.

Valsalva maneuver or by placing the patient in a left lateral decubitus position with the ear undermost for 30 minutes. She collected the fluid and β2-transferrin assay was performed and found to be positive. Re-review of her CT of temporal bone showed an area of bony thinning at the tegmen mastoideum (Figure 11–8).

The diagnosis of encephalocele was now suspected as the cause of her problem. She underwent a left transmastoid and middle fossa repair (Figure 11–9). There were several small "knuckles" of brain seen herniating through the tegmen mastoideum and tympanum. These were repaired in a "sandwich" fashion with a split-thickness calvarial bone graft, temporalis fascia and fibrin glue (Figure 11–10). The remaining craniotomy plate was replaced (Figure 11–11). She healed uneventfully with no further leak of fluid. Her hearing remained stable and her preoperative dizziness is improving with balance therapy.

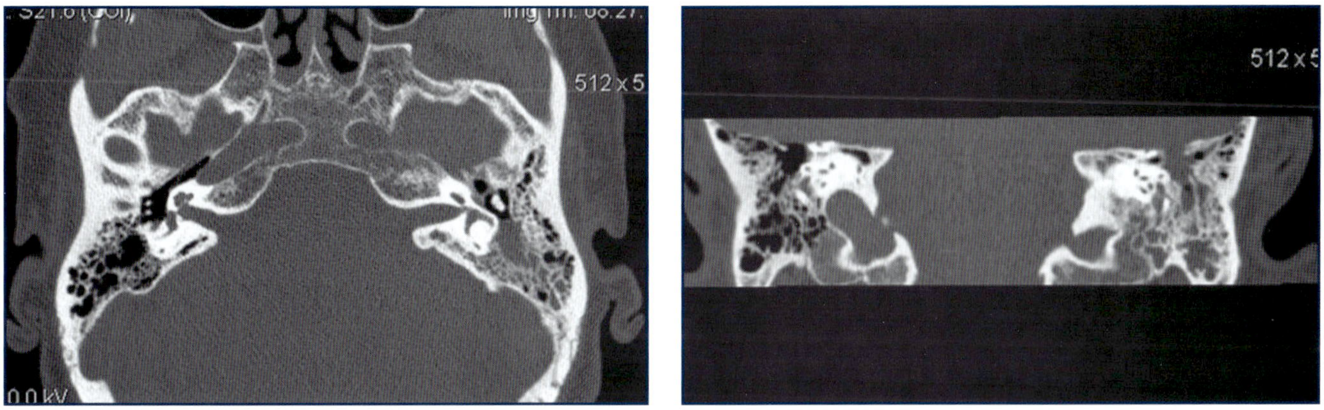

A B

Figure 11–8. Pre-op CT. **A.** Axial image. **B.** Coronal image. Review of this showed an area of thin bone at the tegmen mastoideum.

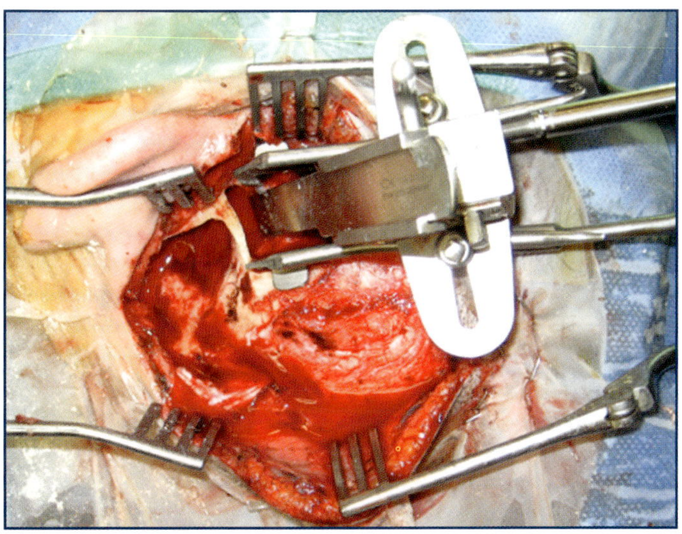

Figure 11–9. Intraoperative view of left combined transmastoid and middle fossa exposure of encephalocele. There were several small "knuckles" of brain seen herniating through the tegmen mastoideum and tympanum.

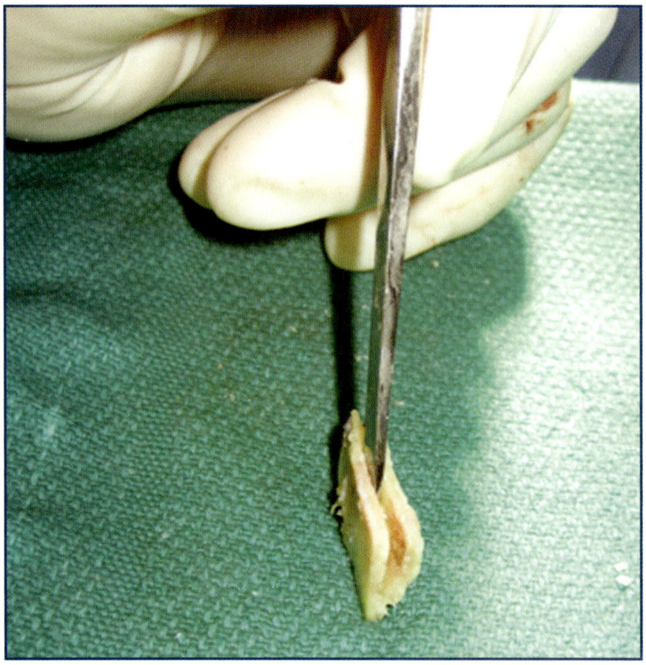

A

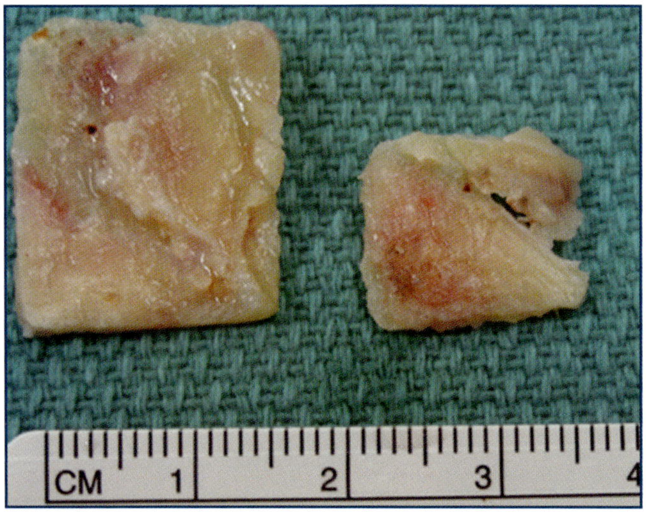

B

Figure 11–10. Intraoperative views. **A.** Split-thickness calvarial graft. **B.** Resulting bone grafts.

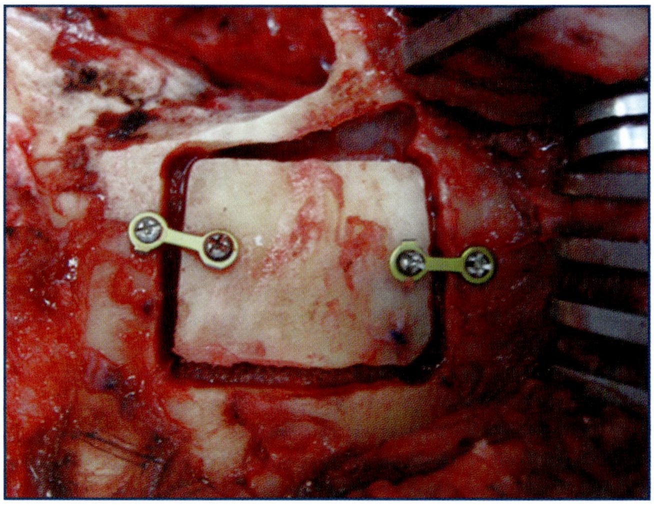

Figure 11–11. Intraoperative views. Replacement of left middle fossa outer table craniotomy bone flap.

CONCLUSIONS/ SUMMARY

The history, physical examination, audiometric, and radiologic evaluation of the patient presenting with CSF otorrhea or rhinorrhea have been reviewed. The index of suspicion increases in patients who are obese, elderly, smoke, or have had antecedent meningitis, otologic surgery, or head trauma involving the temporal bone. The entity of CSF leak and encephalocele should be considered in any patient with unilateral, persistent serous otitis media, even in patients without antecedent temporal bone fracture or meningitis.

The co-operation of a skilled neuroradiologist is essential to help locate the likely source of the CSF leak. Modern computerization allows for close fusion of CT and MR data to precisely align bone and soft-tissue information.

Adjunctive tests such as β2-transferrin and radioisotopic studies are of value when positive, but are of no value when negative. They must be regarded along with the other clinical and laboratory evidence.

The more commonly performed surgical treatments of encephaloceles of the temporal bone have been described. It is important for the surgeon to look for multiple defects in the tegmen and to be prepared to repair every single defect found. Most repairs are done with gross and microscopic visualization alone. Intraoperative navigational assistance has not proven to be of added value in the repair of encephaloceles.

The surgical approach is determined by the nature of the lesion, the location(s) of the leak(s), the amount of discharge, the age and general health of the patient including any concomitant morbidities, especially cholesteatoma, and the amount of residual hearing. The surgeon should be armed with several techniques for repair. The majority of repairs in this series were performed via a transmastoid/ middle cranial fossa combined approach. A "sandwich" technique of soft tissue and bone with or without biologic adhesives has proven sufficient to close the tegmen and dural defect(s) in almost all patients.

In occasional patients, a lumbar drain to decrease the head of CSF pressure during the immediate postoperative period may be beneficial.

Surveillance for re-formation of encephaloceles of the temporal bone includes a thorough history and micro-otoscopic examination. As long as there is no re-accumulation of fluid, radiographic surveillance is rarely needed. If there is any question, an edge-enhanced CT will usually yield sufficient information about the reformation of an encephalocele.

REFERENCES

1. Kuhweide R, Casselman JW. Spontaneous cerebrospinal fluid otorrhoea from a tegmen defect: transmastoid repair with minicraniotomy. *Ann Otol Rhinol Laryngol.* 1999;108:653–658.
2. Lundy LB, Graham MD, Kartush JK, LaRouere MJ. Temporal bone encephalocele and cerebrospinal fluid leaks. *Am J Otol*. 1996;17:456–461.
3. Caboche H. De la hernie cérébrale dans les interventions intracraniennes dirigés contre les otities moyennes suppurées. *Annales des maladies de l'oreille, de larynx, du nez et du pharyn.* 1902;28:278–294.
4. Jackson CG, Pappas Jr DG, Manolidis S, et al. Brain herniation into the middle ear and mastoid: concepts in diagnosis and surgical management. *Am J Otol*. 1997;18:198–206.
5. Gacek RR. Arachnoid granulation cerebrospinal fluid otorrhea. *Ann Otol Rhinol Laryngol*. 1990;99:854–862.
6. Gacek RR. (1992). Evaluation and management of temporal bone arachnoid granulations. *Arch Otolaryngol Head Neck Surg*. 1992;2:118:327–332.
7. Brown NE, Grundfast KM, Megerian CA, O'Malley BW, Rosenberg SI. Diagnosis and management of spontaneous cerebrospinal fluid-middle ear effusion and otorrhea. *Laryngoscope*. 2004;114;800–805.
8. Levy LM, Gulya AJ, Davis SW, LeBihan D, Rajan SS, Schellinger D. (1995). Flow-sensitive magnetic resonance imaging in the evaluation of CSF leaks. *Am J Otol*. 1995; 16:591–596.
9. Schuknecht HF, Zaytoun GM, Moon CN Jr. Adult-onset fluid in the tympanomastoid compartment. *Arch Otolaryngol*. 1982;108:759–765.
10. Bassiouny M, Hirsch BE, Kelly RH, Kamerer DB, Cass SP. Beta-2 transferrin application in otology. *Am J Otology*. 1992;13:552–555.
11. Skedros DG, Cass SP, Hirsch BE, Kelly RH. Beta-2 transferrin assay in clinical management of cerebral spinal fluid and perilymphatic fluid leaks. *J Otolaryngol*. 1993;22:341–344.
12. Kemink JL, Graham MD, Kartush JM. Spontaneous encephalocele of the temporal bone. *Arch Otolaryngol Head Neck Surg*. 1986;112:558–561.
13. Linstrom CJ, Krajewski MJ, Shapiro AL, Caruana S. Outer table graft in middle fossa surgery. *Otolaryngol Head Neck Surg*. 1994;111:70–75.

PART III

Facial Nerve: Testing and Management

CHAPTER 12

Electrical Testing of Facial Nerve

Howard Sander and Seilesh Babu

ELECTRODIAGNOSTIC EVALUATION OF THE FACIAL NERVE

Patients presenting with complete facial nerve paralysis usually require electrical testing of the facial nerve. Management decisions will be made based on these results; therefore, a thorough interpretation of these tests needs to be understood. This chapter reviews electrical testing of the facial nerve and present the common disease processes where the testing provides additional information.

It is important for the otolaryngologist to know that the same testing modality will have different synonyms, depending upon the specialty. Thus, what the neurologist terms *compound muscle action potential* (CMAP) testing will be called *electroneuronography* (ENOG) by the otolaryngologist. It is essentially the same test with 2 different names. This difference in nomenclature should be kept in mind while reading literature regarding electrical testing.

INTRODUCTION

Facial nerve function can be evaluated using several electrodiagnostic studies. The goals of performing these studies include determining the nature, location, and severity of an injury, as well as determining a prognosis for recovery, and documentation of ongoing recovery (Table 12–1). To be maximally beneficial, they must be performed accurately and then interpreted in light of the clinical history and examination.

Electrodiagnostic testing involves two distinct types: nerve conduction studies and needle electromyography. The term "electromyography" and the abbreviation "EMG" are commonly used to refer to all of these tests. Nerve conduction studies to evaluate facial nerve functioning involve electrical nerve stimulation. The evoked electrical response is then recorded usually by electrodes placed on the skin surface, or less commonly, the degree of evoked muscle twitch is visually estimated. Needle electromyography involves recording muscle fiber discharges thorough a needle inserted into a muscle, without administration of any electrical impulse. These are sometimes termed voluntary (needle EMG) and involuntary EMG (nerve stimulation/conduction study).

Table 12–1. Questions Addressed by Facial Nerve Electrodiagnostic Studies

Is a lesion present?
Where is the dysfunction located?
Is the underlying pathophysiology axonal or demyelinating?
How severe is the injury?
Is there anatomic nerve continuity?
What is the prognosis for recovery of function?
Has there been any recovery of function?
Is recovery continuing?
Is the dysfunction part of a generalized polyneuropathy, or is it restricted to the facial nerve?

NERVE CONDUCTION STUDIES

Electroneuronography (ENOG) or Evoked Electromyography (EEMG)

Motor nerve conduction studies of the facial nerve are performed by electrically stimulating the facial nerve with intensity sufficient to excite all the axons in the nerve, leading to depolarization of all the muscle fibers in the target muscle. This is termed a supramaximal stimulus. The associated electrical activity is recorded with surface electrodes and the recorded response is called a compound muscle action potential (CMAP). On occasions, subcutaneously placed needles may also be used for recording.[1] A CMAP is therefore the spatial and temporal sum of the individual muscle fiber action potentials from a muscle. Many commercial EMG systems are available. The recording electrodes are placed on the skin overlying a muscle with one electrode (G1, active electrode) over the muscle belly and a second electrode (G2, reference electrode) over a nearby relatively silent area. The evoked CMAP has two commonly measured characteristics: amplitude and latency.

There is no accepted standard site from which to record. Commonly used sites include the orbicularis oculi, nasalis, nasolabial fold, and orbicularis oris. A ground electrode is also placed at any remote location, such as the forehead or chin, to eliminate ambient artifact. Stimulation is performed with a bipolar stimulator on the skin surface near the stylomastoid foramen either just posterior or anterior to the bottom of the auricle (Figure 12–1). Increasing intensity stimulations are applied to obtain a supramaximal facial nerve CMAP. Extreme care must be taken to avoid simultaneous activation of the masseter muscle, as this large response will create a falsely enlarged combined CMAP. Use of a pediatric stimulator (Nicolet Biomedical, Madison, WI, # 019-733400) with closely spaced prongs (14 mm between tips) also facilitates selective facial nerve activation. In some cases, it may be difficult to determine if the masseter is contributing to the response. The CMAP in these cases should be considered nondiagnostic.

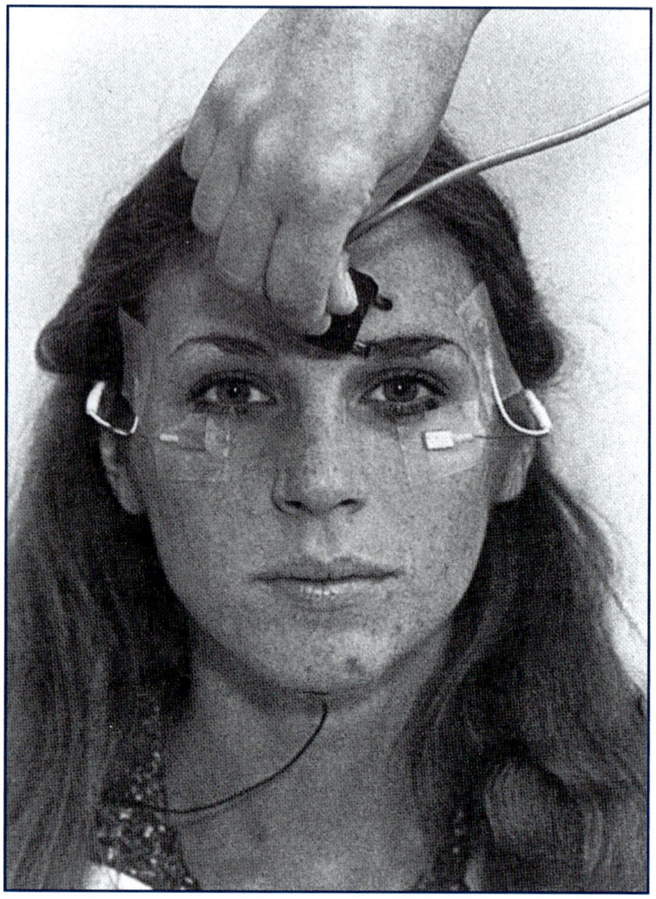

Figure 12–1. Example of electrode placement for performing facial motor nerve conduction studies with recording of the orbicularis oculi facial compound muscle action potential (CMAP, ENOG). The active electrode (G1) is placed on the orbicularis oculi, the reference electrode (G2) is placed on the temple, and a ground electrode is placed on the chin. Stimulation is performed with the cathode just anterior to the mastoid process. (From Kimura J. *Electrodiagnosis in diseases of nerve and muscle: Principles and practice*. 2nd ed. Philadelphia, PA: FA Davis, 1989. Reprinted with permission of Oxford University Press).

The CMAP amplitude is related to the number and size of the depolarizing muscle fibers and (in the absence of muscle or neuromuscular junction disease) is roughly proportional to the number of functioning axons in the nerve. The facial nerve CMAP may have 2 or 3 phases. When there is a third phase with an initially positive (downward) deflection, this indicates that the recording electrode was not positioned over the motor point, and some of the response is volume conducted from a distant location. In practice, the facial CMAP is a combination of responses from several different muscles, and it is very difficult to position the recording electrode precisely over the motor point. Accordingly, the amplitude of the response is measured from the highest peak to the lowest peak to avoid variability associated with the presence of an initial positivity.

The CMAP latency is predominantly an indicator of the functioning of the myelin sheath. As the nerve conduction slows, the latency will be greater. In facial nerve testing, there is insufficient distance to reliably stimulate at two separate points to allow better determination of latency. It is therefore difficult to obtain accurate conduction velocities without needle stimulation and recording.[1] Latency values (in milliseconds) are used instead. Normative latency values have been derived from population-based studies, and side-side latency values are available for some methods.

Changes in the CMAP amplitude and latency may provide information as to the severity of damage that has occurred and aid in determining chance of full recovery.

Bell's Palsy: CMAP Changes

CMAP Amplitude

In Bell's palsy, facial nerve testing with ENOG is performed when complete paralysis is present and both sides of the face are tested. Care should be taken to place the recording electrodes symmetrically. The amplitudes are expressed as a ratio of the affected side over the unaffected side. This CMAP amplitude ratio has been presumed to reflect the percentage of the axons that are still functioning. This should only be considered as a very rough estimate, as area measurements would be more accurate. Furthermore, the ratio in normal controls may be as low as 65%.[2] The CMAP amplitude ratio should not be used if there is facial dysfunction on the contralateral side (eg, prior Bell's palsy). In the first 3 or 4 days following Bell's palsy onset, the response will remain normal despite clinically severe weakness, as Wallerian degeneration will not yet have progressed distally. Axonal degeneration may occur for 2 to 3 weeks following onset. Data derived from large patient populations to predict prognosis for facial nerve recovery are available for 2 weeks following onset. Following 2 weeks, the CMAP amplitude ratio appears to lose its prognostic value. Facial nerve conduction studies should therefore be performed on days 4 to 14 following onset, preferably between days 5 to 10.[3,4] The studies may be performed once, or alternatively some authors suggest that they should be performed serially every 1 to 2 days to determine prognosis. Surgical need for facial nerve decompression may be assessed in this time frame as well.

Many clinical studies have been performed to determine appropriate cutoff values for the CMAP amplitude ratio for prognostication. There is a generally accepted current consensus that if the CMAP ratio falls below 10% at any point within the first two weeks, ie, ≥ 90% degeneration, there is a poor prognosis for recovery, with either incomplete recovery or significant synkinesis developing over 6 to 12 months.[3,5–8] If the CMAP ratio is 10 to 30% there is an intermediate prognosis, with mild-moderate eventual dysfunction, and progression of recovery over 2 to 8 months. If the CMAP ratio is above 30% there is a good prognosis for recovery, with recovery usually occurring within 2 months. It is important to recognize, and to also communicate to patients, that these prognostic indicators are not always correct. Thus, for example, a small percentage of patients with a ratio of less than 10% nonetheless enjoy a full cosmetic recovery, and on occasion a patient with a ratio of 40% may achieve only moderate recovery. Furthermore, as the cutoff values are somewhat arbitrary, patients with borderline values may have a recovery fitting either group.

The rate of decline of the CMAP amplitude has also been shown to have prognostic significance. Axonal degeneration may continue to occur for several weeks following onset. For patients who are evaluated relatively early, a repeat examination, or serial examinations may provide useful information. A patient with an amplitude ratio of 25% on day 5, and 15% on day 6, may decline to 5% by day 8. In this instance, the "moderate prognosis" would be changed to a "poor prognosis." Some authors have recommended that treatment should be altered based upon CMAP amplitude ratios. It has been suggested that facial nerve decompression be considered if the ratio falls below 10% or that the dosage and duration of prednisone therapy be increased in this patient group.[9,10] If surgery is being considered, serial testing should be performed.

The healing process may begin with axonal sprouting followed by axonal growth about 2 to 3 weeks following onset of Bell's palsy. The CMAP amplitude then reflects both the degree of initial injury and also the extent of recovery. If spontaneous recovery does not begin to occur, follow-up nerve conduction and EMG studies in 2 to 4 months should be scheduled. If there is insubstantial recovery, then additional studies (eg, MRI of the cerebellopontine angle) should be considered to exclude other etiologies of facial paralysis such as a mass lesion.

In childhood Bell's palsy, the CMAP amplitude has also be used for prognostication. However, the time course of the response is different than in adults. Additional studies are required to develop standardized guidelines. The acoustic reflex, which evaluates the function of the stapedius muscle, may be helpful in children if there is difficulty in tolerating electrical stimulation.[11]

CMAP Latency

In Bell's palsy, the CMAP latency has not been demonstrated to be helpful in prognostication.[5,8,12,13] This is understandable intuitively, as the site of dysfunction is proximal to the stimulation and recording sites, and Bell's palsy does not cause demyelination along the locations at which the CMAP latency is being measured. Nonetheless, the latency may increase due to degeneration of the fastest conducting axons, but this can occur in both mild and severe cases. Normative latency values are available for different recording sites and for side-side CMAP latency asymmetry.[5,8,12,13]

Nerve Conduction Studies in Generalized Polyneuropathies

Axonal neuropathies usually cause a reduced CMAP amplitude with normal or only mildly slowed conduction. Most metabolic neuropathies, (eg, diabetic, uremic, or HIV neuropathy) are length dependent processes, affecting predominantly the legs. The arm and facial CMAPs are involved only in rare, severe cases. In contrast, mononeuropathy multiplex (eg, polyarteritis nodosa, temporal arteritis, lupus erythematosus, Lyme disease) may cause an axonal facial neuropathy with a low amplitude facial CMAP.[13,14]

OTHER NERVE CONDUCTION STUDIES

Nerve Excitability Test (NET)

The nerve excitability test was originally described in 1962 and had been widely used for prognostication in Bell's palsy.[15] The test involves stimulation of the facial nerve at the level of the stylomastoid foramen with progressively increasing current intensity. The lowest intensity current that elicits a clinically observable twitch is noted. Testing is performed bilaterally. A poor prognosis for recovery is indicated when the side to side difference in threshold intensities exceeds a cutoff value. Reported methods for performing this test have varied considerably, with the stimulus duration ranging from 0.1 to 1 msec, and the cutoff for a poor prognosis ranging from 2 to 5 mA.[12,16] The usefulness of this test is limited because a twitch will be observed even if only a few fibers are unaffected. There are also technical difficulties with adequate skin preparation, and with a masseter response obscuring small facial twitches. The rate of erroneous determination of a good prognosis has been cited as high as 42%.[17] The NET has therefore been replaced by other studies.

Maximal Stimulation Test (MST)

The maximal stimulation test is similar to the NET in that the response is visually graded by the examiner. It employs supramaximal stimulation intensity sufficient to excite all the axons in the underlying nerve. The stimulation is performed bilaterally. Using stimulus duration of 0.6 ms, the stimulus is increased until the patient's tolerance limit or 5 to 8 mA, whichever is higher. The stimulator may be held stationary or slowly moved across the face. The degree of visible muscle contraction is subjectively graded as normal, decreased, or absent. Some grading systems divide "decreased" into mildly decreased and greatly decreased, and one grading system further adds a moderately decreased category.[5,7,12,16,18,19] The response in the distribution of the five facial branches are evaluated: forehead, periorbital region, upper lip and nasal ala, lower lip, and cervical area. May reported results of MST in 37 patients with Bell's palsy and complete facial paralysis who were studied within 10 days of onset. When the twitches on both sides were equal, there was a 92% chance of complete recovery of facial function. In patients with markedly reduced or absent twitches, there was an 86% chance of incomplete facial nerve recovery.[17] The MST has therefore been shown to be capable of accurate prognostication when used by examiners who use the test routinely and in a standardized fashion. However, a major drawback of the MST is the requirement for the examiner to subjectively assess the degree of twitch. It is less likely to be diagnostically useful when used only occasionally by examiners without considerable experience, and there have not been any studies documenting reliability between different examiners.

Electrical recording of muscle activity (CMAP or ENOG) provides a more quantifiable and objective measurement of nerve functioning than the MST, and has largely replaced this test.[6]

NEEDLE ELECTROMYOGRAPHY (EMG)

Routine needle electromyography is performed using either a monopolar or a concentric recording needle. The monopolar electrode compares the electrical environment at the tip of the needle with a separate surface reference electrode. The concentric needle contains a built-in reference electrode near the tip. In the past, monopolar needles had an advantage of being slightly narrower and therefore more comfortable for the patient. Currently, concentric needles are as thin as monopolar needles (usually 26-gauge for extremity recordings), and they produce technically better recordings with considerably fewer artifacts than monopolar needles. Very thin gauge (30G) concentric needles are also now available and are particularly suited for facial muscle electromyography. With use of these fine electrodes, patients usually find facial EMG testing only mildly discomforting. The potentials generated by the muscle fibers are displayed graphically on a monitor and are connected to a speaker for audio interpretation. The electromyographic examination is performed at rest, under mild voluntary activation and during strong contraction. Figure 12–2 is a summary of needle electromyographic findings.

EMG of Resting Muscle

Normal Findings

At rest, a normal muscle will not generate any spontaneous activity outside the endplate region. Therefore no potentials are visible on the monitor and there speakers are silent. If the needle is moved within the muscle, there will be depolarization of the fibers touching the needle causing brief electrical activity, called insertional activity, which ends very shortly following cessation of needle movement.

Fasciculation potentials are another discharge occasionally observed in resting muscle. They may be either a normal finding, or may be related to pathology. These discharges represent the spontaneous discharge of a motor unit potential. They may be accompanied by a clinically observable fasciculatory twitch. As caffeine use and sleep deprivation may provoke these discharges, they should be considered as normal, unless they are accompanied by abnormalities of other tests.

Abnormal Findings

A muscle fiber that has been denervated (detached from an innervating neuron) will have an increased amount of insertional activity, and it will also begin to produce spontaneous discharges at rest, which are recorded as either fibrillation potentials or positive sharp waves. These discharges may be referred to as active denervation, indicating that the muscle fiber generating the potential is currently not attached to an innervating axon. In the setting of acute nerve injury, these potentials develop only after there has been sufficient time for Wallerian degeneration and muscle end plate degeneration to occur. This is a length-dependent process taking 10 to 21 days. In Bell's palsy, active denervation is usually not present until about 10 days following onset. Fibrillation

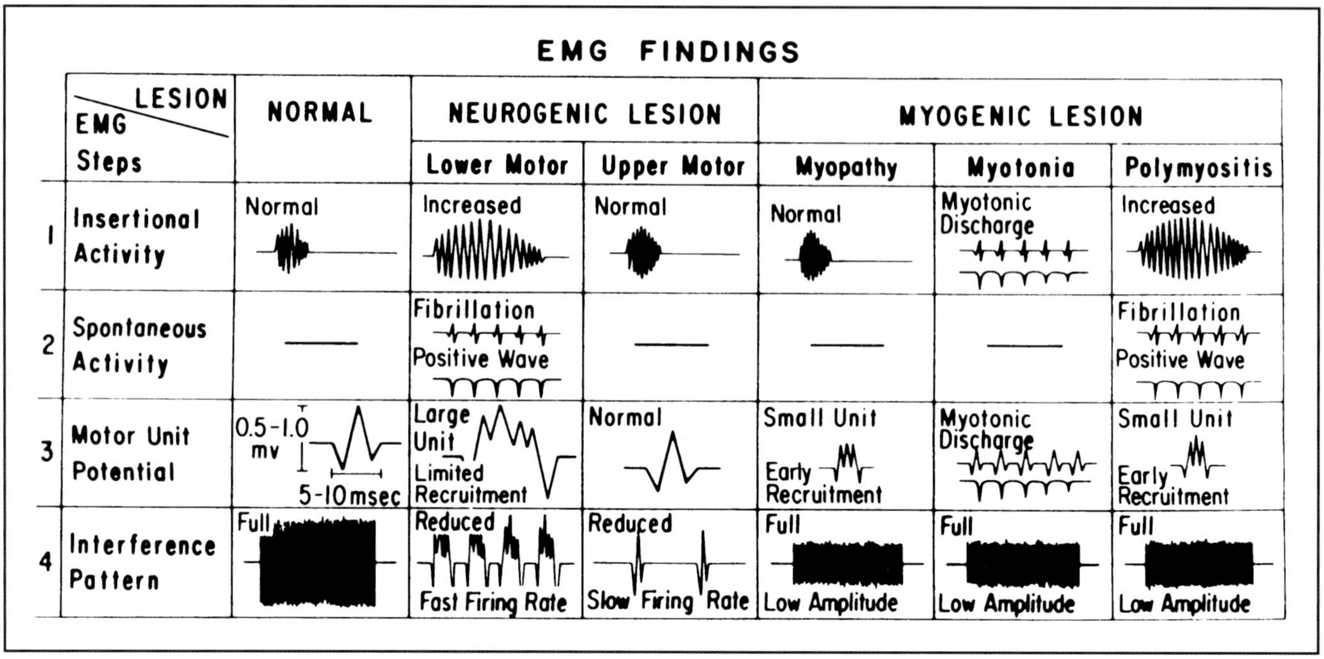

Figure 12–2. Typical findings on needle electromyography (EMG) in lower and upper motor neuron disorders and myogenic illnesses compared with normal findings. A peripheral facial palsy would have the characteristics of a lower motor neuron disorder. (From Kimura J. *Electrodiagnosis in diseases of nerve and muscle: Principles and practice*. 2nd ed. Philadelphia, PA: FA Davis, 1989. Reprinted with permission of Oxford University Press).

potentials are initially positive, brief (<5 ms) duration biphasic or triphasic waves. Positive sharp waves are initially sharply positive (downward deflection) with a long-duration (10–30 ms) negative phase. They both discharge in a regular, slow pattern, and sound similar to the "ticking of a clock."[20] Fibrillation potentials are generated by muscle fibers uninjured by the needle. Positive sharp waves are generated by muscle fibers that have been injured by the recording needle, and cannot produce the repolarization phase. These two discharges have an identical diagnostic significance. Active denervation is most commonly caused by neuropathy. Active denervation may also occur in inflammatory myopathies (eg, polymyositis). In this instance the inflammation causes muscle fiber splitting, and the orphaned fibers may be detached from their nerve supply. These fibers will then develop fibrillation potentials and positive sharp waves (active denervation).

Fasciculation potentials are spontaneously discharging motor unit potentials. Although these potentials occur in normal patients, as described above, they may also occur in association with any neuropathy. In motor neuron diseases, such as amyotrophic lateral sclerosis, they are usually very frequent and widespread.

EMG During Mild Voluntary Muscle Activation

During mild voluntary activation, individual motor unit potentials (MUP) are recorded. A motor unit is defined as a single motor neuron (including its axon and dendrites) and all the muscle fibers it innervates. Muscle fibers of a single motor unit are normally interspersed with fibers belonging to other motor units. An MUP is the summation of the electrical potentials generated by all the muscle fibers innervated by a single neuron that are within the needle recording area. If any MUPs are recorded, there is evidence of nerve continuity (of at least a few axons) from the brain to that muscle. In the setting of trauma, the presence of recordable MUPs can demonstrate that a nerve has not been completely severed. Alternatively, however, the absence of recordable MUPs does not distinguish between severe nerve injury and nerve discontinuity. The morphology (shape) of a MUP is altered in disease. In neuropathic illness, alteration of the MUP morphology indicates that re-innervation has occurred. Early in the process of re-innervation, when only a few muscle fibers have been re-innervated, the MUPs may have a low amplitude with either a normal or a slightly increased duration. With continued re-innervation a single axon innervates many adjacent muscle fibers through collateral sprouting. As adjacent muscle fibers are now innervated by the same motor unit, a recording needle electrode will summate potentials generated by a greater number of fibers. The recorded MUP of a re-innervated motor unit is therefore larger, with a prolonged duration and a high amplitude. The processes of denervation and subsequent re-innervation usually occur over a several month time period. Large MUPs therefore indicate that a chronic neuropathic process is present. Chronic denervation is the term applied to the presence of large MUPs. This term is somewhat misleading, however, because the healing process (re-innervation) must have also occurred for it to be present. In myopathic illnesses the MUPs have a short duration and a low amplitude because the individual muscle fiber membranes generate smaller potentials. The duration of a MUP is therefore helpful in distinguishing neuropathy from myopathy. Polyphasia of the MUP is a less diagnostically useful finding, as 15% of normal MUPs are polyphasic, and polyphasia more occur in both neuropathy and myopathy.

EMG During Strong Voluntary Muscle Contraction

In normal individuals, initially upon mild voluntary contraction, only one or a few MUPs will be recorded on the monitor. In facial muscles, the initial MUPs have a firing frequency of 8 to 10 Hz, which is faster than the 4 to 5 Hz observed in extremity muscles.[22] With increasing volitional effort, the firing rate of individual MUPs increases, and additional MUPs are also recruited. With full voluntary effort, the entire baseline is obliterated by a summation of many MUPs. This is termed a *full interference pattern*. In a muscle that has been denervated, there are fewer MUPs available for force generation. If a nerve has been severed, there will be no MUPs recruited (absent recruitment). In severe, but incomplete neuropathy, only a few axons are functional. In this instance, only a single MUP may discharge (single unit interference pattern) with a substantially increased firing rate (25–40 Hz) in an attempt to generate sufficient force. With mild or moderate neuropathy, there is a gradation of mildly-moderately decreased interference patterns and mildly-moderately increased firing rates (decreased interference pattern). Myopathy has a different pattern. In myopathy many MUPs will be recruited with minimal volitional effort (early recruitment) as the individual muscle fibers are weak and do not generate sufficient force. As the amplitudes of the individual myopathic MUPs are small, the amplitude of the summated interference pattern will be decreased (low-amplitude envelope).

EMG in Bell's Palsy

Electromyography in Bell's palsy cannot be reliably used to predict prognosis. Although one author initially reported encouraging results, these finding have not been replicated.[23,24] In the setting of recent onset Bell's palsy, EMG may however provide useful information. The complete absence of any recordable motor units from any muscle would suggest a more severe lesion. EMG is particularly helpful in following the progression of recovery. As reinnervation occurs, the extent of active denervation (fibrillation potentials and positive sharp waves) will decrease, and prolonged duration MUPs will appear consistent with chronic denervation and re-innervation. The interference pattern will become progressively fuller, giving a rough estimate of the degree of recovery that has occurred. These findings may precede the clinically visible improvement and provide a basis for optimism. Furthermore, if there is no return of function (no recordable MUPs) after several months, other causes of facial paralysis should be sought.

BLINK REFLEX

The blink reflex is the electrophysiologic correlate of the clinically elicited corneal reflex (Figure 12–3). The afferent component of this reflex arc is conveyed via the ophthalmic division of the trigeminal nerve, CN V1. The efferent component is conveyed via the facial nerve. An electrical stimulus is applied to the skin overlying the supraorbital nerve at the supra-

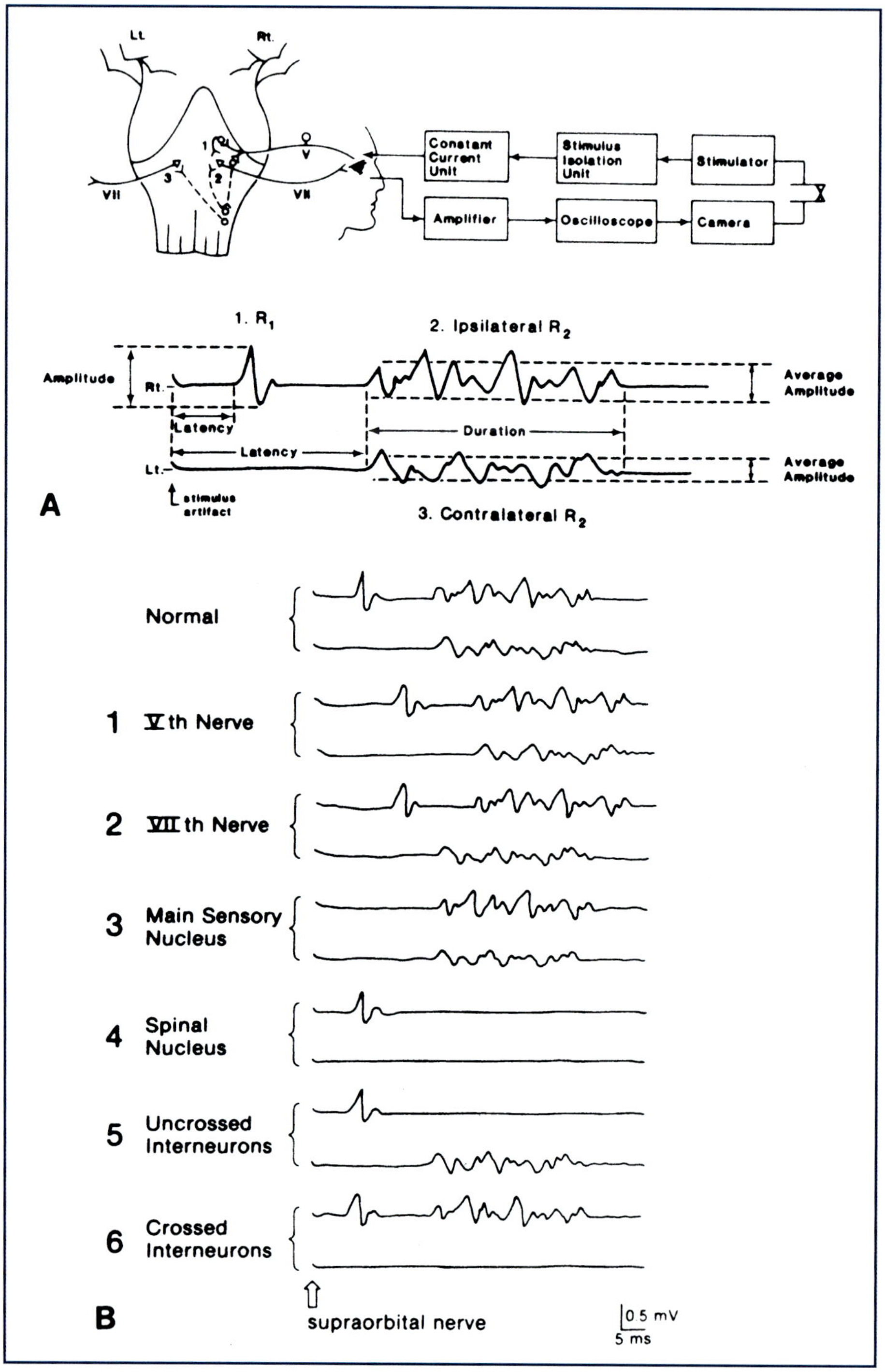

Figure 12–3. Blink reflex summary. **A.** *Top*: schematic of blink reflex pathways with R1 ipsilateral to the stimulation through the pons [1], and R2 bilaterally through the pons and lateral medulla [2 and 3]. *Bottom*: a typical blink reflex elicited by right-sided stimulation. Note an ipsilateral R1 and bilateral R2 responses. **B.** Five basic types of blink reflex abnormalities. *From top to bottom*, the findings suggest conduction abnormality of the: [1] afferent pathway along the trigeminal nerve; [2] efferent pathway along the facial nerve; [3] main trigeminal sensory nucleus or pontine interneurons (pathway 1 in **A**); [4] trigeminal spinal tract and nucleus or medullary interneuronal pathways; [5] uncrossed medullary interneurons to the ipsilateral facial nucleus (2 of **A**); and [6] crossed medullary interneurons to the contralateral facial nucleus (3 of **A**). (From Kimura J. *Electrodiagnosis in diseases of nerve and muscle: Principles and practice.* 2nd ed. Philadelphia, PA: FA Davis, 1989, Reprinted with permission of Oxford University Press).

orbital notch. Recordings electrodes are placed over the orbicularis oculi muscle (Figure 12–4). Following unilateral supraorbital stimulation, a clinically visible blink occurs bilaterally. The recorded electrical response on the ipsilateral side has two components, R1 and R2.

The blink reflex pathway involves the entire extent of the seventh nerve (including the proximal portions), the fifth nerve, the pons, and the medulla. The blink reflex may therefore demonstrate abnormalities related to these sites that are not revealed with traditional motor nerve conduction or electromyography studies.[13,14] A significant benefit of the blink reflex, in comparison to the direct facial motor nerve conduction study, is that the pitfall of activation of the masseter muscle is avoided. Therefore, if a response is obtained, facial nerve continuity is definitively demonstrated.

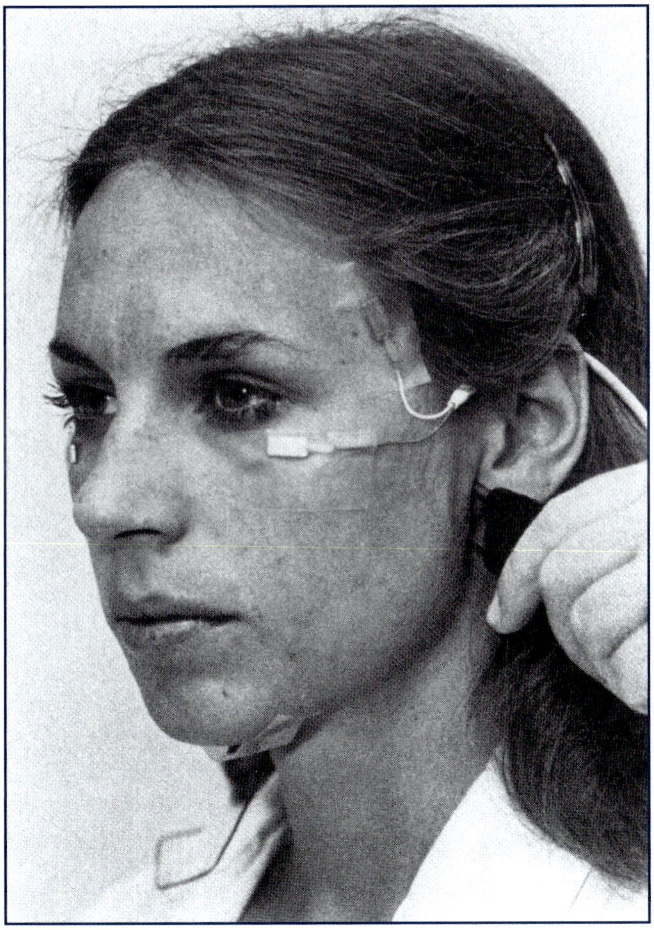

Figure 12–4. Electrode placement for performing a blink reflex study. Unilateral supraorbital nerve stimulation is performed and recordings are obtained from bilateral orbicularis oculi muscles. A ground electrode is placed on the chin. (From Kimura J. *Electrodiagnosis in diseases of nerve and muscle: Principles and practice*. 2nd ed. Philadelphia, PA: FA Davis, 1989. Reprinted with permission of Oxford University Press).

An additional calculation, the R/D ratio, may be helpful in localization of blink reflex abnormalities. This ratio (blink reflex R1 latency divided by the direct facial CMAP latency) may aid in determining if a facial neuropathy is located proximal or distal to the stylomastoid foramen. Care must be exercised in its use, as it can also be altered by trigeminal neuropathy.[5,14]

Blink Reflex in Bell's Palsy

Blink reflex responses are almost always abnormal in Bell's palsy, and change considerably over time. The R1 response of the blink reflex may remain nearly normal for several days and then may decline in amplitude or develop a prolonged latency. Due to this delayed change, the blink reflex alone is not helpful in predicting prognosis early in the course of Bell's palsy. However, the blink reflex is helpful in prognostication after the initial 2 week period, when motor nerve conduction studies alone cannot be used for prognosis.[25–27]

FACIAL NEUROPATHY FROM CAUSES OTHER THAN BELL'S PALSY

The prognostic indicators that have been developed for Bell's palsy cannot be applied to facial neuropathy of other causes. These other lesions have a pathophysiology and temporal progression that differs from Bell's palsy, and large patient data pools have not been collected to allow prognostication. Nonetheless, electrodiagnostic studies can be extremely helpful in these disorders. The testing may help assess the severity of the injury, follow the progression and rate of recovery, and determine the presence of concomitant abnormalities in other nerves. In the setting of traumatic facial neuropathy, the studies may also be able to demonstrate nerve continuity in one or several branches, which may obviate the need for surgery. They may also be helpful in deciding whether to perform selected operative procedures (eg, XII to VII nerve transposition) and in presurgical planning.

OTHER NERVE STUDIES

Synkinesis Testing

Synkinetic facial movements may be documented by a synkinesis study. This may be used in patients with inadequate clinical recovery from facial neuropathy to document that nerve regeneration, although misdirected, is occurring. It may be helpful in an occasional patient to document the presence of a prior peripheral facial neuropathy, when this history is unavailable. Synkinesis is also easily demonstrable in patients with hemifacial spasm. Synkinesis may be demonstrated in two ways.[22] In one method, which is analogous to the blink reflex, the supraorbital nerve is stimulated and recordings are made from the orbicularis oculi and an additional muscle in the lower face (eg, orbicularis oris or mentalis). If synkinesis is present, abnormal blink reflex R1 and R2 components will be recorded from the lower muscle, in addition to the normally appearing R1 and R2 responses from the orbicularis oculi. In another method, the lateral spread response, the recording electrodes are placed as described above, and stimulation is applied over a branch of the facial nerve. The zygomatic and mandibular are independently stimulated. In the presence of synkinesis, a response will be recorded from both muscles, with a delay in latency of the responses from the aberrantly contracting muscle. In hemifacial spasm, the lateral spread response may disappear following successful surgery.

Magnetic Stimulation

Magnetic stimulation of the facial nerve by an appropriately positioned magnetic coil, will cause excitation at the level of the root exit zone. The evoked magnetic evoked potential (MEP) is then recorded from facial muscles. In Bell's palsy, the amplitude of the MEP becomes decreased within days 0 to 4 and often remains abnormal subsequent to full recovery of both clinical function and the electrical CMAP.[28,29] Magnetic stimulation has also been shown to demonstrate abnormalities in facial neuropathy due to Guillain-Barré syndrome, Lyme disease, HIV, herpes zoster, brainstem lesions, and carcinomatous meningitis.[30] There is insufficient experience with this technique, however, to recommend its routine clinical use.

Electrogustometry

This test evaluates the taste fibers in the chorda tympani by application of an electrical stimulation to the tongue until an acidic taste occurs. A ratio of the lowest intensity stimulus (threshold) sufficient to cause the taste on each side is calculated. Although one study reported promising results, this test has not been adopted by others.[31]

Trigeminal Nerve Studies

In the electrodiagnostic evaluation of facial nerve dysfunction, it is occasionally necessary to also evaluate other cranial nerves, most commonly the trigeminal. The blink reflex and the masseter reflex are the most commonly performed study.[13,14]

The masseter reflex is the electrical correlate of the clinically elicited jaw jerk. The afferent and efferent components of this response are conducted via the mandibular division of the trigeminal nerve with central pathways in midbrain and pons. An electronic reflex hammer is used to tap the lower jaw, which triggers a recording from surface electrodes placed over both masseter muscles. Mandibular nerve dysfunction may cause an abnormality of the ipsilateral response. There are also other infrequently used studies to evaluate the trigeminal nerve including the masseter inhibitory reflex and trigeminal somatosensory evoked potentials.[13]

CONCLUSION

Electrodiagnostic testing of the facial nerve can add clinically important information in the setting of facial neuropathy. These tests can aid in diagnosis and prognosis of recovery. The most useful diagnostic tests are the facial motor nerve conduction study with CMAP recording (ENOG) and needle electromyography (EMG). These tests are useful in the face of complete facial paralysis to assist in the discussion of prognosis and possible surgical intervention with the patient.

CASE STUDIES

Case 1: Bell's Palsy With a Good Prognosis

A 50-year-old woman was evaluated for a 10 day history of idiopathic right peripheral facial weakness. The weakness had progressed over several days. Facial motor nerve conduction and blink reflex recordings are revealed in Table 12–2 (Figures 12–5 and 12–6).

The findings were consistent with a right facial neuropathy. A good prognosis was predicted by the

Table 12–2. Needle Electromyography of the Right Orbicularis Oculi and Blink Reflex

	Facial Nerve Conduction Study Orbicularis Oculi CMAP Recording			Blink Reflex Study SON = supraorbital nerve			
	Amplitude (Normal >1.1 mV)	Amplitude Ratio	Latency (Nl <3.1)	Right SON, R1 latency (msec)	Right SON, R2 latency (msec)	Left SON, R1 latency (msec)	Left SON, R2 latency (msec)
Right	1.3	**38%**	**3.1**	12.5	31.4		27.6
Left	3.4		2.6		26.7	11.3	24.6

Findings are consistent with a right facial neuropathy. The CMAP amplitude ratio of 38% shows a good prognosis, as do the recordable blink reflexes.

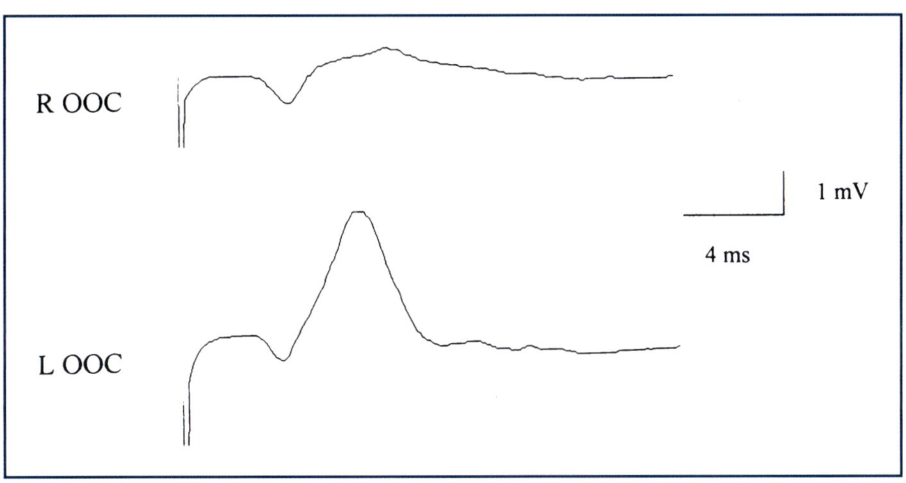

Figure 12–5. Case 1: Facial compound muscle action potentials. The CMAP amplitude ratio is 38%. OOC = orbicularis oculi.

facial CMAP amplitude ratio of 38% and the recordable blink reflexes. At a follow-up examination in 2 weeks there had been considerable interval improvement with only trace residual weakness.

Case 2: Bell's Palsy With a Poor Prognosis

A 30-year-old woman developed left peripheral facial weakness 9 days following delivery by cesarean section. Neurologic examination was otherwise normal. A magnetic resonance imaging study of the brain was normal. She was evaluated 12 days following the onset of the facial weakness. Facial motor nerve conduction and blink reflex recordings are presented in Table 12–3 (Figures 12–7 and 12–8).

With voluntary effort, there was a decreased interference pattern with a fast firing rate, and normal motor unit potential morphology. The findings were consistent with a left facial neuropathy. A poor prognosis was predicted by the facial CMAP amplitude ratio of 5% and the absent blink reflexes. At a follow-up examination in 6 months there had been some improvement, but facial weakness was still present

Case 3: Possible Iatrogenic Facial Nerve Injury

A 56-year-old woman developed ear pain with vesicles in the ear canal. 5 weeks later she developed a severe peripheral left facial palsy. Three weeks following the onset of the palsy, she underwent facial

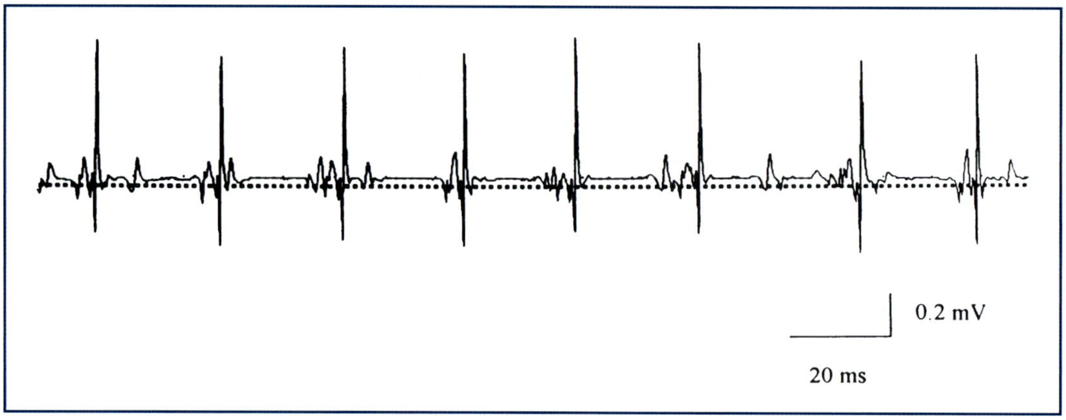

Figure 12–6. Case 1: Needle electromyogram with right orbicularis oculi recording. There is a severely decreased interference pattern.

Table 12–3. Needle Electromyography of the Right Orbicularis Oculi and Orbicularis Oris Muscles Revealed Profuse Active Denervation in the Orbicularis Oris Only

	Facial Motor Nerve Conduction Study Orbicularis Oculi CMAP Recording			Blink Reflex Study SON = supraorbital nerve			
	Amplitude (Normal >1.1 mV)	Amplitude Ratio	Latency (Normal <3.1msec)	Right SON, R1 latency (msec)	Right SON, R2 latency (msec)	Left SON, R1 latency (msec)	Left SON, R2 latency (msec)
Right	1.66	**5%**	1.2	9.6	35.0		36.7
Left	**0.08**		1.5		**Absent**	**Absent**	**Absent**

The findings were consistent with a left facial neuropathy. A poor prognosis was predicted by the facial CMAP amplitude ratio of 5% and the absent blink reflexes.

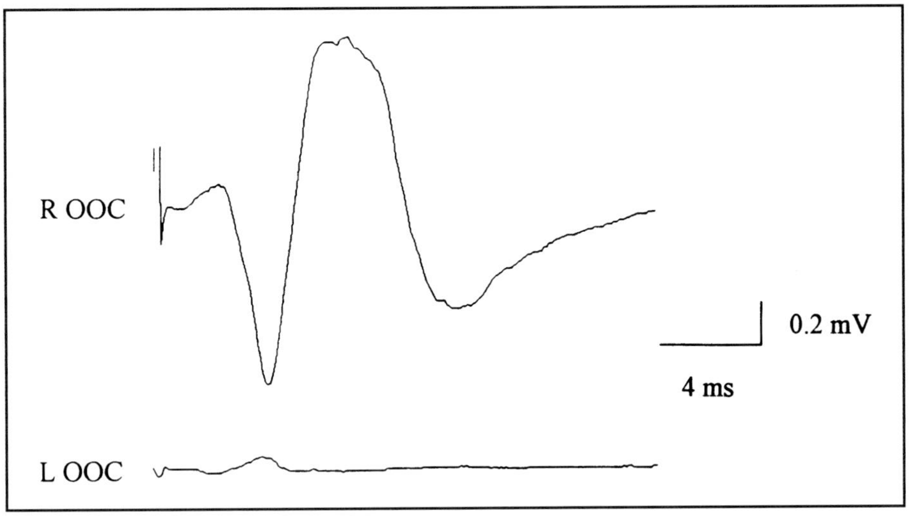

Figure 12–7. Case 2: Facial compound muscle action potentials. The CMAP amplitude ratio is 5%. OOC = orbicularis oculi.

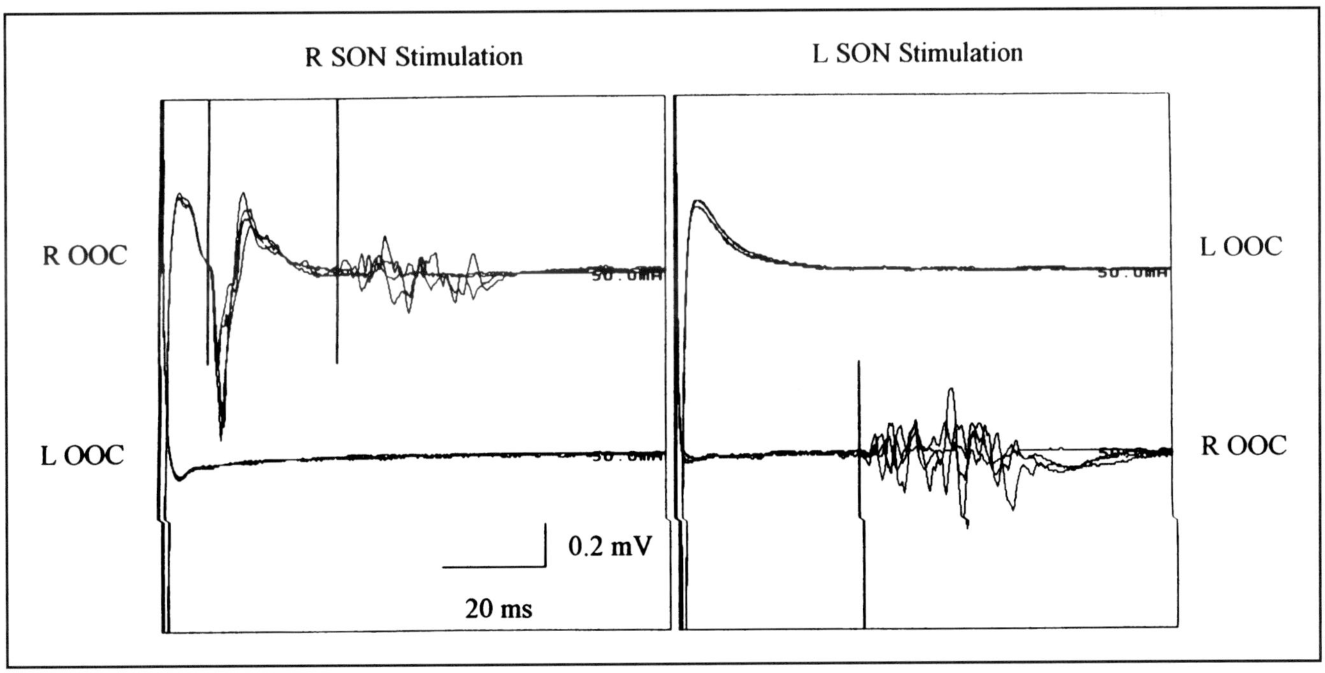

Figure 12–8. Case 2: Blink reflex study. Following right supraorbital nerve (SON) stimulation there is a normal right R1 and R2, but an absent left R2. Following left SON stimulation the left R1 and R2 are absent, and there is a normal right R2. This indicates severe left facial nerve dysfunction. The vertical lines indicate the locations at which the R1 and R2 latencies were measured. Several traces are superimposed to demonstrate reproducibility. OOC = orbicularis oculi.

nerve decompressive surgery. One month following the surgery, she had complete clinical facial weakness. Her surgeon was concerned that the facial nerve might have been injured at the time of the surgery, given the complete lack of visible facial movement and referred her for electrodiagnostic studies.

Facial motor nerve conduction and blink reflex recordings are presented in Table 12–4.

With voluntary effort, both muscles had polyphasic and mildly prolonged motor unit potentials, with a fast firing pattern (Figure 12–9). There was a single unit interference pattern in the orbicularis oculi and a decreased interference pattern in the orbicularis oris.

The absent nerve conduction and blink study responses indicated the presence of a severe facial neuropathy. The recordable motor unit potentials on needle electromyography demonstrated early re-innervation. Facial nerve continuity was therefore demonstrated. Based upon these results the patient was managed conservatively. At a follow-up examination in 6 weeks, facial movements were visible. Repeat electrodiagnostic studies are presented in Table 12–5.

The interference pattern was normal in the orbicularis oculi and decreased in the orbicularis oris (Figure 12–10). The firing rates were fast in both muscles. These studies indicated ongoing re-innervation. At a follow-up examination in 9 months following the onset of the facial palsy, the patient had experienced moderate recovery with a House-Brackmann Grade of III/VI.

Table 12–4. Needle Electromyography of the Right Orbicularis Oculi and Orbicularis Oris Muscles at Rest Revealed Profuse Active Denervation

	Facial Motor Nerve Conduction Study Orbicularis Oculi CMAP Recording			Blink Reflex Study SON = supraorbital nerve			
	Amplitude (Normal >1.1 mV)	Amplitude Ratio	Latency (Normal <3.1msec)	Right SON, R1 latency (msec)	Right SON, R2 latency (msec)	Left SON, R1 latency (msec)	Left SON, R2 latency (msec)
Right	1.3	0%	1.6	10.0	26.7		27.9
Left	**Absent**		**Absent**		**Absent**	**Absent**	**Absent**

The absent nerve conduction and blink study responses indicated the presence of a severe left facial neuropathy.

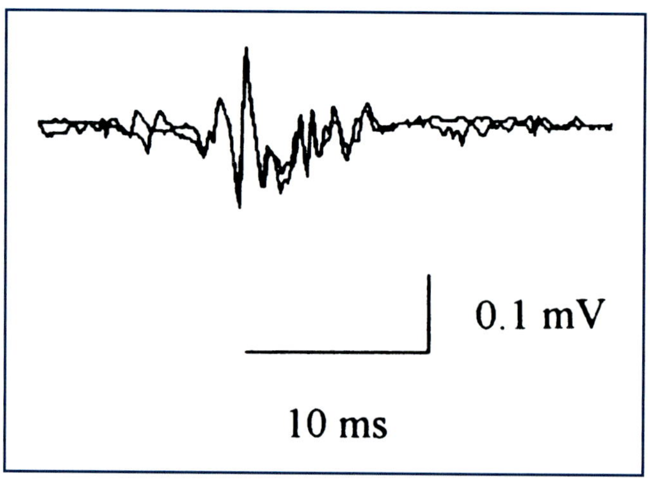

Figure 12–9. Case 3: Polyphasic, mildly prolonged duration (12 msec) motor unit potential recorded from left orbicularis oculi. (Duration normal upper limit is 11 msec.) Several traces are superimposed.

Table 12–5. Needle Electromyography Revealed Mild Active Denervation Only in the Left Orbicularis Oris Muscle

	Facial Motor Nerve Conduction Study Orbicularis Oculi CMAP Recording			Blink Reflex Study SON = supraorbital nerve			
	Amplitude (Normal >1.1 mV)	Amplitude Ratio	Latency (Normal <3.1msec)	Right SON, R1 latency (msec)	Right SON, R2 latency (msec)	Left SON, R1 latency (msec)	Left SON, R2 latency (msec)
Right	1.2	**50%**	1.9	9.3	29.7		30.7
Left	**0.6**		2.5		43.6	22.8	37.2

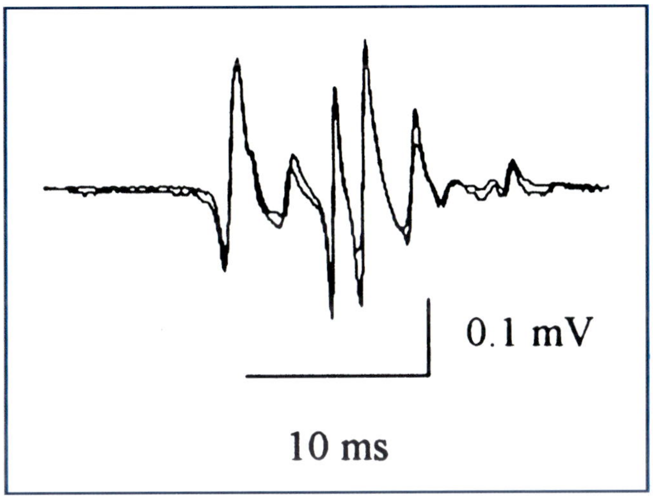

Figure 12–10. Case 3: Polyphasic, prolonged duration (18 msec), high amplitude motor unit potential recorded from left orbicularis oris. Several traces are superimposed.

REFERENCES

1. Jori J, Szekely L, Kiss JG, Toth F. The prognostic value of facial nerve conduction velocity in patients with Bell's palsy. *Clin Otolaryngol.* 1998;23:520–523.
2. de Medeiros JL, Nobrega JA, de Andrade LA, Juliano Y. Facial nerve electroneurography. Variability in normal subjects. *Arq Neuropsiquiatr.* 1996;54:393–396.
3. de Medeiros JL, Nobrega JA, de Andrade LA, Juliano Y. Facial nerve electroneurography. Variability in the early stage and comparison between interpretation methods. *Arq Neuropsiquiatr.* 1996;54:397–401.
4. Esslen E. Electromyography and electroneuronography. In: Fisch U. *Facial Nerve Surgery*. Birmingham, UK: Aesculapius; 1977:93–100.
5. Dumitru D. *Electrodiagnostic Medicine*. Philadelphia, PA: Hanley & Belfus; 1995:689–740.
6. Fisch U. Maximal nerve excitability testing vs electroneuronography. *Arch Otolaryngol.* 1980;106:352–357.
7. Marenda SA, Olsson JE. The evaluation of facial paralysis. *Otolaryngol Clin North Am.* 1997;30:669–682.
8. Oh SJ. *Clinical Electromyography: Nerve Conduction Studies*, 2nd ed. Baltimore, MD: Williams and Wilkins; 1993: 501–506.
9. Fisch U. Prognostic value of electrical tests in acute facial paralysis. *Am J Otol.* 1984;5:494–498.
10. Fisch U. Surgery for Bell's palsy. *Arch Otolaryngol.* 1981; 107:1–11.
11. Qiu WW, Yin SS, Stucker FJ, Hoasjoe DK. Neurophysiological evaluation of acute facial paralysis in children. *Int J Pediatr Otorhinolaryngol.* 1997;39:223–236.

12. Aminoff MJ. *Electromyography in clinical practice*. 3rd ed. New York, NY: Churchill Livingstone;1998:511–522.
13. Kimura J. *Electrodiagnosis in Diseases of Nerve and Muscle*. 2nd ed. Philadelphia, PA: FA Davis; 1989:252:307–331.
14. Kimura J. Conduction abnormalities of the facial and trigeminal nerves in facial neuropathy. *Muscle Nerve*. 1982; 5:S139–S144.
15. Campbell EDR, Hickey RD, Nixon KH, Richardson AT. Value of nerve-excitability measurements in prognosis of facial palsy. *Br J Med*. 1962;2:7–10.
16. Adour KK. Facial nerve electrical testing. In: Jackler RK, Brackmann DE, eds. *Neurotology*. St. Louis, MO: Mosby; 1994:1283–1290.
17. May M, Blumenthal F, Klein SR. Acute Bell's palsy: prognostic value of evoked electromyography, maximal stimulation, and other electrical tests. *Am J Otol*. 1983;5:1–7.
18. Adour KK, Sheldon MI, Kahn ZM. Maximal nerve excitability testing versus neuromyography: prognostic value in patients with facial paralysis. *Laryngoscope*. 1980;90: 1540–1547.
19. Adour KK. Facial paralysis. In: Ballenger JJ, Snow Jr JB. *Otorhinolaryngology*. Baltimore, MD: Williams & Wilkins; 1996:1153–1165.
20. Daube JR. AAEM minimonograph #11: needle examination in clinical electromyography. *Muscle Nerve*. 1991;14: 685–700.
21. Sander HW, Tavoulareas GP, Chokroverty S. Heat sensitive myotonia in proximal myotonic myopathy. *Neurology*. 1996;47:956–962.
22. Preston DC, Shapiro BE. *Electromyography and neuromuscular disorders: clinical electrophysiological correlations*. Boston, MA: Butterworth-Heinemann; 1998:337–351.
23. Granger CV. Toward an earlier forecast of recovery in Bell's palsy. *Arch Phys Med Rehabil*. 1967;48:273–278.
24. Granger CV. Prognosis in Bell's palsy. *Arch Phys Med Rehabil*. 1976;57:33–35.
25. Kimura J, Giron LT, Young SM. Electrophysiological study of Bell palsy: electrically elicited blink reflex in assessment of prognosis. *Arch Otolaryngol*. 1976;102:140–143.
26. Kimura J. Clinical uses of the elicited blink reflex. *Adv Neurol*. 1983;39:773–786.
27. Kimura J. Blink reflex in facial dyskinesia. *Adv Neurol*. 1988;49:39–63.
28. Glocker FX, Magistris MR, Rosler KM, Hess CW. Magnetic transcranial and electrical stylomastoidal stimulation of the facial motor pathways in Bell's palsy: time course and relevance of electrophysiological parameters. *Electroencephalogr Clin Neurophysiol*. 1994:93;113–120.
29. Rimpilainen I, Eskola H, Laippala P, Laranne J, Karma P. Prognostication of Bell's palsy using transcranial magnetic stimulation. *Acta Otolaryngol Suppl*. 1997;529:111–115.
30. Rosler KM, Magistris MR, Glocker FX, Kohler A, Deuschl G, Hess CW. Electrophysiological characteristics of lesions in facial palsies of different etiologies. A study using electrical and magnetic stimulation techniques. *Electroencephalogr Clin Neurophysiol*. 1995:97;355–368.
31. Peiris OA, Miles DW. Galvanic stimulation of the tongue as a prognostic index in Bell's palsy. *Br Med J*. 1965:2;1162.

CHAPTER 13

Acute Facial Palsy: Diagnostic Assessment and Treatment

Chris Linstrom and Brian Duff

All that palsies is not Bell's.

INTRODUCTION

The patient presenting with facial paresis or paralysis may at first seem a daunting task to the clinician. A carefully taken history will serve to guide the clinician toward an estimate of the cause and severity of the problem, its investigation, and treatment.

This chapter reviews the pertinent anatomy and physiology of the facial nerve and facial movement with an emphasis placed on the care of the eye, specifically of the cornea. A review of the common etiologies of acute facial dysfunction and a plan of treatment for acute facial paralysis are given, along with several clinical case examples. Chapter 12 reviewed electrodiagnostic testing.

RELEVANT ANATOMY AND PHYSIOLOGY

The facial nerve (CN VII) is a composite nerve with primarily motor function to the muscles of facial expression (branchial motor) but also, through the nervus intermedius of Wrisberg, carrying general sensory and special sensory fibers (taste) and preganglionic parasympathetic fibers (visceral motor) for lacrimation and salivation (to the submandibular and sublingual glands). The geniculate ganglion represents the nucleus of the sensory root of the facial nerve.

The facial nerve may be detected in embryonic life as early as the third week of gestation, when the embryo is 3 mm long. This collection of neural crest cells also gives rise to the VIIIth (acoustic) cranial nerve and thus is called the facioacoustic primordium and takes the longest intraosseous course of any cranial nerve.[1] There are several segments of the facial nerve. The meatal segment extends from the porus of the internal auditory canal to the meatal foramen. The meatal foramen is the narrowest (0.68 mm) portion of the facial canal. The shortest segment, the labyrinthine segment (3–5 mm), extends from the meatal foramen to the geniculate ganglion. In this region, the greater superficial petrosal nerve (GSPN) carrying fibers to the lacrimal gland leaves anteriorly from the ganglion by means of the hiatus of the facial canal. The Schirmer test for tear secretion is useful to assess the function of the GSPN. Adequate tear secretion implies a site of lesion distal to the geniculate ganglion.

The tympanic segment courses in a posterior direction to the first genu at the geniculate ganglion. The facial nerve then enters the medial tympanic cavity and is superior to the oval window niche where the bone of the facial canal can be thin and dehiscent in as many as 55% of individuals. The distal tympanic segment lies just anterior and inferior to the lateral semicircular canal, where the nerve curves through its second genu and begins its vertical descent. Most intratemporal traumatic injuries occur in the perigeniculate region and labyrinthine segment.

The mastoid segment of the facial canal is the longest of all segments (10–14 mm). It extends from the pyramidal process to the stylomastoid foramen, where it branches at the pes anserinus (goose's foot) into two main divisions, the temporofacial (superior) and cervicofacial (inferior) branches, to travel between the superficial and deep lobes of the parotid to innervate the muscles of facial expression via five named rami (branches): temporal (frontalis muscle), zygomatic (orbicularis occuli muscle), buccal (buccinator and orbicularis oris muscles), (marginal) mandibular (platysma, depressor anguli oris), and cervical (occipitalis) via the posterior auricular branch).

Proximal to the point of ramification into these five named rami, the facial nerve gives off three and sometimes four small branches:

1. The nerve to the stapedius muscle (within the facial canal).
2. The posterior auricular (to the occipitalis).
3. The nerve to the posterior belly of the digastric.
4. The lingual branch which the corda tympani joins to carry afferent special sensation (taste) for the anterior two-thirds of the tongue.[2–4]

The nervus intermedius exits the brainstem near the motor nucleus of the facial nerve. Cell bodies for lacrimation, salivation, and vasomotor fibers destined for the nasal mucosa arise in the superior salivatory nucleus and join the facial nerve after it has passed the abducens nucleus (VI), traveling together until the nerve reaches the geniculate ganglion. The greater superficial petrosal nerve (GSPN) takes off at this point, carrying preganglionic parasympathetic fibers for the pterygopalatine ganglion and eventually innervating the lacrimal, minor salivary and mucosal glands of the palate and nose.

A small named contribution to the facial nerve, the chorda tympani, carries special sensory fibers for taste from the anterior two-thirds of the tongue. Its cell bodies are located in the geniculate ganglion. These special sensory afferent fibers will eventually synapse in the medulla in the nucleus solitarius of the tractus solitarius. General sensation for the tongue is mediate by the lingual nerve (V3).[4]

FACIAL PARALYSIS: HISTORY TAKING

It is of utmost importance to concentrate on the time course of facial paralysis. Paresis or paralysis of the face occurring over a matter of minutes (ie, trauma) or hours (Bell's palsy) is usually quite different from that occurring over a period of years (cholesteatoma involving the otic capsule, other inflammatory conditions of the temporal bone and facial nerve, facial nerve neuroma or, rarely, acoustic neuroma). What was the overall general health of the patient at the time of facial dysfunction? Does the patient have any other metabolic disorders, such as diabetes? Did the paralysis occur during pregnancy? What was at first thought to be Bell's palsy may in fact be something completely different after a careful history has been obtained.

Has the patient ever had an episode of paresis or paralysis similar to the current one on the same or opposite side of the face? Are there any additional findings that the patient has noticed, has been told about or remembers from a prior episode, for example, fissuring of the tongue (lingua plicata) as in Melkerson-Rosenthal syndrome? Was facial paralysis accompanied by vesicular lesions around the ear or soft palate (herpes zoster oticus)? Were there any other otologic complaints such as pain, aural discharge, tinnitus, or vertigo associated with loss of facial nerve function? Did facial paralysis occur in the context of otologic surgery? If so, it is important to hear from the referring surgeon or to determine from the operative report the exact nature of the disease being treated, the surgical procedure and the suspected site of injury to the facial nerve.

Trauma to the temporal bone resulting in facial paralysis requires special consideration. If the nature of the trauma is remembered by the patient or an observer or is well documented, this may aid in estimating the likely nature and extent of facial nerve injury. Usually, facial nerve function is not well documented as more life-threatening injuries are stabilized.

If the patient with traumatic facial paralysis had been observed initially with facial movement, one can safely assume that at least part of the facial nerve was intact and functioning. If the patient subsequently loses facial function completely, one would treat as they would for Bell's palsy: anti-inflammatory agents (steroids) first with surgical decompression of the nerve if indicated.

If, however, the trauma patient does note have adequate history of facial nerve movement initially and has complete paralaysis, one must consider injury or transection of the nerve. The temporal bone should be imaged with an edge-enhanced CT that will yield the greatest amount of anatomic information of the bone/air/soft tissue interfaces. Further management will be based on this result and the overall health of the patient. A patient in a coma on a respirator is obviously not a candidate for a facial nerve exploration and decompression. However, the same patient may be much more functional two to three months hence and still have a facial nerve paralysis. In this case, he or she may be able to endure a facial nerve decompression to definitively manage the nerve, as indicated.

CORNEA PROTECTION

Facial paralysis is much more than a cosmetic deficit. Because eyelid closure is dependent upon an actively functioning orbicularis occuli, facial nerve dysfunction for any reason places the cornea at risk. With every eyeblink, two very important actions happen to the tear film:

1. The tears are wicked from a superolateral point of production in the lacrimal gland in an inferomedia direction toward the superior and inferior lacrimal puncta and is
2. Everted, much as a sheet is turned upside down in a dryer.

These two active functions ensure that the tear film is kept fresh and actively moving across the globe to lubricate the cornea. With facial paralysis, this active function is severely impeded or ceases, thus placing the cornea at risk for exposure. If there is a concomitant corneal afferent sensory deficit (V1), especially in patients after resection of large posterior fossa tumors involving the Vth nerve, the cornea is now at severe risk for exposure keratitis, corneal abrasion, corneal ulceration, and eventually enophthalmitis. If left untreated, the patient ultimately may lose sight in the affected eye.

Because of the grave potential risk to the globe, it is important that the clinician focus carefully on the eye, especially on the health of the cornea. Awareness of the grave consequences of exposure keratitis will ordinarily suffice for both the doctor and patient to keep the eye moist. It is wise to enlist the collaboration of an ophthalmologist experienced in the care of the anterior chamber to help in the care of these patients. Treatment for the eye is discussed later.

PHYSICAL EXAMINATION/ EVALUATION OF FACIAL NERVE FUNCTION

A complete general head and neck exam should be performed with attention to the potential contributory pathologies such as a lesion in the parotid, base of the tongue, retromolar trigone, or nasopharynx. Not all pathology involving the facial nerve occurs within the temporal bone. Once the general ENT exam has been performed and is negative, a careful examination of the facial nerve should be performed.

A thorough exam will reveal which part of the face has impaired movement. The patient must be instructed not to bite, but to simply try to move the face. Can the patient raise the eyebrow (while the examiner holds down the contralateral "normal" side)? Is there active eyelid closure? Or is there simply passive relaxation of the upper lid with a Bell's reflex (upward rotation of the globe, protecting the cornea)? Is there an active close-lipped smile? Do the extremes of the face (frontalis, depressor anguli oris,) move? Where is the greatest deficit: upper face versus lower face versus the whole face? Is there synkinesis?

The clinician needs to identify active movement of the face only. It is a common fault to mistake relaxation of the levator (innervated by CN III) with active eyelid closure. This is not active eyelid closure. Even a newborn baby will demonstrate "crow's feet" formation at the lateral margins of the orbit while crying and this pattern alone indicates active contraction of the orbicularis oculi, not relaxation of an adymanic upper lid. The examiner must elicit true active motion as opposed to passive relaxation.

Most facial nerve grading systems are based on the clinical observation of facial nerve function and not upon objective measures of linear displacement, velocity, or acceleration.

Two of the more commonly used systems are: The House-Brackmann (H-B) and the Fisch Classification Systems.[5–8] The former has been approved by the American Academy of Otolaryngology-Head and Neck Surgery (AAO-HNS) for general use in describing facial nerve function. Although it is commonly used to describe facial function at any time along the course of facial dysfunction, it was actually devised to describe a state of function after medical or surgical intervention, that is, later on in the course of disease. Nonetheless, the House-Brackmann System is easy to learn and to apply to the patient (Table 13–1). The face may be divided into an upper face containing the eye and a lower face. The dividing line in this system is an actively closing eye (H-B III) and an eye that cannot close on its own (IV). Patients with normal facial function in all divisions of the nerve are termed H-B I; patient with flaccid/adynamic hemifacial function are termed VI. Mimimal paresis of the nerve but with active eyelid closure and no synkinesis is termed II. Tone only of the face without active facial movement is termed V. Any amount of synkinesis downgrades the patient to a H-B III.

The ease of application of this system is also its greatest disadvantage. Not all H-B IIIs are the same; not all IIs are the same. There may be marked differences in the appearance of two "hemifaces" within the exact same classification "bin," especially in patients in which the deficit is predominantly in the upper versus the lower face. Nonetheless, the H-B system has proven to be of great utility in the evaluation and management of facial paralysis.

The second most commonly used system has been developed by Professor Fisch.[7,8] He has recognized the problem of sorting out facial function by non-arithmetic "bins" and has tried to achieve a point-based grading system that may yield greater predictability for recovery of acute facial dysfunction. In his system, the hemi-face is divided into five regions: frontal, eyelid, mid-face (buccal), mouth, and lower face, corresponding roughly to those regions innervated by the respective branches of the facial nerve: temporalis; zygomaticus; buccal; ramis mandibularis and cervicalis.

Table 13–1. House-Brackmann (H-B) Classification of Facial Nerve Function

Grade	Clinical Description
I	**Normal** facial function in all divisions both at rest and with active motion.
II	**Mild Dysfunction** Rest: normal symmetry and tone slight weakness noted. Active motion: Mild dysfunction, usually at the extremes of the face; (+) active eyelid closure.
III	**Moderate Dysfunction** Rest: Obvious difference between the two sides. Active motion: Greater dysfunction; (+) active eyelid closure with forced movement.
IV	**Moderately Severe Dysfunction** Rest: Obvious, disfiguring asymmetry Active motion: (–) active eyelid/ incomplete closure (passive eyelid closure only)
V	**Severe Dysfunction** Rest: Asymmetry at rest; tone only Active motion: Barely perceptible motion. (–) active eyelid closure
VI	**Total Paralysis** Rest and active motion: Flaccid, adynamic face.

Twenty points are awarded for each of the 5 facial regions, totaling 100 points. Synkinesis subtracts points from the final score. A larger overall grade is better than a smaller grade and is thought to predict greater return. Although this grading system takes a bit longer to calculate, it is intuitive and does attempt to use a clinical metric, that is, regional observation, to predict outcome. However, it is not truly arithmatic in that the final grading system is ultimately subjective in design and cannot undergo strict mathematic functional analysis.

OBJECTIVE MEASUREMENT OF FACIAL FUNCTION

Many attempts have been made to measure facial nerve function in an objective way and thereby to remove observer bias from the calculation. Various methods have been quite ingenious in the way facial function is measured.

Linear measurement of facial displacement may be made using surface electrodes and an electromyographic recording and measuring system.[9,10] Neely et al[11] and Holman et al[12] used a subtracted-image, computer-assisted technique that measures the degree of facial surface deformation (per expression, per time segment) expressed as a summation of all pixels in the subtracted area. Light reflectance was taken as a two-dimensional marker of the three-dimensional surface deformation occurring during facial expression.

Still another system uses normal facial shadows of the various regions of the face to calculate linear regional displacement, using variations of luminance produced by changes of facial expression.[13,14]

Landmark-based systems apply some type of fixed marker to the face with measurement of facial movement from repose performed either by hand or via a video/computer digital interface. Yet another ingenious system actually views the face *en face* and from 45 degrees left and right via a mirror placed behind the patient and measures facial movement from these 3 angles. Digital systems assign Cartesian co-ordinates (x, y) to facial markers (reflective or non-reflective, depending upon the program) and are capable of advanced computations such as linear displacement in the x and y planes, velocity (rate of change of linear displacement), and acceleration (rate of change of velocity).[15–17]

These systems are advanced, eloquent, and supremely "believable" in that the data they generate is not subject to observer bias. Unfortunately, almost all have the built-in burden of advanced computation and are never real time. Some require over an hour of computer time to compute the data analysis for one requested movement, for example, closed lip smile. A somewhat general analogy would be a standard hearing test versus an auditory brainstem reflex test (ABR). The former is immediate but the examiner may be fooled, especially if there is a problem with masking. The latter yields more subtle information but requires advanced computation and is not real-time. Thus, the clinical utility of objective facial nerve function systems is limited, but as a research tool they are superb. With faster "super computers" an objective, real-time metric of facial function may one day be possible.

TOPOGNOSTIC (SITE-OF-LESION) TESTING

Testing the various branches of the facial nerve for the presence or absence of function has been performed in an effort to locate the site of the lesion. The supposition for these tests is that decreased function at a given site identifies the approximate site of pathology and that the nerve proximal to this site is functioning. These suppositions are not always true. Topognostic testing has been shown to correlate poorly with the chronological return of function. The accuracy of defining the absolute site of lesion is also quite low. For these reasons, topognostic testing has largely been replaced by electrical testing of the facial nerve and radiographic imaging of the temporal bone. Perhaps the test of greatest utility is the Schirmer test because it may help identify the eye at risk for exposure keratitis. These tests are reviewed for mostly historical interest and summarized in Table 13–2.

The greatest potential use of topognostic testing remains in cases of temporal bone trauma in which the patient retains a slight amount of facial movement and in which there is a discrete area of injury

Table 13–2. Topognostic Testing of the Facial Nerve

Clinical Test	Branch of the Facial Nerve
Tearing (Schirmer test)	Greater superficial petrosal nerve
Acoustic reflex testing	Stapedial branch
Salivary secretion test via cannulation of Warthin's duct	Lingual branch
Blink test	Reflex arc of VI (afferent) and VII (efferent)
Taste test	Chorda tympani branch

to the nerve, identified on a CT scan. In these cases, topognostic testing may give clinical clues to the precise area of injury. In the majority of cases, however, the face is flaccid and adynamic. Topognostic sites in these cases are also severely affected.

EVALUATION

Audiogram

All patients with facial paralysis, regardless of the suspected cause, should have an audiogram with a minimum battery of tests, performed separately for each ear, of pure tones, bone conduction (masked appropriately), word discrimination, and immittance with reflex decay, if the level of hearing permits.

Otoacoustic emission testing (OAE) and auditory brainstem response testing (ABR) may be considered if the patient is unresponsive or cannot otherwise co-operate with a behavioral audiogram. If facial nerve neuroma is suspected as a part of retrocochlear pathology, the ABR may be helpful as part of the test battery to determine if hearing can be preserved in the management of a neoplasm affecting the facial nerve.

Electrical Testing of the Facial Nerve

Electrical testing of the nerve has been covered in Chapter 12. A basic overview is provided here with routine electrical tests that are utilized.

Minimal Excitability Test

This test employs a portable, battery-powered, transcutaneous stimulator of the facial nerve. A Hilger® stimulator or a similar device is placed on the face near the stylomastoid foramen of both the normal (reference) and affected sides. The lowest stimulus intensity that excites all branches of the nerve on the unaffected side is considered the electrical baseline. A 2.0- to 3.5-mA difference between the normal and affected sides indicates impending denervation of the affected side. Advantages of this technique are its portability, relatively low electric current requirements and relatively less discomfort for the test subject. The disadvantage is that the metric is subjective: the tester must judge that all branches are either moving or not. In addition, the test may excite larger branches easier than smaller branches and give a false picture of the overall function of the nerve.[18]

Maximal Excitability Test

This test is performed by using a transcutaneous electrical device to maximally saturate and stimulate both the unaffected and affected sides of the face. A subjective determination is made that the affected side is: (1) Equal to the normal side; (2) 50% diminished (minimally affected) when compared to the normal side; (3) 75% diminished (markedly affected) when compared to the normal side; or (4) 100% diminished (completely affected), absence of electrical stimulation. The advantage of this test is its ease of application. The obvious disadvantage is that it is a subjective test and lacks a metric to quantify the amount of facial dysfunction.[19]

Supramaximal Tests: Electroneuronography (ENOG) and Evoked Electromyography (EEMG)

This is a supramaximal stimulation of the facial nerve and may be used to measure the integrity of working axons within the nerve and to prognosticate degeneration as well as return. It is of clinical value when a nerve is in "evolution," that is, within 2 to 3 weeks after the onset of facial paralysis and after Wallerian degeneration should have occurred (48–72 hours after onset of paralysis). It is of little value after this time due to dyssynchrony of fibers within an affected nerve.

When used during the "window of opportunity" from the onset of clinical paralysis, this test has been shown to separate those patient who will be expected to have good to excellent clinical recovery of facial nerve function from those who will be expected to have less than complete recovery or to have clinical sequelae such as synkinesis. A degeneration of the affected side of 90% or greater is used to separate these two groups: patients who retain at least 10% of electrical function on ENOG testing are thought to have better clinical return than those with ≤10% electrical function.

Because of its ability to offer an objective metric and its relative ease of application, this test now supersedes almost all others in clinical use. It has become the mainstay of clinical practice. Its main drawback is its technical application: an inexperienced technician may erroneously stimulate the masseter (CN V) thereby giving falsely encouraging results. These false positive results occur mainly in children and in patients with very thin necks. It is important to watch the face as it is being stimulated to assure that only the branches of the facial nerve are being stimulated.[7]

Electromyography (EMG) of the Facial Nerve

EMG is performed as voluntary and spontaneously generated facial motor responses are measured and compared on the affected side and to the unaffected side. The greatest utility of EMG is in the measurement of facial nerve integrity and the prognostication of expected return of function in cases of significant neuropraxia, such as acoustic neuroma dissection, or possible neurotmesis in temporal bone fracture.

Ten to fourteen days after the onset of clinical paralysis, EMG recordings reflect the dynamic resting membrane potentials of postsynaptic elements. In this phase, the muscle membrane, deprived of "trophic" substances that are normally transported through the axon, undergoes changes that destabilize the resting potential. These changes produce spontaneous depolarizations reflected in the EMG as fibrillation potentials and are interpreted as indicators of persistent denervation.

Successful re-innervation generates high-frequency polyphasic potentials that increase in amplitude and duration and replaces fibrillation potentials. These polyphasic potentials may be used to measure the course of re-innervation.[20]

Of these tests, electroneuronography (ENOG) and needle electromyography (EMG) are by far the more utilized in a clinical setting. These give real-time information about the status of the nerve and help to both follow the course of facial paralysis in electrical evolution and to offer prognosis about the likelihood of recovery.

In practice, in a patient with acute *complete* facial paralysis, most otologists will rely upon the ENOG (cMAP) and possibly EMG findings to guide the decision between medical treatment (steroids and antivirals) versus surgical decompression of the facial nerve.

Radiographic Evaluation

For cases of idiopathic facial paralysis *without* accompanying hearing loss, radiographic imaging is usually not indicated because it will not affect either the clinical decision-making process or the eventual outcome of the patient. In this case, because idiopathic facial paralysis (Bell's palsy) results in inflammation of the nerve especially at the meatal foramen, it is expected that an MRI of the temporal bone/brain will demonstrate enhancement of the nerve. If the MRI shows enhancement of the nerve, this does not exclude a retrocochlear neoplasm. It does, however, commit the patient to a probable follow-up MRI after inflammation would be expected to have subsided, about six months later. If the hearing is stable and symmetric, it is unnecessary to obtain an MRI in the *acute* phase because inflammation will make the scan positive. Most patients with idiopathic facial paralysis would be expected to recover at least some function. In demographic studies, Peitersen[21,22] described the natural history of untreated (but observed) idiopathic facial paralysis. No one with truly idiopathic (Bell's) palsy was left with a flaccid, adynamic face. Approximately 71% had near perfect recovery; 29% had imperfect recovery of either a facial region or of synkinesis. One of the important findings of this study is that all patients had some recovery of facial function. Those who had no recovery did not strictly have Bell's palsy and were further studied to exclude retrocochlear neoplasia, including facial nerve neuroma. For these rare patients, a retrocochlear imaging study would be appropriate after some observation period, not during the acute inflammatory phase.

Facial paralysis occurring in the context of acute or chronic inflammatory or infectious disease should be investigated as one would image the underlying disease, usually with a CT of the temporal bone. The expected course of the intratympanic facial nerve is easy to follow in the normal temporal bone. Its expected location may be lost in inflammatory or infectious disease, thus pinpointing the likely site of facial nerve involvement.

Temporal bone trauma is best investigated with a CT of the temporal bone as well. With edge-enhanced studies the temporal bone may be imaged in any plane. In facial nerve trauma, one wants to best detail the bony architecture as it affects the normal and expected pathway of the intratympanic facial nerve. If there is complete loss of hearing along with facial paralysis, one would expect to find a transverse or mixed fracture of the temporal bone involving the otic capsule. If the otic capsule has been spared and if the patient has a conductive pattern of hearing loss, one would expect a longitudinal fracture of the temporal bone. Rarely, a discrete fracture line may be seen to point to the geniculate ganglion with no other findings. Because the geniculate is "tethered" by the branching of the greater superficial petrosal branch, it is a likely site of injury and should be carefully inspected.

DIFFERENTIAL DIAGNOSIS

It is important for the clinician to think broadly as he or she takes the patient's history. The most common causes of acute facial paralysis will be Bell's (idiopathic), herpes zoster oticus, infectious/inflammatory conditions including Lyme disease, and temporal bone trauma. Other conditions are included for the sake of completion but are rare to see.

TREATMENT OPTIONS

Medical

The mainstay of medical care for acute facial paralysis is lubrication and passive protection of the cornea and the administration of exogenous steroid. Any oral form of steroid may be chosen with the dosage equivalent of approximately one mg/kg of prednisone up to 60 mg/kg per day. Regardless of the cosmetic deficit, the patient must be instructed that the real problem at hand is ongoing exposure of the eye and every effort must be taken to ensure that the cornea is kept moist.

There is controversial evidence from acute and convalescent serological studies that idiopathic facial paralysis may be linked to a herpetic infection, especially herpes simplex type 1. One may consider the addition of antiviral medications such as acyclovir or amicyclovir into the medical treatment of acute idiopathic facial paralysis. In known herpetic infections, such as Ramsey Hunt syndrome (herpes zoster oticus), antiviral medications would be indicated along with steroids, usually for 5 to 7 days. The patient's hepatic function may need to be monitored for higher or longer dosing regimens.

Rarely, acute facial paralysis may be part of a polyneuropathy involving both the VIIth and VIIIth cranial nerves, as is occasionally seen in Ramsey Hunt syndrome. These patients may require acute hospitalization and sedation to control vertigo.

In addition to artificial tears and salves, many other nonsurgical techniques are readily available to help in acute facial paralysis. The affected eye may be taped shut or may be covered with a "Feuchtkammer" (German: moisture-chamber) made of clear plastic. This is somewhat bulky but changes the local milieu of the cornea from dry to moist and may be required acutely in exposure keratitis. Patching the eye is less desirable because the levator (CN III) remains functional and unopposed and may keep the eyelid open underneath the patch, especially during sleep. The lower lid may be suspended with a thin adhesive tape such as a Steri-Strip. A small fusiform piece of adhesive tape placed above the tarsal crease may help to keep the upper lid in a somewhat ptotic position, thus providing improved passive closure of the eyelid. All of these "first-aid" techniques are medical in nature and can be performed in the office.

Surgical Therapy for the Eyelid

Most patients will do very well with a temporary tarsorrhaphy or a gold or platinum weight properly placed to counterbalance the levator. The technique of lid-loading is straightforward, easy to learn, and may be performed under straight local anesthesia in an office-based procedure room. However, it is important for the non-ophthalmologist to know his or her limits. The Asian paralytic eyelid or an eyelid with in-turning lashes for any reason is a very difficult eyelid to treat. These paralytic eyelids often do poorly with standard, simple surgical techniques and should be referred immediately to an oculoplastic surgeon.

Lid Loading

Over time, the paralytic eyelid will become more at risk for exposure because the levator oculi (CN III) is unopposed and usually normal. Various techniques and materials for upper lid loading have been developed in an effort to counteract the tonic retraction of the unopposed levator.[23]

The most important technique is lid loading with either a pure (24 kt or 99.98% pure gold or platinum bar, 0.6 g to 1.6 g). The bar to be implanted is either taped or affixed to the paralytic eyelid via temporary fixative, usually tincture of benzoin or double-sided adhesive tape. The patient is placed in a sitting position and is asked to relax the eyelid. The patient makes a decision about the weight of greatest comfort; the surgeon decides the weight of best closure. Topical corneal anesthesia may be provided with drops (tetracaine 0.5%) and the lid is injected with 1% lidocaine with epinephrine 1:100,000,. This outpatient procedure may be done under straight local anesthesia with or without intravenous sedation. Most patients will require a 1.0 to 1.2 g weight. The gold or platinum bar is implanted in a small pocket made at or above the level of the tarsal crease and is suture-fixated to the pretarsal soft tissue. A layered closure of the orbicularis oculi and skin must be performed because the foreign body (gold or platinum bar) crosses an incision line. When the eyelid is relaxed, gravity will allow the upper lid to close. It is important for the patient to be told that this technique provides better passive closure in the sitting or standing position, less so in the supine position. When facial function returns, the eyelid may feel excessively heavy because the now functioning orbicularis oculi is reinforced with the weight. At this time, with consultation from the ophthalmologist, the weight may be removed. Of interest, in a series of patients who had acute facial paralysis from various causes and who had a gold weight inserted, only about one-third (34%) decided to have the gold weight removed after recovery of facial function. The remainder felt more confident with the complete closure the eyelid weight provided.[24]

Tarsorrhaphy

Tarsorrhaphy is a static technique to offer corneal protection. It does not aid in wicking the tear film across the globe. Although it has been the mainstay of treatment of the acutely paretic eyelid for many years, it has largely fallen into disfavor because other dynamic techniques are readily available.

In certain instances, a lateral and/or medial tarsorrhaphy must be performed in order to narrow the area of corneal exposure and still allow frontal vision. The typical patient is elderly with a facial and trigeminal nerve weakness. The technique may be performed either with temporary silk suture or with permanent scarring. The superior and inferior tarsus are sutured close either medially or laterally. The occasional patient may require both medial and lateral tarsorrhaphies. In this case, the field of vision will be severely limited. The permanent technique is performed by removing a small (2 mm × 3–4 mm) strip of skin and mucosa from the upper and lower lids in the area of the intended tarsorrhaphy (lateral and/or medial). One or two mattress sutures are placed (with or without silicon bolsters) to approximate the raw surfaces which will result in healed apposition of the upper and lower lids. The indication for permanent tarsorrhaphy is in the patient in whom an insensate cornea and paretic eyelid place the eye at extreme risk.

Palpebral Spring

A palpebral spring may be thought of as an open safety pin under the upper eyelid. Because the levator (CN III) is almost always normal and unopposed, the eyelid will have normal opening forces. These opening forces are opposed by a spring, made from biocompatible material (usually gold), and inserted under the upper lid to force it into the closed position. This technique, although straightforward and relatively simple, in most cases requires revision due to slippage of the spring or due to the changing needs of opposing force as the eyelid recovers motor function. In large measure, it has been replaced by lid-loading techniques.

Canthoplasty for Ectropion Repair

The paralytic lower eyelid may become ptotic over time and lead to further exposure of the cornea. Epiphora may become an additional problem due to sagging of the paralytic lower lid. This is especially so in patients age 55 and over in whom the normal supportive and elastic properties of the face have already weakened. For patients with facial paralysis who are over 50 years of age, ectropion formation should be anticipated and the lower lid supported with a small lateral canthoplasty. This technique is easy to understand and master. The arch of the upper lid is drawn downward for about 6mm. A line 4–5 mm medial to the lateral canthus is also drawn. The lower lid is injected with the same local anesthetic as the upper lid. The incisions to be made are grasped with straight hemostats placed in the inferior fornix and the small triangle so clamped is removed as a wedge resection. The inferior tarsal plate is supported with a 5-0 suture of 5-0 clear nylon that is sutured to the lateral canthal tubercle. The skin is closed with interrupted sutures of 5-0 fast-absorping gut.

Surgical: Facial Nerve

Decompression of the facial nerve in the acute time period remains controversial. The main questions to be answered are these:

1. In the acute situation, does facial nerve decompression *significantly* improve the outcome of facial paralysis over standard medical management?
2. Which patient should be selected for facial nerve decompression?

As a preface to the long and convoluted history of decompression versus medical management alone, it must be realized that the paucity of well-designed, prospective, randomized clinical studies with large numbers of patients is a major problem for the "jury." This "lack of evidence" has led to confusion and to significant change from "decompression before sunset" in days gone by (not that long ago) to a "let's watch and wait" attitude. The important work of Peitersen in studying the natural history of untreated idiopathic facial paralysis should loom large in the mind of any surgeon contemplating decompression of the facial nerve for Bell's palsy.[21,22] A further confounding factor is that the metric for the most part is *subjective*, that is, the House-Brackmann or Fisch classification systems. There is no universal, easy-to-apply objective measurement system of facial movement or expression.[7,24]

Electrical testing of the facial nerve is of value while the nerve is *in evolution*, that is, within about the first 10 to 14 days of onset of facial paralysis. It is of little or no value after this time due to the lack of synchronous axonal firing.

For surgeons interested in this field, the seminal work of Professor Fisch must be carefully studied and mastered, acknowledging that the numbers of patients both observed and treated are not large. In addition, to be recalled is that the outcome grading of facial movement was better by the surgeon and worse by the person with the problem, that is, the patient. In general, based upon his work in patients with *idiopathic* facial paralysis, a window of opportunity of approximately 2 weeks exists from the onset of clinical paralysis (not paresis) and electrical degeneration ≥90% by ENOG (cMAP) testing in which decompression of the facial nerve and especially of the meatal segment of the facial nerve will beneficially affect the clinical outcome of the nerve. Both the time window (2 weeks, not 3 weeks?) and indication for decompression remain controversial in cases of acute idiopathic facial paralysis. The decompression is performed with transmastoid and middle cranial fossa approach to remove the bone of the fallopian canal, especially at the meatal foramen.[7]

Of less controversy are cases of traumatic facial paralysis and, for some surgeons, herpes zoster oticus (HZO). The natural history of facial function after HZO is bleak for patients with both clinical and electric paralysis. Approximately 50 to 60% of patients with facial paralysis due to HZO will have adverse sequalae: lack of re-innervation and/or synkinesis. Because of its poor natural history, the case for surgical decompression may be greater in cases of HZO than for idiopathic facial paralysis.

Temporal bone trauma may be treated as Bell's palsy, depending on the timing of the observation of the face, as previously described. Surgical exploration will be dictated by the history and electrical testing.

Surgical Technique for Facial Nerve Exploration and Decompression

Middle Cranial Fossa Approach

This approach can be used to expose the IAC, labyrinthine portion of the facial nerve, geniculate ganglion, and tympanic segment. A posteriorly based trapdoor incision is made superior to the ear and a skin flap is elevated. Temporalis fascia is harvested for closure of the dural defect. Next, the temporalis muscle and periosteum are elevated exposing the temporal root of the zygoma, which approximates the floor of the middle cranial fossa. A medium cutting burr is used to develop a bone flap above the temporal root of the zygoma with care taken to control any bleeding from branches of the middle meningeal artery. Dura is then elevated from posterior to anterior off of the floor of the middle fossa until the petrous ridge, arcuate eminence, and GSPN are encountered. A medium diamond bur is used for drilling posterior to the arcuate eminence until the otic capsule and blue line of the superior semicircular canal are identified. The IAC is revealed by removing bone in a line 60 degrees anterior to the superior semicircular canal. The facial nerve is in the anterosuperior portion of the IAC and is followed anteriorly to the labyrinthine segment and geniculate ganglion. The tegmen tympani is removed to expose the tympanic segment of the facial nerve. The final thin layer of bone over the nerve is thinned down to an eggshell and carefully picked away with a microinstrument. After adequate exposure, a sickle knife or small blade is used to slit the perineurium and epineural sheath thus decompressing the facial nerve. For closure, a bone plate or artificial material is used to cover the tegmen and IAC defect. Previously harvested temporalis fascia seals the dural defect and bone plug is replaced. The temporalis muscle and skin are then closed in layers.

One advantage to the middle cranial fossa approach is that it completely exposes the IAC and labyrinthine segment of the facial nerve. Although this approach ideally preserves hearing, conductive hearing loss can occur from temporal lobe herniation or ossicular chain disruption. Drilling injury may cause sensorineural hearing loss if the cochlea is damaged or vestibular dysfunction if the semicircular canals are violated. Finally, cerebrospinal fluid leak and AICA injury are other serious risks of the middle cranial fossa approach.

Transmastoid Approach

The transmastoid approach is useful for exposing the facial nerve from the geniculate ganglion to the stylomastoid foramen. First, a postauricular incision is made and a complete mastoidectomy is performed. The facial recess is exposed with a small diamond bur. The tympanic segment of the facial nerve lies anterior to the lateral semicircular canal. The fallopian canal is then exposed to the stylomastoid foramen which is found at the anterior margin of the digastric ridge. The nerve is exposed by removing the posterior half of the fallopian canal and retrofacial air cells, if necessary. The geniculate ganglion is exposed with a 1-mm diamond bur. Again, the final layer of bone is removed with blunt elevators and incision of the perineurium is performed with a small sickle knife or blade. The wound is closed in layers and a drain is placed for 24 to 36 hours.

This approach provides great exposure of the mastoid and tympanic segments of the facial nerve. Unfortunately, the labyrinthine segment cannot be addressed without risking violation of the ampulla of the lateral semicircular canal. Also, the incus must be temporarily removed in order to assess the geniculate ganglion, which puts the patient at risk for a conductive hearing deficit.

Exploration of the facial nerve by means of the translabyrinthine approach is performed when hearing and vestibular function is lost. This approach offers access to the entire intratemporal course of the facial nerve with substantially decreased morbidity.

Surgical Outcomes

The need for facial nerve decompression has to be weighed against the potential risks of surgical complications such as hearing loss, dizziness, facial nerve injury, and meningitis.

Facial nerve function was retrospectively analyzed in 27 patients with facial paralysis secondary to Bell's palsy and ENoG findings of greater than 90% degeneration within 2 weeks· Fourteen patients underwent MCF decompression while the remaining 13 patients were managed nonsurgically. The authors reported significant improvements in outcome with MCF decompression.[25] However, in this study, the degree of improvement was not clearly stated. Fisch's study also indicated a 50% rate of spontaneous recovery if the degeneration exceeded 90% on ENoG.[26] This result was further supported by similar findings that showed recovery to House-Brackmann Grade I or II in 50% of patients with >90% degeneration within 2 weeks after the onset of facial paralysis.

A multi-institutional review of 59 patients with complete facial paralysis was reported.[27] Twenty-six patients underwent surgical decompression while 33 patients were managed conservatively. HB grade I or II recovery was noted in 23 of 26 patients in the surgical group and 14 of 33 patients in the nonsurgical group. They concluded that surgical decompression was superior to conservative management. However, in this study, a majority of patients who were managed conservatively showed recovery to HB grade III or better. The results further indicate that HB grade I, II, or III is achieved in 25 of 26 patients undergoing surgical decompression and in 31 of 33 patients with conservative management. Thus, although 92% of patients treated with surgical decompression and 45% of patients treated with medical treatment achieved HB grade I or II; when considering HB grade III or better facial nerve function, the results in the two treatment groups were similar (96% with surgery, 94% of patients without surgery).

In conclusion, based on the published literature, the management of complete facial paralysis secondary to Bell's palsy remains controversial. A thorough discussion is warranted with patients regarding the risks and benefits of both surgical decompression and nonsurgical management of complete facial paralysis. Patients need to be aware of the potential implications of both treatment modalities in order to make an informed decision.

Delayed Surgical Procedures

Brow Ptosis Treatment

The various techniques described above may be used for patients with chronic facial paralysis. Patients with chronic facial paralysis and brow ptosis may have severe limited field vision on the affected side. The paretic eyelid may retract under the ptotic brow (lateral hooding) and cause poor natural toilet of the cornea. All of these factors may predispose the eye to blepharitis, chronic conjunctivitis and further infection. In the chronic state, the needs and level of activity of the patient must be taken into account. The vision in both the affected and unaffected eyes should be carefully evaluated.

When indicated, the ptotic brow may be lifted with a variety of straightforward techniques (endoscopically, directly above the brow line, or through a re-created forehead crease). The lifted brow will now be in a more neutral position just above the level of the superior orbital rim and allow the upper lid to be seen. The upper lid may require lid loading at this time to counterbalance the chronic retraction of the levator oculi. The lower lid may have undergone ectropion formation that may require correction. An experienced ophthalmologist must be consulted to help thoroughly evaluate the vision in both eyes and to assist in the overall needs and goals of the patient.

Facial Reanimation Techniques

Many techniques exist for facial reanimation. The surgical catalogue is far too great to mention in detail for the purposes of this summary. The interested reader is referred to applicable texts on facial plastic and reconstructive surgery and to oculoplastic surgery.

Synkinesis after return of facial function may be improved with the selective use of botulinum toxin (Botox®) to temporarily, chemically denervate unwanted facial movement. If desired, a more permanent selective denervation may be achieved either chemically (with phenol, absolute alcohol) or surgically.

There is no surgical technique of facial reanimation that will equal a working, normal facial nerve. Reconstructive procedures are in essence attempts to regain facial symmetry (static procedures) or isolated and/or regional facial movement (dynamic procedures) but never possess the subtlety of mimetic facial expression from a normal, functioning facial nerve. This fact must be clearly understood by the patient (and physician) so that reasonable goals and expectations may be achieved. It is always better to underplay intended surgical results and have a delighted patient than to overstate them and have a disappointed one. Neither physician nor patient should yield to magical, unrealistic thinking.

In guiding the patient toward facial re-animation, it is important for the clinician to understand the history and biology of the disease, the likelihood or lack of same that the facial nerve may regain function and the time that has elapsed from the causative event. It is important to allow a reasonable period of 6 to12 months for native function to return, if it is expected to do so. Electromyography of the facial nerve may aid in the decision making process.

In cases in which the nerve has been severely damaged and/or unlikely to return, attention should be directed to re-innervation of the distal nerve via substitution (XII–VII), cross-facial innervation from the contralateral native VII, and/or muscle transfer or transposition, either with a single muscle (eg, temporalis, gracilis free transfer) or group of muscles (temporalis, masseter) or dynamic or static sling techniques (eg, tensor fascia lata or alloderm from the temporalis to the lateral commissure), depending upon the age, needs and goals of the patient.

One size definitely does not fit all and it is foolhardy for the physician to suggest or impose one technique for every patient. One "face" will not work for all. The physician must carefully attend to the history and time course of the paralysis and the functional needs and goals of the patient. Consultation with other physicians and surgeons in related disciplines, especially ophthalmology, may be required to achieve the best overall plan for the patient. With all of these techniques, the best plan for restoring facial function for the individual suffering with facial paralysis may be reached.

CASE EXAMPLES

Bell's Palsy (recurrent)

A 13-year-old female presented with a seven-day history of left facial paralysis, the second time for this patient. A prior episode of facial paralysis on the same side had occurred about 2 years prior. There were no other contributing findings: no fissuring of the tongue and no vesicles around the ear or in the nasopharynx. The hearing was WNL by tuning fork and audiometric examination. The left ipsilateral and right contralateral acoustic reflexes were absent, as expected. She had no facial movement on the left and a good Bell's reflex. She was graded as VI/VI by the House-Brackmann classification system. An ENOG was obtained and showed complete degeneration of the left facial nerve at 100%. A nonenhanced CT of the petrous temporal bones was normal.

Because she had recurrent facial paralysis, her parents were informed that a surgical decompression of the left facial nerve would be advisable in order to increase the chances of a good outcome and to help prevent recurrent episodes of left facial paralysis. The patient underwent surgical decompression of the complete facial nerve via a transmastoid and middle cranial fossa approach. She healed well and has a very slight weakness of the left ramis mandibularis as her only sequalae. She has been followed for over 10 years and has had no subsequent episodes of facial paralysis.

Herpes Zoster Oticus

A 32-year-old male presented in with right facial paralysis of 2 week's duration. He had no active eyelid closure and severe right facial dysfunction, VI/VI HB score. The facial paralysis was preceded by an eruption of blisters around his right ear and lower face, in the distribution of right CN VI. On the day of presentation, he was approximately 8 days out from the onset of facial paralysis.

The otoscopic examination was normal. He had a few healing blisters around the right ear, none in the oro- or nasopharynx. The tuning fork test at 512 Hz was normal, as was his level of audition.

An ENOG was obtained which showed 64% degeneration (or 36% function) of the VII nerve on the right. He was treated with prednisone 60 mg/day × 10 days with a tapering dose thereafter. He had already been treated with famicyclovir 2 g per day × 7 days.

He was using artificial tears during the day and lubrication at night, but still had excessive dryness of the right eye during the day. He underwent a right upper lid gold weight insertion (1.2 g) under local anesthesia approximately 1 week after presentation. Serial ENOGs revealed degeneration of the right facial nerve in the range of 40 to 60%. At the second week after presentation, a slight twitch of motion was detected in the right frontalis region. He will finish his prednisone and be observed with no other intervention. Substantial recovery of facial function is expected.

Temporal Bone Trauma (gunshot wound)

A 27-year-old male was seen in the ER with an acute gunshot wound to the right side of the face. He was brought to the hospital in an unconscious state, was intubated and treated by the trauma team for vascular injuries to the right and left carotid arteries. The entry site of the bullet was seen on the right cheek with x-ray findings of shrapnel in the temporal bone. He did not suffer a stroke. When he regained consciousness, it was apparent that the right side of his face was not moving.

He was cleared by the vascular team and anesthesia and underwent a right tympanoplasty with mastoidectomy, evacuation of shrapnel of the mastoid, right and left necks and a modified right neck dissection. The right facial nerve was injured by the bullet and a reparative neuroma was found. This was excised. The proximal and distal ends of the facial nerve were found and freshened, for a distance of about 2.5 cm. A right greater auricular nerve graft was prepared and was sutured in an end-to-end fashion with 2 anastomoses. This patient also had a right upper lid gold weight placed.

He additionally sustained significant injuries to his right external auditory canal and right temporomandibular joint and has had to have subsequent surgery to repair these sites. He regained function to an H-B III/VI level with significant synkinesis. After removal of the injured tympanic ring and a wide meatoplasty, he closed the conductive deficit on the right ear to within 10 dB.

SUMMARY

The patient presenting with acute, subacute, or chronic facial paralysis may challenge the treating physician. Because of its complex nature as a combined nerve and its long course through the temporal bone, many different etiologies may result in facial nerve compression and paralysis. A few important points may be gleaned:

1. A thorough and careful history will usually point toward the correct pathway of investigation for facial paralysis.
2. The facial nerve must be viewed in light of the whole patient and especially the function of the inner ear.
3. Regardless of the cosmetic concerns the patient may have, it is the affected eye and specifically the cornea that are of prime concern. Attention should be focused upon eye care. In many cases, ophthalmologic intervention will be required, most especially in the patient with a concomitant afferent sensory deficit.
4. Once a facial nerve completely loses function, it is highly likely that recovery will be less than complete and may include sequalae such as synkinesis or regional paresis. The patient must be so instructed.
5. The surgeon should have at his or her disposal several easy, straightforward medical and surgical techniques to help in the care of the eye, the upper, and the lower face. The best techniques are based on recovery of the nerve itself. Substitution of any other technique may yield acceptable function and cosmesis, but will never supplant a native, working nerve, however imperfectly the nerve may function. Because of concerns regarding ongoing synkinesis, re-animation with isolated muscle transposition or substitution is becoming more widespread. Dynamic

re-animation techniques ordinarily yield better functional results than static techniques.

6. It is almost every treating physician's belief that for acute idiopathic facial paralysis steroids offer a better outcome than nothing.
7. Surgical decompression for idiopathic facial paralysis remains controversial for several reasons:
   a. Large outcome studies are lacking and objective evidence demonstrating the statistically significant benefit of decompression versus observation in appropriately matched patients is either nonextant or not compelling. Such a study would need to be prospective, randomized with sufficiently large numbers of properly matched patients with no treatment versus medical treatment alone versus surgery alone versus medical treatment and surgery to definitively answer the question of which method(s) of treatment would yield the best outcome.
   b. Facial nerve outcomes based on subjective analyses are fraught with observer bias and are, for this reason, unconvincing. Treating surgeons tend to award higher outcome scores than do patients.

Timely surgical decompression of the facial nerve in the appropriate patient with both clinical and electrical degeneration of the nerve remains a viable option and should be offered to the patient. Time is of the essence and in most studies the "window of opportunity" to help with surgical intervention is no greater than approximately two weeks from the onset of paralysis. If the treating physician does not perform surgical decompression, the patient should be sent to a surgeon who does so that this critical time period will not lapse.

Traumatic injury to the facial nerve is the most compelling reason for surgical decompression.

REFERENCES

1. May M. *The Facial Nerve*. New York, NY: Thieme; 1986:3–17.
2. Anson BJ, Donaldson JA. *Surgical Anatomy of the Temporal Bone*. Philadelphia, PA: WB Saunders Co; 1981:510–515.
3. Donaldson JA, Duckert LG, Lambert PM, Rubel EW. *Surgical Anatomy of the Temporal Bone*. 2nd ed. New York, NY: Raven Press; 1992:366–376.
4. Pauwels L, Akesson EJ, Stewart PA. *Cranial Nerves: Anatomy and Clinical Comments*. Toronto, Canada: B.C. Decker; 1988.
5. House JW. Facial nerve grading systems. *Laryngoscope*. 1983;93:1056–1069.
6. House JW, Brackmann DE. Facial nerve grading system. *Otolaryngol Head Neck Surg*. 1985;93:146–147.
7. Fisch U. Surgery for Bell's palsy. *Arch Otolaryngol*. 1981; 107:1–11.
8. Fisch U: Prognostic value of electrical tests in acute facial paralysis. *Am J Otol*. 1984; 6:494–498.
9. Burres SA. Facial biomechanics: the standards of normal. *Laryngoscope*. 1985:95;708–714.
10. Burres SA. Objective grading of facial paralysis. *Ann Otolaryngol Rhinol Laryngol*. 1986;95:238–241.
11. Neely JG, Jekel JF, Cheung J. Variations in maximum amplitude of facial expressions between and within normal subjects. *Otolaryngol Head Neck Surg*. 1994;110:60–63.
12. Holman ML, Neely JG, Joaquin AH. Computer-assisted clinometric tool for the study of facial expression: a pilot validity study. *Laryngoscope*. 1996;106:135–138.
13. Meier-Gallati V, Scriba H, Fisch U. Objective scaling of facial nerve function based on area analysis (OSCAR). *Otolaryngol Head Neck Surg*. 1998;118:545–550.
14. Scriba H, Stoeckli S, Veraguth D, Pollack A, Fisch U. Objective evaluation of normal facial function. *Ann Otolaryngol Rhinol Laryngol*. 1999;108:641–644.
15. Linstrom CJ, Silverman CA, Susman WM. Facial-motion analysis with a video-and computer system: a preliminary report. *Am J Otolaryngol*. 2000;21:123–129.
16. Linstrom CJ, Silverman CA, Colson D. Facial motion analysis with a video and computer system following treatment of acoustic neuroma. *J Otol Neurotol*. 2002;23:572–579.
17. Linstrom CJ. Objective facial motion analysis in patients with facial nerve dysfunction. *Laryngoscope*. 2002;112: 1129–1147.
18. Lewis BI, Ardour KK, Kahn JM, Lewis AJ. Hilger facial nerve stimulator: a 25-year update. *Laryngoscope*. 1991; 101:71–74.
19. Gates GA. Nerve excitability testing: technical pitfalls and threshold norms using absolute values. *Laryngoscope*. 1993;103:379–385.
20. Sillman JS, Niparko JK, Lee SS, Kileny PR. Prognostic value of evoked and standard electromyography in acute facial paralysis. *Otolaryngol Head Neck Surg*. 1992; 107:377–381.
21. Peitersen E. The natural history of Bell's palsy. *Am J Otol*. 1982;4:107–111.
22. Peitersen E. The natural history of Bell's palsy. *Acta Otolaryngol Suppl*. 1992;492:122–124.
23. Kartush JM, Linstrom CJ, McCann PM, Graham MD. Early gold weight eyelid implantation for facial paralysis. *Otolaryngol Head Neck Surg*. 1990;103:1016–1023.

24. Linder TE, Pike VE, Linstrom CJ. Early eyelid rehabilitation in facial nerve paralysis. *Laryngoscope*. 1996;106:1115–1118.
25. Marsh MA, Coker NJ. Surgical decompression of idiopathic facial palsy. *Otolaryngol Clin N Am*. 1991;24:675–689.
26. Fisch U, Esslen E. Total intratemporal exposure of the facial nerve: pathologic findings in Bell's palsy. *Arch Otolaryngol*. 1972;95:335–341.
27. Gantz BJ, Rubinstein JT, Gidley P, Woodworth GG. Surgical management of Bell's palsy. *Laryngoscope*. 1999;109:1177–1188.

PART IV

Inner Ear Pathology

CHAPTER 14

Congenital Hearing Loss

Dan Sdrulla and Seilesh Babu

IMPACT OF HEARING LOSS

Profound hearing loss has an effect on speech and language development, learning ability, reading and arithmetic skills, and eventual income potential. There are approximately 400,000 students who have hearing deficits requiring special learning classes with overall costs estimated at $121 billion.[1]

INTRODUCTION

Early identification of newborn and pediatric hearing loss and appropriate intervention provides the best opportunity for counseling, habilitation, and development. Additionally, early enrollment in services for a child with hearing impairment reduce health care, special education, and other service costs for families and taxpayers.

Congenital hearing loss is the most common sensory deficit, with an incidence of between 1 per 1,000 and 1 per 2,000 affected infants. It can be a result of environmental and genetic factors. Half of these patients have environmental risk factors, such as exposure to infectious agents or ototoxic medications. The other half of patients with congenital hearing loss is caused by genetic defects, the majority of which are isolated (nonsyndromic). Approximately 25% of genetic causes are associated with other known birth defects, termed syndromic.[2]

ENVIRONMENTAL RISK FACTORS FOR HEARING LOSS

The dissemination of high-risk criteria for neonates and infants in 1990 did not notably alter the mean age at diagnosis (Table 14–1). About 50% of children with SNHL do not have risk factors, with only 10% of neonates having 1 or more of the high-risk criteria that prompt an evaluation. These rates are among the reasons cited for the need for universal neonatal hearing screening. The goals of such screening are to identify children who are deaf or hard of hearing and to start intervention by age 6 months.

Table 14–1. High-Risk Criteria for Neonates (birth to 28 days)

Family history of congenital or early SNHL
Congenital infection known to be associated with SNHL
Craniofacial anomalies
Birth weight of more than 1500 g (<3.3 lb)
Hyperbilirubinemia over the exchange level
Exposure to ototoxic medications
Bacterial meningitis
Low Apgar scores at birth
Prolonged mechanical ventilation
Findings of a syndrome associated with SNHL

GENETIC INHERITANCE

Hereditary deafness is a highly heterogeneous disease with multiple genes responsible for auditory dysfunction. Mutations of several different genes can cause identical clinical phenotypes and different mutations in one gene can cause variable phenotypes. Hereditary hearing loss can be transmitted in several inheritance patterns, including autosomal dominant, autosomal recessive, X-linked inheritance, and mitochondrial inheritance.

These are briefly described below.

Autosomal Dominant

Autosomal dominant (AD) inheritance exhibits a vertical pattern of transmission because only one altered gene is necessary. There is a 50% chance of transmission. Parents usually exhibit findings associated with the mutated gene.

Autosomal Recessive

Autosomal recessive (AR) inheritance is the most common transmission pattern in hereditary hearing loss. Both copies of the mutated gene must be present and the risk is that 25% of the offspring will manifest the disease. Parents, who may be asymptomatic, each carry the recessive gene which may be then passed along. This mode of transmission has a horizontal pattern.

X-linked

The X-linked inheritance involves genes located on the X chromosome, which will affect males more because they only possess one copy of that chromosome. Females may carry the mutated gene on one X chromosome without any expression. The carrier mother's sons and daughters will have a 50% chance of inheritance, with the daughters having a 50% chance of becoming a carrier of the mutation.

Mitochondrial Inheritance

Mitochondrial inheritance is caused by mutations in the mitochondrion DNA, which is only passed on from mothers because only ova carry mitochondrial DNA.

Other Genetic Defects

Exciting developments in genetic mapping have revealed approximately 2 dozen abnormal genes that lead to deafness, but are nonsyndromic. In some, the molecular or structural defect has been identified (eg, collagen in the basilar membrane, structural defect in a membrane-gating protein). These genes have been classified according to their mode of inheritance: AD (*DFNA1* through *DFNA11*), AR (*DFNB1* through *DFNB12*), X-linked recessives (*DFN1* through *DFN6*), or mitochondrial (12Sr RNA and tRNA-Ser UCN). Some of the genes exhibit variable penetrance. They are discussed briefly later.

CLINICAL PRESENTATION

Universal newborn screening has drastically increased the numbers of patients being diagnosed at an early age. These patients are usually asymptomatic except for the fact that they may have failed their hearing screening tests. Children may present with loss of cooing by the age of 6 to 9 months and with frank language delay. Older children may have hearing difficulties identified by the caregiver. Those with a mild hearing loss will hear loud sounds, such as yelling or phone ringing, but they do not hear most conversational speech. These concerns should prompt immediate evaluation. Little justification supports delaying the diagnosis while language delay or behavioral problems are ruled out, especially because hearing loss may be the cause of these problems.

EVALUATION

A complete history should include prenatal, perinatal, postnatal, and family history. Risk factors during pregnancy, including toxic medications, infections, or medical issues need to be pursued. Family history needs to be investigated, especially for family members with hearing loss at a young age. Constructing a pedigree may be helpful as well.

PHYSICAL EXAMINATION

Physical exam should focus on looking for features associated with congenital infection or syndromic hearing loss. Note hair color, the presence of a white forelock, and facial and skull shape. Eyes should be examined for color of the iris, position of the canthum, intercanthal distance, cataracts, and other retinal findings. The ear is evaluated for preauricular pits, skin tags, shape and size of the pinna for microtia, abnormality of the ear canal including atresia, and abnormalities of the tympanic membrane or ossicles. The neck is examined for branchial anomalies and thyroid enlargement. The oral cavity is inspected for any cleft abnormalities. Thorough inspection of the skin for areas of hyper- or hypopigmentation and café-au-lait spots should be performed. Except for the hearing loss, the physical examination is usually normal.

AUDIOLOGIC EVALUATION

Universal Hearing Screening

The Joint Committee on Infant Hearing (JCIH) recommends hearing screening in all infants by age 1 month and those who fail the initial test should have a thorough audiologic evaluation by age 3 months, with appropriate intervention by age 6 months.

Specific Hearing Tests

Auditory Brainstem Response Testing (ABR)

ABR testing records neuronal electrical activity from the ear to the central auditory cortex. An automated ABR (AABR) is recommended for universal newborn hearing screening. Sound clicks are presented to each ear, and 2 electrodes placed on the scalp record brain-wave activity. An internal template of what the waveforms should resemble is used to determine if the baby passes the test (waveforms match) or not (waveforms do not match). People with relatively little training can perform the ABR test quickly and inexpensively. It has a sensitivity and specificity of about 100% and 96%, respectively.

AABR testing cannot be used to distinguish conductive hearing loss from sensorineural hearing loss. In neonatal screening, the false-positive rate is 10 to 15% because amniotic fluid and cellular debris may obstruct the ear canal. Repeat testing is recommended for this reason to allow the debris or fluid to clear.

If any question arises as to the accuracy of the AABR, formal ABR testing is recommended.

Otoacoustic Emission Testing

Otoacoustic emission (OAE) testing has been discussed in Chapter 5. The concept of OAE is that the normal sounds produced by the inner ear can be recorded and their absence may point to hearing loss. OAE testing can be performed quickly and inexpensively by personnel with relatively little training making it a suitable screening tool for newborn hearing screening. An earphone is placed over the ear of a resting neonate, and the machine produces and records the evoked response. The sensitivity and specificity reported with evoked OAE are 100% and 82%, respectively. Automated ABR or OAE are used for universal hearing screening as the initial test.[3]

Audiometry

Routine audiometry can be performed in older children who can raise their corresponding hand when a sound is heard. Pure tone sounds can be presented so that specific volumes at specific frequencies can be documented. Conductive and sensorineural hearing loss can be differentiated, and speech recognition can also be tested. The only limits to the sensitivity and specificity of the test are the patient's ability to understand the instructions and his or her willingness to cooperate. Pure-tone audiometry can be performed as a quick and easy screening test, but in older, cooperative patients.

Behavioral (visual reinforcement) and conditioned play audiometry can be completed in children as young as 6 months. Children can be conditioned to look at a puppet or a light show when a pure sound stimulus is presented or their name is called from one side of the room. If the evaluators are reliable, they can judge whether the child is cooperative and responding to cues other than the sound stimulus. In general, this test is fairly successful for identifying hearing loss in children. Disadvantages are that it requires considerable time and equipment, it cannot be used to distinguish CHL from SNHL, and it succeeds only if the child is cooperating.

EVALUATION AND WORKUP

Depending on the patient's history and physical findings, laboratory blood work may help to determine the etiology of deafness if a genetic syndrome is suspected. A child with hearing loss should at least have thyroid and renal function evaluation with thyroid function tests, BUN/creatinine levels, and urinalysis. An electrocardiogram (EKG) may be useful for prolonged QT interval and cardiac arrhythmias found in Jervell and Lange-Nielsen syndrome.

Other laboratory studies that may be included as deemed necessary are complete blood count (CBC), electrolytes, blood sugar, fluorescent treponemal antibody absorption (FTA-ABS), and genetic evaluation with chromosomal studies.

Imaging studies include computed tomography (CT) of the temporal bone to identify potentially surgically reparable causes of conductive or sensorineural hearing loss and may also be used to identify the less dysplastic, and presumably better-hearing, ear when considering auditory habilitation. CT abnormalities are found in up to 30% of individuals with hearing loss and thus are an important component of the evaluation. The most common finding is enlarged vestibular aqueduct, followed by Mondini malformation. Enlarged vestibular aqueduct (EVA) suggests the diagnosis of Pendred syndrome, but may be also found in branchio-oto-renal syndrome or as an isolated finding.

CT scanning and MRI may help in identifying a malformation of the cochlea or the cochlear nerve. Such information may be critical when cochlear implantation is considered in profoundly deaf individuals.

CONGENITAL AURAL ATRESIA

Congenital aural atresia (CAA) is defined by the absence of the external auditory canal. Microtia refers to malformation of the auricle. CAA occurs in 1/20,000 births and is more common in males. It is usually unilateral; however, bilateral cases do exist. CAA is mostly sporadic. Syndromic associations such as Treacher Collins, Goldenhar, branchio-oto-renal, and Crouzon syndromes occur.

Embryology

The auricle and the middle ear develop between the 3rd and 6th week of development. This accounts for the ossicular abnormality (with malleus and incus) and microtia findings of the auricle. The external auditory canal (EAC) develops during the 8th week from the first branchial groove with recanalization occurring during the 21st week of development. Abnormalities in this process result in various presentations of microtia and aural atresia.

Imaging

High-resolution CT scan (HRCT) should be obtained in order to evaluate the status of the inner ear, the extent of temporal bone pneumatization, the course of the facial nerve and the presence of the oval window/stapes footplate. Additionally, one should also assess the thickness of the atretic bone, soft tissue contribution to the atresia, size/status of the middle ear cavity, and the presence/absence of congenital cholesteatoma.

Jahrsdoerfer et al[4] developed a grading system based on CT findings.[4] It provides each anatomical structure such as presence of stapes, oval window, middle ear space, and normal facial nerve either 1 or 2 points, with the presence of stapes footplate being the only one with 2 points. 10 points are the maximum. This scheme is also used to indirectly estimate the likelihood of success if surgical correction is performed. If the patient has an 8 or 9, this correlates with an excellent candidate for reconstruction. On the other hand, if their score is 6 or less, then the patient is a poor candidate for the surgery.

Treatment

The goals of treatment are hearing improvement and creating the appearance of a patent, skin-lined ear canal. Hearing improvement can be accomplished with a Soft-Band Baha, an implanted Baha, or atresiaplasty.[5]

Atresiaplasty is a technically difficult surgery with potential risks of meatal stenosis, continued hearing loss, worsening hearing, facial nerve injury, and recurrent otorrhea. It is usually planned in stages along with microtia repair at the age of 5 or 6 years old. The success rate of surgery is dependent on the experience and expertise of the surgeon.

Unilateral atresia may be observed or offered amplification during early childhood. Bilateral atresia needs urgent attention for hearing amplification in the form of Soft-Band Baha.

SYNDROMIC HEARING LOSS

Autosomal Dominant Syndromes with Hearing Loss

These are less frequent causes of hearing loss than autosomal recessive disorders. Examples include Waardenburg, neurofibromatosis, branchio-oto-renal, Tietze, Hermann, Leopard, Kearns-Sayre, Crouzon, Forney, achondroplasia, Duane, and Marfan syndromes. The common ones are detailed below. A more thorough and detailed description of these and many other syndromes can be found in other genetic textbooks.

Waardenburg Syndrome

Waardenburg syndrome (WS) is the most common cause of autosomal dominant syndromic hearing loss. The disease was named for Petrus Johannes Waardenburg, a Dutch ophthalmologist who noticed that people with two different colored eyes frequently had hearing problems. It is estimated to account for 2% of all cases of congenital hearing loss in the United States.

WS has 4 types: Type I features are lateral displacement of the medial canthi which gives an appearance of a widened nasal bridge (dystopia canthorum), high nasal root, hyperplasia of the medial portion of the eyebrows, heterochromia irides, white forelock, and sensorineural deafness. WS Type II, which is the most common type, has features of type I without the dystopia canthorum and has a higher incidence of sensorineural hearing loss. Type III also has features of upper limb malformations and is called Klein-Waardenburg syndrome. Type IV is similar to type II, but has the addition of Hirschsprung's disease.

WS has been localized at gene locus 2q35 or 2q37.3, which codes for *PAX3*. PAX3 is a DNA-binding protein that is important in determining the fate of neural crest cells in the developing nervous system.[6] *PAX3* mutations cause WS type I and WS type III. Some cases of WS type II are caused by mutations in *MITF*. WS type IV has been linked to mutations in *EDNRB, EDN3,* and *SOX10*.[7] *EDNRB* is postulated to play an essential role in the development of the two neural crest-derived cell lineages, epidermal melanocytes and enteric neurons. SOX10 belongs to the family of transcription factors that bind DNA and regulate its transcription. Interaction of these three genes has been suggested.

Branchio-Oto-Renal Syndrome

Branchio-oto-renal (BOR) syndrome is the second most common type of autosomal dominant syndromic hearing loss, which consists of branchial derived anomalies (in 60%), otologic anomalies, and renal malformation (in 15%). Auricular malformations, preauricular pits (in 80%), and ossicular malformations may occur causing a conductive hearing loss, along with sensorineural hearing loss. Kidney function is usually normal.

BOR is caused by mutations in *EYA1* and *SIX1* genes. These genes must play a role in both the development of the inner ear and kidney.[8]

Neurofibromatosis 2

Neurofibromatosis 2 (NF2) is caused by a mutation in the *NF2* gene on chromosome 22 and is characterized by the development of multiple tumors, including vestibular schwannomas, meningiomas, gliomas, and ependymomas. The hearing loss associated with vestibular schwannomas is potentially treatable with early surgical intervention.

Stickler Syndrome

Stickler syndrome has findings of progressive myopia, retinal detachment, blindness, abnormal epiphyseal development, midface hypoplasia, irregularities of the vertebral bodies, cleft palate deformity, and variable sensorineural hearing loss.

It is caused by mutations in *COL2A1*, *COL11A2*, or *COL11A1*. The classic phenotype is associated with mutations in COL2A1, a fibrillar collagen that is arrayed in quarter-staggered fashion to form fibers similar to those of *COLI*. These may also be responsible for findings in Alport's syndrome.

Treacher Collins Syndrome

Treacher Collins syndrome is a disorder of craniofacial development, with slanting of the eyes and inferior displacement of the lateral canthi with respect to the medial canthi, coloboma of the lower lids, micrognathia, microtia and other deformity of the ears, hypoplastic zygomatic arches, and macrostomia. Conductive hearing loss and cleft palate are often present.

The *TCOF1* gene has been localized on chromosome 5 and identified to play a role in nucleolar-cytoplasmic transport resulting in abnormal protein coding.

Autosomal Recessive Disorders

Usher Syndrome

Usher syndrome is named after ophthalmologist Charles Usher (1914) who characterized the hereditary nature of hearing loss and blindness caused by retinitis pigmentosa.[9] The disorder is responsible for up to 10% of cases of congenital deafness, making it the most common autosomal recessive disorder.

Vision impairment may be difficult to identify in children as fundoscopic examination is limited before age 10. Electroretinography can reveal early retinal abnormalities in young children but is not routinely available. Loss of vision is progressive, and 50% of individuals develop complete blindness before age 50 years.[10] Hearing loss is generally present at birth, and 85% of affected individuals eventually become totally deaf. Vestibulocerebellar ataxia is present in a high percentage of individuals with severe deafness.

Clinically, three different types can be distinguished based on the severity of the hearing loss and extent of the vestibular system involvement. Type 1 patients have profound congenital deafness, absent vestibular response, and the onset of retinitis pigmentosa in the first decade of life. Type 2 patients have normal vestibular response. Type 3 patients have more variable presentation of progressive hearing loss, vestibular response, and delayed onset of retinitis pigmentosa.

Six genes have been identified in Usher syndrome with 11 different loci. The *MYO7A*, which encodes myosin 7A, represents a unique molecular motor for hair cells. The *CDH23* gene encodes cadherin 23, which is an adhesion molecule maybe important for cross-linking of stereocilia. It may also be involved in maintaining the ionic composition of the endolymph. Studies have suggested that myosin 7A, and cadherin 23, along with another protein harmonin, which is coded by the *USH1c* gene, form a transient functional complex in stereocilia.[11]

Pendred Syndrome

Pendred syndrome is represented by congenital hearing loss and multinodular goiter. It is a common syndromic form of deafness, accounting for approximately 8% of cases. The goiter usually does not present at birth, but develops later in life due to abnormal organification of iodine. A positive potassium perchlorate discharge test may be helpful in identifying this organification defect. Patients are usually euthyroid but can be hypothyroid.

Hearing loss is bilateral and most prominent in higher frequencies, often with positive recruitment suggestive of a cochlear site of lesion. It may be fluctuating or progressive. A Mondini cochlear malformation and enlarged vestibular aqueduct are often identified along with Pendred syndrome.

Mutations of the gene *PDS* (*SLC26A4*) on chromosome 7q31 account for most cases of Pendred syndrome.[12] This gene encodes pendrin, which is an anion transporter found in the inner ear, thyroid, and renal tissue. Mutations in this gene can also be found in nonsyndromic deafness DFNB4 and many cases of enlarged vestibular aqueduct syndrome.

Jervell and Lange-Nielsen Syndrome

Jervell and Lange-Nielsen syndrome accounts for 1% of all cases of recessive hearing loss, and is characterized by EKG changes of prolonged QT interval, torsade de pointe arrhythmias, syncopal attacks, and even sudden death.[13] The hearing loss is bilateral and severe with temporal bone findings of atrophy of the organ of Corti and spiral ganglion, along with large periodic acid-Schiff (PAS)–positive hyaline deposits throughout the membranous labyrinth. Atrophy of sensory cells within the utricle and saccule is also evident.

A screening EKG may show prolonged QT interval, but the sensitivity is not high. Children with a family history of sudden death, sudden infant death syndrome (SIDS), syncopal episodes, or prolonged QT interval should be closely examined.

Two genes, *KVLQT1* and *KCNE1*, have been identified that may be associated with this syndrome. They may encode for a potassium channel in the inner ear.

Cockayne Syndrome

Cockayne syndrome is associated with dwarfism, retinal atrophy, and deafness. Other characteristics include kyphosis and ankylosis, prognathism, sunken eyes, mental retardation, and carious teeth. Evidence points to degenerative changes of the spiral ganglion, cochlear nucleus, and olivary nucleus.[14]

Alström Syndrome

Alström syndrome is associated with progressive hearing loss, retinitis pigmentosa, diabetes mellitus, and obesity. Hearing loss is bilateral and progressive.

Refsum Disease

Refsum disease is a recessive-inherited disorder characterized by retinitis pigmentosa, ichthyosis, polyneuritis, cerebellar ataxia, and hearing loss. Affected individuals often do not survive past the second decade of life. Visual loss typically occurs in patients older than 20 years. Progressive SNHL occurs in more than 50% of patients.[15] Degeneration of the organ of Corti and stria vascularis has been reported in histopathologic studies.

Hurler Syndrome

Hurler syndrome is a lysosomal storage disease caused by an enzymatic deficiency that results in accumulation of the mucopolysaccharides heparin sulfate and dermatan sulfate. It is characterized by mental retardation, dwarfism, kyphosis, hepatosplenomegaly, and hearing loss. Hearing loss is generally mixed with prominence of sensory loss in the higher frequencies. Temporal bone studies have demonstrated PAS-positive material within the substance of the mesenchyme with degeneration of the organ of Corti.[16] Generally, survival is rare past the second decade of life for the autosomal recessive disorder.

Oculocutaneous Albinism

Oculocutaneous albinism is an autosomal recessive disorder that is due to defects in the biosynthesis and distribution of melanin. Patients demonstrate lack of pigmentation in the skin, eyes, and hair. Hearing loss varies in degree of severity.

X-Linked Disorders

Alport's Syndrome

Alport's syndrome represents the most common form of hereditary nephritis, with an incidence of 1 case per 200,000 individuals. It is mostly an X-linked hereditary disorder of basement membranes.[17] Autosomal recessive as well as autosomal dominant inheritance has also been observed. Hematuria, posterior cataracts, corneal dystrophy, and dislocation of the lens characterize the condition. The hematuria is often accompanied by red cell casts, indicating that the renal lesion is a glomerulitis. Although the disease is more common in females, boys are affected more severely than girls, commonly progressing to end-stage renal failure during their second or third decade of life. Untreated males die by age 30 years. Symptoms typically appear during the first decade of life.

Hearing loss is usually bilateral and symmetric, but progressive SNHL, with higher frequencies most prominently affected, has also been noted.

Mutations in three different type 4 collagen genes (*COL4A3*, *COL4A4*, and *COL4A5*) have been identified. These collagens are essential for the basement membrane and can be found in the basilar membrane, parts of the spiral ligament, and stria vascularis of the inner ear. It is suggested that the loss of integrity of the basement membrane might affect adhesion of the tectorial membrane resulting in hearing loss.

Norrie Syndrome

Norrie syndrome is an X-linked disease that has ocular symptoms and hearing loss. The ocular symptoms include pseudotumor of the retina, retinal hyperplasia, hypoplasia, and necrosis of the inner layer of the retina, cataracts, and phthisis bulbi. The sensorineural hearing loss is progressive. Mental retardation may also be present.

NDP gene, coding for norrin, has been identified in association with this disease. The norrin protein may aid in vascularization of the cochlea and retina.

Hunter Syndrome

Hunter syndrome is similar to Hurler syndrome in its clinical presentation except that it is x-linked instead of autosomal recessive. Hunter syndrome is a milder form and the hearing loss may be conductive, sensorineural, or mixed.

Fabry Disease

Fabry disease is caused by accumulation of sphingolipid within endothelial, smooth muscle, and ganglion cells. Hearing loss is typically bilateral with a predominant sensorineural high-frequency loss. Histopathologic studies of affected temporal bones include atrophy of the spiral ligament and accumulation of sphingolipid in vascular endothelial and ganglion cells of the auditory system.

Oto-Palato-Digital Syndrome

Oto-palato-digital syndrome includes cleft palate, fishmouth, clinodactyly, prominent forehead, hypertelorism, and antimongoloid palpebral fissures. Hearing loss is conductive because of ossicular malformations.

NONSYNDROMIC HEARING LOSS

As research continues, new genetic loci are being discovered that can result in nonsyndromic hearing issues. The severity of hearing loss ranges from severe to profound and the inheritance can be autosomal dominant, autosomal recessive, and X-linked forms. The recessive forms seem to be prelingual and more severe compared to the other types.[18]

Signal Transduction in Hearing Loss

Signal transduction along the hearing pathway requires maintenance of basement membranes, support structures, connecting proteins, and ionic concentrations. Any protein that becomes defective along this pathway may lead to potential hearing loss.

Ionic concentration is maintained by gap junction genes that code for proteins (called connexins) that allow ions to migrate to the stria vascularis and into the endolymph. Four connexins have been implicated (*with the genes that code for it*): connexin 26 (*GJB2*), connexin 31 (*GJB3*), connexin 30 (*GJB6*), and connexin 43 (*GJA1*).[19] *GJB2* is the first nonsyndromic sensorineural deafness gene to be identified and is estimated to account for 50% of recessive nonsyndromic hearing loss. 80 different recessive and 6 different dominant mutations have been found in *GJB2* coding. The most frequent mutation that has been identified so far is the 35delG (one guanosine residue deletion from nucleotide position 35).[20] Diagnostic testing is available for this mutation; however, there are so many other causes of this mutation that its specificity is quite low.

Transcription factor genes have also been implicated in some causes of hearing loss. These include *POU3F4*, *POU4F3*, *EYA4*, and *TFCP2L3*. *POU3F4* is responsible for X-linked mixed hearing loss, consistent with stapes fixation. This may also lead to the perilymph gusher that may be noted during stapes surgery. The others have been implicated in autosomal dominant hearing loss.

There are other proteins that are critical for the stereocilia of the cochlea to function well. These include myosins, otoferlin, actin-polymerization protein, harmonin, and cadherin. Myosins are molecular motor proteins that bind to actin and that hydrolyze ATP to generate the force to move across actin filaments that are coded by myosin genes (*MYO3A*, *MYO6*, *MYO7A*, *MYO15*). Otoferlin (encoded by *OTOF*) acts in calcium triggered synaptic vesicle transfer. It may the next most common cause for recessive nonsyndromic hearing loss not caused by connexin 26. Harmonin and cadherin organize multiprotein complexes in specific subcellular domains. They anchor and cluster transmembrane proteins and recruit signaling molecules and may be implicated in Usher type I syndrome.

Abnormalities of the basement membrane have been discussed. Defects in the structure of the tectorial membrane may result in hearing loss as well. *TECTA* encodes alpha tectorin, a component of the tectorial membrane and *COL11A2* encodes type XI collagen. Abnormalities of these can lead to disorganized collagen fibrils of the tectorial membrane. These types of mutations seem to exhibit symptoms of Ménière's syndrome, including vertigo, tinnitus, and aural pressure.

CHROMOSOMAL ABNORMALITIES WITH HEARING LOSS

Trisomy 21

Trisomy 21, or Down syndrome, is the most common chromosomal disorder in the world with an incidence of 1 per 1,000 births. Clinical features include a broad short trunk, epicanthal folds, muscular hypotonia, congenital heart disease, and mental retardation. Hearing loss can be conductive, sensorineural, and mixed with 75% of patients have some type.[21] Histopathologic temporal bone findings include residual mesenchyme in the middle ear, endolymphatic hydrops, and a wide angle of the facial nerve genu.

Trisomy 13

Trisomy 13 results in severe congenital malformations that are not compatible with life beyond the first year. Clinical features include microcephaly, cleft lip and palate, polydactyly, low-set malformed pinna, cardiac defects, scalp defects, and mental retardation. Temporal bone analysis reveals cystic changes within the stria vascularis, shortened length of the cochlea, saccular degeneration, and anomalies of the semicircular canals.

Trisomy 18

Trisomy 18 is another chromosomal abnormality that is not compatible with life, with most infants not surviving more than 4 to 6 months. Clinical features include malformed pinna, micrognathia, prominent occiput, intestinal defects, and mental retardation. Temporal bone findings reveal damage to the stria vascularis.[22]

COUNSELING

The genetic counseling team consists of clinical/medical geneticist, genetic counselor, social worker, and psychologists. The risk and benefit of genetic testing should be explained to the family. Three genetic tests are currently available: GJB2, SLC26A4, and EYA1. Genetic information may help predict whether the hearing loss progress or not or whether a cochlear implant may be useful. Genetic testing can also provide a deaf individual or the parents of deaf child information when making reproductive choices for future children.

Other members of the team will include otolaryngologist, otologist, audiologist, speech and language therapist, teachers, parents, and, of course, the patient.

TREATMENT FOR NEWBORN SNHL

Once a hearing loss is identified, the decision must be made regarding treatment choices.

Amplification

The goal of amplification is to use any residual hearing to at least orient patients to surrounding environments and to maximize auditory language development. Hearing amplification can generally be implemented successfully during the first 6 weeks of life. Available hearing amplification devices include conventional analog hearing aids, digital hearing aids, bone conduction hearing aids, and bone-anchored hearing aids (especially for those with aural atresia).

Assistive Listening Devices

These devices aid in reducing the signal-to-noise ratio to decrease the background noise. These include FM amplification devices. Telephone devices are also available to aid in communication. Some hearing aids may be coupled with telephones. Telecommunication devices help deaf people who are unable to use a standard telephone. Television viewing is significantly enhanced with closed captioning for the hearing impaired. Signaling devices substitute visual signals for auditory signals and detect environmental sounds, such as doorbells, telephones, alarm clocks, fire alarms, or crying babies.

Educational Methods

Numerous educational methods are currently used for children with hearing impairment. These methods include auditory-oral training, cued speech, and total communication. Auditory-oral training stresses acquisition of speech and language through enhancement of residual hearing mostly with lipreading skills and amplification. The cued speech approach is a visual-oral system that uses hand cues to supplement information received from lip-reading. Hand cues alone are ambiguous, necessitating development of appropriate lipreading skills for language comprehension. Manualism is a system of communication that stresses use of the manual alphabet (finger spelling) and sign language for communication. American Sign Language (Ameslan) has been the language of the deaf population in the United States for more than a century. The total communication method emphasizes manual, oral, and aural modes of communication. This method urges early use of residual hearing while accepting sign language as a normal means of communication. Speech and use of spontaneous expression are also encouraged.

No single educational program is correct for all children with hearing impairment, but, rather, decisions should be individualized for each child. Parents must be able and willing to participate in the language education that they chose for their child, and be extremely involved. School failures and behavior problems are not inherent to deafness but frequently result from a frustrated child who has no ability to communicate and no ability to connect with others.

Surgical Options

Certain children with hearing loss may have a conductive hearing loss and treatment options may include surgical intervention either for ossicular abnormalities or stapes fixation. Unilateral conductive hearing loss usually may be managed conservatively. Bilateral conductive hearing loss may require intervention either with amplification, bone anchored implants, or surgery in the form of ossicular chain reconstruction or stapedotomy. An informed discussion needs to be had with the patient and family due to the increased risk of complete hearing loss from surgical intervention either due to malformed inner ear or increased perilymph pressure resulting in perilymph gusher or even cerebrospinal fluid (CSF) leak.

SUMMARY

Communication is the most important loss in deafness. Communication is necessary for socialization and integration into family and society. All interventions must have the goal of optimizing the child's ability to successfully communicate and interact.

Early diagnosis of hearing loss is now possible allowing immediate intervention. The genetic cause of hearing and balance issues is evolving and it may become possible to not only intervene with amplification, but also with treatment of the underlying cause of the hearing loss.

REFERENCES

1. Arnos KS. (2003). The implications of genetic testing for deafness. *Ear Hear.* 24(4):324–331.
2. Friedman T, Schultz J, Ben-Yosef T, et al. Recent advances in the understanding of syndromic forms of hearing loss. *Ear Hear.* 2003;24(4):289–302.
3. Jacobson JT, Jacobson CA, Spahr RC. Automated and conventional ABR screening techniques in high-risk infants. *J Am Acad Audiol*. 1990;1(4):187–195.
4. Jahrsdoerfer RA, Yeakley JW, Aguilar EA, Cole RR, Gray LC. Grading system for the selection of patients with congenital aural atresia. *Am J Otol*. 1992;13(1):6–12.
5. Wazen JJ, Spitzer J, Ghossaini SN, Kacker A, Zschommler A. Results of the bone-anchored hearing aid in unilateral hearing loss. *Laryngoscope*. 2001;111(6):955–958.
6. Ishikiriyama S, Tonoki H, Shibuya Y. Waardenburg syndrome type I in a child with de novo inversion (2) (q35q37.3). *Am J Med Genet*. 1989;33(4):505–507.
7. Waardenburg PJ. A new syndrome combining developmental anomalies of the eyelids, eyebrows, and nose root with pigmentary defects of the iris and head hair and with congenital deafness. *Am J Hum Gen*. 1951;3:195–253.
8. Coppage KB, Smith RJ. Branchio-oto-renal syndrome. *J Am Acad Audiol*. 1995;6(1):103–110.
9. Belal A Jr. Usher's syndrome (retinitis pigmentosa and deafness). A temporal bone report. *J Laryngol Otol*. 1975; 89(2):175–181.
10. Usher CH. On the inheritance of retinitis pigmentosa, with notes of a case. *London Hosp Rep*. 1914;19:130–136.
11. Kimberling WJ, Moller C. Clinical and molecular genetics of Usher syndrome. *J Am Acad Audiol*. 1995;6(1):63–72.
12. Illum P, Kiaer HW, Hvidberg-Hansen J. Fifteen cases of Pendred's syndrome. Congenital deafness and sporadic goiter. *Arch Otolaryngol*. 1972;96(4):297–304.
13. Friedmann I, Fraser GR, Froggatt P. Pathology of the ear in the cardioauditory syndrome of Jervell and Lange-Nielsen (recessive deafness with electrocardiographic abnormalities). *J Laryngol Otol*. 1966;80(5):451–470.
14. Gandolfi A, Horoupian D, Rapin I. Deafness in Cockayne's syndrome: morphological, morphometric, and quantitative study of the auditory pathway. *Ann Neurol*. 1984;15(2):135–143.
15. Refsum S. Heredopathia actica polyneuritis formis. *Acta Psych Scand*. 1946;38:301–303.
16. Konigsmark B. *Genetic and Metabolic Deafness*. Philadelphia, PA: WB Saunders Co; 1976.
17. Wester DC, Atkin CL, Gregory MC. Alport syndrome: clinical update. *J Am Acad Audiol*. 1995;6(1):73–79.
18. Gürtler N; Lalwani AK. Etiology of syndromic and nonsyndromic sensorineural hearing loss. *Otolaryngol Clinic North Am*. 2002;35(4):891–908.
19. Chang, EH, Van Camp G, Smith RJ. The role of connexins in human disease. *Ear Hear.* 2003;24(4):314–323.
20. Van Laer L, Cryns K, Smith Richard J, Van Camp G. Nonsyndromic hearing loss. *Ear Hear*. 2003;24(4):275–288.
21. Igarashi M, Takahashi M, Alford BR. Inner ear morphology in Down's syndrome. *Acta Otolaryngol*. 1977;83(1-2): 175–181.
22. Miglets AW, Schuller D, Ruppert E, Lim DJ. Trisomy 18. A temporal bone report. *Arch Otolaryngol*. 1975;101(7): 433–437.

CHAPTER 15

Cochlear Implants, Osseointegrated Bone Conduction Hearing Devices, and Other Implantable Devices

Seilesh Babu, Paulette McDonald, and Eric Sargent

INTRODUCTION

The cochlear implant is an electronic prosthesis that stimulates cells of the auditory spiral ganglion to provide a sense of sound to persons with hearing impairment. Although many thousands of patients have now been implanted, these represent only a fraction of the hearing-impaired individuals worldwide who would potentially benefit from implantation but do not have access to one because of failure to recognize appropriate individuals or socioeconomic reasons.

Although the individual response of a patient to a cochlear implant is highly variable and depends on a number of physical and psychosocial factors, the trend toward improved performance with increasingly sophisticated electrodes and programming strategies has caused the indications for cochlear implantation to be dramatically expanded (Table 15–1). Originally, cochlear implants were thought of primarily as an aid to some sound perception for the profoundly hearing impaired. Now, it is common to find implanted patients have better unaided hearing levels and perform at levels that exceed those obtained by conventionally aided patients. Through the 1970s, devices were implanted only in adults with profound hearing loss under the FDA guidelines of the time. In 1980, the age limit was lowered to 2, and later declined to 18 months. Currently the limit for implantation is 12 months of age. Over time, the adult indications have been broadened to include patients with severe hearing

Table 15–1. Current Pediatric and Adult Cochlear Implantation Guidelines

Pediatric	Adult (>18 years)
12–24 months: Bilateral profound sensorineural (SRT ≥ 90 dB) **≥24 months:** Severe to profound sensorineural hearing loss. Limited auditory skill development in conjunction with appropriate amplification and intervention. An educational program that supports listening and speaking for communication. No medical contraindications.	Severe-to-profound bilateral sensorineural hearing (SRT ≥ 70 dB) A score of 50% or less on sentence recognition tests under best-aided conditions (HINT testing in quiet wearing best fit hearing aids). No medical contraindications.

loss who obtain some benefit from conventional amplification.

Successful cochlear implantation requires a collaborative effort not only from the patient and family, but from a multispecialty team that includes school personnel (in the case of children), audiologist, speech/hearing therapists, and otolaryngologic surgeon. A motivated and properly counseled patient is the most important link in the chain. A deaf patient is not a surgical "problem" who responds to the simple intervention of an implant surgeon. A patient's preoperative expectations largely shape their postoperative satisfaction and use of the implant. All patients and families require proper attention and counseling by an implant team before embarking on a life-changing journey.

AUDITORY TESTS USED TO ESTABLISH CANDIDACY

For adults and children able to reliably respond, standard tests of pure-tone and speech audiometry are used to initially determine likely candidates for cochlear implantation. For children, the speech reception threshold should equal or exceed 90 dB; for adults, the speech reception threshold should equal or exceed 70 dB. If the patient can detect speech with best-fit hearing aids in place a speech recognition test in a sound field of 55 dB (HL) sound pressure level is then performed.

There are a number of speech recognition tests in current use. One of the most commonly used is the Hearing In Noise Test (HINT), a test of speech recognition in the context of sentences.[1] In cochlear implant evaluation, the test is performed in a sound field without noise while the patient is wearing appropriate bilateral amplification. Several versions exist for this testing and each center may find the most appropriate one to utilize to determine candidacy.

Many cochlear implant clinics now use the AzBio Sentences test.[2] Unlike the HINT test, which utilizes the male voice alone, the AzBio includes a variable number of prerecorded sentences presented by both male and female voices. Scores range from 1–100% based on the percent of words correctly identified.

CHILDREN

Severe to profound hearing loss sustained prior to the development of language, whether congenital or acquired, is estimated to occur in 0.5 to 4 in 1,000 births. The most common cause of childhood deafness is genetic (33–50%) with a large number of these cases being single gene mutations. Twenty five to thirty three percent of childhood deafness is due to "non-genetic" or environmental causes. The remaining 25 to 33% are sporadic for which the etiology is not determined. A large proportion of "sporadic" cases will likely prove to be genetic in origin as technology and testing improves.[3]

Meningitis causes about 9% of childhood deafness and can make implantation difficult (see *labyrinthitis ossificans*, below).[3] Of the organisms that commonly cause meningitis (from most common to least common: *H. influenzae*, *S. pneumoniae*, and *N. meningitis*), the organism with the highest incidence of hearing loss is *S. pneumoniae* (31%). Factors that will likely reduce the frequency of deafness caused by meningitis include the increased use of immunization against *H. influenzae* and *S. pneumoniae.*

It has long been known that 3 factors are important in determining the outcome of pediatric implant patients: (1) Age at onset of deafness and duration of deafness before implantation; (2) Progression of hearing loss; and (3) Educational setting. Generally, earlier implantation favors more rapid development of oral communication ability. Placement in a school setting that stresses oral (versus signed) communication is important for the best outcome of implantation. However, many variables remain unknown, as at least 50% of the variance in postimplant performance cannot be predicted from these factors.

A period of hearing aid use to determine the development of aided communication ability is a critical criterion for determining candidacy in young children.

After determining that audiologic criteria have been met, parental expectations and attitudes should be carefully assessed. Unrealistic expectations on the part of the family will frustrate the efforts of the child and the implant team. When counseling families, the need for long-term therapy, the variable outcome of implantation, and the limitations of implantation should be stressed.

Imaging with magnetic resonance imaging (MRI) using FSE T2-weighted images should be performed prior to implantation to evaluate the cochleovestibular apparatus and internal auditory canals. Imaging will reveal the absence or abnormal caliber of the internal auditory canal and/or cochlear dysplasia. This may alter the choice of the implanted ear or raise other issues.

In pediatric or young adult patients with progressive hearing loss, neurofibromatosis II should be excluded with an MRI scan before proceeding with implantation. Although computed tomography (CT) remains a tool for evaluating cochlear patency, occasionally this modality will erroneously suggest a patent scala tympani that proves to be obstructed with bone or fibrous tissue at the time of surgery. MRI offers the ability to better examine the fluid spaces of the cochlea and is increasingly being thought of as the best modality for imaging the cochlea. Both studies may need to be performed for complete evaluation of the cochlea and other auditory structures.

Although 12 months is currently the FDA age limit on implantation, there may be factors that cause the implant team to proceed at an even earlier age. In particular, a child deafened by meningitis may develop *labyrinthitis ossificans* (filling of all the cochlear duct—usually the scala tympani starting near the round window—with bone) that may necessitate special techniques to implant and render the result of implantation suboptimal. For patients at risk for labyrinthitis ossificans, implantation at the time initial ossification or fibrosis is identified may be indicated. Implant teams may follow patients newly deafened by meningitis with serial imaging and implant at the first sign of replacement of the scala tympani with fibrous tissue or bone. Otherwise, implantation in cases of post-meningitic deafness is usually recommended after a six-month period to allow for the possible recovery of aidable hearing in at least one ear.

Children with active middle ear disease should be implanted with caution only after they have been free of middle ear infections.

ADULTS

Hearing loss is the third most common self-reported health problem in adults over the age of 65.[4] Although the most common cause of hearing loss in adults is noise damage, other causes include Ménière's disease, otosclerosis, temporal bone trauma, autoimmune hearing loss, and ototoxic drug exposure.

As in children, adult candidacy can only be determined after performing tests for speech recognition under best-aided conditions. If patients present to the cochlear implant team with inadequate or malfunctioning aids, a trial of more appropriate hearing aids should be undertaken before determining implant candidacy. There is no upper age limit for implantation.

After meeting the audiologic criteria for implantation outlined above, an adult desiring implantation should have an accurate understanding of the possible outcomes. When counseling patients, the implant team must stress the broad range of auditory experience achieved by cochlear implant users. Although rare, some patients may perceive only improved awareness of environmental sounds and improved speech reading ability. Others will be "transparent" users, able to converse with hearing individuals with little evidence of hearing loss, use a telephone, and perform well in other difficult hearing environments. Although increasing numbers of implant users perform like the latter group, most fall into an area between the two extremes.

One of the strongest predictors of performance include duration of deafness and age at implantation. Yet, as with children, these factors account for only part of the variance in cochlear implant performance.[5] Generally, patients implanted soon after the onset of profound hearing loss perform better than those implanted later. Other factors that favor good performance in adult cochlear implant candidates include lip-reading ability and residual hearing before implantation.[6,7] Poor prognostic indicators include implantation of patients as adults with hearing loss that occurred prior to the development of speech and patients who rely primarily on signing for communication.

As in children, imaging of the cochleovestibular structures prior to implantation is mandatory in adults. The MRI may detect cochlear malformations or ossification of the cochlea that mandate a change in the choice of which ear is implanted or the technique used. CT imaging may also be indicated based on the history, physical, and type of hearing loss.

Adults deafened by meningitis are treated in a similar manner to children. Because of the fairly high rate of recovery of hearing in at least one ear following meningitis, an observation period of at least 6 months should be allowed to pass before implantation. As in children, identification of incipient obliteration of the cochlea by fibrous tissue or bone may cause implantation to be recommended early. Thus, serial imaging may be indicated for surveillance.

SURGICAL TECHNIQUE

Because cochlear implantation increases the risk of meningitis, especially in children less than 6 years of age, the CDC recommends age-appropriate vaccination with a polyvalent anti-streptococcal vaccine at least 2 weeks prior to implantation.[8]

Similar to the indications for cochlear implantation, aspects of the surgical approach to cochlear implantation have changed over time while the outlines of implantation remain the same. This surgery is done with continuous facial nerve monitoring. A preoperative broad-spectrum antibiotic is administered.

Before prepping, the position of the implant is marked on the periosteum through the skin with methylene blue using the metal implant dummy as a guide. The C-shaped incision is made 5 mm behind the postauricular crease and carried to the level of the temporalis fascia superiorly. If the scalp is thick, a small curvilinear, posteriorly oriented limb is made in the superior part of the incision to allow for relaxation of the tissues. Often it is found that a minimal postauricular incision is adequate for exposure, but requires some adjustment in technique in creating a pocket to place the implant. Inferiorly, the incision is deepened to the subcutaneous layer while leaving the periosteal layer intact. The scalp is elevated posteriorly for 2 to 3 cm, leaving periosteal tissue intact. An incision in the periosteum is made superiorly along the temporal line and posteriorly at the edge of the mastoid bone, roughly outlining the defect that will be created. The periosteum is then elevated forward, with its broad attachment to the concha left intact to create a flap that will be used to cover the electrode array. This also allows a stepwise, layered closure to reduce the risk of electrode exposure in the unlikely event of wound dehiscence.

Unlike a mastoidectomy in chronic ear surgery where the edges of the mastoid cavity are "saucerized," the mastoid defect in cochlear implantation may be kept small and relatively tight with sharp edges to help retain the electrode in the mastoid cavity. Other differences in surgical technique for cochlear implantation include not needing to identify the sigmoid sinus and allowing some pneumatized bone to remain. It is also extremely useful to thin the bone on the posterior aspect of the posterior external auditory canal to facilitate drilling the facial recess and insertion of the implant electrode into the middle ear. The other aspects of the technique are similar to a "traditional" mastoidectomy such as identification of the tegmen tympani, fossa incudis, and horizontal semicircular canal.

The middle ear is exposed through a conventional facial recess approach, leaving a buttress between the incus and the facial recess (Figure 15–1). However, adequate exposure of the round window may require sacrifice of the chorda tympani nerve. Removing the incus and incus buttress allows exposure of the round window without loss of the chorda tympani nerve. With the increasing incidence of bilateral implantation, sparing the chorda will likely become a more important quality of life issue. The facial recess is enlarged as much as possible, while leaving a bony covering on the facial nerve.

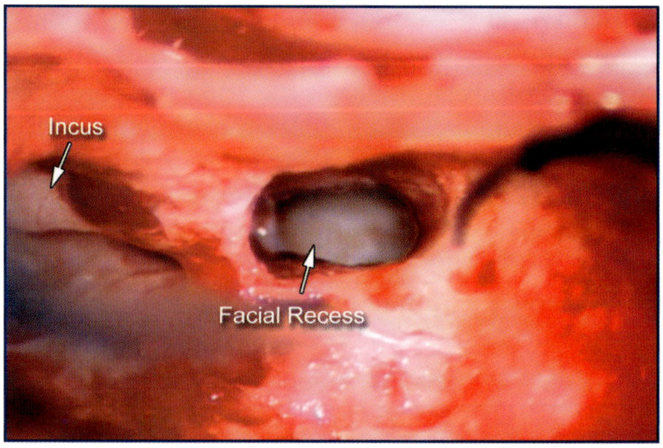

Figure 15–1. Right mastoidectomy with facial recess opened. Long process of incus points to the facial recess. Medial border is the facial nerve; lateral border is the chorda tympani nerve.

The cochleostomy is drilled anterior and inferior to the lip of the round window (Figure 15–2). The lip of the round window can be drilled away to facilitate localization. In patients with otosclerosis obliterating the round window or other anatomical variations that obscure its location, the round window can be found less than 2 mm from the inferior edge of the oval window. The cochleostomy should expose the *scala tympani* without breeching the basilar membrane. A cochleostomy roughly the size of a 1 mm diamond bur is performed to easily admit the electrode. The endosteum of the scala tympani is "blue-lined" and the membrane is opened with a pick. Alternative technique to cochleostomy may be an incision through the round window and direct placement through this opening. The angle and stiffness of the electrode may make this difficult to place in certain patients and with certain implant electrodes. Newer, smaller, and less rigid electrodes may make this easier in the future.

After drilling the cochleostomy, a pocket is made behind the mastoid to accept the implant and a well for the body of the implant is drilled, keeping the anterior edges of the well sharp to prevent forward migration of the implant. A crude but effective retractor for this purpose can be made by inserting the metal implant dummy in the pocket and using the Wietlaner retractor against the metal dummy to elevate the scalp. This, along with rotating the patient toward the surgeon, usually allows sufficient exposure of the site for the well without extending the incision. A trough is drilled extending from the cochlear implant well to the mastoid to allow the electrode to travel this path.

Although many surgeons use tie-down sutures anchored to periosteum of the surrounding skull or forego tie-down sutures entirely, the author uses 1-0 silk sutures through tie-down holes drilled in the bone. A simple way to do this is to use a cutting bur to drill troughs above and below the well and using the 1-mm diamond bur used for the cochleostomy to connect the troughs to the well; 2 holes above and 1 hole below are typically made to anchor the silk suture in three places. If a minimal incision and subperiosteal pocket is utilized instead, usually a single silk suture can be used to secure the implant in the subperiosteal pocket by tightening the tissue around the implant. Care is taken to place the knot of the suture on the side of the device so that there is no chance for erosion of the electrode.

After ensuring hemostasis in the operative field, the wound is irrigated with Bacitracin irrigation and meticulously cleaned of bone debris. The cochlear implant is opened onto the operative field. Monopolar cautery is disconnected to reduce the risk of shunting current through the cochlea if it is inadvertently used later. The electrode is inserted into the cochlea under direct vision (Figure 15–3). Several

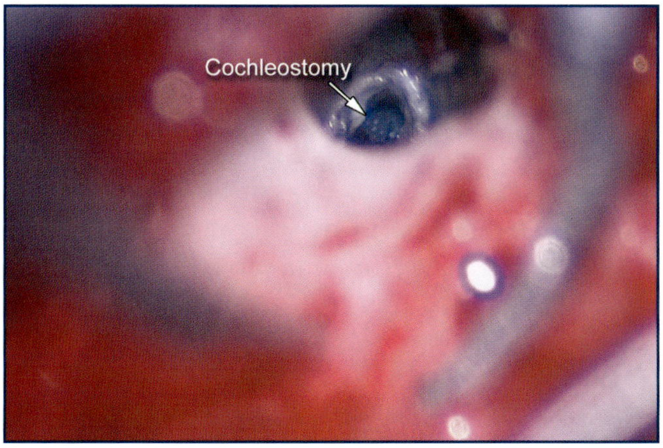

Figure 15–2. Left facial recess opened. Cochleostomy opened anterior and inferior to round window.

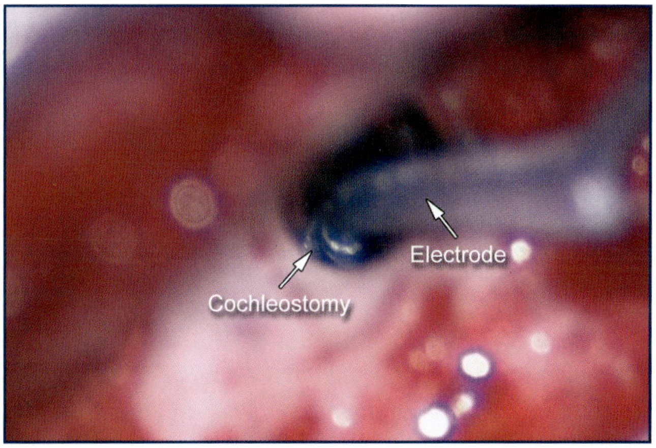

Figure 15–3. Left cochleostomy with cochlear implant electrode in place.

techniques are used in insertion of the implant: using insertion tool or advanced off-stylet technique. After electrode insertion, the cochleostomy is packed with fascia and the ground electrode is placed in a pocket medial to the temporalis muscle.

The periosteal flap is then sutured to cover the electrodes that have been tucked into the mastoid cavity. The subcutaneous layer is similarly sutured and the skin is sutured with fast-absorbing 5-0 catgut suture. A compression dressing is placed.

POSTOPERATIVE CARE

Most patients under the age of 65 are discharged after recovering from anesthesia. Patients who are elderly or have multiple comorbidities are typically observed overnight. The dressing is removed the following day. Showering, washing the incision, and shampooing the hair are allowed on postoperative day 3.

The first postoperative visit is scheduled for one week. Cochlear implant programming is started 3 to 4 weeks after surgery.

BILATERAL IMPLANTATION

The benefits of binaural hearing are well known. Lacking the head shadow effect, monaural patients lose much of the ability to determine the direction of a sound source. Monaural patients also lose the ability to suppress the interference of background noise afforded by binaural hearing. For these reasons bilateral cochlear implantation has been an area of considerable research effort that is gaining popularity in clinical practice. Much of the barrier to the wider acceptance of bilateral implants is financial: third-party payers vary widely in their policies for coverage. The typical payer will only cover a 2nd implant if the patient demonstrates minimal benefit from the first implant. One group in which this may be critical is patients with auditory dyssynchrony, who are often noted to perform much better with binaural implants than with one (Charles Berlin, personal communication, 2006).

COMPLICATIONS

Cochlear implants are not contraindicated in cases of cochlear dysplasia, such as common cavity or enlarged vestibular aqueduct malformations. However, the surgeon should be prepared for a cerebrospinal fluid (CSF) leak due to an incomplete partition between the cochlea and internal auditory canal. The family should be informed of the potential risk of CSF leak and meningitis and the variable performance of patients with dysplastic cochleas who undergo implantation.

Infections, although rare, are typically treated with incision and drainage if there is fluctuance followed by prolonged culture-based intravenous or oral antibiotics. In a 2007 retrospective review of 268 pediatric cochlear implants, Hopfenspirger et al found an infection rate of 8.2%.[9] Because the cochlear implant can harbor biofilms that allow persistence of bacteria even after clinical resolution of infection, a small number of implant patients will require explantation of the device. Surgeons have described cutting the electrode at the cochleostomy while removing the rest of the implant and leaving the intracochlear electrode to maintain cochlear patency.

SPEECH CODING STRATEGIES

Intensity

Coding the intensity of a sound transmitted by a cochlear implant to the VIIIth nerve is very different from the coding of sound intensity by the inner hair cells (IHCs) of a healthy cochlea. In bypassing the hair cells, electrical stimulation causes the loss of important intensity cues. The outer hair cells lose their ability to actively modulate the dynamics of the basilar membrane in response to different sound intensities. Inner hair cells lose their ability to fire heterogeneously (which depends mainly on the type of synapse between IHC and nerve) due to the synaptic transmission of the electrical impulse to the VIIIth nerve by the implant being bypassed. In addition, hair cell refractory effects are eliminated.

The net effect is a perception of sound intensity that rises from inaudible to uncomfortable within a very narrow range of electrical stimulation in the implanted patient, typically between 3 to 20 dB. Thus, compression of the cochlear implant signal is always required.[10]

Spectral Processing

The complex nature of speech sounds requires processing the cochlear implant signal to represent the spectrum of frequencies that make up a sound (a vowel, for example) at different points along the basilar membrane and this is termed *spectral processing*.

The cochlear implant speech processor utilizes various coding strategies using known signal processing theories. These strategies improve speech perception by mimicking the way the cochlear nerve fibers respond to the frequency and amplitude of the speech signal. The internal electrode of the cochlear implant transmits sound in the form of electric impulses to the cochlear neurons.

First, the processor analyzes incoming sound to determine its component frequencies (*formants*). The component frequencies of the sound are mapped to specific electrodes at different positions in the cochlea (*place coding*). The electrodes along the array approximate the characteristic frequencies of the hair cells that would be stimulated in a healthy cochlea. The healthy cochlea has the functional equivalent of approximately 28 "bands" or "filters" in the range of frequencies important for human speech. This presents a limiting effect of the relatively small number of "bands" on a cochlear implant electrode (typically less than 8). Another problem that can occur is a misassignment of frequencies to electrodes in relation to their area of the cochlea to which they correspond. For example, an electrode triggered by the computer to fire an impulse in response to a 2000 Hz sound may actually be driving the part of the cochlea that corresponds to 3000 Hz.

Second, pitch can be represented in the repetition rate of pulses by the electrode (*temporal coding*). This can be useful in low frequencies that could not otherwise be stimulated by the implant directly (as they are coded in the apical cochlea where the electrode typically will not reach). Cochlear implant users can use repetition rates less than about 300 Hz to perceive low-frequency pitch. Above 300 Hz, increasing repetition rates do not cause a perceived change in pitch in cochlear implant patients.

In the healthy cochlea a complex pattern of responses is evoked from speech sounds in which some neurons respond more vigorously than others. This response contributes to the quality, or timbre, of complex sounds. In other words, the more sound energy that falls close to the characteristic frequency (CF) of the neuron, the higher the firing rate of the neuron (*phase locking*). The distribution of the spectral shape is represented by the relative firing rate the neurons as a function of the CF which is also called the "place" code for spectral shape. Multiple areas of the cochlea will be stimulated during a complex sound due to the fundamental frequency of the sound and its associated higher frequency harmonics. In the healthy auditory system, the missing low frequency fundamental of a complex sound can be interpolated (*resolved*) by central processing by analysis of the unresolved harmonics. Current cochlear implant processing strategies do not make use of this function.

The CF is only true for low level complex sounds but is not so in the case of sounds with moderate to high intensities. This is due to the restricted dynamic range of certain cochlear nerve fibers. As the discharge rate changes this determines the dynamic range at any given frequency of a cochlear nerve fiber and tells us changes in intensity. When the incoming signal is over 40 dB sound pressure level (SPL) the discharge rate saturates and no longer cause changes in stimulus intensity.

Keeping this theory in mind, speech-processing strategies were designed. In current cochlear implant systems, as the signal enters the microphone it is preamplified with emphasis placed on the high frequency portion of the signal. Adaptive Gain Control (AGC) compresses the dynamic range of speech in to a narrow range, which is usable to the implant patient. AGC also reduces the distortion of loud sounds.

The signal is then digitized and sent through processing filter bands that divide sound in to a corresponding pitch range. Each filter is assigned to one of the electrodes along the array and represents one channel. The output of each filter is determined by the electrical signal that is delivered to a single electrode. In some schemes the analog waveform at the filter output is used to drive the electrode; in other schemes the waveform at the output of the filter is used to trigger current pulses into groups of pulses which are then delivered to the electrode. The number of cycles determines the rate of stimulation. When the signal occurs *N* numbers of electrodes are stimulated and one cycle of stimulation is completed. The number of cycles/second creates the rate of stimulation. It has been shown that temporal processing can be increased with high rates of stimulation. Depending on the cochlear implant manufacturer adjacent electrodes maybe simultaneously stimulated or sequentially stimulated.

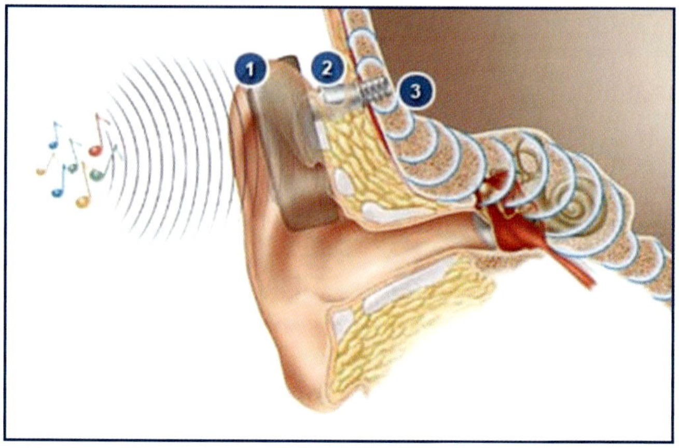

Figure 15–4. Right BAHA in place showing the 3 components: (1) Sound Processor; (2) Abutment; (3) Titanium implant. Sound is able to be conducted along the skull to the cochlea to bypass the external and middle ear structures.

OSSEOINTEGRATED BONE CONDUCTION HEARING DEVICES

Osseointegrated bone conduction hearing devices utilize bone conduction to bypass any abnormality of the external or middle ear to directly stimulate the cochlea. The generic term BAHA is still utilized to describe these implants and is used in this chapter, but future nomenclature may change. The BAHA (Cochlear Corp.) was first described in Europe in 1977 and became FDA approved for conductive hearing loss in 1996 and for single-sided deafness (SSD) in 2002.[11] A competitor, the Ponto (Oticon Medical), was approved by the US FDA in 2009.

Typical hearing aids rely on air conduction and a functioning middle ear. In cases where the middle ear function may be blocked, damaged, or occluded, the BAHA system may be a better option as it bypasses the middle ear altogether. Instead, sound is sent around the damaged or problematic area, naturally stimulating the cochlea through bone conduction. Once the cochlea receives these sound vibrations, the organ "hears" in the same manner as through air conduction; the sound is converted into neural signals and is transferred to the brain, allowing a BAHA recipient to perceive sound.

The BAHA consists of three parts: (1) the titanium screw that is implanted into the skull (which is similar to dental implants); (2) an external abutment that fits into the screw; and (3) the sound processor that attaches onto the abutment (Figure 15–4). The titanium implant is placed during a minor surgical procedure and over time integrates with the bone behind the ear (Figure 15–5).

Osseointegration

An essential process must occur that bonds the titanium fixture to bone termed osseointegration.[12] This allows a more efficient transfer of sound. This process may take several weeks to become solid. The hearing aid device may then be used, usually waiting 4 to 6 weeks after implantation.

BAHA Candidates/Indications

Conductive or Mixed Hearing Loss

Patients with conductive and mixed hearing loss are candidates for the BAHA. Specifically, patients who have undergone surgical resection of cholesteatoma who have not had an improvement in their conductive hearing loss will benefit from the BAHA. They may have a mastoid cavity that becomes moist and drains therefore making it difficult for them to wear a traditional hearing aid. They would find numerous advantages to the BAHA. It is also beneficial for patients who suffer from pathology of the outer and

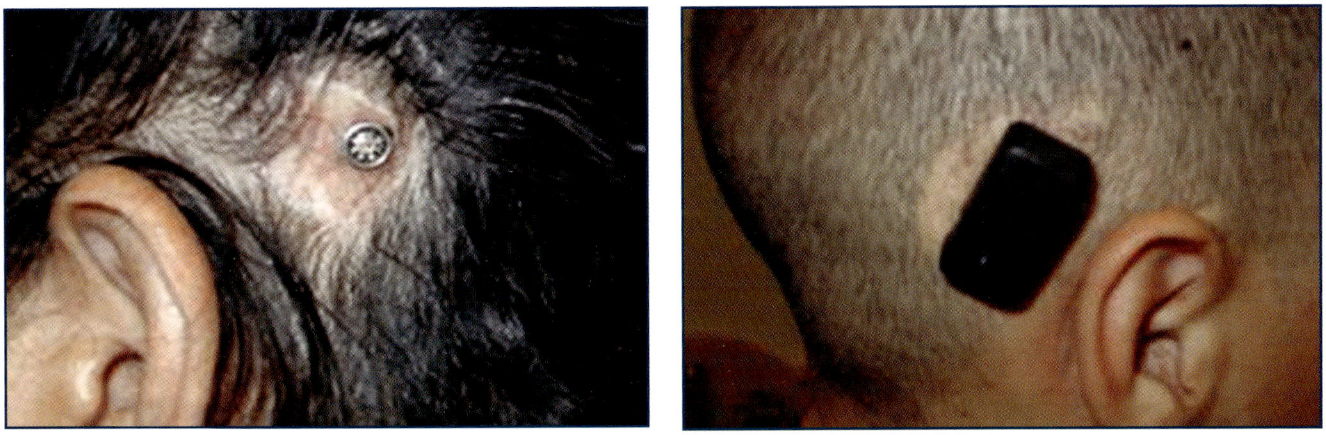

A B

Figure 15–5. A. Left BAHA implant and abutment in place after 8 weeks. **B.** Right BAHA implant with sound processor in place.

middle ear preventing sound conduction. Patients with congenital aural atresia, ossicular discontinuity, and otosclerosis are candidates for this option.

Single-Sided Deafness

Single-sided Deafness (SSD) is also an indication for a BAHA. This affects approximately 55,000 people per year and is due to various etiologies including viral causes, Ménière's disease, acoustic neuromas, or trauma. Hearing solutions are necessary to allow hearing in background noise, as well as safety issues when driving or bicycling. These solutions rely on the ability to route the sound signal to the contralateral ear. This is traditionally accomplished with a contralateral routing of signal (CROS) hearing aid. Recently, the BAHA has become an alternative for these patients. It is placed on the deaf side and, through bone conduction, transfers the signal to the contralateral cochlea.[13] The BAHA system provides the opportunity to hear and understand sounds with binaural ability where previously the head shadow prevented this. Recent studies have shown that patients prefer the sound and speech clarity achieved with the BAHA when compared to the CROS and the unaided condition.[14]

Sound Processors

There are 2 manufacturers for the bone anchored implants: Cochlear Corporation produces the BAHA and Oticon Medical produces the Ponto. Each company has several sound processors available for the amount of amplification required as well as directional microphones. Patients should be educated on the various bone conduction options to make as informed of a decision of implant choice as possible. Test trial of the various products should be available for the patient to appreciate the differences.

Audiologic Criteria

Conductive or Mixed Hearing Loss

Patients with conductive hearing loss need good sensorineural hearing for successful BAHA outcome. On an audiogram, this is measured by bone-conduction thresholds which are better than 45 dB hearing level in the affected ear for ear level devices and 65 dB hearing level for the body-level device.

Unilateral Sensorineural Hearing Loss

Criteria for candidacy for BAHA in unilateral hearing loss are: (1) Profound hearing loss as measured by air-conduction pure-tone threshold worse than 90 dB hearing level; (2) Poor discrimination score less than 15%; and (3) Normal hearing on the contralateral side measured as pure-tone thresholds better than 20 dB hearing level.[14] Occasionally, some patients do not meet these criteria perfectly, but will still do very well with a BAHA implant.

Other criteria are age older than 5 years old, ability to maintain wound site, and manual dexterity to attach and remove hearing device to abutment. Patients less than 5 years old may benefit from a soft-band BAHA that is held in place by a headband instead of surgical implantation.

Baguley et al performed a meta-analysis of published studies on unilateral hearing loss and concluded that there is a benefit of contralateral hearing amplification (either with a BAHA or CROS aid) over the unaided condition. Speech discrimination in noise and subjective questionnaire measures of auditory abilities showed an advantage for BAHA over CROS and over unaided conditions. However, these studies did not find significant improvements in auditory localization with either aid. Interestingly, these studies only had 1-month trial of the CROS and then followed by the BAHA, potentially allowing bias to be introduced in the patients who liked the BAHA over the CROS aids.[15]

BAHA Evaluation Process

The evaluation process requires collaboration of the otolaryngologist and the audiologist. The degree and type of hearing loss and possibility of candidacy for the BAHA implant is determined. The BAHA simulation is then performed which involves testing aided patients with a test BAHA device that is fit behind the affected ear by a band. This allows the patient to experience the quality of sound that the BAHA offers. Most patients seem to note an improvement in their hearing that was better than the actual simulation. Once determined safe to use the external processor, the patient meets with the audiologist to be fitted with BAHA and to be counseled about its use and care, snapping the BAHA on and off, use of the directional microphone, and the use of the BAHA with other devices, such as the telephone, mp3 players, and FM systems. Evaluation of various manufacturers implants and processors can be done so that the patient can make as informed decision.

Surgical Technique

The procedure to place the BAHA device is a short outpatient procedure that can be done under local anesthesia with intravenous sedation. Occasionally, general anesthesia is performed. Sometimes, the procedure is performed in conjunction with a surgery that will cause unilateral hearing loss or the required conductive loss (ie, acoustic nerve resection).

The postauricular site is prepared with hair shaving, draping, and surgical prepping. Antibiotic coverage for skin flora is recommended prior to skin incision. The BAHA implant should be placed 5 to 6 cm posterior and superior to the tragus at a 45-degree angle. This will allow placement of the hearing device without contacting the auricle.

Traditional technique involves the use of a dermatome to create a split-thickness skin graft. Some surgeons have switched to a single skin incision that may be vertical or curvilinear. With either technique, the key to success in the procedure is wide undermining and removal of the subcutaneous tissue. Hair follicles may be removed to decrease risk of infection; however, this will leave a wound that is devoid of hair. An approximately 2-cm radius of tissue needs to be excised to the level of the periosteum.

A cruciate incision is made in the periosteum. 3- and 4-cm pilot drill guides are used to measure the appropriate implant length. Once the appropriate length is determined, a countersink opening is made, and the BAHA is implanted.

Meticulous wound closure is critical. The edges of the skin may be tacked to the periosteum to allow better healing around the abutment. The skin graft is placed back into position and the skin closed with absorbable sutures. A dermal punch is used to create an opening in skin graft. If a single incision is made, the skin edges are closed with suture and either the abutment is placed in the middle of the incision or may be allowed to exit through a separate dermal punched hole. The skin is closed with either nylon sutures or absorbable skin sutures. A bolster dressing, healing cap, and pressure dressing are applied. Patients are discharged with instructions to leave bolster dressing and healing cap in place until 5 to 7 day follow-up visit.

One of the authors (SB) has been doing 6mm punch biopsy incision through the skin with placement of the implant and abutment through this small opening. The procedure is relatively fast and the healing is remarkable as no sutures are needed to close the incision.

Postoperatively, the patient is instructed to keep the area around the abutment clean and dry. Gentle debridement may be performed with hydrogen peroxide, antibiotic ointment, and occasionally steroid cream to keep the area healthy and decreased risk of granulation tissue.

In pediatric patients or certain others, a "sleeper" or second receptacle is inserted for use should the initial receptor fail or be damaged. This is to serve as a reserve in case something happens to the primary implant. Recently, most BAHA implants are done in a single-stage procedure. A double stage procedure is carried out for children or for certain medical reasons. The first stage involves creating a skin graft and placing the implant (and possible sleeper implant). Then, time is allowed for the skull to thicken and osseointegration to occur. After osseointegration (may take 3–6 months), the second stage is performed by elevating the skin graft and attaching the abutment.

BILATERAL BAHA IMPLANTS

Patients with bilateral conductive hearing loss will benefit from one BAHA implant. Some studies have shown an even better response with bilateral implantation.[13] A 1997 prospective study with children with bilateral conductive hearing loss showed a benefit from bilateral BAHA implantation in terms of improved sound localization and better speech recognition in noise.[16]

OTHER IMPLANTABLE OPTIONS

Other products are being introduced to the market to provide bone conduction hearing amplification in a more cosmetic fashion. A fully implanted device under the skin allowing transcutaneous transmission of sound through magnetic coupling is emerging and should be available in near future. Sound quality and skin breakdown issues will need to be addressed.

Another product is the SoundBite Hearing system as a nonsurgical option for bone conduction via the patient's teeth. It consists of a custom-fit hearing device placed on the upper teeth and a behind-the-ear (BTE) microphone unit.

TOTALLY, PARTIALLY, AND SEMI-IMPLANTED HEARING DEVICES

In addition to cochlear implants and osseointegrated devices, there are 3 implantable hearing devices currently approved by the FDA. Semi- and fully implantable hearing aids have been developed to overcome specific problems that arise with conventional hearing aids, mainly feedback at high gains in the high frequencies, the occlusion effect, and distortion. Feedback is defeated in all 3 because they mechanically stimulate the ossicular chain. Elimination of feedback allows higher gains at high frequencies than are allowed in conventional hearing aids. All of these devices claim increased clarity of sound and elimination of distortion compared to conventional hearing aids and are generally supported by subjective surveys of patients that show increased satisfaction compared to the patients' preoperative conventional hearing aids. None of the devices are currently approved for use in the treatment of conductive hearing loss and none are MRI safe.

Vibrant SoundBridge (MED-EL Corp)

Approved by the US FDA in 2000 for patients older than 18 with moderate to severe hearing loss, the Vibrant SoundBridge (MED-EL Corp) uses an electromechanical floating mass transducer clipped and cemented to the incus through a mastoid/facial recess approach to mechanically drive the ossicular chain. When not in use, the mass of the device introduces a negligible 3 dB conductive hearing loss. It is considered a semi-implantable device, as it requires an externallyplaced processor held to the scalp by a magnet. The current Amade processor offers 16 programmable bands and 8 channels of compression.

In conventional placements in healthy ears with normal anatomy, the gain provided by the implant averages 28 dB. While SRTs remain unchanged in patients with the implant compared with a best fit conventional hearing aid, the device is said to provide better high frequency hearing than conventional hearing aids because of the elimination of feedback.[17,18]

There are now many reports of placement of the Vibrant floating mass transducer in the round windows of patients with chronic ear disease whose anatomy precludes clipping to an ossicle (as in the case of absent ossicles) or in the oval window. With this placement, mean gains of 37 dB (4-frequency PTA) have been reported.[19]

Esteem (Envoy Medical Corp)

In 2010, the Esteem (Envoy Medical Corp) was approved by the FDA for patients older than 18 with mild to severe sensorineural hearing loss and speech discrimination >40%. It is the first totally implantable hearing device in the US. Implantation requires cementing separate piezoelectric transducers to the body of the incus and capitulum of the stapes through a mastoid/facial recess approach. Input to the system is provided by the transducer on the incus, which acts as a microphone. Signal from the transducer on the incus is sent to a sealed processor, with an integrated battery, implanted in the mastoid. The 2-channel processor filters, compresses, and amplifies the signal. The signal is then sent to the active transducer on the stapes to electromechanically drive the stapes. Because a connection between the input (incus) and output (stapes) would introduce feedback, the incus and stapes are surgically disarticulated. The implanted battery has an expected life of 4.5 years when "on" continually, 6.5 years when used 16 hours per day, and 9 years when used 8 hours per day. When not in use, however, patients with the device have maximal conductive loss due to ossicular discontinuity.

Phase 1 trials of the device reported a high rate of surgical revision required to achieve benefit. Four of seven patients in the initial group required revision before benefiting. Two achieved no benefit from the device.[20] A Phase 2 trial in 57 patients demonstrated improvement in SRTs from 41 dB with conventional hearing BTEs to 29 dB after implantation. The revision rate (3/57) was much lower.[21] The company cites a 5% revision rate and 2% explantation rate and in regulatory filings notes an approximately 11 dB improvement in SRT compare to preoperative testing under best-aided condition. While the initial success rate of the surgery has improved considerably with refinement of technique and intense training of surgeons by the company, higher revision rates—usually for minor issues—have been anecdotally reported. The multistep procedure remains technically demanding and time consuming. The device and surgery remain very expensive and it is financially out of reach of many individuals who would be candidates.

The auditory benefits of the Esteem have been well established. For example, in a report of 5 patients with profound high-frequency hearing loss, the Esteem provided an average functional gain of 20 dB compared to the conventional high-gain BTE hearing aids worn by the patients before implantation. Word recognition improved from 69% with BTE hearing aids to 88% after implantation.[22]

Maxum (Ototronix Corp)

The Maxum (Ototronix Corp), the 2nd generation of the SOUNDTEC implant, is a middle ear prosthesis/external processor that utilizes a titanium-sealed magnet cemented to the incudostapedial joint. The processor has 12 programmable channels and 10 channels of compression. It is approved for patients older than 18 with moderate to severe hearing loss and word recognition of >40%. After a healing period, a deep earmold coil/processor assembly is fitted to the patient and activated. In Phase 2 trials, the device provided an average of 8 dB (low frequencies) to 10 dB (high frequencies) of functional gain and a 5% increase in speech discrimination compared to patients' conventional hearing aids. The device relies on the external coil assembly held approximately 2 mm from lateral to the tympanic membrane. The mass of the magnet adds a small 4 dB conductive hearing loss.[23]

Unlike the Vibrant SoundBridge and the Envoy Esteem, the implantation of the Maxum is minimally invasive and can be performed under local anesthesia with or without sedation. The approach requires elevating the eardrum in a manner typical of most middle ear surgery and exposure of the incudostapedial joint. The magnet is glued to the incudostapedial joint and the tympanomeatal flap is replaced. Positioning the external coil assembly in proper orientation and close proximity to the implanted magnet is critical to its performance.

CONCLUSIONS

Cochlear implantation is one of the greatest sources of professional satisfaction in otology due to the dramatic impact on a patient's quality of life. Identifying candidates for implantation in adults is straightforward. In children, especially neonates, prompt identification of deafness allows earlier implantation and better success. The surgical technique is relatively easily learned and, when properly applied following the principles of gentle tissue handling, yields excellent results with few complications.

Bone anchored hearing aids (BAHA) also provide a significant benefit to patients suffering from conductive hearing loss and single sided deafness. It is a relatively easy procedure, but requires meticulous wound care to be effective.

In the future, other implantable hearing devices may prove to be beneficial as well.

REFERENCES

1. Nilsson M, McCaw V, Soli S. *Minimum Speech Test Battery for Adult Cochlear Implant Patients: User Manual*. Los Angeles, CA: House Ear Institute; 1996.
2. Spahr AJ, Dorman MF, Litvak LM, et al. Development and validation of the azbio sentence lists. *Ear Hear*. 2012; 33(1):112–117.
3. Grundfast KM, Lalwani AK, eds. *Pediatric Otology and Neurotology*. Philadelphia, PA: Lippincott-Raven Publishers; 1998.
4. Havlik R. *Aging in the eighties: impaired senses for sound and light in persons age 65 and over.* Preliminary data from the supplement on aging to the National Health Interview Survey: United States, January–June 1984. Advance data from vital and health statistics. DHHS (PHS) publication no. 125. Hyattsville, MD: National Center for Health Statistics; 1986:86–1250.
5. Gantz BJ, Tyler RS, Knutson JF, et al. Evaluation of five different cochlear implant designs: audiologic assessment and predictors of performance. *Laryngoscope*. 1988; 98:1100–1106.
6. Cohen NL, Waltzman SB, Fisher SG, et al. A prospective, randomized study of cochlear implants. *N Engl J Med.* 1993;328:233–237.
7. Gantz BJ, Woodworth GG, Abbas PJ, Knutson JF, Tyler RS. Multivariate predictors of audiological success with multichannel cochlear implants. *Ann Otol Rhinol Laryngol*. 1993;102:909–916.
8. CDC. Pneumococcal vaccine for cochlear implant recipients. *MMWR*. 51:931.
9. Hopfenspirger, MT, Levine, SC, and Rimell FL.Infectious complications in pediatric cochlear implants. *Laryngoscope*. 2007 Oct;117(10):1825–1829.
10. Moore BCJ. Coding of sounds in the auditory system and its relevance to signal processing and coding in cochlear implants. *Otol Neurotol*. 2003;24:243–245.
11. Tjellstrom A, Hakansson B, Lindstrom J, Branemark PI, Hallen O, Rosenhall U, Leijon A. Analysis of the mechanical impedance of bone-anchored hearing aids. *Acta Oto-Laryngol*. 1980;89(1–2):85–92.
12. Spitzer JB, Ghossaini SN, Wazen JJ. Evolving applications in the use of bone-anchored hearing aids. *Am J Audiol.* 2002;11(2):96–103.
13. Wazen JJ, Spitzer JB, Ghossaini SN, et al. Transcranial contralateral cochlear stimulation in unilateral deafness. *Otolaryngol Head Neck Surg*. 2003;129(3):248–254.
14. Wazen JJ, Spitzer J, Ghossaini SN, Kacker A, Zschommler A. Results of the bone-anchored hearing aid in unilateral hearing loss. *Laryngoscope*. 2001;111(6):955–958.
15. Baguley DM, Bird J, Humphriss RL, Prevost AT. The evidence base for the application of contralateral bone anchored hearing aids in acquired unilateral sensorineural hearing loss in adults. *Clin Otolaryngol*. 2006;31(1):6–14.
16. Priwin C, Granstrom G. The bone-anchored hearing aid in children: a surgical and questionnaire follow-up study. *Otolaryngol Head Neck Surg*. 2005;132(4):559–565.
17. Sziklai I, Szilvássy J. Functional gain and speech understanding obtained by Vibrant Soundbridge or by open-fit hearing aid. *Acta Otolaryngol*. 2011 Apr;131(4):428–433
18. Luetje CM, Brown SA, Cullen RD. Vibrant Soundbridge implantable hearing device: critical review and single-surgeon short- and long-term results. *Ear Nose Throat J*. 2010 Sep;89(9):E9–E14.
19. Beltrame AM, Martini A, Prosser S, et al. Coupling the Vibrant SoundBridge to cochlea round window: auditory results in patients with mixed hearing loss. *Otol Neurotol*. 2009; 30(2):194–201.
20. Chen DA, Backous DD, Arriaga MA, et al. Phase 1 clinical trial of the Envoy system: a totally implantable middle ear device for sensorineural hearing loss. *Otolarngol Head Neck Surg*. 2004;131(6): 904–916.

21. Kraus EM, Shohet JA, Catalano PJ. Envoy Esteem totally implantable hearing system: phase 2 trial, 1-year hearing results. *Otolaryngol Head Neck Surg*. 2011;145(1):100–109.
22. Shohet JA, Kraus EM, Catalano PJ. Profound high-frequency sensorineural hearing loss treatment with a totally implantable hearing system. *Otol Neurotol*. 2011; 32(9):1428–1431.
23. Hough JVD, Matthew P, Wood MW, et al. Middle ear electromagnetic semi-implantable hearing device: results of the Phase II SOUNDTEC direct system clinical trial. *Otol Neurotol*. 2002;23(6):895–903.

CHAPTER 16

Tinnitus

Michael Hoa and John Zappia

INTRODUCTION

Tinnitus is relatively common with up to 25% of the population experiencing it for some extended period.[1] In addition, tinnitus-like sounds can be observed in a large portion (64%) of healthy, young individuals when placed in a quiet environment for twenty minutes, possibly illustrating that this noise may be a continuum in which its level is below perception in the majority of the population.[2]

Tinnitus is defined as the perception of sound with no identifiable source outside the individual. Tinnitus is a symptom and not a true medical diagnosis. The experience, for both those who have it and those that attempt to treat it, can be frustrating.

Only a minority of patients has a cause that is identifiable, medically significant, or truly curable. The evaluation is focused toward determining if any of these are in fact the case. For the remainder and majority, careful reassurance is usually all that is necessary. For the minority that has incurable and disruptive tinnitus, although there is no true symptomatic cure, there are a variety of treatment options.

EVALUATION

The goals in the evaluation of the patient with tinnitus are to identify medically significant problems, identify treatable problems, and determine the severity in the patients without truly treatable causes. Fortunately, medically significant causes of tinnitus are rare. For most, after a simple evaluation, either reassurance in the majority or palliative treatment in the minority is undertaken. The assessment of the tinnitus patient typically consists of a history, physical examination, and basic audiogram although in certain situations further evaluation is necessary.

History

The quality of the tinnitus may give insight into its cause. Bilateral symptoms are much less likely to represent significant pathology and as a result, much less likely to warrant an extensive workup. Pulsatile features guide one toward vascular causation. Clicking or tapping components signify myoclonus of either middle ear or palate. In patients with hearing loss, tinnitus frequently tends to correspond to the loss: with roaring nature suggesting low-frequency problems, hissing with broad loss, and ringing or whistling associated with high-frequency loss. Complex sounds such as music or voice can be associated with psychiatric disorders or temporal lobe tumors.

Tinnitus that has been present for a long period of time is less likely to represent serious issues. A careful review of events at the time of onset is important. Medical issues, medications, trauma, or any other systemic or personal issues can be valuable. The pattern or timing will be insightful. Diurnal patterns or association with particular events such as sodium intake or noise exposure are important.

Associated symptoms are important information to recognize. Aural complaints such as hearing loss and fullness are useful. Hyperacusis is uncommon and can be associated with endolymphatic hydrops. Hyperacusis, with or without tinnitus, can be associated with psychiatric problems and can be difficult to treat or control. Facial weakness, double vision, or evidence of any adjacent cranial nerve weakness will require further evaluation for mass lesions or neurologic problems. Headaches or any evidence of sensory or motor deficits will have the same implications. Anxiety, depressive symptoms, or sleep disruption are associated with more significant tinnitus and can be difficult to sort out causation/association factors.

The patients' medical history is important. Some diseases, such as diabetes, anemia, thyroid problems, and hypertension can be associated with tinnitus. Known anxiety, depressive, or psychotic disorders are known aggravating factors and occasionally true causes of tinnitus.

Additional past historical information that can be important includes exposure to noise or ototoxic agents. Trauma, either at the time of onset of symptoms or prior, can help identify problems. Another important part of the history is previous otologic diseases or surgery.

Current and past medication usage is important. As mentioned above, salicylates, quinine, and aminoglycosides are the most notable ones that can contribute to tinnitus (Table 16–1).

Table 16–1. Drugs Associated with Tinnitus

Drug Class	Specific Medications
Analgesics	Aspirin, NSAIDs
Antibiotics	Aminoglycosides, chloramphenicol, erythromycin, tetracycline, vancomycin, vibramycin
Chemotherapy & Antiviral drugs	Bleomycin, interferon, pegylated interferon-alpha-2b, cisplatin, mechlorethamine, methotrexate, vincristine
Heavy metals	Mercury, arsenic, lead
Loop diuretics	Furosemide
Other	Chloroquine, quinine, quinidine

Physical Examination

An otologic examination includes inspection of the external auditory canal, tympanic membrane, and assessment of the middle ear. Occasionally, movement of the tympanic membrane will be seen. Twitching movement will be consistent with middle ear myoclonus. Movement of the tympanic membrane with respiration suggests patulous eustachian tube. Tuning fork testing including Weber and Rinne will help identify hearing loss and enhance the audiogram findings. Cranial nerves should be tested particularly those adjacent to VIII. A general head and neck exam is necessary. Variation of the symptoms, particularly with pulsatile tinnitus, with head movement or gentle neck compression can be useful. Cessation of tinnitus with either of these maneuvers may be indicative of a venous origin for the patient's tinnitus and may help to direct further evaluation. Observation of palatal twitching will suggest palatal myoclonus. This will usually need to be done with a nasopharygoscope through the nose as opening the mouth to observe will frequently suppress the movement. Auscultation of the head, neck, and external auditory canal with an appropriate insert will detect any objective tinnitus and is particularly important in pulsatile tinnitus

The ophthalmologic exam is occasionally important to check for papilledema in benign intracranial hypertension. As many otolaryngologists would not be comfortable with this, ophthalmologic consultation is likely necessary.

Audiologic Testing

As knowledge of a patient's hearing is critical when suffering from tinnitus, all receive a basic audiogram consisting of pure tone audiometry, speech recognition testing, and word recognition score. For the majority of tinnitus patients, the basic audiogram, in addition to the history and physical examination, supply enough information to complete the evaluation.

Tympanometry may supply additional information about the tympanic membrane and middle ear. The stapedial reflex assesses the integrity of the pathway from the VIIIth nerve to the brainstem, as well as checking for ossicular fixation which will be limited in a disorder such as otosclerosis.

Audiometric brainstem response (ABR) testing is utilized most commonly in assessment of patients with unilateral symptoms and/or hearing loss to assess retrocochlear status. With the advent of MRI scanning, questions about its sensitivity (the probability that a person with an acoustic neuroma will have an abnormal ABR) have arisen.[3] Decisions about their relative merit are based on the fact that MRI is the gold standard but is significantly more expensive.

Imaging

Magnetic resonance imaging (MRI) of the brain and posterior fossa has an occasional role as part of the work up of a tinnitus patient. It is indicated primarily for patients with unilateral symptoms and/or those with asymmetric sensorineural hearing loss. It is also important in patients with reasonable suspicion of intracranial problems such as one with an affected adjacent cranial nerve (Figure 16–1). If the high frequency hearing level in the 2 to 4 kHz range is worse than 55 dB, then the accuracy of ABR is limited. Some controversy exists in tinnitus patients with better high frequency hearing as to whether ABR is the most time and financially efficient evaluation modality. Figure 16–2 is an evaluation paradigm for a patient with unilateral, nonpulsatile tinnitus.

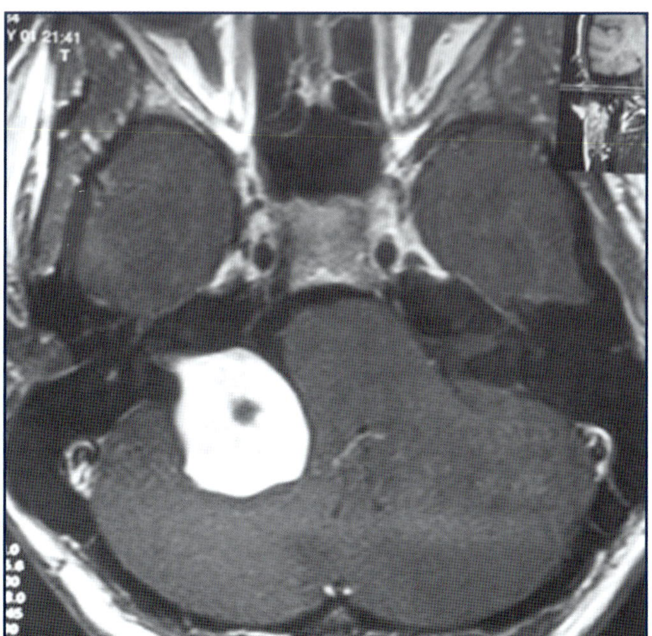

Figure 16–1. T1-weighted MRI image demonstrating right vestibular schwannoma which can occasionally be diagnosed from a patient presenting with unilateral tinnitus.

CAT scan imaging is most valuable in looking for pathology within the temporal bone. It is most commonly indicated in patients with unilateral, pulsatile tinnitus. Frequent pathologic abnormalities identified on the CAT scan concern the position and bony coverage of the jugular bulb and internal carotid artery.[4]

For unilateral pulsatile tinnitus, MRA/MRV is also useful. There is discussion whether MRA/MRV or CAT of the temporal bone should be the first study considered in the patient with subjective pulsatile tinnitus. The final conclusion is pending but generally it has been reported that the CAT scan is more likely to be abnormal but that MRA/MRV is more likely to find significant problems.[4]

Angiography is necessary in a select few patients. Those with objective pulsatile tinnitus will almost invariably require an arteriogram even if it is not the first test ordered. It will also be useful in patients with subjective pulsatile tinnitus who have an abnormality defined on another study such as an MRA or in those with normal evaluation but a strong suspicion of a vascular source. In particular, angiography is helpful in diagnosing transverse sinus dural AV fistulas which may not be found on MRA.[4] Angiography can be diagnostic as well as therapeutic when combined with an intervention such as coiling in patients with appropriate diagnoses such as arteriovenous malformations.

Additional Evaluation

As already mentioned, evaluation beyond the history, physical and basic audiogram is rarely necessary. Serologic testing including CBC, TSH with/without TFTs, FTA, glucose, electrolytes, and calcium, and magnesium for metabolic causes such as anemia, thyroid problems, syphilis, diabetes, and myoclonus can be indicated. Ophthalmologic evaluation for papilledema or lumbar puncture for CSF

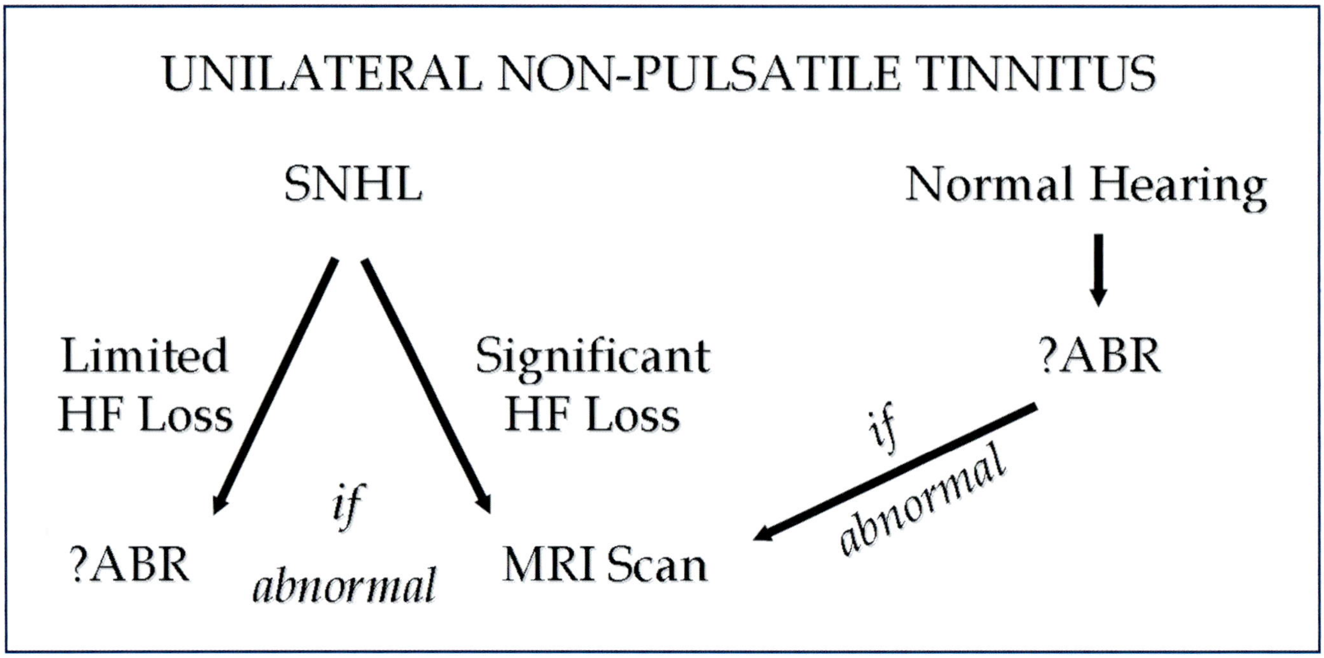

Figure 16–2. Algorithm for the workup of nonpulsatile tinnitus.

pressure is useful when benign intracranial hypertension is suspected.

Tinnitus Analysis

Beyond obtaining a history, questionnaires can be used to analyze and quantify tinnitus. The Tinnitus Reaction Questionnaire (TRQ) consists of 26 items measuring the general distress resulting from the tinnitus with a score of 0 representing no distress and 104 being maximum disruption.[5] The 25-item Tinnitus Handicap Inventory (THI) can give insight into the functional and emotional effect of tinnitus with 0 being no distress and 100 being maximum handicap.[6] These questionnaires can help both the patients and the clinician understand the level of tinnitus disturbance.

Tinnitus can be indirectly analyzed by matching. In this technique, an external sound is presented to the tinnitus patient and the pitch, character and loudness adjusted until it is felt to be similar, or match, the sound that the individual is experiencing. This can help the clinician understand the exact sound the patient is experiencing. Although it can supply some information, we do not routinely perform matching as there is not a clear relationship between the loudness and the disturbance of the tinnitus.[7]

CLASSIFICATION

Ideally, tinnitus should be classified by location and etiology. Unfortunately, this information is known in only a minority of patients, making this type of classification generally impossible. Previous classifications have made attempts to divide the tinnitus in some useful ways. Central versus peripheral has been proposed and makes theoretical sense but is difficult to determine in the majority of patients. Vibratory versus nonvibratory differentiates sounds being generated mechanically such as blood flowing through a vessel or muscles twitching (vibratory) with sound information being generated electrically within the auditory system. Sometimes the vibratory causes can be detected by the examiner.

Probably the more useful classifications are objective vs. subjective and pulsatile vs. nonpulsatile. Objective tinnitus/sounds, which represent only about 1% of patients, are those that can be heard by the examiner. There is significant overlap of these two classifications because the majority of patients with objective tinnitus have pulsatile tinnitus. Although the percentage of pulsatile tinnitus that is objective is higher than nonpulsatile, it still remains that most pulsatile tinnitus cannot be heard by the examiner.

A classification that is commonly used is based on whether the etiology is known: Identifiable versus idiopathic (Figure 16–3). The identifiable category is divided into vascular and nonvascular (Table 16–2). The idiopathic category is divided by the presence or absence of sensorineural hearing loss. This classification seems to be more applicable in addressing tinnitus and tinnitus patients.

Identifiable Causes: Vascular

Glomus tumors, either jugulare or tympanicum, can result in pulsatile tinnitus with a middle ear mass usually visible on examination (Figure 16–4). Dural

Table 16–2. Identifiable Causes of Tinnitus

Vascular	Glomus tumor
	AV malformation
	Internal/External carotid artery stenosis
	Persistent stapedial artery
	Ectopic intratympanic carotid artery
	Dehiscent jugular bulb
	Jugular venous hum
	Venous diverticulum
	Vascular compression of CN VIII
	Hypertension
Nonvascular	Medications
	Acoustic neuroma
	Intracranial neoplasms (Temporal lobe)
	Metabolic disorders
	TMJ dysfunction
	Middle ear disease
	Ménière's disease
	Sudden Sensorineural Hearing Loss
	Psychiatric

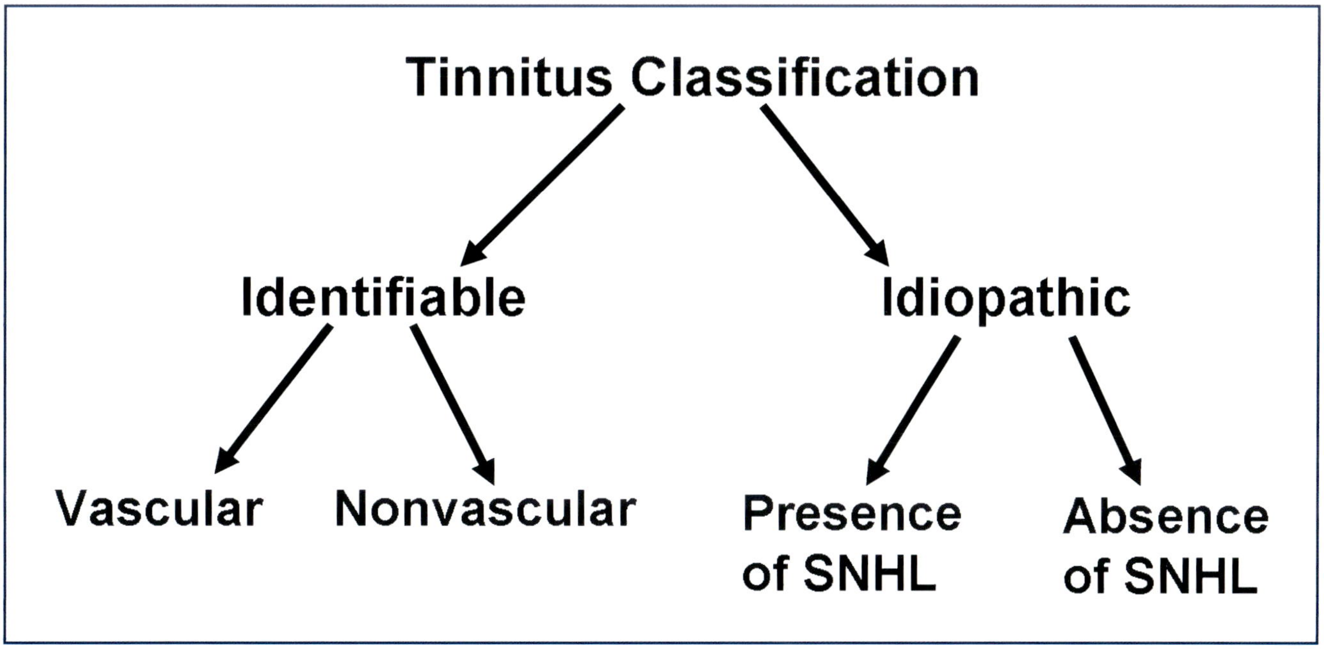

Figure 16–3. Suggested tinnitus classification.

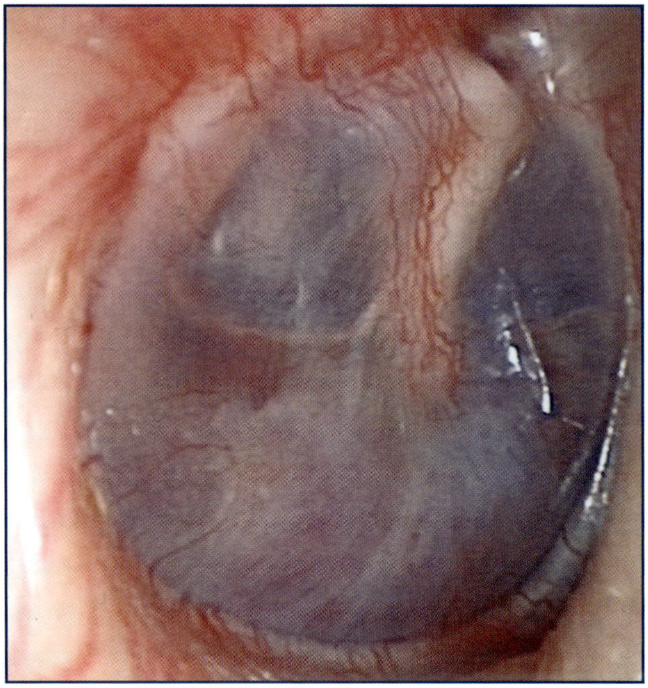

Figure 16–4. Image of glomus tympanicum which can be a cause of pulsatile tinnitus.

arteriovenous malformations can usually be auscultated by the examiner. Treatment of these is frequently endovascular although some may require an open procedure depending on size and location. Stenosis anywhere along the carotid arteries can create turbulent flow resulting in pulsatile tinnitus. This is most commonly due to atherosclerosis in the elderly but can also be due to fibromuscular dysplasia in young to middle age females. Treatment decisions ultimately will depend on the hemodynamic significance of the stenosis. Rarely, the stapedial artery of the second branchial arch, will not fully involute and can be large enough to produce auditory pulsations. These small vessels are only occasionally seen on examination or vascular studies.

Minor anatomic variants can create symptoms in some patents. Either the carotid artery or the jugular vein can be high or within the middle ear space. This proximity can result in pulsatile tinnitus particularly if either is not bone covered. Diverticuli of the sigmoid sinus have been identified as a cause of pulsatile tinnitus that will resolve with reduction of the outpouching surgically.[8]

Compression of the VIIIth nerve in the cerebellopontine angle is a potential cause of tinnitus although in this case the tinnitus is nonpulsatile in spite of the vascular cause. Microvascular decompression is curative in these cases. Pulsatile tinnitus can also be associated with hypertension due either to the higher and turbulent flow and/or the associated atherosclerotic narrowing. A venous hum is a potential vascular cause resulting from the pulsing noise occasionally created by the walls of the jugular vein.

Identifiable Causes: Nonvascular

There are a variety of identifiable nonvascular causes of tinnitus. The most medically significant are tumors near the acoustic nerve. Acoustic neuromata will commonly result in unilateral, nonpulsatile tinnitus and usually will be accompanied by hearing loss. Other symptoms can be associated with cerebellopontine angle masses and can lead one to appropriately suspect and evaluate a person appropriately. Tumors of the temporal lobe can cause more complex tinnitus such as music or voice and must be considered.

Medications can cause tinnitus, which is usually bilateral. The salicylates are the most recognized entity. High doses of salicylates will create tinnitus that is usually reversible after discontinuance, but can be permanent. This problem is less commonly encountered as the use of dose aspirin therapy has decreased. Quinine is used less frequently, but can create tinnitus. Narcotic use/abuse, such as Vicodin, has been reported to create sensorineural hearing loss and its use should be questioned although this information may not readily be offered by the patient.[9] One of the more recognized ototoxic medication classes, the aminoglycosides, can cause nonpulsatile tinnitus that is usually bilateral and accompanied by sensorineural hearing loss. There can be some recovery from its toxicity after discontinuation, but frequently it is permanent.

Metabolic disorders should be considered. Entities that can create high blood flow states such as anemia, hypertension, and hyperthyroidism can result in pulsatile tinnitus. End organ and small blood vessel damaging entities such as diabetes mellitus and hypertension are associated with increased rates of sensorineural hearing loss and nonpulsatile tinnitus.

Common otologic problems are usually obvious and should not be overlooked. External auditory canal problems, such as cerumen impactions, can result in tinnitus. Tinnitus will frequently accompany middle ear pathology such as effusions, tympanic membrane perforations, and otosclerosis. These are easily identified with a physical examination and an audiogram. Ménière's disease is characterized by the tetrad of hearing loss, fullness, vertigo, and tinnitus and is usually suspected from the history.

Clicking or tapping sounds can be a feature of myoclonus. Palatal myoclonus results from spasms of the soft palate, most likely involving the tensor veli palatini muscle. The movement of the palate and eustachian tube will result in a clicking sound and sometimes a feeling associated with the disorder. The twitching of the palate will more readily be viewed transnasally with an endoscope as the muscular activity is frequently suppressed with mouth opening. The tensor tympani muscle can be involved. If it acts alone it is called middle ear myoclonus. This movement of the malleus can sometimes be seen on examination of the ear as well as with tympanometry. Electrolyte abnormalities associated with muscle hyperactivity such as potassium, calcium, and magnesium should be considered. As multiple sclerosis has been linked, an MRI scan of the brain can be useful in the evaluation of these patients. If symptoms persist, treatment with muscle relaxants such as Valium, Soma, or baclofen can be curative. Occasionally surgical transection of the middle ear muscle tendons is indicated. This may reduce or eliminate the symptoms, but hyperacusis may result.

A more recently recognized cause of pulsatile tinnitus is benign intracranial hypertension (BIH), also called pseudotumor cerebri. It is more common in middle-aged, overweight females. The cause of the elevated cerebrospinal fluid is not known but may be due to central venous compression. Headaches and visual symptoms, secondary to pressure on the optic nerve, are common and important symptoms to recognize. Fundoscopic examination showing papilledema is strongly suggestive. Lumbar puncture with an opening pressure of more than 200 mm water is diagnostic. When indicated, medical treatment includes diuretics or acetozolamide (Diamox) to reduce CSF pressure. For severe forms with problematic headaches or visual compromise, ventricular shunting is available.

Patulous eustachian tube is an unusual entity that can result in low pitched tinnitus, abnormal perception of one's own voice (autophony), and abnormally loud perception of breathing sounds. A sense of aural fullness and hearing loss are also frequently present. Diagnosis is usually suspected clinically. Examination of the nasopharynx endoscopically will frequently reveal an abnormally patent eustachian tube orifice. Patulous eustachian tube can be associated with certain metabolic situations such as recent weight loss, cancer, or dehydration although in many there is no clear etiology. Treatment of the underlying metabolic problem can be curative; that is, weight stabilization in weight loss situations or hydration in dehydration situations. Medical treatment is moderately successful and includes nasal congestion with nasal topical medications including estrogen or chlorine. Tympanostomy tubes can be successful at altering the acoustics of the middle ear to lessen the fullness and autophony. Surgery of the eustachian tube can be very successful in problematic cases not responsive to conservative management. In the past, controlled scarring or obliteration of the eustachian tube lumen had been performed but this tended to create additional problems and was discussed in very limited situations. More recently, eustachian tuboplasty has been successful in narrowing the lumen without obliteration and has a high success rate with minimal morbidity.

Psychiatric problems are frequently encountered in tinnitus patients. There is an unusually high incidence of anxiety and depression in patients with bothersome tinnitus.[10] This is important because if treatment is undertaken, the psychiatric problem is frequently as or more important to address than the tinnitus symptom alone. Occasionally, a psychiatric problem alone is the cause of the tinnitus. Psychotic disorders can result in severe simple tinnitus or complex tinnitus such as voices that can be associated with other symptoms such as hyperacusis.

Idiopathic

The vast majority of tinnitus patients do not have an identifiable or curable cause for their tinnitus. These patients are typically nonpulsatile and most commonly bilateral. Ninety percent have at least some hearing loss, usually sensorineural. A small percentage of these people have normal hearing. The presence of hearing loss would seem to suggest some level of "damage" in the auditory system. In most cases the only implication is that a hearing aid is a consideration in the treatment of those with hearing loss and not in those with normal hearing. There is some evidence that those with a hearing loss may have more subjective disruption.[11]

TREATMENT

The lack of correlation of measured tinnitus intensity on tinnitus matching and overall disruptiveness of tinnitus does reinforce the idea that there are two aspects to tinnitus. The first is the physical symptom. The clinician must reinforce with the patient that there is a very real symptom, but it is the tolerance or perception of the tinnitus that becomes problematic. An interesting study by Knobel[12] revealed that 68% of healthy individuals had tinnitus-like perceptions when asked to listen specifically for sounds in a sound-proof booth for five minutes. In contrast, only 20% heard these perceptions when performing a problem-solving task while in the booth. This seems to suggest that focus and attention play an important role in the perception of tinnitus. In the treatment of tinnitus this focus/attention aspect may be the more important issue. The all too true cliché in tinnitus care is that there are many treatment options but no true cure for most tinnitus patients, although a few minutes on the Internet may convince one otherwise. The treatment will depend on the patient's particular situation and the clinician's experience. Medications and masking are the most common interventions but there are many other options.

Reassurance

In patients in the idiopathic group, the most common necessary intervention is reassurance.[13] Once the necessary evaluation is complete, it should be reinforced that there is no medically serious problem present and that the tinnitus is unlikely to worsen. For those who find the tinnitus disruptive or limiting, treatment options should be explored.

Masking

In most patients, tinnitus can be suppressed with the presentation of an external sound. Many tinnitus patients already understand this masking concept and realize that environmental and household sounds can reduce tinnitus perception. Items like fans or radios are known to be beneficial. Readily available environmental noise generators produce natural sounds like oceans and rain showers that are not only maskers but have the added benefit of being psychologically soothing.

One of the more useful and commonly utilized masking devices is the hearing aid. These are especially well suited for the patient with problematic hearing loss and tinnitus. Ear level maskers that generate a broadband sound in a hearing aid shell, create a mobile device that can be valuable in unilateral or bilateral tinnitus. In bilateral cases, patients can either wear one masker if they experience contralateral inhibition or two maskers if they do not. Occasionally, a person will desire the benefit of a hearing aid, but will not get the adequate masking. In this situation an ear level device, with both a hearing aid and masker component, called a tinnitus instrument, is available. Programming a tinnitus instrument requires some experience to ensure the masker is adequate to suppress the tinnitus, but not so intrusive to hamper the hearing aid function.

In most patients with tinnitus, their candidacy for masking can be inferred from their history. In those where there is uncertainty, minimum masking level evaluation (MML) can be useful.[14] In this technique, a band of noise in the 3 to 12 kHz range is presented. If tinnitus is suppressed at or below 3 dB SL, then masking is very likely to be successful. If presentation levels above 10 to 15 dB SL are necessary, then masking will probably not be a good choice. The occurrence of residual inhibition (persistence of suppression after discontinuance of stimulus) is also a good prognostic sign.

Medications

Many medications have been considered and used in the treatment of tinnitus. At this time there are no FDA approved medications for the treatment of tinnitus. Some medications are oriented specifically for treatment of the tinnitus and others address some of the secondary issues that may occur, such as sleep disruption.

The most successful medication in the treatment of tinnitus is lidocaine. Its value was discovered incidentally in cardiac and pain clinics in patients who coincidently reported tinnitus reduction while receiving intravenous lidocaine for other reasons. It has been demonstrated to significantly reduce tinnitus in 75% of treated patients. The mechanism of action is unknown but it is most likely centrally mediated. This theory is strongly supported by Baguley et al[15] who treated 16 patients who had undergone translabyrinthine resection of an acoustic neuroma and were experiencing tinnitus. Twelve of the 16 patients reported significant reduction of their tinnitus with lidocaine use. Unfortunately the benefit is uniformly short-lived and lidocaine has little value in its clinical setting.

Lidocaine's success led to the investigation of oral equivalent medications including tocainide, mexiletine, and flecainide. These medications showed some promise although studies did not clearly define their benefit and the potential side effects (bone marrow suppression, cardiac) are considerable. The presumed central effect of lidocaine created an interest in anti-seizure medications. Phenytoin and carbemazepine have been studied and utilized with sporadic success. Potential side effects in these medications are also a serious consideration.

Vasodilators are likely the oldest group of medications used is the in the treatment of tinnitus. Niacin has been frequently utilized. There has been little formal evaluation of its clinical benefit. It may have value in the elderly and those with small vessel disease. Alternately, its benefit may be a result of its vitamin status as vitamin B_3. Other vasoactive medications that have been discussed include papaverine, dipyridamole, histamine, and trental. Like niacin, all have some reported clinical benefit although no significant support in the literature.

A variety of studies have documented the high incidence of depression and depressive symptoms in patients with problematic tinnitus. Thus, with good reason, antidepressants are likely the most often utilized medications for tinnitus treatment. The most commonly evaluated and utilized medications are the tricyclic antidepressants: amitriptyline and nortriptyline. Dosing is usually begun at a low level of 10 to 25 mg daily and slowly increased until therapeutic response. Some patients may require dosages of 75 mg per day. There are potentially three ways these medications may be beneficial. There can be direct reduction of the amplitude of the tinnitus, there can be sleep enhancing effects (which is a common association in problematic tinnitus), and there can be anxiety reducing effects.

A revealing study of nortriptyline use in 92 patients with disabling tinnitus was reported by Dobie et al.[16] They found that 38 (41%) met the criteria for major depression. There was significant tinnitus reduction in 43% of nortriptyline patients (vs 30% in control) and there was a global benefit in 67% of nortriptyline patients (vs 40% in control). The statistical significance of the global benefit suggests that nortriptyline has more benefits than just tinnitus reduction. They concluded that female gender, sleep disruption, and depressive symptoms were predictors for success and that the presence of musculoskeletal complaints significantly reduced the chances of success.

Benzodiazepines have been used with some success for tinnitus reduction, as well. One report suggested that alprazolam controlled tinnitus in 76% of patients with only 5% placebo response.[17] Although it seems benzodiazepines have a role, many practitioners have not had this level of success. The concerns in the use of these medications are their addictive potential and the possibility of recurrence with discontinuation. Intuitively, it might be suspected that benzodiazepines' success would be related to their known anxiety reducing effects, but it may be more complex. They may be valuable in their role as a γ-aminobutyric acid (GABA) agonist as there is animal evidence that benzodiazepines can reduce hyperactivity in the inferior colliculus suggesting GABA agonism.[18] There is evidence that tinnitus may be at least partially caused by a reduction of inhibition in neurons in the ascending auditory pathway in which GABA has a role as an inhibitory neurotransmitter.[19] Recently, there has been interest in GABA agonists as possible treatment agents.

Although some success has been found with gabapentin, formal studies have not proven its value.[20] Acamprosate, which is used in the treatment of alcoholism, is another GABA agonist that has been studied. An encouraging report suggested that half of the patients undergoing treatment in this controlled study experienced over 50% reduction in their tinnitus.[21] There has not been any follow-up to this information.

There is some evidence that transtympanic therapy may have a role. Gentamicin has proven beneficial in control of Ménière's disease with a good chance (63%) of tinnitus reduction.[22] Intratympanic steroids exclusively for tinnitus are not universally accepted although one study reported 60% of patients with either sudden sensorineural or noise-induced hearing loss experienced a reduction after treatment.[23]

A variety of supplements have been utilized in tinnitus treatment with little scientific data to substantiate the effects. The most commonly discussed is ginkgo biloba. In spite of its popularity, its benefit has not been proven.[24] Melatonin, a hormone secreted by the pineal gland and felt to be important in circadian rhythms, has been reported to be effective in treatment of tinnitus and in sleep enhancement.[25] Multiple B vitamins including B_1 (thiamine), B_3 (niacin), B_6, B_{12}, and folic acid have been discussed. Minerals including zinc and magnesium have been used for tinnitus treatment. Their roles as antioxidants and/or simple supplementation are theoretical reasons for their value.

Tinnitus Retraining Therapy

Tinnitus retraining therapy (TRT) is a program of treatment aimed at reducing the perception and disruptiveness of tinnitus and hyperacusis. This program consists of two modalities: auditory retraining and directive counseling. The auditory retraining involves prolonged exposure to low level sound with the use of ear level devices that are worn regularly, typically for months. The sound is presented below masking levels in an attempt to create permanent changes in the central auditory system, resulting in altered and reduced perception. The directive counseling is designed to lessen the negative connotations associated with tinnitus.[26,27]

Although the initial reports were good, the actual data and results were difficult to interpret. In practice, many have found that compliance in these intense programs and overall success does not seem to be as good as initially reported.

A newer approach based on the TRT model is the Neuromonics® treatment. This treatment consists of 2 parts: counseling and progressive auditory treatment. The importance of the counseling is recognized in both this and other TRT programs. The Neuromonics® stimulus is carefully programmed based on the patient's audiogram and initially consists of music with embedded white noise. The white noise is designed to suppress the tinnitus. Over a period of two months, the white noise is withdrawn from the stimulus. The desired result is that the patient's tinnitus loses the disruptiveness through the counseling and the perceptual changes induced by the stimulus.[28,29]

Other Therapies

Many other therapies for tinnitus have been utilized. One of the more successful therapies is the relaxation techniques. Biofeedback is the method of controlling involuntary functions such as heart rate and body temperature. Some clinicians have found this to be useful in selected tinnitus patients.[30,31] Yoga and Tai Chi have also been reported to be useful. Botulinum toxin injections around the auricle reportedly can be valuable in tinnitus treatment.[32] Muscle relaxation around the ear may be the mechanism of improvement.

Diet seems to be valuable in some cases. There is likely an overall benefit to adhering to a generally healthy diet. Specific entities such as caffeine, and less commonly sodium, have been reported by patients to be aggravating factors. Recently, a study by Sutbas and colleagues[33] suggested lipid reduction therapy by diet and or medication could result in significant tinnitus reduction. These authors suggested that the incidence of hyperlipidemia was higher in patients who experienced tinnitus relief.

Goldstein and colleagues[34] have suggested that ultra-high-frequency vibration therapy may be a potentially viable therapy for patients with problematic tinnitus. Transcranial magnetic stimulation has been performed with some success in tinnitus treatment. However, one recent study did not find benefit with transcranial stimulation.[35] Interestingly, when transcranial temporal stimulation was combined with prefrontal stimulation in another study, there was long-term benefit suggesting a benefit to addressing the attention or emotional aspect of tinnitus.[36]

Electrical stimulation has always been thought to have potential value. Basic research has suggested that positive current pulses can be inhibitory.[37] Cochlear implantation has supplied additional information and it has been reported that up to 86% of implanted patients experience some suppression of their tinnitus.[38,39]

Psychiatric

As previously mentioned, there is an unusually high incidence of anxiety and depression in patients with bothersome tinnitus. This frequently needs to be addressed either indirectly with counseling and/or low dose antidepressants or with more formal psychiatric or psychological evaluation. In many patients it is difficult to determine if the somatic complaint of tinnitus is the primary or secondary problem although most sufferers firmly believe that it is the former. Any patient expressing suicidal ideation needs immediate evaluation regardless of whether the clinician thinks that the patient may be exaggerating or acting out. In an occasional patient there is a true psychotic disorder suggesting that treatment is well beyond the scope of the otologist.

CONCLUSION

Evaluation of the tinnitus requires a systematic approach. The nature of the tinnitus will strongly guide the work up, with unilateral symptoms and pulsatile features being the most important characteristics guiding the decision making. After an initial evaluation including the history and physical examination, most patients can be appropriately reassured and no further intervention is necessary. Some tinnitus sufferers are limited by their symptoms and require intervention. At present there is unfortunately no true cure but there are many options depending on the patient's particular situation. Secondary issues such as anxiety and sleep disruption frequently are present in the more affected individuals and need to be addressed as part the treatment regimen.

REFERENCES

1. Seidman MD, Jacobson GP. Update on tinnitus. *Otolaryngol Clin North Am*. 1996;29(3):455.
2. Tucker DA, Phillips SL, Ruth RA, Clayton WA, Royster E, Todd AD. The effect of silence on tinnitus perception. *Otolaryngol Head and Neck Surg*. 2005;132(1):20–24.
3. Zappia JJ, O'Connor CA, Wiet RJ, Dinces EA. Rethinking the use of auditory brainstem response in acoustic neuroma screening. *Laryngoscope*. 1997;107(10):1388–1392.
4. Shin EJ, Lalwani AK, Dowd CF. Role of angiography in the evaluation of patients with pulsatile tinnitus. *Laryngoscope*. 2000;110,1916–1920.
5. Wilson PH, Henry J, Bowen M, Haralambous G. Tinnitus Reaction Questionnaire: psychometric properties of a measure of distress associated with tinnitus. *J Speech Hear Res*. 1991;34(6):197–201.
6. Newman CW, Jacobsen GP, Spitzer JB. Development of the Tinnitus Handicap Inventory. *Arch*. 1996;122,143–148.
7. Meikle MB, Vernon J, Johnson RM. The perceived severity of tinnitus. Some observations concerning a large population of tinnitus clinic patients. *Otolaryngol Head Neck Surg*. 1984;92(6):689–696.
8. Otto KJ, Hudgins PA, Abdelkafy W, Mattox DE. Sigmoid sinus diverticulum: a new surgical approach to the correction of pulsatile tinnitus. *Otol Neurotol*. 2007;28(1):48–53.
9. Friedman RA, House JW, Luxford WM, Gherini S, Mills D. Profound hearing loss associated with hydrocodone/acetaminophen abuse. *Am J Otol*. 2000;21(2):188–191.
10. Zöger S, Svedlund J, Holgers KM. Relationship between tinnitus severity and psychiatric disorders. *Psychosomatics*. 2006;47:282–288.
11. Savastano M. Tinnitus with or without hearing loss: are its characteristics different? *Eur Arch Otorhinolaryngol*. 2008;265(11):1295–1300.
12. Knobel KAB, Sanchez TG. Influence of silence and attention on tinnitus perception. *Otolaryngol Head Neck Surg*. 2008;138:18–22.
13. Sismanis A. Tinnitus. *Curr Neurol Neurosci*. 2001;1(5):492–499.

14. Tyler RS, Conrad-Armes D, Smith PA. Postmasking effects of sensorineural tinnitus: a preliminary investigation. *J Speech Hear Res*. 1984;27:466–474.
15. Baguley DM, Jones S, Wilkins I, Axon PR, Moffat DA. The inhibitory effect of intravenous lidocaine infusion on tinnitus after translabyrinthine removal of vestibular schwannoma: a double-blind, placebo-controlled, crossover study. *Otol Neurotol*. 2005;26(2):169–176.
16. Dobie RA, Sakai CS, Sullivan MD, Katon WJ, Russo J. Antidepressant treatment of tinnitus patients: report of a randomized clinical trial and clinical prediction of benefit. *Am J Otol*. 1993;14(1):18–23.
17. Johnson RM, Brummett R, Schleuning A. Use of alprazolam for relief of tinnitus. A double-blind study. *Arch Otolaryngol Head Neck Surg*. 1993;119(8):842–845.
18. Szczepaniak WS, Moller AR. Effects of baclofen, clonazepam, and diazepam on tone exposure- induced hyperexcitability of the inferior colliculus in the rat: possible therapeutic implication for pharmacological management of tinnitus and hyperacusis. *Hear Res*. 1996;97:46–53.
19. Krnjevic K. Significance of GABA in brain function. In: Tunnicliff G, Raess BU, eds. *GABA Mechanisms in Epilepsy*. New York, NY: Wiley Liss; 1991:47–87.
20. Piccirillo JF, Finnell J, Vlahiotis A, Chole RA, Spitznagel E Jr. Relief of idiopathic subjective tinnitus: is gabapentin effective? *Arch Otolaryngol Head Neck Surg*. 2007; 133(4):390–397.
21. Azevedo AA, Figueiredo RR. Tinnitus treatment with acamprosate: double-blind study. *Braz J Otorhinolaryngol*. 2005;71(5): 618–623.
22. Hoffer ME, Kopke RD, Weisskopf P, et al. Use of the round window microcatheter in the treatment of Ménière's disease. *Laryngoscope*. 2001;111:2046–2049.
23. Hoffer ME, Wester D, Kopke RD, Weisskopf P, Gottshall K. Transtympanic management of tinnitus. *Otolaryngol Clin North Am*. 2003;36(2):353–358.
24. Drew S, Davies E. Effectiveness of Ginkgo biloba in treating tinnitus: double blind, placebo controlled trial. *Br Med J*. 2001;322:73.
25. Rosenberg SI, Silverstein H, Rowan PT, Olds MJ. Effect of melatonin on tinnitus. *Laryngoscope*. 1998;108(3):305–310.
26. Bartnik G, Fabijanska A, Rogowski M. Our experience in treatment of patients with tinnitus and/of hyperacusis using the habituation method. In: Hazell JWP, ed. *Proceedings of the Sixth International Tinnitus Seminar* Cambridge, *U.K.* London, UK: T.H.C; 1999:415–417.
27. Sheldrake JB, Hazell JWP, Graham RL. Results of tinnitus retraining therapy. In: Hazell, JWP, ed. *Proceedings of the Sixth International Tinnitus Seminar, Cambridge, U.K.* London, UK: T.H.C; 1999:292–296.
28. Hanley PJ, Davis PB. Treatment of tinnitus with a customized, dynamic acoustic neural stimulus: underlying principles and clinical efficacy. *Trends Amplif*. 2008;12(3): 210–222.
29. Davis PB, Paki B, Hanley PJ. Neuromonics tinnitus treatment: third clinical trial. *Ear Hear*. 2007;28:242–259.
30. Grossan M. Treatment of subjective tinnitus with biofeedback. *Ear Nose Throat J*. 1976;55(10):314–318.
31. House JW. Treatment of severe tinnitus with biofeedback training. *Laryngoscope*. 1978;88(3):406–412.
32. Stidham K R, Solomon PH, Roberson JB. Evaluation of botulinum toxin A in treatment of tinnitus. *Otolaryngol Head Neck Surg*. 2005;132(6):883–889.
33. Sutbas A, Yetiser S, Satar B, Akcam T, Karahatay S, Saglam K. Low-cholesterol diet and antilipid therapy in managing tinnitus and hearing loss in patients with noise-induced hearing loss and hyperlipidemia. *Int Tinnitus J*. 2007;13(2),143–149.
34. Goldstein BA, Lenhardt ML, Shulman A. Tinnitus improvement with ultra-high-frequency vibration therapy. *Int Tinnitus J*. 2005;11(1):14–22.
35. Lee SL, Abraham M, Cacace AT, Silver SM. Repetitive transcranial magnetic stimulation in veterans with debiliting tinnitus: a pilot study. *Otolaryngol Head Neck Surg*. 2008;138:398–399.
36. Kleinjung T, Eichhammer P, Landgrebe M, et al. Combined temporal and prefrontal transcranial magnetic stimulation for tinnitus treatment: a pilot study. *Otolaryngol Head Neck Surg*. 2008;138:497–501.
37. Aran JM, Cazals Y. Electrical suppression of tinnitus. *Ciba Found Symp*. 1981;85:217–231.
38. Miyamoto RT, Wynne MK, McKnight C, Bichey B. Electrical suppression of tinnitus via cochlear implants. *Internat Tinnitus J*. 1997;3(1): 35–38.
39. Quaranta N, Wagstaff S, Baguley DM. Tinnitus and cochlear implantation. *Int J Audiol*. 2004;43(5):245–251.

CHAPTER 17

Endolymphatic Hydrops and Medical Management of Dizziness

Sean Wise and Eloy Villasuso III

INTRODUCTION

Patients frequently come to the otolaryngologist looking for help with problems regarding dizziness and balance. Some of the most common causes of vertigo that the otolaryngologist will encounter are benign paroxysmal positional vertigo, endolymphatic hydrops, vestibular neuritis, and migraine-associated vertigo. This chapter discusses endolymphatic hydrops, which refers to increased hydraulic pressure within the inner ear. This pressure accumulation may cause the following symptoms: (1) fluctuating hearing loss (2) episodic vertigo with nausea and vomiting, (3) tinnitus, and (4) aural fullness. Endolymphatic hydrops often is used synonymously with Ménière's disease.

Classic Ménière's disease (MD) is characterized by this tetrad of symptoms. When these four symptoms present in a pattern, a diagnosis of MD can be made. Ménière's disease is also frequently associated with nausea, vomiting, headaches, and fatigue. The vertigo attacks of MD often last from 20 minutes to a few hours. After an attack the patient often returns to normal activities with little sequalae. Other associated symptoms that patients with MD frequently report include diplacusis, pressure in the head, and positional symptoms. The prognosis for patients with MD is highly variable; some patients will have only mild symptoms while others may progress to severe sensorineural hearing loss and vestibular dysfunction.

PATHOPHYSIOLOGY OF ENDOLYMPHATIC HYDROPS

The exact pathophysiology of Ménière's disease remains elusive. It is histologically characterized by distention of the endolymphatic chambers of the inner ear. Merchant et al[1] reported on the presence of endolymphatic hydrops in all Ménière's disease patients, but also noted that not all patients with endolymphatic hydrops suffered from Ménière's disease. It is debatable whether the endolymphatic hydrops itself causes symptoms or if the hydrops is another manifestation of the underlying etiology. Theorized etiologies have included vascular, viral, infectious, autoimmune, allergic, anatomic (obstructive), and genetic origins. Disorders of endolymphatic homeostasis are also frequently considered. It is speculated that distention of the endolymphatic membranes, particularly in the cochlea and the saccule, may result in hearing loss and vertigo as a consequence of mixing of the perilymph and endolymph and a resultant abnormal depolarization of the nerve endings. Repetitive cycles of distention may eventually lead to damage to the delicate membranes and to the permanent hearing loss and vestibular dysfunction seen in the late stages of the disease. Such effects may be magnified within the relatively constricted regions of the apex. This may explain the low-frequency hearing loss commonly encountered in MD.

CLINICAL PRESENTATION

The most important aspect of evaluating a patient with dizziness is the history. Classic Ménière's disease is characterized by unilateral aural fullness, tinnitus, and decreased hearing often preceding an episode of vertigo that may last several hours. Some patients with MD may present with only unilateral aural fullness, tinnitus, and decreased hearing but no vertigo. These patients may be diagnosed with cochlear Ménière's disease or atypical Ménière's disease. Such patients will usually have an associated low-frequency sensorineural hearing loss, which may fluctuate. In time, some of these patients may develop the vestibular symptoms as well. Conversely, some patients may have episodic vertigo without aural fullness, tinnitus or hearing loss. These patients have vestibular Ménière's disease or atypical Ménière's disease. This diagnosis is more difficult to make because the hallmark of MD includes some cochlear symptoms. It is sometimes difficult to distinguish this presentation from a recurrent vestibulopathy of different origin. The majority of patients are somewhere between these two extremes. Those patients labeled with atypical Ménière's disease are treated based on their symptoms.

When taking the history of a vestibular patient, one must investigate the pattern, severity, and frequency of previous episodes. Over the course of a lifetime, many patients with MD may experience variability in the type of dizziness affecting them, and some episodes may exhibit characteristics consistent with vestibular neuronitis or benign paroxysmal positional vertigo (BPPV).

The vertiginous attack of Ménière's disease may be preceded by cochlear symptoms, or the cochlear symptoms may be concurrent with the vertigo. During such an attack, patients will typically experience a persistent vertigo sensation that lasts 20 minutes to a few hours which may be accompanied by nausea, vomiting, and headaches. Sometimes, as the vertigo resolves, all the other symptoms resolve as well and the patient feels fine. At other times, the patient may experience a persistent headache or "foggy" feeling that may last hours after the attack. The tinnitus, aural fullness, and decreased hearing may resolve completely after an attack or return to baseline. Some patients may not be able to effectively lateralize the cochlear symptoms, and describe only a fullness or heaviness in their head and nonlocalizing tinnitus. Bilateral disease may be considered in such patients. Antonio and Friedman[2] summarize that over time, about one third of patients with Ménière's disease will develop symptoms in the contralateral ear. Although possible, it is uncommon for a patient to initially present with bilateral Ménière's disease. Patients are frequently able to provide more information on cochlear symptoms and localization after they have been educated on the symptoms of MD and given instructions to keep a symptom diary. This can prove to be extremely helpful in follow-up evaluation.

It is also important to review the patient's complete history with special attention to ocular disorders such as uveitis or interstitial keratitis, which may lead to alternative diagnoses such as Cogan's syndrome or syphilis. Vestibular disorders are often multifactorial, and contributions from cardiovascular, musculoskeletal, neurological, pulmonary, and psychiatric disease may also play a role in the patient's overall dizziness.

There is a small, familial tendency to MD, as well as possibly a small female preponderance. While it can occur at any age, it most often presents in midlife. Occasionally, a patient with otosclerosis will describe Ménière's type dizziness. Stapes surgery should be regarded with caution in these patients as the increased endolymphatic pressure may predispose them to a perilymphatic gusher or saccular injury, with increased risk of sensorineural hearing loss.

Differential Diagnosis of Ménière's Disease

The differential diagnosis of any patient with dizziness is extensive. The characteristic dizziness of MD may be caused by a variety of conditions, and the diagnosis of MD remains one of exclusion. Ménière's disease is idiopathic, whereas Ménière's syndrome has a cause (ie, trauma, autoimmune dysfunction, or medications).

The most common cause of dizziness or episodic vertigo that may mimic MD is migraine-associated vertigo, also referred to as migraine-associated dizziness or vertiginous migraine. Because many of the symptoms overlap, it may be difficult to distinguish these two entities. There is no gold standard test to diagnose either condition. Many patients with migraine-associated vertigo do not meet all of the criteria for migraine as defined by the International Headache Society classification for migraine. Many Ménière's patients will likewise fall into possible or probable categories, as defined by the Committee on Hearing and Equilibrium (1995)[3] guidelines for diagnosing Ménière's disease. Differentiating migraine-associated vertigo from MD often requires a high level of suspicion and clinical judgement. In 2006, Shepard[4] summarized how patients with Ménière's disease also suffer more from migraines than the general population. Patients should be questioned about migraine-type symptoms such as unilateral, throbbing, pulsating, severe headaches with associated phonophobia, photophobia, nausea, and vomiting. Migraine patients may also have auras such as flashing lights, jagged lights, scotomas, or visual changes before the headaches. Auras can also take the form of disorientation, paresthesias, muscle weakness and other sensory disturbances. The migraine patient may also have otologic symptoms of tinnitus, fluctuating hearing loss, and pressure in the head. The dizziness may come as part of the aura, and the patient may or may not have an associated headache. These patients often complain of more persistent symptoms of rocking and swaying sensations with nausea, rather than discrete episodes of vertigo. This rocking and swaying sensation tends to be more constant and can last days, weeks or even months. Migraine patients tend to be more sensitive to visual stimuli such as patterns of lines, and have increased motion intolerance, such as carsickness. Many of these patients will have had a previous history of migraines, though many have been without headaches for many years. There is also a strong familial tendency for migraines. A basilar migraine is most likely to produce Ménière's type symptoms.

Delayed endolymphatic hydrops is a Ménière's type dizziness that may occur many years after an initial insult leading to a unilateral sensorineural hearing loss. Patients may develop ipsilateral or contralateral Ménière's symptoms of tinnitus, aural fullness and episodic vertigo. Some commonly associated insults and etiologies include congenital inner ear anomalies, trauma, sudden sensorineural hearing loss, and meningitis. Gianoli[5] reviewed many of the diagnoses to consider in the vertigo patient (Table 17–1).

Diagnosing Ménière's Disease

The most important aspect of diagnosing a vestibular patient is the history and physical examination. This may be supplemented with further audiovestibular tests. There is no gold standard diagnostic test for Ménière's disease.

In 1995, the Committee on Hearing and Equilibrium updated the American Academy of Otolaryngology-Head and Neck Surgery guidelines for the diagnosis and evaluation of therapy in Ménière's disease.[3] The diagnosis of Ménière's disease is divided into four categories: *certain, definite, probable,* and *possible*. MD is an idiopathic condition. Therefore, before a diagnosis of Ménière's disease can be made, all other possible etiologies must be excluded. *Certain MD* is defined as definite Ménière's disease with histopathologic confirmation. Thus, this category is not

Table 17–1. Differential Diagnosis of Ménière's Disease

Ménière's trauma	Acoustic trauma, post-otologic surgery (fistula), head trauma (temporal bone fracrues), barotrauma
Otologic	BPPV, labyrinthitis, vestibular neuronitis, otosclerosis, vestibular schwannoma (acoustic neuroma), perilymphatic fistula
Central etiologies	Migraine associated vertigo, multiple sclerosis, meningiomas, Chiari malformations, symptomatic arachnoid cysts, disorders of spinal fluid pressure
Obstructive lesions	Endolymphatic sac tumors tumors of the posterior fossa or cerbellopontine angle
Metabolic disorders	Diabetes mellitus, thyroid disease, dialysis patients, Paget's disease, leukemia, hyperlipidemia
Autoimmune disorders	Autoimmune inner ear disorder, lupus, Cogan's syndrome
Infectious etiologies	Syphylis, meningitis, Lyme disease, post mumps

typically clinically useful. *Definite Ménière's disease* is defined as two or more definitive episodes of vertigo lasting at least 20 minutes with audiometrically documented hearing loss on at least one occasion with tinnitus or aural fullness in the suspected ear. *Probable* Ménière's disease is defined as one definitive episode of vertigo and audiometrically documented hearing loss with tinnitus or aural fullness in the suspected ear. *Possible* MD is defined as episodic vertigo without documented hearing loss, or sensorineural hearing loss with disequilibrium. Definite MD is easily recognized, although most patients will fall into the probable and possible categories.

In patients with Ménière's, it is not uncommon that all audiovestibular testing will yield unremarkable results. This does not exclude Ménière's disease, but it is important before making a diagnosis of Ménière's disease to exclude all other possible etiologies.

Audiogram

Adhering to the Academy guidelines, this is the only test that will contribute to a diagnosis of Ménière's disease. However, most often the audiogram will be normal, placing the patient in the possible category by the current guidelines. The audiogram may reveal normal age related changes such as bilateral, symmetric, high frequency sensorineural hearing loss. The most useful diagnostic scenario is the presence of a low-frequency sensorineural hearing loss. When present, it is typically asymmetric for the affected ear but may be bilateral in cases of bilateral disease. The determination of low-frequency sensorineural hearing loss and asymmetry is open to clinical discretion, but the rationale should be justifiable for each case. Patients with long-standing Ménière's disease often exhibit a progression from a low-frequency sensorineural hearing loss initially, which later involves the higher frequencies resulting in a moderate flat sensorineural hearing loss. Battista found that it is infrequent for patients with migraines to have a significant sensorineural hearing loss, and if present, this rarely progresses.[6] Currently, there is no test to track or monitor the progression of MD. Audiograms are used to monitor the sensorineural hearing loss associated with MD and should be obtained on a regular basis. This should be accomplished annually for stable patients, as needed for any sudden changes in hearing and before and after any significant interventions.

Electronystagmogram (ENG)

The ENG assesses vestibular function. It is frequently normal in Ménière's disease. ENGs provide information as to the patient's current vestibular function, which then needs to be placed into the context of the patient's history; they do not yield diagnoses. Patients with long-standing MD may exhibit a unilateral vestibular weakness. Interestingly, migraine patients may also exhibit a unilateral vestibular weakness. Ménière's disease patients rarely have oculomotor abnormalities, while patients with migraine-associated vertigo may have some abnormal testing on that portion of the ENG, suggesting central involvement. The direction of the spontaneous nystagmus during or after an attack of Ménière's is not a reliable indicator of the site of the lesion. An irritative phase may occur during the attack (fast phases directed toward involved ear) followed by a paretic phase (fast phases directed toward opposite ear). Patients with a vestibular weakness and a history of chronic imbalance in between their episodes of vertigo may benefit from vestibular rehabilitation.

Auditory Brainstem Response (ABR)

This examination assesses the peripheral auditory pathways from the cochlea to the brainstem. This test is performed to evaluate for possible retrocochlear pathology, such as a vestibular schwannoma mimicking Ménière's type dizziness. It may be also be abnormal in cases such as multiple sclerosis and auditory neuropathy. An abnormal ABR exam is an indication for further testing with magnetic resonance imaging (MRI) of the internal auditory canals (IACs) and brain with and without contrast. A normal ABR exam does not sufficiently rule out a retrocochlear lesion, as a small vestibular schwannoma may be missed.

Electrocochleography (ECoG)

This examination is used specifically to identify endolymphatic hydrops. It uses a similar technique as the ABR, and utilizes wave I of the ABR. A comparison is made between the summating potential (SP) and the action potential (AP). If the ratio of these two potentials (SP/AP) exceeds a set limit, a diagnosis of endolymphatic hydrops may be supported. The test can be done with several different recording mechanisms, with variations in the placement of the recording electrode and stimuli. Each of these variations will affect the interpretation of results. The electrode may be placed in a far field location, at the meatus, in the external auditory canal, on the tympanic membrane or transtympanically on the cochlear promontory. In general, the closer to the cochlear promontory that the recording electrode is placed, the more accurate the reading and the smaller the SP/AP ratio needs to be to diagnose endolymphatic hydrops. Stimuli may be clicks or tone bursts. Hain and Rudisill[7] noted a sensitivity of 60 to 70% for an abnormal ECoG in Ménière's disease. Kim et al[8] reported an abnormally elevated ECoG in 67% of definite Ménière's disease patients, and 52% for probable and possible Ménière's disease patients. The test may be more useful if the patient is having symptoms at the time of testing. However, it is often not practical to schedule the test when the patient develops symptoms. It is useful to record any symptoms the patient may be experiencing at the time of testing. Results need to be interpreted in the context of the clinical picture. Patients with a history highly suggestive of MD may exhibit normal ECoG results. Occasionally, abnormal results are obtained from the contralateral, asymptomatic ear. Such findings may suggest bilateral hydrops, or potential future risk for the development of symptoms in the currently asymptomatic ear. The test is also limited in patients with significant sensorineural hearing loss. False positive results may occur in the case of perilymphatic fistula.

Vestibular Evoked Myogenic Potential (VEMP)

Vestibular evoked myogenic potentials (VEMPs) have been developing an increasing following over the last several years. The VEMP is a vestibulocolic reflex. A brief loud sound stimulates neurons in the saccule, which conducts via the inferior vestibular nerve to central pathways that lead to an inhibition of the tonically contracted sternocleidomastoid muscle. Following the path of the signal may provide information regarding middle ear status, saccule function, inferior vestibular nerve function, labyrinthine integrity, and status of the lower central pathways. As, endolymphatic hydrops affects the saccule, one would expect to see changes in the VEMP in patients with MD. Characteristics of the VEMPs include latency, amplitude, and threshold. Murofushi et al[9] reported abnormal amplitudes in 51% of patients with Ménière's disease, but only one had a prolonged latency. Rauch et al[10] reported on other abnormal VEMP findings in Ménière's disease, including elevated thresholds in both the affected and unaffected ear and a change in the frequency tuning when compared to normal controls. As with electrocochleography, an elevated VEMP in the unaffected ear may be an early sign of contralateral disease, which may manifest itself in the future. An absent VEMP may be indicative of inferior vestibular nerve involvement by either a vestibular neuritis or vestibular schwannoma. Rauch[11] reported that a lowered VEMP threshold, 20 dB less than normal patients, can be seen in cases of superior canal dehiscence syndrome. Central lesions such as multiple sclerosis as described Murofushi et al,[9] or basilar migraines as described by Liao,[12] may cause a prolonged latency or delay in the VEMP as it travels through the lower central pathways. An abnormal VEMP should prompt an MRI of the IACs and brain with and without contrast. An exception may occur in cases of suspected superior canal dehiscence syndrome in which computed tomography (CT) of the temporal bones would be indicated.

Glycerol Dehydration Test

The Glycerol dehydration test is based on the notion that decreasing the endolymphatic pressure of the inner ear will relieve symptoms, particularly on the audiogram. The patient performs a baseline audiogram and is then given glycerol or a diuretic, such as furosemide, to decrease the endolymphatic pressure. The audiogram is then repeated and the puretone averages and speech discrimination scores are compared pre- and postdehydration. An improvement of >10 dB or >15% in the speech discrimination score is considered significant. This test is not commonly used.

Magnetic Resonance Imaging (MRI)

It is uncommon for a patient with classical MD to be identified as having an underlying vestibular schwannoma or posterior fossa tumor. However, patients with unilateral aural symptoms such as hearing loss, especially a documented asymmetric sensorineural hearing loss; unilateral tinnitus; dizziness, or a documented vestibular weakness; fullness or pressure unexplained by other etiologies; and headaches or migraines may have an underlying posterior fossa lesion. Consequently, an MRI examination with and without contrast of the IACs and brain is warranted. An MRI of the IACs with and without contrast is the gold standard to rule out any posterior fossa, internal auditory canal or cerebellopontine angle lesion. Patients with Ménière's disease should also have an MRI of the IACs and brain with contrast to rule out retrocochlear pathology before undergoing any surgical intervention.

Many patients with vestibular symptoms often have seen other physicians who may have already obtained an MRI of the brain with or without contrast. Careful review of those films with attention to the internal auditory canals and cerebellopontine angles may reveal significant findings. Often, in a brain MRI with contrast there are insufficient cuts through the internal auditory canals, but close examination of axial and coronal planes may yield sufficient views to conclude that there is no cerebellopontine angle lesion. Many brain MRIs ordered by primary care physicians and neurologists are without contrast. Careful evaluation of the T2 fast spin echo images may provide adequate information to reveal any filling defects due to mass effect from a tumor. Newer modalities such as construction interference steady-state (CISS) sequencing provide excellent detail of the cochlear vestibular bundle as well as the facial nerve and vasculature of the cerebellopontine angles without the use of contrast. Such modalities are particularly useful in those patients for whom gadolinium contrast is contraindicated, such as those with significant kidney disease, allergy or pacemaker. Some newer pacemakers are now MRI compatable. Better images of the cochlea are also now being obtained with the 3-tesla magnets in the newer MRIs. Two studies, one by Nagawana et al[13] and another by Carfrae et al,[14] have looked at the cochlear partitions to try to identify endolymphatic hydrops, obtaining images 4 hours after the administration of intravenous gadolinium and observing its uptake in the cochlea. Such strategies can potentially delineate the perilymphatic space from the endolymphatic space to allow for observation of hydrops, but these techniques are still under investigation.

Nephrogenic systemic fibrosis (NSF) is a rare condition developing from a reaction to gadolinium which can be rather devastating. Patients with poor renal function may be at higher risk. NSF is characterized by swelling, thickening and tightening of the skin and can be fulminant in some cases. It is becoming increasingly important to check renal function in patients prior to the administration of gadolinium.

Nonspecific white matter changes in a younger patient with a history of headaches may be a sign of migraines, demyelinating disease such as multiple sclerosis, or infectious or inflammatory processes. In older patients, nonspecific white matter changes are usually secondary to chronic small vessel ischemia.

Computed Tomography (CT)

CT imaging provides excellent bony detail of the temporal bones. It is not commonly ordered in the workup of Ménière's disease. If the patient is unable to obtain an MRI due to pacemaker or other implanted materials, a high resolution CT scan of the temporal bones with and without contrast may be used to evaluate for retrocochlear lesions. One needs to pay special attention to the internal auditory canals noting any bony erosion or expansion or significant asymmetry of the IACs between the two sides. If suspicious areas are identified, an air contrast CT may be necessary. Some patients with Ménière's disease are noted to have an anterior sigmoid sinus and a more acute angle at the vestibular aqueduct, which may alter flow through the endolymphatic duct to the endolymphatic sac, thereby altering endolymphatic homeostasis. CT scan may be considered preoperatively before endolymphatic sac surgery. CT of the temporal bones in a plane parallel to the superior semicircular canal can be diagnostic for superior canal dehiscence syndrome.

Bloodwork

Bloodwork for the vestibular patient should include complete blood count (CBC), complete metabolic panel, thyroid stimulating hormone (TSH), lipid profile, and fluorescent treponemal antibiody absorption testing (FTA-Abs). This may be expanded to include autoimmune bloodwork and Lyme disease titers should the history and physical warrant such considerations.

Rotary Chair Testing and Computerized Dynamic Posturography

These tests are not useful for diagnosing Ménière's disease. Nonetheless, they may be obtained during the evaluation of a challenging vestibular patient to identify areas of abnormalities. In patients with a history of chronic imbalance, such testing may provide information suggestive of an uncompensated vestibulopathy or other chronic condition that may benefit from surgical intervention or vestibular rehabilitation.

Treatment of the Acute Attack

The treatment of Ménière's disease is prophylactic in nature, with the primary goal being to decrease the frequency and intensity of the attacks. In contrast to migraines, there is no abortive medication for an acute attack of Ménière's disease.

Treatment is symptomatic, and includes vestibular suppressants such as meclizine or diazepam. These agents may reduce the brain's response to vestibular signals and can decrease symptoms, but generally only mask the vertigo. Many vestibular suppressants may cause drowsiness, dry mouth, and blurred vision. Caution in angle-closure glaucoma, prostatic hypertrophy, pyloric or duodenal obstruction, and bladder neck obstruction needs to be observed. Meclizine decreases the excitability of the labyrinth and blocks conduction in vestibular-cerebellar pathways. These effects are associated with relief of nausea and vomiting. Other similar medications include dimenhydrinate and scopolamine. Benzodiazepines, such as diazepam (Valium), act as antiemetics and vestibular suppressants by binding to specific receptor sites which potentiate the effects of gamma-aminobutyric acid (GABA), facilitating inhibitory GABA neurotransmission and other inhibitory transmitters. Treatment with a compounded sublingual formulation of 1–2 mg of lorazepam (Ativan), has been noted to provide some relief in acute attacks with the sublingual route providing rapid onset of action even when not able to tolerate medication by mouth due to nausea and vomiting.

Anti-nausea medication such as promethazine (Phenergan) or prochlorperazine (Compazine) oral or per rectum, and ondansetron (Zofran), which is available sublingual, are prescribed for the nausea and vomiting as needed. These medications have an antidopaminergic agent that blocks postsynaptic dopaminergic receptors in the brain and reduces stimuli to the brainstem reticular system. This may explain their mechanism of action in the relief of nausea and vomiting. Should nausea and vomiting lead to dehydration, a visit to the emergency room for intravenous (IV) fluids and more aggressive nausea management and vestibular suppression is recommended.

If the patient has been having increasing frequency and intensity with clustering of attacks, increasing the diuretic to twice a day for a couple of days may return the patient to their baseline. In such instances, a short course of oral steroids may also help return them to their baseline. Occasionally, as the steroids are tapering, symptoms may flare up again in which case a 2-week high-dose steroid taper, 60 mg a day for one week tapered over the second week, may return the patient to their baseline. Antacid medication should be prescribed along with steroids. When the patient suffers an attack, they must always be aware that should they develop any other neurological symptoms not typical of their usual attacks, they should seek emergency medical evaluation to rule out the possibility of stroke. If a patient's attacks differ from their usual attacks, are of short duration and positional in nature, consideration should be given to the possibility of acute benign paroxysmal positional vertigo, common in patients with Ménière's disease.

Patients may also suffer from a significant sensorineural hearing loss without vertigo that does not recover in a few hours. In such circumstances, consideration should be given to immediate treatment with a short course of oral steroids with continued adherence to their baseline medical treatment regimen. If the hearing still does not improve, an audiogram should be obtained. If hearing loss is confirmed, one may proceed with a 2-week steroid taper with a follow-up audiogram. If the hearing loss persists, consideration should be given to intratympanic steroids.

Crisis of Tumarkin is a variant of Ménière's disease where patients suffer a drop attack, losing all muscular tone and falling to the floor suddenly, without loss of consciousness and often without warning. Patients suffering from drop attacks need aggressive management of their Ménière's disease to prevent injury from falls. As with Ménière's disease, the exact etiology of these crises are unknown. Other pathology must be ruled out before such spells can be attributed to Ménière's disease.

Medical Management of Ménière's Disease

It is very challenging to treat a condition without understanding the underlying pathophysiology. Coelho and Lalwani[15] provide an excellent review of the many possible medical and surgical treatments for Ménière's disease. Treatment is based on symptoms and primarily directed toward the control of vertigo. The second goal of treatment is to preserve hearing. Some treatments have proven effective and are well established. Other treatments are less mainstream but are used successfully. There are few well-designed, randomized, double-blind, placebo-controlled trials in the study of Ménière's disease.

Most otolaryngologists will institute lifestyle modifications, a low salt diet and a diuretic. Patients are often counseled to avoid caffeine, alcohol, nicotine, stress, fatigue, monosodium glutamate, and any known allergens in an effort to control symptoms. Some women may note increasing symptoms around their menses, possibly associated with water retention. Guidelines for a low salt diet typically recommend less than 1.5 to 2 g of sodium per day. Such therapies are effective for most patients with Ménière's disease. Some patients may notice an exacerbation of their symptoms when eating food outside the home or with increased salt consumption. A few patients may opt for natural homeopathic diuretics, which may be of benefit for mild symptoms.

Diuretics

Diuretics are used in the treatment of Ménière's disease based on the theory that there is an imbalance in endolymphatic homeostasis leading to increased endolymphatic pressure (hydrops). Diuretics serve to lower the endolymphatic pressure, albeit the exact mechanism is unknown. One of the more common diuretics used is Dyazide (hydrochlorothiazide 25 mg/triamterene 37.5 mg). Hydrochlorothiazide is a potassium wasting diuretic while the triamterene is a potassium sparing diuretic. Some otolaryngologists will prescribe hydrochlorothiazide 25 mg along with a potassium supplement (eg, KCl 10 mEq per day). Patients should be counseled regarding the alternatives, risks, benefits, and complications of diuretic therapy, especially hypokalemia. Routine bloodwork should be checked after beginning diuretic therapy and on a yearly basis. Patients who subsequently complain of leg cramps or palpitations should have their electrolytes evaluated to ensure they are not hypokalemic. Should the patient develop such symptoms, they should be instructed to hold the diuretic until the bloodwork results are known. In the meantime, they may increase their intake of foods that are high in potassium, such as bananas. If they are found to be hypokalemic and symptoms are mild, they may be given oral potassium replacement therapy and have the bloodwork rechecked. For severe symptoms or significant hypokalemia, emergency medical attention should be sought. Many patients may come to the physician already on a diuretic for hypertension or other reasons. In such cases, consulting with the primary care physician and adjusting the dose may be beneficial. Patients with sulfa allergies may be started on triamterene alone, but they should not take potassium supplements as triamterene may cause hyperkalemia. Many patients allergic to sulfa tolerate hydrochlorothiazide without any difficulty.

Thirlwall and Kundu[16] reviewed the literature to assess the efficacy of diuretic therapy in patients with Ménière's disease. They did not find any articles that met the inclusion criteria of randomized controlled trials. Despite the lack of well-designed trials, diuretic therapy is generally considered to be an effective, standardized therapy for the treatment of patients with Ménière's disease.

It is important to counsel the patient that diuretic therapy is a long-term treatment course. They should remain on medication until they are symptom-free for a minimum of 6 to 12 months. Many patients are noncompliant and stop the medication once they are feeling better, only to relapse. If relapse occurs, the medication should be restarted. It has been noted that many patients experience a remission of their vertigo after a period of about two years, although a few patients will continue to suffer from MD for many years beyond this.

Steroids

Steroids may be used to treat exacerbations of MD. Patients with Ménière's disease often suffer from a regular cycle of attacks. When the regular cycle of attacks increases in frequency and intensity, and begin to cluster, steroids may sometimes return them to their baseline. A brief trial with an oral steroid such as methylprednisolone (eg, Medrol Dosepak) may be beneficial. Attacks may be vertiginous in nature or simply manifest as prolonged episodes of decreased hearing without vertigo. Both circumstances should be treated. Changes in the frequency and intensity of tinnitus and fullness may herald vertigo and hearing loss, but such symptoms may be observed until there is actual vertigo or hearing loss. Patient adherence to their baseline regimen should be encouraged. For more severe symptoms or incomplete resolution after a Medrol Dosepak, a 2-week high dose steroid taper may be effective. The exact mechanism of action of steroids in Ménière's disease is unclear. Steroids have many potential beneficial effects including anti-inflammatory properties, diuretic effects, and neuroprotective properties. All of these may contribute to their beneficial effect in Ménière's disease. Some patients respond well to steroids and may require low dose steroids for long periods of time to maintain adequate control. This observation may suggest that in some cases, Ménière's disease may be autoimmune or allergic in nature.

Steroids have a significant number of expected side effects which the patient should be made aware of, including insomnia, weight gain, anxiety, restlessness, gastrointestinal complaints, and peptic ulcer disease. Gastrointestinal prophylaxis should be given when high-dose steroids are used. More infrequent complications of steroids may be reviewed with the patient as well, to include aseptic necrosis of the hip, cataracts, and with prolonged use, hypothalamic pituitary adrenal axis suppression. Steroids are contraindicated in patients with glaucoma, and their treating ophthalmologist should be contacted before instituting such therapy.

Allergy Management

Allergic evaluation and management should be considered in selected patients who give a history of bilateral symptoms, symptoms related to certain foods or seasons, or a history of more traditional allergic symptoms. Some of these patients respond less effectively to traditional treatment, but tend to respond well to steroids.

Other Treatments

Betahistine (Serc) is a vasodilator that is used in Europe and Latin America. It is possible that a vascular etiology may be involved in Ménière's disease. In such patients, vasodilator therapy may be beneficial. James and Burton[17] conducted a literature review on the use of betahistine and Ménière's disease. They found no studies that met the highest quality standard set for the review. Nonetheless, most available trials do suggest a reduction in vertigo frequency, but without significant effects on hearing loss. No serious adverse effects have been identified. Betahistine is not approved for use in the United States by the Federal Drug Administration. Adult dosing may be initiated at 8 mg two to three times a day, and increased up to a maximum of 16 mg three times a day.

Lipoflavinoids are a nonprescription vitamin supplement that may reduce the symptoms of Ménière's disease, although there is no good evidence to support this. The mechanism of action is unknown, but may possibly relate to changes in the microcirculation.

Treatment of Migraine-Associated Vertigo

These patients tend to have more chronic symptoms and abortive migraine medications have not proven very effective. The first steps toward controlling migraines should involve lifestyle modifications to include the avoidance of dietary triggers, developing a regular sleep cycle and avoiding sudden exposure to bright lights, stress or other known triggers. These patients are best treated by migraine prophylactic medications such as beta blockers (eg, propranolol), calcium channel blockers (eg, verapamil), anti-epileptic medications (eg, topiramate), or antidepressants such as a tricyclics (eg, nortriptyline) or selective serotonin-reuptake inhibitors (eg, venlafaxine). These patients should have a neurology consult and preferably have their migraines managed by a migraine subspecialist.

Managing Anxiety

Patients with vestibular disorders often suffer from elevated anxiety. Anxiety is often increased due to the patients overwhelming concern about their next attack. Many of the medications used in the treatment of MD, such as diazepam, meclizine, and promethazine, have sedative effects. The patient should be counseled with regards to their anxiety, and if they have a known or suspected underlying anxiety disorder, referral to a mental health specialist may be beneficial. Some mild sedatives taken on an as-needed basis may be quite beneficial for these patients.

Auditory Rehabilitation

Many patients with Ménière's disease develop a significant sensorineural hearing loss. While the hearing loss is fluctuant, it is difficult to fit appropriate amplification. These patients may receive limited benefit from a hearing aid. As time passes, the hearing stabilizes and many of these patients will be good candidates for hearing aids. Appropriate amplification may assist some patients with their tinnitus as well.

Vestibular Rehabilitation

Vestibular rehabilitation does not play a role in the acute attack of MD. Shepard summarized that vestibular rehabilitation may be beneficial in patients with a history of chronic imbalance and head movement sensitivity in between acute attacks of vertigo.[4] Such therapy may also benefit patients with a unilateral vestibular weakness on ENG. Also, those with multifactorial dizziness with contributions from a neurological or musculoskeletal disorder may benefit from therapy. Older patients often have chronic imbalance that may benefit from a course of vestibular rehabilitation. Exacerbations of benign paroxysmal positional vertigo, which do not respond to in office canalith repositioning maneuvers, would also benefit from a course of vestibular rehabilitation. Patients undergoing vestibular ablation procedures such as intratympanic gentamicin, vestibular neurectomy or labyrinthectomy may also benefit from vestibular rehabilitation should they have difficulty compensating after their procedure.

Other Office-Based Treatments

Office-based management of Ménière's disease may involve several minor surgical procedures such as myringotomy tube placement, intratympanic dexamethasone, and intratympanic gentamicin. The Meniett device (Medtronic Xomed, Jacksonville, FL) is used to treat Ménière's disease based on the theory that positive pressure reduces the endolymphatic hydrops and reduces symptom intensity and frequency. To use this device, patients must have a myringotomy tube placed in the affected ear. Patients then place the device in the affected ear and it automatically generates a series of sound pressure waves, which transmit through the myringotomy tube to the labyrinth. Gates et al[18] published their long-term follow-up with the Meniett device with 67% of patients reporting significantly improved vertigo control. The automated Meniett device is expensive and may not be covered by insurance companies. There also is a manual version: the P-100 (Enttex, Hanover, Germany) which is inexpensive.

Tinnitus and Aural Fullness

Oftentimes treatment of the Ménière's disease will lead to decreased symptoms with regards to tinnitus and aural fullness. When these symptoms are the patient's primary complaints, medical management should be optimized. Fluctuating tinnitus may be difficult to deal with. However, if the patient has a constant baseline tinnitus that is bothersome, they may benefit from tinnitus retraining therapy or the Oasis device (Neuromonics, Bethlehem, PA). There is no role for surgical therapy for these symptoms.

Future Directions

One should keep up to date in areas of electrodiagnostic testing with VEMPs as well as radiologic advances, including enhanced imaging with MRI. As knowledge of genetics increases, perhaps some of the underlying genetic causes of Ménière's disease may be elucidated to allow for more directed therapies in the future.

Summary

Ménière's disease is a poorly understood condition which can lead to serious patient disability. Our lack of understanding makes it a frustrating problem for both patients and physicians to manage. It is important to provide support for these patients as many of them feel misunderstood. One should use the treatments outlined throughout this chapter as a ladder to help these patients manage their disease and symptoms in a minimally disruptive and invasive manner, proceeding to the next step only as the previous ones fail. There needs to be good communication between the physician and their patient to decide when to move to the next step. It is unlikely that a single etiology will be found to explain symptoms in this vast group of patients. One hopes that as our understanding of the disease process evolves and we are able to identify the cause of disease in individual patients, we will be able to tailor a more specific treatment for the individual patient with overall improvement in treatment outcomes. Fortunately, most patients will respond to the management strategies outlined above. For those who do not, there are surgical interventions that provide significant control of vertigo.

REFERENCES

1. Merchant SN, Adams JC, Nadol JB Jr. Pathophysiology of Ménière's syndrome: are symptoms caused by endolymphatic hydrops. *Otol Neurotol*. 2006;26:74–81.
2. Antonio SM, Friedman R. Ménière's disease. In: Jackler RK, Brackmann DE eds. *Neurotology*. Philadelphia, PA: Elsevier Mosby; 2005:621–638.
3. Committee on Hearing and Equilibrium. Guidelines for the diagnosis and evaluation of therapy in Ménière's disease. American Academy of Otolaryngology-Head and Neck Surgery Foundation, Inc. *Otolaryngol Head Neck Surg*. 1995;113(3):181.
4. Shepard NT. Differentiation of Ménière's disease and migraine-associated dizziness: a review. *J Am Acad Audiol*. 2006;17(1):69–80.
5. Gianoli GJ. DDX: Fluctuating vestibular disease. In: Goebel JA, ed. *Practical Management of the Dizzy Patient*. Philadelphia, PA: Lippicott Williams and Wilkins, 2001: 211–224.
6. Battista RA. Audiometric findings of patients with migraine-associated dizziness. *Otol Neurotol*. 2004;25(6): 987–992.
7. Hain TC, Rudisill H. ECOG testing (Eloectrocochleography). Last updated Dec. 31, 2007. Retrieved January 31, 2008, from http://www.dizziness-and-balance.com.
8. Kim HH, Kumar A, Battista RA, Wiet RJ. Electrocochleography in patients with Ménière's disease. *Am J Otolaryngol*. 2005;26(2):128–131.
9. Murofushi T, Shimizu K, Takegoshi H, Cheng PW. Diagnostic value of prolonged latencies in the vestibular evoked myogenic potential. *Arch Otolaryngol Head Neck Surg*. 2005;127(9):1069–1072.
10. Rauch SD, Zhou G, Kujawa SG, Guinan JJ, Herrmann BS. Vestibular evoked myogenic potentials show altered tuning in patients with Ménière's disease. *Otol Neurotol*. 2004;25(3):333–338.
11. Rauch SD. Vestibular evoked myogenic potentials. *Curr Opin Otolaryngol Head Neck Surg*. 2006;14(5):299–304.
12. Liao LJ, Young YH. Vestibular evoked myogenic potentials in basilar artery migraine. *Laryngoscope*. 2004;114(7): 1305–1309.
13. Naganawa S, Komada T, Fukatsu H, Ishigaki T, Takizawa O. Observation of contrast enhancement in the cochlear fluid space of healthy subjects using a 3D-FLAIR sequence at 3 tesla. *Eur Radiol*. 2006;16(3):733–737.
14. Carfrae MJ, Holtzman A, Eames F, Parnes SM, Lupinetti A. 3-Tesla delayed contrast magnetic resonance imaging evaluation of Ménière's disease. *Laryngoscope*. 2008; 118(3):501–505.
15. Coelho DH, Lalwani AK. Medical management of Ménière's disease. *Laryngoscope*. 2008;118(6):1099–1108.
16. Thirlwall AS, Kundu S. Diuretics for Ménière's disease or syndrome. *Cochrane Database Syst Rev*. 2006;3:CD003599.

17. James AL, Burton MJ. Betahistine for Ménière's disease or syndrome. *Cochrane Database Syst Rev.* 2001:CD001873.
18. Gates GA, Verrall A, Green JD Jr, Tucci DL, Telian SA. Meniett clinical trial: long-term follow-up. *Arch Otolaryngol Head Neck Surg.* 2006;132(12):1311–1316.

CHAPTER 18

Migraine-Related Vertigo

Eric Sargent

INTRODUCTION

Migraine, defined as a benign recurring headache and/or neurologic dysfunction with pain-free interludes, is extremely common: >10% of Americans (~6% of men, 15–17% of women) suffer from the condition. Furthermore, migraine varies widely between patients in frequency, duration, and disability.[1] In migraine aura presenting as vertigo with or without headache, reported symptoms may vary from intense rotational vertigo to (commonly) a sense of linear rocking and swaying. In the absence of a reliable objective test for the condition, the diagnosis of migraine-related vertigo is based on clinical history and the exclusion of other organic processes.[2]

The pathophysiology of migraine may be an abnormal sensitivity of neurovascular reactions to stimuli. Calcium channel function and cell membrane sensitivity, particularly in smooth muscle and certain neurons, have been implicated in the increased vasoreactivity reported in migraineurs. Migraine is considered hereditary in 75 to 95% of cases. Discovery of gene loci for familial hemiplegic migraine supports the hypothesis of a genetic basis of migraine.[3] Of three known "migraine genes," one codes for components of a neuronal calcium channel called the P/Q channel, one encodes a neuronal sodium/potassium ion pump, and a third encodes a neuronal sodium channel. These genes can also carry mutations associated with epilepsy. Collectively, such disorders are now known as "channelopathies," acknowledging their shared foundation in disordered ion channel function.[4]

The International Headache Society (IHS) has categorized migraine into two major types: migraine without aura (common migraine) and migraine with aura (classic migraine).[5] A subclassification of migraine with aura, termed *basilar migraine*, was the first described symptom complex of migraine-related vertigo. Its presentation suggests dysfunction in the distribution of the basilar artery resulting in two or more of the following: visual symptoms in both eyes, dysarthria, vertigo, tinnitus, decreased hearing, double vision, ataxia, bilateral paresthesias, bilateral pareses, or decreased level of consciousness.

Recognition of migraine by the otolaryngologist or otologist is important because many migraine sufferers will present with migraine-related dizziness, whether or not headache is associated with the symptoms. Such manifestations have been labeled as a type of *migraine aura without headache* by the International Headache Society classification system. Previous terms have included migraine equivalent, migraine accompaniment, or acephalgic migraine.[5]

Despite many reports in the literature, the recognition of migraine-related dizziness as a diagnostic entity has been controversial due to the lack of reliable objective tests to diagnose migraine. Unsteadiness, disequilibrium, or episodic vertigo occurring alone or as an aura to the headache characterizes its presentation. It has been described under several labels: vertiginous migraine equivalent, episodic giddiness, benign recurrent vertigo, recurrent vestibulopathy, Bickerstaff's syndrome, syncopal migraine, and migraine vestibulopathy. The character of dizziness associated with migraine differs in reports, with the spectrum of presentations spanning from predominantly true vertigo to predominantly nonvertiginous dizziness to a combination of both.

Like migraine in general, the diagnosis of migraine-related dizziness is based on clinical history and the exclusion of other organic processes. Unfortunately, the protean nature of migraine-related dizziness, coupled with the lack of reliable objective tests, often complicate and delays diagnosis, occasionally prompting what proves eventually to be unnecessary labyrinthine surgery. Treatment of migraine-related dizziness with already established antimigraine pharmacotherapy has been effective in numerous published reports.

DIAGNOSIS

Like other disease entities without objective confirmatory tests, vertiginous migraine (without headache) is a diagnosis of exclusion. Illnesses that should specifically be excluded are seizure disorder, demyelination, and cerebrovascular disorders. The isolated Ménière's syndrome tetrad (unilateral tinnitus, aural fullness, fluctuating hearing loss, and episodic vertigo) can usually be determined. However, one must remember that the incidence of migraine is twice as common in Ménière's patients. Many patients thought to have "pure" Ménière's syndrome on closer questioning also report neurocognitive symptoms outside the tetrad (eg, sound and/or light sensitivity, binaural fullness, vague headache or pressure, stupor ["brain fog" aka "migraine stupor"]). These "Ménière's" patients often have a gratifying response to antimigraine treatment.

Audiovestibular testing in patients who ultimately respond to antimigraine therapy follows few rules. Unilateral or bilateral vestibular hyporeflexia, unilateral or binaural hearing loss (either typical low-frequency Ménière's type or atypical high frequency loss) has been observed in many patients successfully treated with migraine preventive medication. Similarly, electrocochleography does not seem to predict success or failure of antimigraine therapy in these patients: marked unilateral or bilateral abnormalities have been noted in many patients with the condition treated by the author.

One relatively reliable indicator is bilateral caloric hyperreflexivity. Patients with vertiginous migraine often have dramatic vestibular hypersensitivity (as many other migraineurs have auditory or visual hypersensitivity) reflected in their symptoms as "motion sickness" (often lifelong) and in vestibular testing with summed total slow-phase eye-velocity on air-caloric testing that easily exceeds 150°/sec. As other CNS pathological entities, such as demyelination, also may cause this finding, their exclusion is critical.

TREATMENT

When other otologic or neurologic causes of dizziness have been excluded or, if in the case of Ménière's syndrome and some patients with positional nystagmus migraine is suspected to be the cause or strongly associated, anti-migraine treatment is initiated. Fortunately, for many patients education about the condition and dietary modification is all that is required. Reassurance is important in all cases. Patients are often happy to be given a diagnosis after what, for many, is a frustrating, prolonged, expensive, and fruitless process of evaluation, testing, and perplexing visits to primary care physicians, neurologists/neurotologists, and psychiatrists.

About half of migraine patients can identify dietary, environmental, and hormonal triggers of migraine. The common feature of foods that trigger migraine is a high level of tyramine, which is naturally present in aged food. These foods include cured or smoked meats, aged cheeses, avocado, guacamole, bananas, and dried fruit. Other common food triggers include chocolate, citrus fruit, monosodium glutamate, aspartame, beer, and wine.

Migraine may also be precipitated by environmental changes: barometric pressure changes, perfumes, exercise, and bright or flickering light, among many others. Many patients with migraine and migraine-related vertigo without headache often experience seasonal variation of symptoms, as do classic "Ménière's syndrome" patients.

If dietary and environmental modification fails to adequately control migraine-related vertigo, preventive therapy with medication may be initiated. There are no firm indicators of when medication should be used and, as in patients with migraine headache, migraine-related vertigo is usually undertreated. Generally, if patients have recurring symptoms that, in their opinion, interfere significantly with their daily routines preventive therapy should be considered.

There are no formal guidelines available for the treatment of isolated migraine-related vertigo. However, the guidelines for the prevention of migraine promulgated by the US Headache Consortium are a valuable tool.[6] Among the principles of care recommended by the consortium, and adapted by the author, these are most applicable to the patients that will be seen by neurotologists:

1. Initiating therapy with the lowest effective dose of a given medication and increasing the dose over time until clinical benefits are observed in the absence of adverse effects or until limited by adverse effects.
2. Giving medication a sufficient trial (2–3 months in many cases).
3. Avoid interfering medications.
4. Use long-acting formulations where possible to improve compliance.
5. Monitor therapy regularly.
6. Re-evaluate therapy in stabilized patients and taper and/or discontinue medication after a symptom-free period.
7. Select medication that treats both the migraine-related vertigo and comorbid conditions (for example, migraine-related vertigo patients with disturbed sleep and depression may benefit from a tricyclic antidepressant).
8. Avoid medications that should be used with caution in or are contraindicated by comorbid conditions (for example, beta-blockers in asthmatics or unstable diabetics).
9. Beware of drug interactions.
10. Use preventive drugs in pregnant women or women who intend to become pregnant with special care and only if absolutely necessary.

The most common drugs mentioned in articles by neurotologists for migraine-related vertigo are tricyclic antidepressants, beta-blockers, calcium channel blockers, and Topomax. Each has proponents and detractors. Table 18–1 summarizes specific recommendations, contraindications, and potential side effects of these medications. The American Headache Consortium ranks the preventive medications based on their established clinical efficacy, significant adverse events, safety profile, and clinical experience.

CONCLUSION

The diagnosis of migraine-related vertigo is generally one of exclusion, especially in the absence of a typical headache. However, the physician who approaches dizzy patients with an open mind and tries to integrate symptoms into a unified diagnosis will find that these patients often have a rapid and gratifying response to treatment.

Table 18–1. Medical Treatment for Migraine-Related Vertigo (both abortive and prophylactic medications are described)

Drug (Class)	Frequency of Adverse Reactions	Comments
Amitriptyline (Tricyclic Antidepressant) (Efficacious doses in clinical trials: 30–150 mg/day)	Frequent	Drowsiness, weight gain, and anticholinergic adverse events are common; long-term weight gain can be troublesome. Particularly useful in patients with coexistent depression.
Nortriptyline (Tricyclic Antidepressant) (Efficacious doses in clinical trials not established. Clinical experience suggests similar to Amitriptyline)	Frequent	Better tolerated than amitriptyline.
Atenolol (Beta-Blocker) (Efficacious doses in clinical trials: 100 mg/day) **Propranolol** (Efficacious doses in clinical trials: 80 to 240 mg/day)	Infrequent	Adverse events include tiredness, fatigue, and dizziness. May not be accepted by active patients (eg, athletes). Particularly helpful in patients with coexistent anxiety/panic attacks and essential tremors (propranolol). When propranolol is used in conjunction with Rizatriptan, a lower dose of rizatriptan should be given. Should not be used in patients with coexistent asthma, cardiac insufficiency, or Raynaud's disease. May exacerbate depression.
Verapamil (Calcium-Channel Blocker) (Efficacious doses in clinical trials: 240 mg/day)	Occasional	Constipation common. Do not use if conduction block is present. Alternative to beta-blockers in athletes. Recommended in patients with coexistent stroke, or for prolonged or atypical migraine aura. Monitor liver function regularly as dose is increased.
Topiramate (Antiepileptic, mechanism unknown) (Efficacious doses: not established in placebo-controlled trials)	Occasional	Occasional CNS adverse events (sedation and cognitive impairment). Kidney stones and weight loss with topiramate. Sedation could occur at doses of topiramate required to achieve efficacy.

Source: Adapted from the US Headache Consortium, 2006.

REFERENCES

1. Stewart WF, Shechter A, Rasmussen RK. Migraine prevalence. A review of population-based studies. *Neurology*. 1994;44(6 suppl 4):S17–S23.
2. Le T, Burch C, Sargent E. Intracranial blood flow velocities and CO_2 reactivity in diagnosing migraine-related dizziness. *Otolaryngol Head Neck Surg*. 2004;131:736–739.
3. Ophoff RA, Terwindt GM, Vergouwe MN, et al. Familial hemiplegic migraine and episodic ataxia type-2 are caused by mutations in the Ca^{2+} channel gene CACNL1A4. *Cell*. 1996;87:543–552.
4. Dodick DW, Gargus JJ. Why migraines strike. *Sci Am*. 2008;299:56–63.
5. Headache Classification Committee of the International Headache Society. Classification and diagnostic criteria for headache disorders, cranial neuralgias and facial pain. *Cephalgia*. 1988;8:19–73.
6. http://www.aan.com/professionals/practice/pdfs/gl0090.pdf; 2006.

CHAPTER 19

Surgical Therapy for Vertigo

Michael LaRouere

INTRODUCTION

Ménière's disease is effectively managed by a low salt diet and diuretic therapy. Almost two-thirds of patients exhibit a marked reduction of their vertigo symptoms following this protocol.[1] Additional medical treatment strategies include vestibular suppressants such as Valium or oral steroids. Valium, used either for acute symptoms or prophylactically, has been in use for decades.[2] In patients who continue to have symptoms despite dietary and diuretic therapy, Valium in a dose of 2 mg three times a day may further reduce vertigo symptoms. Likewise, intermittent bursts of oral steroids may reduce vertigo symptoms both acutely and occasionally for prolonged periods of time. In addition, hearing improvement has been reported following oral steroid administration and sudden drops in hearing appear to best respond to this treatment modality.[3]

If medical management fails to control spells of vertigo associated with Ménière's disease, then more aggressive therapy may be warranted. Medical failure can vary from patient to patient. Numerous factors are taken into consideration, such as the frequency and severity of vertigo episodes, the patient's age, overall health status, and their occupation. The hearing status of the affected ear is ascertained as well as the risk of bilateral disease. Ménière's disease has been shown to occur bilaterally in up to 40% of patients.[4] Furthermore, the likelihood that bilateral disease will develop occurs earlier in the course of the disease process.

SURGICAL MANAGEMENT

Surgical therapy for vertigo can be classified into two categories: vestibular preservation and vestibular ablative techniques. Vestibular preservation treatments include intratympanic perfusion with steroids and endolymphatic sac surgery. Vestibular ablative techniques include those that preserve hearing (vestibular nerve section, intratympanic gentamicin, and intramuscular streptomycin) and those procedures that sacrifice hearing (labyrinthectomy and translabyrinthine vestibular nerve section).

Vestibular Preservation Techniques

Intratympanic Steroid Perfusion

Intratympanic perfusion of the middle ear with steroids has received much attention. Intratympanic steroids have been used to treat both the hearing loss and spells of vertigo associated with Ménière's disease.[5] Intratympanic steroid use for sudden sensorineural hearing loss not associated with Ménière's disease has gained acceptance as well.[6] The exact mechanism of action of steroids on the inner ear is not clear. The duration of the effects of intratympanic steroids appears variable. The most ideal frequency of steroid administration is not known, although the only reported deleterious effect has been that of tympanic membrane perforations.[5] As of this writing there is no prescribed dose, type of steroid, or mechanism of injection that is universally accepted. Commonly, 10 to 24 mg/mL of dexamethasone is injected via a spinal needle through an eardrum anesthetized with phenol. Approximately 0.2 to 0.5 cc is infiltrated. In many patients, one to two injections are done over a period of 1 month. Some patients require injections every 2 or 3 months in order to obtain relief of their symptoms. In our practice the only adverse effect has been persistent tympanic membrane microperforations. All patients treated in this manner continue on a low sodium diet and diuretic therapy.

Endolymphatic Sac Surgery

Endolymphatic sac surgery has been met with roller coaster excitement over the past 30 years. Ever since Portmann[7] described endolymphatic sac surgery in 1926, this procedure has had its proponents and its critics. Initial reports of endolymphatic sac surgery estimated that 70% of patients had a marked reduction or elimination of their vertigo spells.[8] In 1981 Thomsen and co-workers[9] reported that endolymphatic sac surgery and mastoidectomy (their placebo) were equivalent in reducing the vertigo attacks associated with Ménière's disease. In a 1989 Glasscock article,[10] the authors abandoned sac surgery due to its low rate of complete vertigo control. Some recent studies have shown endolymphatic sac surgery to be effective in 85% of patients 2 years postoperatively.[11] Our experience has mirrored these recent studies. For many years, endolymphatic sac surgery was the initial procedure performed for patients with Ménière's disease. This was then replaced by the vestibular nerve section. Currently, both endolymphatic sac surgery and intratympanic perfusion therapies are the initial procedures of choice for patients who fail medical therapy.

Endolymphatic sac surgery can be done through a variety of techniques including endolymphatic sac with subarachnoid shunt, endolymphatic sac with mastoid shunt, or wide bony decompression of the endolymphatic sac (Figure 19–1). All three approaches have yielded similar results in that 70 to

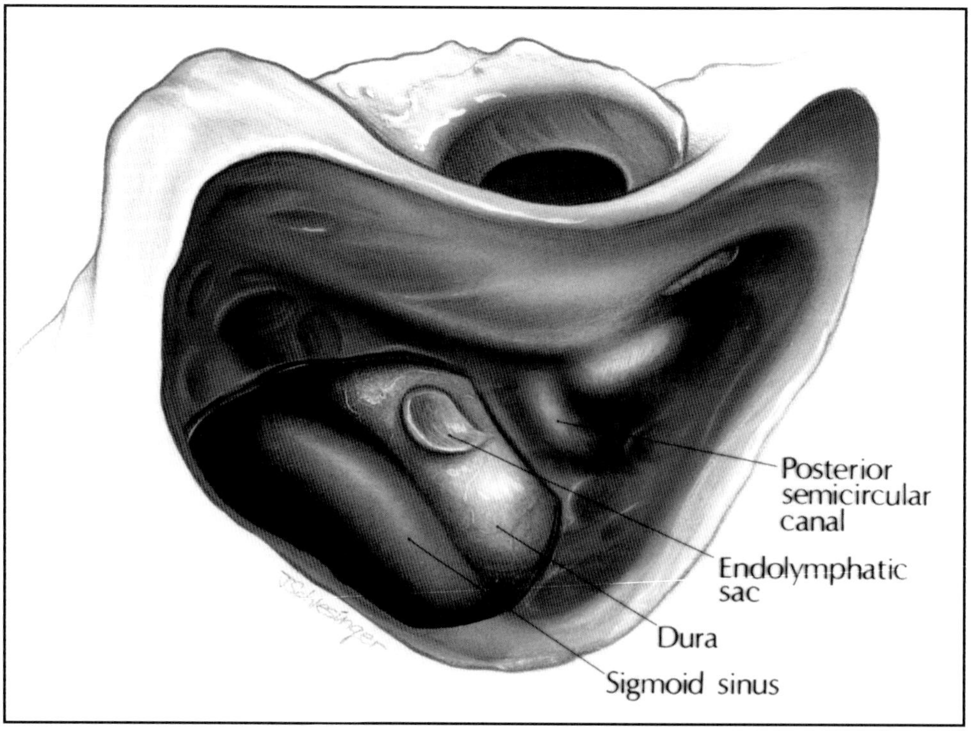

Figure 19–1. Left mastoidectomy performed with wide bony decompression of the endolymphatic sac.

80% of patients have a marked reduction or elimination of their vertigo spells. It has been our preference to perform a wide bony decompression of the sigmoid sinus and posterior fossa dura including the endolymphatic sac. The endolymphatic sac can be identified by following a line parallel to the horizontal canal and perpendicular to the posterior canal toward the sigmoid sinus (Donaldson's line). The sac can be found inferior to this line along the posterior fossa dura. Care must be taken to avoid injury to the posterior semicircular canal and the facial nerve. In our experience, by not shunting the endolymphatic sac, the rate of sensorineural hearing loss has been near zero. Vertigo control has been 85% at two years and many patients have demonstrated hearing stabilization or improvement.[11]

Recently, a quality of life study by Kato et al[12] examined the effect of endolymphatic sac surgery on three domains that determine quality of life: physical, emotional, and social well-being. The authors found that 87% of patients reported significant improvement in quality of life scores after endolymphatic sac decompression without shunting.[12]

Interestingly, in Glasscock's 1989 article[10] in which he abandoned sac surgery, 71% of his patients were "very pleased" with the results of their surgery. In Pillsbury's re-review of Thomsen's mastoidectomy "sham" study data,[13] 71% of the endolymphatic sac/mastoid shunt group improved where as 47% of the placebo group improved using 1985 Academy guidelines for the treatment of Ménière's disease. It is also compelling to note that endolymphatic sac surgery, done in the past in non-Ménière's disease patients, has met with little success arguing against the placebo effect of this procedure being the sole mechanism of action.

Currently, a wide bony decompression of the endolymphatic sac is offered to patients with relatively good hearing who have failed maximum medical treatment. Revision endolymphatic sac decompressions are occasionally performed for those patients who initially did well for several years and then had a recurrence of their vertigo spells. Like Paparella,[14] it has been our experience that about 90% of patients show improvement after revision sac decompression if they showed initial sustained improvement following their first surgery. Conversely, revision sac decompression in patients who initially failed sac surgery has generally been met with failure.

Vestibular Ablative Techniques

Intratympanic Gentamicin

The use of intratympanic aminoglycosides has evolved similar to endolymphatic sac surgery. Shuknecht,[15] introduced the use of high dose streptomycin for the treatment of Ménière's disease in 1956. Graham et al[16] introduced titration streptomycin therapy for bilateral Ménière's disease in 1984. In 1991, Magnusson and Padoan[17] introduced low dose intratympanic gentamicin. Prior to this, the ototoxic effect of this medication outweighed its vestibulotoxic benefit. Nedzelski[18] reported the vertigo control rate of patients treated with intratympanic gentamicin to be 83%; however, when trying to achieve total ablation of the vestibular system there was a 27% rate of sensorineural hearing loss, 10% of this being a profound loss. Because of this information many have altered their technique with careful titration of gentamicin causing partial ablation of the vestibular system with a concomitant lower risk of sensorineural hearing loss. With aminoglycosides, gentamicin in particular, the vestibulotoxic effect is cumulative. Thus, the amount and frequency of administration of gentamicin should be approached cautiously. Our current protocol involves intratympanic injection of gentamicin via a spinal needle after phenol has been applied to the tympanic membrane. The injection site is just superior to the round window. Occasionally, a control hole is made in the anterior portion of the tympanic membrane to release pressure. Between 0.2 to 0.5 cc of a buffered 27.5 mg/mL solution of gentamicin is slowly injected. Injections are performed every two to four weeks until symptoms have dissipated or hearing declines. Our results mirror those of Nedzelski[18] in that 85% of patients with Ménière's disease show a marked reduction or elimination of their vertigo spells. There is a very low (5%) risk of sensorineural hearing loss if patients have normal hearing pre-treatment. If patients have a pre-existing sensorineural hearing loss our numbers approach those of Nedzelski's in that 30% demonstrate further hearing loss due to intratympanic gentamicin.

The greater number of treatments further increases the risk of sensorineural hearing loss. There also appears to be a small subset of patients who have a genetic susceptibility to aminoglycosides and could potentially lose hearing with just one injection.

Vestibular Neurectomy

Vestibular neurectomy has long been the gold standard for treatment of unilateral Ménière's disease in a good hearing ear. Silverstein and Kemink both reported success rates of greater than 95% for the control of vertigo following vestibular nerve section.[19,20] The risk of sensorineural hearing loss in experienced hands is less than 1%. The approach used for vestibular nerve section has changed throughout the years. Initially, a middle cranial fossa approach was used. Despite high success rates regarding vertigo control, the risks of facial nerve injury and sensorineural hearing loss remained high. Neurotologists then switched to a retrolabyrinthine approach.[21] The success rate of vertigo control was high. Facial nerve and hearing results were excellent, but there remained a relatively high risk of cerebrospinal fluid leakage. Today, most surgeons perform vestibular nerve section via retrosigmoid approach with overall excellent results (Figure 19–2). Recently, we have been performing totally endoscopic retrosigmoid vestibular nerve section. In addition to overall good results (97% vertigo elimination, less than 1% sensorineural hearing loss, and 0% facial nerve weakness) our operative time is reduced and our length of hospitalization has been reduced by one-third. With vestibular nerve section, the patient must weigh the risk of a craniotomy. The patient must also be aware of the risk of postoperative disequilibrium. This occurs with all ablative procedures including vestibular nerve section, intratympanic gentamicin, and labyrinthectomy. Usually, the postoperative disequilibrium is mild; however, in some reported series the disequilibrium has been moderate to severe in over 25% of patients.[22]

Labyrinthectomy

Labyrinthectomy continues to be the preferred procedure for those patients with unilateral Ménière's disease and poor hearing. The benefit of the proce-

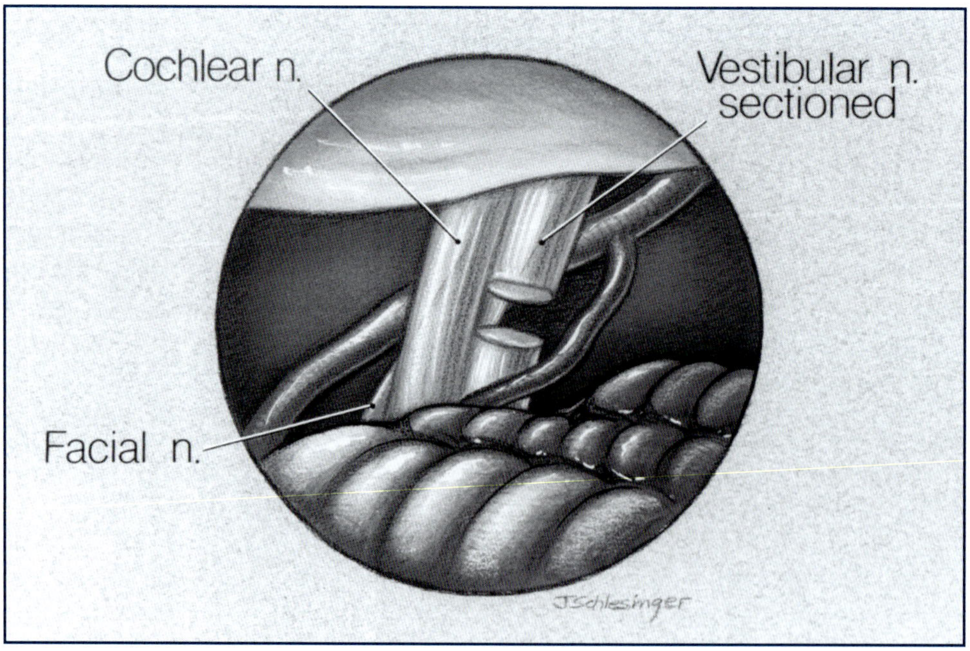

Figure 19–2. Endoscopic retrosigmoid vestibular nerve section.

dure is complete removal of the neuroepithelium of the vestibular system. The obvious negative is the hearing loss that occurs as the result of this approach. This hearing loss may be assisted with the use of a CROS hearing aid or a bone-anchored hearing implant (BAHA). Two techniques of labyrinthectomy are currently used: transcanal and transmastoid. The transcanal approach, as advocated by Armstrong, which can be performed under local anesthesia, has over a 90% success rate; however, there is a risk of retained neuroepithelium and continued dizziness.[23]

The transmastoid approach allows for direct visualization of the labyrinth with a lower risk of leaving behind neuroepithelium (Figure 19–3). A quality of life study by Diaz et al[24] shows transmastoid labyrinthectomy to be an excellent procedure for severe Ménière's disease. Ninety-eight percent of patients had improvement in total quality of life score after labyrinthectomy. Patients did not report a significant loss of quality of life in terms of their hearing loss.[24]

Translabyrinthine vestibular nerve section appears to offer limited benefit over transmastoid labyrinthectomy for vertigo control. The risks, including facial weakness and CSF leak, seem to outweigh its advantages. If a patient fails labyrinthectomy it is more likely that Ménière's disease has surfaced in the contralateral ear or there was a failure to remove all neuroepithelium.

Current Treatment Protocols

There are multiple options for the treatment of vertigo in patients who fail maximum medical treatment. Currently, in our practice, intratympanic steroids are used if diet therapy and diuretic use fail. Subsequently, either endolymphatic sac decompression or intratympanic gentamicin is recommended. In those patients with pre-existing sensorineural hearing loss, endolymphatic sac surgery is favored due to the slight risk of hearing loss with gentamicin injections. If endolymphatic sac surgery fails either intratympanic gentamicin or vestibular nerve section is recommended if the hearing is intact. Retrosigmoid nerve section is now done with an endoscopic approach. In patients with poor hearing and unilateral Ménière's disease transmastoid labyrinthectomy is recommended.

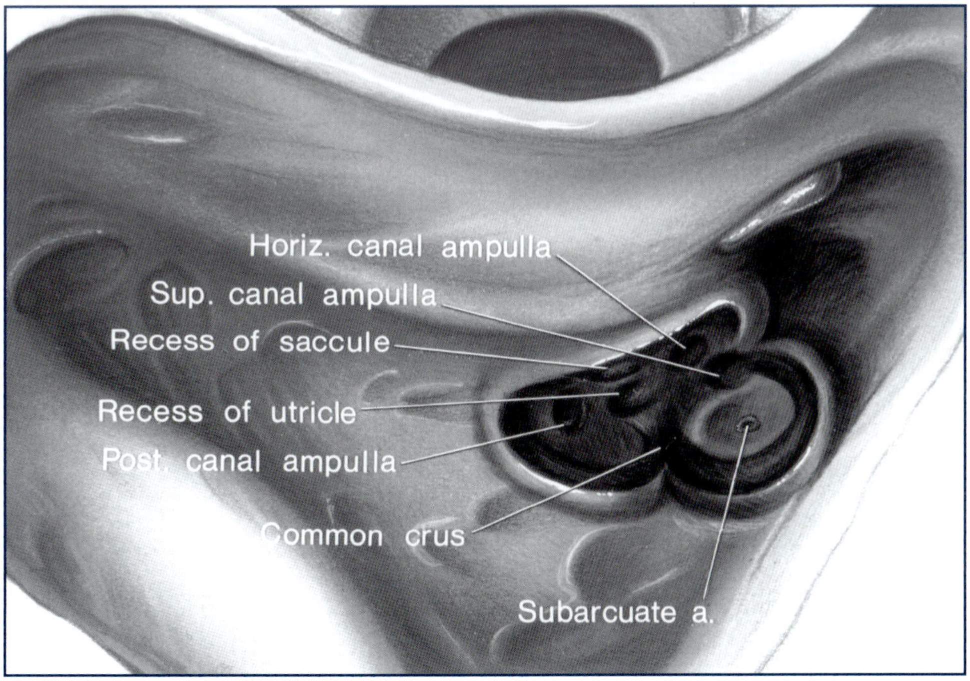

Figure 19–3. Left transmastoid labyrinthectomy performed.

Difficult Treatment Situations

Difficult situations arise when patients present with Ménière's disease in an only hearing ear or in patients with bilateral disease who are refractory to maximum medical treatment. In patients with bilateral disease either bilateral sequential endolymphatic sac decompressions can be performed or intramuscular streptomycin can be given. Intratympanic gentamicin injections can be performed; however, one must tread cautiously due to the risk of sensorineural hearing loss. Likewise, in patients with an only hearing ear who are refractory to medical treatment, intratympanic steroids may be used. Endolymphatic sac surgery or vestibular nerve section can also be performed. These procedures are preferred to intratympanic gentamicin in the case of an only hearing ear. One must check vestibular function on both sides prior to ablative surgery as the risk of bilateral vestibular loss (and oscillopsia) can be high.

Patients are counseled as to the above treatment options for Ménière's disease. In the end it is both the educated patient and the doctor's decision as to which treatment option fits best.

REFERENCES

1. Gantz BJ, Godley PW. Ménière's disease: medical therapy. In: Gates GA, ed. *Current Therapy in Otolaryngology Head and Neck Surgery*. 6th ed. St. Louis, MO. 1998:79–80.
2. McCabe GI, Sekitari T, Kyu JH. Drug effects on postlabyrinthectomy nystagmus. *Arch Otolaryngol*. 1973;98: 310–313.
3. Hayes GB, Barna BP, Kinney SE, et al. Autoimmune endolymphatic hydrops: five-year review. *Otolaryngol Head Neck Surg*. 1988;98:221–225.
4. Balkany T, Sires B, Arenberg I. Bilateral aspects of Ménière's disease. An underestimated clinical entity. *Otolaryngol Clin North Am*. 1980;12:603–609.
5. Hamid M, Treene D. Issues, indications and controversies regarding intratympanic steroid perfusion. *Curr Opin Otolaryngol Head Neck Surg*. 2008;16(5):434–440.
6. Haynes DS, O'Malley M, Cohen S, Waterford K, Labadie RF. Intratympanic dexamethasone for sudden sensorineural hearing loss after failure of systemic therapy. *Laryngoscope*. 2007;117(1): 3–15.
7. Portmann G. Saccus endolymphaticus and operations for drainage of same for relief of vertigo. *J Laryngol Otol*. 1927;42:809–927.
8. Smith WC, Pillsbury HS. Surgical treatment of Ménière's disease. *Am J Otol*. 1988;9:39–43.
9. Thomsen J, Brettlau P, Tos M, Jonsen JJ. Placebo effect in surgery for Ménière's disease. *Arch Otolaryngol*. 1981; 107:271–277.
10. Glasscock ME, Jackson CG, Poe DS, Johnson GD. What I think of sac surgery in 1989. *Am J Otol*. 1989;10:230–233.
11. Gianoli GJ, LaRouere MJ, Kartush JM, Wayman J. Sac vein decompression for intractable Ménière's disease: two-year treatment results. *Otolaryngol Head Neck Surg*. 1998;188:22–29.
12. Kato BM, LaRouere MJ, Bojrab DI, Michaelides EM. Evaluating quality of life after endolymphatic sac surgery: the Ménière's disease outcomes questionnaire. *Otol Neurotol*. 2004;25;339–344.
13. Pillsbury HC, Arenberg I, Ferraro J, Ackley R. Endolymphatic sac surgery: the Danish sham surgery study: an alternative analysis. *Otolaryngol Clin North Am*. 1983;16: 123–127.
14. Paparella MM, Sajjadih H. Endolymphatic sac revision for recurrent Ménière's disease. *Am J Otol*. 1988;9:441–447.
15. Schuknecht HP. Ablation therapy for the relief of Ménière's disease. *Laryngoscopy*. 1956;66:859.
16. Graham M, Sataloff R, Kemink J. Titration streptomycin therapy for bilateral Ménière's disease: a preliminary report. *Otolaryngol Head Neck Surg*. 1984;92:440.
17. Magnusson M, Padoan S. Delayed onset of otologic effects in Gentamicin treatment of Ménière's disease. Rational for extremely low dose therapy. *Acta Otolaryngol (Stockholm)*. 1991;11:671–676.
18. Nedzelski J, Chiong C, Fradet G, et al. Intratympanic Gentamicin instillation as treatment of unilateral Ménière's disease: update of an ongoing study. *Am J Otol*. 1993;14: 278–282.
19. Silverstein H, Morrell H. Retrolabyrinthine vestibular neurectomy. *Otolaryngol Head Neck Surg*. 1982;90:778–782.
20. Kemink JL, Hoft JT. Retrolabyrinthine vestibular nerve section: analysis of results. *Laryngoscope*. 1986;96:33–36.
21. McElveen JT, House JW, Hitselberger WE. Retrolabyrinthine vestibular nerve section. A viable alternative to the middle fossa approach. *Otolaryngol Head Neck Surg*. 1984; 92:136–140.
22. McElveen JT, Shelton C, Hitselberger WE, et al. Retrolabyrinthine vestibular neurectomy. A re-evaluation. *Laryngoscope*. 1988;98:502–506.
23. Shuknecht HP, Armstrong BW. Transtympanic vestibulectomy for Ménière's disease. *Laryngoscope*. 1959;699: 1071–1074.
24. Diaz RC, LaRouere MJ, Bojrab DI, Zappia JJ, Sargent EW, Shaia WT. Quality of life assessment of Ménière's disease patients after surgical labyrinthectomy. *Otol Neurotol*. 2006;28:74–86.

CHAPTER 20

Intratympanic Treatment: Hearing Loss and Dizziness

David Healy, Jr., Michael Hoffer, and Ben Balough

INTRODUCTION

Intratympanic (IT) medical therapy has been a controversial modality since its inception. Although IT treatments have been utilized for over half a century, only recently have they received increasing attention. During the last decade there have been several dozen peer reviewed examinations of this therapeutic modality. For all the medications and indications considered, basic questions remain including best medicine, total dose, dosing regimen, delivery method, and endpoint of therapy. However, as the therapy is relatively easy to administer in an office setting, the numbers of patients receiving intratympanic therapy will increase.

Many disorders may be treated with IT therapy, but the bulk of the basic science work and of the clinical evidence (at least based on popularity) have focused on the following three therapies: (1) gentamicin for the treatment of Ménière's disease (MD), (2) steroids for the treatment of MD, and (3) steroids for the treatment of sudden hearing loss and/or tinnitus. The history and background of gentamicin investigations are discussed, as well as the basic science behind IT medicine administration and specific uses of gentamicin and steroid administration to the inner ear.

GENTAMICIN

History of IT Gentamicin

Streptomycin was discovered in 1943 and quickly became an important antibiotic against severe systemic gram-negative infections and tuberculosis. The most common systemic side effect of this medication was temporary imbalance without vertigo or nystagmus. Higher systemic doses increased the chance of permanent imbalance and, occasionally, deafness. These early observations led to animal and cadaver studies which confirmed the vestibulotoxic and cochleotoxic effects of high-dose streptomycin.

It did not take long for otolaryngologists to try to use the vestibulotoxicity of streptomycin to clinical advantage. Fowler may have been the first to use systemic streptomycin to alleviate vertigo attacks in patients with MD that was refractory to traditional medical management. He and others used between 2 to 4 grams of IM streptomycin per day in patients with unilateral or bilateral MD, typically until onset of severe imbalance, and reported that vertigo attacks could be well controlled without loss of hearing.[1] Often, and especially with higher dosing, vertigo control came with the troubling symptoms of permanent, severe imbalance, and oscillopsia.

Schuknekt appears to be the first to have used IT administration of streptomycin. He conceived of this idea after noting that intratympanic formalin will readily pass into the inner ear and prevented post-mortem degeneration of the inner ear membranous structures in patients. He correctly theorized that streptomycin could also pass into the inner ear and devised a cat animal model that demonstrated clinical and pathologic vestibulotoxicity with intratympanic streptomycin. Based on these results he devised a clinical trial of intratympanic streptomycin administration to patients with uncontrolled unilateral MD. He administered variable amounts of streptomycin (between 0.125 and 0.5 g), either hourly or over 4 hours, over a variable amount of days. Three patients who received 1 or 2 days of treatment, achieved only brief control of their vertigo, but did not lose any hearing. An additional, five patients subsequently received streptomycin for 3 days or longer. These patients had permanent resolution of their vertigo episodes, but at the cost of deafening the ear. Schuknekt coined the term, "chemical labyrinthectomy" to describe this phenomenon. He concluded that intratympanic streptomycin at therapeutic dosage cannot preserve hearing, and should be considered for patients who are not good surgical candidates, but would otherwise be a candidate for inner ear ablation.[2]

Intratympanic and systemic streptomycin (and later gentamicin) were not the only methods by which investigators attempted to chemically ablate the inner ear. Investigators attempted direct injection of streptomycin and other vestibulotoxic substances into the labyrinth, usually through a lateral semicircular canal fenestra. Chemical ablation via the lateral semicircular canal approach eventually fell into disfavor due to added technical difficulty and variable and unpredictable results. Chemical ablation via systemic administration of aminoglycoside also fell into disfavor due to the untoward effects of bilateral vestibulopathy, nephrotoxicity, and unpredictable results.

Nedzelski advocated using gentamicin rather than streptomycin for its theoretical reduction in cochleotoxicity.[3] He reported on 50 patients with MD in whom he treated with microcatheter administration of streptomycin over 5 hours, 4 times in 48 hours. He reported vertigo control in 96% of his patients, with 24% experiencing various degrees of hearing loss. Beck and Schmidt[2] reported on their 10 year experience with intratympanic streptomycin and gentamicin. They theorized that the dosage could be titrated to impede the secretory epithelium of the vestibular apparatus without destroying the sensory cells, thus achieving vertigo control while maintaining caloric response. More importantly, risk of deafness could potentially be eliminated. By reducing the dosage delivered and titrating, they were able to achieve excellent rates of vertigo control (92%) while also achieving respectable hearing preservation rates (15% hearing loss with no cases of deafness).

By the early 1990s, two schools of thought emerged, dubbed the "shotgun" approach, and the "low-dose" approach. The shotgun approach, championed by Nedzelski and others, was characterized by daily IT injections to a fixed endpoint or to a clinical threshold that heralded damage to inner ear.[3] Proponents of this approach attempted to achieve adequate vestibular ablation to achieve long-term vertigo control. The low-dose approach, championed by Magnusson and others, was characterized by weekly IT injections, also to a fixed endpoint or to clinical effect. Proponents of this approach tried to achieve vertigo control while minimizing damage to hearing and potentially preserving caloric response as well.[4]

IT gentamicin gained widespread popularity in the treatment of MD in the 1990s, and continues to be commonly performed throughout the United States and Europe. Gentamicin gained popularity over streptomycin due early clinical data that showed less hearing loss with gentamicin, and because it was both easier and cheaper to obtain (streptomycin at this point being restricted for use in multidrug resistant tuberculosis). Today, gentamicin is usually instilled via IT injection or through a tympanostomy tube to the round window niche. These injections are repeated over a variable amount of time, typically between daily to weekly injections, until a clinical endpoint is achieved or until there is a decline in hearing. There continues to be a widespread variability in dosing methods, timing of delivery, clinical endpoint of therapy, and concentration of gentamicin. This variability stemmed from a lack of both clinical evidence and basic science models that point to the most effective regimen.

Mechanism of Action

The theoretical purpose of aminoglycoside as a therapy in MD is its toxicity against the vestibular apparatus, which causes a reduction in vestibular function. Ideally, aminoglycoside would act to reduce vestibular function, and thus alleviate the patient's symptoms of vertigo, while preserving hearing. There are two general theories to explain the mechanism of action: direct toxicity to vestibular hair cells, and direct toxicity to the endolymph producing apparatus.[5,6]

Multiple theories have been developed to explain aminoglycosides' direct toxicity to hair cells. These include disruption of calcium-dependent cytokine production, causing disruption of hair cell membrane integrity.[7] Other possible mechanisms include increased superoxide production, hair cell transduction blockage, glutamate decarboxylase inhibition, ornithine decarboxylase inhibition, and free radical damage.[8] Aminoglycoside may also act to inhibit production of endolymph, restoring the balance between endolymphatic and perilymphatic pressure. This would also act to alleviate all symptoms of endolymphatic hydrops. Additionally, aminoglycosides are theorized to cause selective damage to the dark cells of the cochlear stria vascularis and planum semilunatum in the cristae ampullares of the semicircular canals, which are involved in ionic regulation and endolymph production.[9] This theory that vestibular dark cells and, thus, endolymphatic flow, are the targets by which aminoglycoside alleviates vertigo is of significant clinical interest because it suggests that it is not necessarily important to ablate the vestibule to achieve vertigo control in MD. This idea can explain why patients with intact caloric responses can still achieve significant vertigo control after intratympanic aminoglycoside administration.[9]

Mechanism of Differential Toxicity

Vestibular hair cells are thought to be more sensitive than cochlear hair cells to the aminoglycosides gentamicin and streptomycin. Other aminoglycosides, such as amikacin are considered to be relatively more cochleotoxic and thus are not used transtympanically. The best evidence for this is the simple clinical observation that patients undergoing systemic gentamicin or streptomycin therapy experience vestibulopathy much more commonly than hearing loss. Vestibulopathy is typically temporary, but can be permanent and severe. This notion of differential toxicity, however, has been difficult to demonstrate in animal studies. Moreover, there is evidence from temporal bone studies that have shown more damage to the cochlea than to vestibular structures in patients who have undergone gentamicin therapy for MD.[8] Furthermore, radiolabeling of gentamicin demonstrates widespread dispersion throughout the inner ear shortly after delivery; hair cells, supporting cells, spiral ganglia, and other neural elements. Hoffer et al[10] reported on early and irreversible damage to the inner hair cells of the Chinchilla cochlea by apoptosis prior to demonstrating vestibular hair cell damage.

An interesting possibility is that type I hair cells may be more sensitive to ototoxic effects than type II hair cells, which could theoretically ameliorate the more profound symptom of vertigo (driven by type I hair cells) while preserving cochlear function.[8]

Pharmacokinetics of Gentamicin

Gentamicin is an aminoglycoside antibiotic with a molecular mass of 477 grams per mole. Like others of its class it is comprised of an amino group and a sugar and is produced by gram positive bacteria. Those derived from the *Micromonospora* genus have the *-icin* suffix whereas those from *Streptomyces* end with *-mycin*. They act by inhibiting the 30S ribosome and also inhibit calcium and magnesium channels in cell membranes.

Gentamicin needs to travel from its delivery point within the oval window niche to the target hair cells within the vestibule in sufficient concentration to create the desired clinical effect of vertigo control. It must accomplish this without concentrating within the cochlea in sufficient quantity to cause clinically important hearing loss. Dosing regimens are designed with this in mind. Pharmacokinetic models to describe this have improved much over the past decade, but still only partially describe what is truly happening.

Gentamicin likely travels across the oval window membrane via passive diffusion, due to its sufficiently small size. There is probably high variability in this process that is clinically important. Cadaver studies have shown that up to 20% of round window niches have a second three-layered mucosal membrane veil that could potentially prevent the medicine from contacting the round window at all. Additionally, obstructing fat or fibrous tissue within the round window niche has also been reported.[10] In the one published in vivo study of perilymphatic drug concentration of gentamicin in humans after middle ear application, high concentrations of drug were present (up to 16 mg/L) after relatively short times (<30 minutes) after application. Cerebrospinal fluid levels were not found and relatively low, 0.4 mg/L, levels were found in serum.[11]

Once gentamicin crosses the round window, the situation becomes more complex. If passive diffusion accounted for its movement to the target cells, then it would need to diffuse down the scala tympani, around the helicotrema, back down the scala vestibuli, across the vestibule, and finally to the ampullae of the semicircular canals. Certainly there is something more complex at work. In fact, gentamicin most likely readily diffuses across the inner ear membranes, readily achieving concentrations within the scala vestibuli, cochlear duct, and vestibule. This has been shown in animal studies demonstrating very early uptake throughout the inner ear, spiral ligament, and spiral ganglion cells.

A study using a guinea pig model that measured gentamicin concentration gradient along the scala tympani demonstrated that the gradient created is probably not due to diffusion alone, but also due to slow movement of perilymph toward the cochlear apex. This has the undesirable effect of slightly increasing gentamicin concentration distally along the cochlea.[12]

A chinchilla model was used by Hoffer and colleagues to elucidate the pattern of cochlear uptake of gentamicin as a function of time using both IT and microcatheter (MC) methods.[13] It also analyzed the effect on hearing and surveyed cochlear damage by pathologic section and immunehistochemical staining for antibodies against cleaved caspase-7 and caspase-3, which are markers for apoptosis. This model showed that with the intratympanic method of delivery, a highly variable concentration of gentamicin was created with a fairly reliable but variable peak concentration of 24 hours from delivery. In contrast, the MC delivery method showed a highly reproducible, and lower, concentration of gentamicin from 24 to 72 hours after delivery, suggesting better control with this method. Surprisingly, this study also demonstrated apoptotic damage of spiral ganglion cells prior to any evidence of hair cell damage with IT administration of the medicine which could mean that IT gentamicin administration has the potential to permanently damage hearing upstream of the hair cells before producing any relief in MD.[14]

Salt et al[15] devised a mathematical model that compared various methods of delivering IT gentamicin. The model was based on previous animal studies that attempted to elucidate the pharmacokinetics of IT gent delivery. This model demonstrated a theoretical risk of building toxic levels of gentamicin at critical points within the cochlea for speech (500 Hz–4 kHz) when gentamicin is administered with less than 3 days between treatments. The authors concluded that "single shot" therapy with greater than 3 days between treatments may decrease hearing loss complications.[15–17]

Clinical Trials

There are no randomized controlled clinical trials or case/control trials for IT gentamicin therapy. All clinical trials are case series without controls. Level of evidence is thus level 4 (case series) and strength of recommendation concerning IT gentamicin for MD is currently grade C. Ménière's disease treatment protocols typically measure vertigo control according to AAO-HNS Committee on Hearing and Equilibrium guidelines for grading vertigo control.[18] Table 20–1 demonstrates the Grade A–F scale. Occasionally, clinical trials also attempt to assess other sequelae such as hearing loss, tinnitus, and aural fullness. A significant difficulty with clinical trials that attempt to determine efficacy of Ménière's treatment is the natural history of Ménière's disease. Commonly, vertigo attacks can improve without treatment of any kind as periods of remission are not

Table 20–1. Summary of Reporting Guidelines for Vertigo Control in Ménière's Disease

Numerical Value*	Class
0	A (complete control of definitive spells)
1 to 40	B
41 to 80	C
81 to 120	D
>120	E
Secondary treatment initiated due to disability from vertigo	F

*Numerical value = (X/Y) × 100, rounded to the nearest whole number, where X is the average number of definitive spells per month for the 6 months 18 to 24 months after therapy and Y is the average number of definitive spells per month for the 6 months before therapy.

Source: Committee on Hearing and Equilibrium guidelines for the diagnosis and evaluation of therapy in Ménière's disease.[18]

uncommon. Thus, a clinical trial without controls will not account for this finding. Another difficulty is that clinical researchers attempt to show hearing preservation with IT gentamicin protocol, but hearing tends to worsen over time in MD. Finally, the variable nature of Ménière's with fluctuation in levels of hearing and even frequency and severity of vertigo can make clinical trials difficult.

Selected Clinical Trials

Beck[19] was the first to report positive results using a titration technique. These investigators used 30 mg of gentamicin, presumably every one or two days (patients were hospitalized) until the onset of inner ear disturbance, whether it be vestibular dysfunction or hearing loss. These investigators achieved a vertigo control rate of 92% with a hearing loss rate of 15% without any cases of deafness.[19]

Atlas and Parnes[9] advocated weekly (as opposed to daily) intratympanic injections of pH buffered 26 mg/mL gentamicin for up to 4 injections, or until evidence of cochleovestibulopathy was obtained.[9] Their goal was to achieve adequate vertigo control while reducing hearing loss; 68 patients were enrolled in this clinical trial. At first injection, they performed oto-endoscopy through a myringotomy to ensure no round window obstruction, and placed a tympanostomy tube. Only once did they need to lyse mucosal bands that obstructed the round window. Typically, they would re-inject more gentamicin at the 10-minute mark to ensure that the round window remained bathed in gentamicin solution for thirty minutes. They reported 84% Class A and 6% Class B vertigo control, with no patients becoming deafened. 8% experienced deterioration of their PTA over a 6-month period, which is potentially due to progression of the disease itself. They also noted that 8 of 12 patients with >50% preservation of caloric response and 11 of 12 with 10 to 50% preservation had Class A vertigo control. They concluded that eradication of caloric response is not always necessary to achieve good vertigo control, particularly if there is concern for bilateral disease development.

Harner and Driscoll[20] studied the efficacy of single-injection IT gentamicin in the control of vertigo for Ménière's disease refractory to medical management. They theorized that "chemical alteration" with a single dosing of gentamicin, rather than "chemical ablation" with higher dosing regimens, could effectively control vertigo while preserving hearing. In a prospective non-controlled study of 56 patients with at least 2 years of follow-up, they performed single-dose injection (0.5–0.75 mg 40 mg/mL gentamicin), which was repeated at the one-month mark if adequate vertigo control was not achieved on the first injection. They achieved Class A or B control of vertigo in 82% of patients. They quoted a deafness rate of less than 1% of patients. Long-term follow-up of audiometric data revealed a range of hearing changes: both improvement and worsening of hearing, which is consistent with the natural history of Ménière's disease. On average, postinjection hearing remained unchanged (56 dB PTA preinjection, 57 dB postinjection). They concluded that low-dose intratympanic Gentamicin can effectively control vertigo symptoms with excellent hearing preservation rates.

Hoffer[21] used a microcatheter delivery system along with aggressive vestibular therapy in a 2-year clinical trial of 27 patients with MD. A round window microcatheter (Durect Corp, Cupertino, CA) filled with 10 mg/mL gentamicin was placed into the round window niche in these patients. The medicine was instilled into the round window either by 1 microliter/hour continuous infusion, or via 3 separate injections through the microcatheter over 14 days. Thorough vestibular and audiometric testing was carried out during and after treatment, and the patients were followed for a 2-year period. One patient demonstrated a mild and temporary reduction in vestibular function by caloric response, and there were no cases of deafness. 92% of patients demonstrated Class A vertigo control at 2-year follow-up.

Diamond et al[22] performed a systematic review of intratympanic gentamicin in Ménière's disease in 2003. Thirty-five clinical trials met the study's guidelines for inclusion in the systematic review; none of these had a proper control group for comparison. Overall, Class A or Class B vertigo control was achieved in 89% of patients (study range 73–100%). Hearing worsened in 26% (study range 0–90%), and subjective improvement in tinnitus was achieved in 57% of patients (no grading scale). The study divided dosing regimens into multiple daily, single daily, and weekly regimens. Multiple daily dosing regimens achieved vertigo control rates averaging 94%, with hearing loss rates of 26%. Daily dosing regimens achieved vertigo control rates of 84%, with hearing loss rates of 32%. Weekly dosing regimens achieved vertigo control rate of 87%, with hearing loss rates averaging 21%. Many studies did not achieve the minimum of two-years follow-up recommended by the AAO-HNS Committee on Hearing and Equilibrium. The authors cite lack of standardization, lack of control groups and blinding, and lack of speech discrimination scores as sources of potential bias. They conclude that no regimen can be considered the best. Because of this they suggest that the simplest technique with the highest level of patient tolerability is the most ideal.[22]

Chia et al[6] performed a meta-analysis of 27 clinical trials of injected gentamicin.[6] In this meta-analysis, the trials were categorized into multiple daily dosing, daily dosing, low-dose technique, continuous microcatheter, or titration technique. Vertigo control rates and hearing loss rates were tabulated. The researchers concluded that the titration technique produces the best vertigo results with comparable hearing loss results to other methods. The "low-dose" techniques demonstrated worse vertigo results without improvement in hearing loss rates. A more recent meta-analysis by Huon et al looked at all studies from 1995 through 2011.[23] They noted that while the quality of the published studies had increased recently, large-scale randomized controlled trials remain needed to confirm the predictive factors for the effectiveness of IT gentamicin injection in treating MD.

Recommended Method for IT Gentamicin Administration

The wide variety of technique used in administering gentamicin reported in clinical trials makes it impossible to recommend a specific technique. Some guidelines can be offered based on the combination of current clinical practice, basic science models, and results from clinical trials. Whatever technique is used, the goal is to apply gentamicin to the round window in sufficient concentration and over a sufficient amount of time that it achieves a therapeutic effect while avoiding both local and systemic side effects, especially hearing loss.

A commonly used technique is the intratympanic injection, which is easily administered in clinic under microscopy. A tuberculin syringe with a 1.5" 27-gauge needle allows easy visualization and patient comfort. The desired amount of aminoglycoside is injected over the round window through the posterosuperior quadrant of the tympanic membrane. There are two common doses of gentamicin for injection. The standard intravenous preparation of gentamicin is 40 mg/mL, which can be buffered with 8.4% sodium bicarbonate so that discomfort on injection is reduced. 1.5 mL of gentamicin mixed with 0.5 mL of sodium bicarbonate at these concentrations will produce a final concentration of 26.6 mg/mL gentamicin. Other groups utilize the pediatric dosing vial which comes at a concentration of 10 mg/mL. Approximately 0.3 to 0.5 mL of solution is usually adequate to bathe the round window in solution.[4,8] Some groups advocate also placing a "ventilation" puncture to allow middle ear space air to ventilate out as it is displaced by medication. The authors have not found this to be necessary. Another reasonable alternative is to place a tympanostomy tube and inject through this, which would avoid the pain of piercing the tympanic membrane. Typically, patients will remain lying flat with the injected ear up for 10 minutes to one hour. Our practice is to wait 20 minutes. This procedure is generally well-tolerated by patients, who should be told to expect brief pain on injection, followed by possible vertigo or disequilibrium. Warming the medication can help in this regard (preventing a cold caloric response). Less common side effects include hemorrhage, prolonged disequilibrium and ataxia, allergic response, and tympanic membrane perforation (especially in an irradiated or otherwise damaged tympanic membrane). It is also critical that all patients who are given intratympanic aminoglycoside understand that permanent hearing loss is possible, even from a single injection.[13]

Depending on the views of the group administering the gentamicin, this procedure is repeated at regular intervals until a vestibular effect is seen. Recently, a number of groups have advocated simply injecting the medicine once and not repeating this injection if the patient appears clinically better or free from attacks and such is our practice. These groups would wait at least one month between injections.[24]

Role of IT Gentamicin in Ménière's Disease?

Generally, IT gentamicin is reserved for unilateral disease that has failed conservative and generally other nonablative treatment. Conservative management includes salt restriction, increased hydration, and avoidance of triggers, including potential allergic triggers, alcohol, caffeine, tobacco, and stress. Pharmacologic management includes diuretics and vasodilators for preventive strategies, and steroids (systemic and intratympanic), vestibular suppressants, and anti-nausea medications for acute attacks.[24]

Devices that create low amplitude positive pressure impulses to the middle ear are theorized to improve endolymphatic hydrops, and thus, the symptoms of Ménière's disease. The Meniett Device (Medtronic Xomed, Jacksonville FL) and the P-100 (Enttex, Hannover, Germany) are examples of this. Clinical trials have demonstrated efficacy in these devices in terms of vertigo control, but not hearing loss. These devices are considered another nonablative therapy choice in the treatment of Ménière's. Placement of a tympanostomy tube is necessary for these devices.

When these measures fail, the choices are either ablative or nonablative surgery, or IT gentamicin. Nonablative surgical therapies are endolymphatic sac decompression or shunt. Ablative surgery consists of vestibular nerve section or labyrinthectomy depending on remaining hearing.

Kaylie et al[25] performed a retrospective chart review comparing surgery to IT gentamicin for vertigo control, hearing preservation, and quality of life indices. The authors found that vertigo control for IT gentamicin is better than ELS patients, comparable to nerve-section patients, and worse than labyrinthectomy patients. Their surgical patients suffered a similar rate of hearing loss to IT gentamicin.

Summary of Intratympanic Gentamicin

IT gentamicin is a viable treatment option for MD that has failed medical therapy. Despite a significant volume of work over the last twenty years questions remain regarding the best dose of medicine, dosing regimen, method of administration, and end point for therapy. In addition, current Ménière's disease outcome standards limit the analysis because those who require retreatment within two years are considered treatment failures. However, many patients with this disease would appreciate being symptom-free (or nearly free) at the cost of an occasional booster if it meant avoiding a surgical procedure.

The place in the "batting order" for treatment of Ménière's disease with IT gentamicin therapy varies widely and is all too often based on biases transmitted from teachers to students but can be tailored to fit the needs of an individual patient. There are very few outcomes based studies to demonstrate if IT gentamicin therapy should come before or after micropressure therapy or before or after endolymphatic sac procedures. Local bias as well as medical financing and the availability of specialists capable of performing nerve sections all play roles in determining the final "line-up." Over the past 15 years our practice has been striving to define the patient characteristics and disease details so that an objective order of treatment can be determined for every patient. Despite our work and that of a number of other groups, this goal has not yet been reached.

INTRATYMPANIC STEROID TREATMENT

Intratympanic steroid injection for inner ear disease was first reported in the literature in 1982 by Sakata et al[26] as a therapy for tinnitus. In 1986, Sakata et al[27] reported on its use in the treatment of MD. Since then, IT steroids have been used against an array of inner ear conditions, including idiopathic sudden sensorineural hearing loss (SSHL), MD, autoimmune hearing loss, noise-induced hearing loss, tinnitus, and Cogan's syndrome. Currently, it is commonly used in the treatment of SSHL, tinnitus, and MD, and there is an increasing body of literature investigating this treatment modality. IT steroid therapy has the theoretical advantage of concentrating steroid at the site of insult and thus maximizing its beneficial effect while avoiding systemic side effects. Despite this, controversy still surrounds IT steroid injection for inner ear disease, and clinical trials have yet to prove its efficacy against currently accepted therapies.

Corticosteroids are potent anti-inflammatory medications with mechanisms of action similar to the human body's endogenous corticosteroid cortisone, produced in the cortex of the adrenal gland. Steroids have a systemic and topical anti-inflammatory effect, and are widely used for a broad range of inflammatory conditions. Interest in steroid as an intratympanic therapy began when systemic steroid therapy showed promise against inner ear disease. IT steroid delivery has the advantage of increased local concentration and activity, while avoiding the many acute and chronic systemic side effects. Acute side effects of systemic steroids include sleeplessness, headache, nausea, peptic ulcers, glaucoma, abdominal discomfort, impaired wound healing, and electrolyte disturbance. Chronic side effects include weight gain, diabetes mellitus, osteonecrosis, cataracts, loss of muscle mass, and tendon rupture.[28] Dexamethasone and methylprednisolone are the most commonly used drugs for IT steroid therapy. Dexamethasone is a synthetic corticosteroid with potent anti-inflammatory properties and without the sodium retaining properties of endogenous steroid. In general terms, steroids act to decrease inflammation. A central point in the use of IT steroids for the treatment of inner ear disease is the notion that inflammation (or inflammatory mediators) is at least part of the pathophysiologic process. Investigators have also suggested other mechanisms by which steroids could impart their salient effect on the inner ear, such as ion homeostasis.

Mechanism of Action

There are at least three proposed mechanisms by which steroids can act against inner ear disease: decrease inflammation, improve ion homeostasis, and increase labyrinthine circulation.

Steroids act intracellularly to inhibit proinflammatory cytokines, thus decreasing inflammation. A key assumption in the theoretical efficacy of steroids is that some or all of the inner ear dysfunction is a product of inflammation. Inflammation has been demonstrated in numerous inner ear disorders, including hydrops, ototoxicity, ischemic injury, meningitis, labyrinthitis, and systemic inflammatory disease.[29]

Steroids also act to modulate ion homeostasis through several mechanisms. Its anti-inflammatory action can have salutary effect on ion homeostasis by suppression of pro-inflammatory cytokines NF-KB and TNF-alpha, which can cause loss of endothelial barrier integrity. Steroids can also bind to mineralocorticoid receptors, impacting sodium-potassium ATPase and epithelial sodium channels, important ion transport channels for stria vascularis function. Aquaporin channels, found almost exclusively in the inner ear, affect water transport and inner ear fluid dynamics, are partially regulated by endogenous steroid.[28] Through action on these different sites, steroids can have a restorative effect on inner ear ion transport mechanisms.[30]

Disturbances of cochlear blood flow and their effects on strial function have also been implicated as an underlying cause for Ménière's disease as well as SSNHL. A variety of substances have been shown to modulate cochlear blood flow in animals. Among these are corticosteroids offering another mechanism of action to support its potential beneficial effects on MD and SSNHL.[31]

Pharmacokinetics

Diffusion of steroid across the round window and through the perilymph and endolymph of the inner ear to its target sites approximates the pharmacokinetics of gentamicin, and the reader is encouraged to refer to the previous discussion of gentamicin pharmacokinetics. There are, however, some notable and important differences. Diffusion across the round window membrane is via an active transport mechanism rather than passive diffusion that occurs with gentamicin. Steroid also acts intracellularly, so measurements of extracellular steroid concentration will not necessarily correspond with steroid efficacy.[32]

Parnes et al[33] studied the pharmacokinetics of 3 different steroids (hydrocortisone, methylprednisolone, and dexamethasone) in a guinea pig model. After bathing the round window membrane in steroid for 30 minutes, perilymph and endolymph were sampled for concentration of steroid at different points in time. Blood sampling was done as well. Similar sampling was performed after systemic steroid administration (both oral and intravenous). This study showed that IT steroid achieved much higher inner ear steroid concentration than systemic administration. The highest steroid concentrations were found in endolymph. Also, IT steroid achieved peak concentration within 2 hours, and lasted in measurable quantity between 6 and 24 hours. The authors concluded that IT steroid achieved much higher levels of inner ear steroid concentration while avoiding clinically significant systemic steroid concentration. Other animal studies have confirmed high levels of inner ear steroid with IT steroid administration. In this study, methylprednisolone consistently demonstrated higher perilymph concentration than the other two steroids. Because of this, these authors argued that methylprednisolone is preferred for IT steroid administration. Others have argued that the sustained high concentration may also be due to its failure to pass intracellularly and thus, act at the target receptor site. For this reason, dexamethasone has been argued to be superior to methylprednisolone despite its lower perilymph concentration.[28]

Plontke et al[34] demonstrated steroid concentration gradients along the scala tympani after IT steroid administration using a guinea pig model. The authors noted that over time this concentration gradient would equilibrate, but clearance of inner ear steroid was still too rapid to achieve therapeutic concentration at the apical cochlea. They noted that this effect may cause variability in clinical outcomes of IT steroid therapy.

IT Steroid in the Treatment of SSHL

Patients with idiopathic sudden sensorineural hearing loss (SSNHL) present as an emergency to the otolaryngologist, and treatment options need to be discussed with the patient. SSNHL is defined as new-onset unilateral hearing loss that occurs within 72 hours.[35] There are two main theories to explain the etiology of SSHL: viral and vascular causes. Autoimmune and metabolic dysfunctions are also considered possible explanations for SSNHL. Regardless of the underlying insult, the efficacy of steroids in the treatment of SSHL would hinge on inflammation or ion homeostasis being an important part of the inner ear disturbance, and this remains unproven.

Clinical Evidence for the Efficacy of Systemic Steroids in SSNHL

In a landmark study in 1980, Wilson et al[36] demonstrated efficacy of systemic steroid in the treatment of SSNHL. In this double-blinded controlled trial, 33 patients received oral steroid (either methylprednisolone or dexamethasone and various doses) and 34 received placebo. Hearing recovery (defined as recovery of hearing within 50% or more of the pre-hearing loss speech reception score or average pure-tone score) was 61% in the steroid group compared to 32% in the placebo group. A cohort of 52 controls who refused steroid (and were not included in the statistical analysis) achieved a recovery rate of 58%. The authors defined a "steroid effective zone" of hearing loss that ranged between 40 dB and 90 dB mid-frequency loss. They found that losses less than this spontaneously recovered, and losses greater than this did not recover regardless of treatment. The authors recommended oral steroid for treatment of SSHL within this steroid effective zone. This study has been cited as the best clinical evidence for the efficacy of steroid in SSHL, however, others have noted important weaknesses in the study. For instance, it is not a randomized clinical trial, and the steroid doses given varied significantly between patients. It should also be noted that one RCT comparing steroid to placebo found no difference in hearing outcomes.[37] Despite these shortcomings, oral steroid is commonly offered as treatment for SSHL.

A 2008 Cochrane Collaboration review of clinical trials investigating steroids for SSHL identified only the 2 trials (Wilson et al, 1980, and Cinamon et al, 2001)[36,37] as randomized controlled trials. In their review, they concluded that the value of steroids in the treatment of SSHL is unclear due to both low methodologic quality of trials and their contradictory results.[38]

Other modalities are used in the treatment of SSHL, including anti-viral medication, hemodilution agents, vitamins, minerals, herbal preparations, batroxobin, carbogen, and hyperbaric oxygen. Unfortunately, clinical trials have not proven efficacy of these various therapies, and steroid is still commonly regarded as the best therapy for this condition.

Recently the American Academy of Otolaryngology-Head and Neck Surgery published a clinical practice guideline which summarizes the currently available knowledge on sudden hearing loss and made recommendations for evaluation and treatment.[39] In that, confirmation of the nature and degree of hearing loss were emphasized, as well as the need for education and to screen for retrocochlear disease. The use of IT steroid was specifically mentioned as a salvage modality for those failing to respond to initial management. Regarding initial management; the panel recommended that oral steroids may be considered equally as well as hyperbaric oxygen citing better evidence to support the later than the former. Antivirals, anti-thrombotics, vasodilators, and antioxidants were discouraged.

Clinical Studies of IT Steroids in SSHL

Clinical trials comparing IT steroid vs. oral steroid in the treatment of SSHL are appearing in the literature. The evidence from several published studies is controversial. Ho et al[40] investigated the efficacy of IT dexamethasone in patients with SSHL who failed 10 days of conservative therapy. Thirty-nine patients who met criteria for SSHL were enrolled in the study and received aggressive conservative therapy (methylprednisolone, nicametate, vitamin B, fludizepam, and carbogen). After 10 days, 29 patients were considered failures of conservative medical management and were randomized into an IT steroid arm (1 mg/mL dexamethasone IT weekly for 3 weeks), or a control arm (continued medical management). The authors reported that in the IT dexamethasone group, 53% had at least 30 dB improvement of hearing compared to 7% of control group (time course not reported). Meanwhile, Ahn et al[41] evaluated IT dexamethasone (0.3 mL on days 1, 3, and 5) with systemic methylprednisolone, compared to methylprednisolone alone in a randomized controlled trial with 120 patients. They found that the addition of IT dexamethasone was no better than systemic steroid alone (73% vs 70% recovery).

There are several reports that were based mainly on literature review which also do not convincingly support the use of IT steroids. Doyle et al[28] reviewed IT steroid therapy for inner ear disease, finding only retrospective case series and uncontrolled prospective cohort studies.[27] The authors concluded that only a weak recommendation can be made supporting IT steroid therapy for SSHL. They cite the ease of administration and low side effect profile as salient reasons to consider IT steroid therapy for SSHL. Alles et al[42] performed a literature review of IT steroid for inner ear disease, evaluating available clinical trials for internal and external validity, comparability, appropriate diagnostic and prognostic criteria, and methodology. The authors concluded that clinical trials to date do not support a gold standard treatment for both SSHL and MD.

Conlin and Parnes[43,44] performed a systemic review and meta-analysis of clinical trials investigating therapies for SSHL. They found positive clinical studies for systemic steroid, IT steroid, batroxobin, magnesium, vitamin E, and hyperbaric oxygen. Unfortunately, none of these studies were considered valid randomized controlled trials, and they noted many inconsistencies and limitations to all studies, concluding that all therapies for SSHL are unproven, and none can be considered the gold-standard. Rauch et al published a paper on a large multicenter, randomized, placebo-controlled study sponsored by National Institutes of Health (NIH) for evaluation of oral versus transtympanic steroid treatment for SSNHL.[45] In this prospective, randomized, non-inferiority trial, 250 patients were enrolled and received either oral or transtympanic steroids. The hypothesis of inferiority of intratympanic methylprednisolone to oral prednisone for primary treatment of sudden sensorineural hearing loss was rejected. Thus, the authors concluded that treatment of patients with idiopathic sudden sensorineural hearing loss with intratympanic steroid treatment was not inferior to oral steroid treatment.

Another multicenter trial by Battaglia, Burchette, and Cueva[46] examined comparing intratympanic steroid, systemic steroid, and a third group where both oral and IT steroids were administered for SSNHL. This was a double-blinded, placebo controlled, randomized study and demonstrated greater hearing improvement at four weeks for the combination therapy group than either of the other two. The study does suffer from small numbers (16–18) of patients in each group but does provide some of the best evidence to date of IT steroid benefit. They have recently completed a follow-up study with larger numbers. Once again combination therapy was more effective than either therapy alone. The main benefit is in improved word recognition scores in the combination group.

In general, there does appear to be some evidence for a positive effect of IT steroids on SSHL; however, good RCT data is sparse. In most cases the use of IT steroids for SSHL is likely based more on the fact that there are no good RCT suggesting that any other therapy is more beneficial and the likelihood of doing harm is very low. However one study using microcatheter administered intratympanic steroids resulted in a single patient losing residual hearing.[47] However, it is important to note that this patient suffered from acute acoustic trauma rather than idiopathic sudden hearing loss.

Ménière's Disease

IT steroid has gained acceptance as a therapy for acute MD attacks because of its relative ease of administration and the theorized advantage of correcting the underlying insult within the inner ear as it is occurring. However, the basic science and clinical evidence for these remains thin.

Similar to SSNHL, the underlying pathophysiology of MD remains debated. However, there is both clinical and laboratory evidence that immune-mediated inflammation plays a role in MD, making steroid a potentially effective treatment.

The longitudinal flow theory advanced by Guild in 1927 has been accepted as an important etiology for MD. Briefly, endolymph created at the cochlear duct moves toward the endolymphatic sac where it is absorbed. Blockage of flow results in endolymphatic hydrops which causes the symptoms of MD. This theory is now being challenged on multiple fronts. Salt and Ma[48] demonstrated that longitudinal flow of endolymph occurs at such a slow rate (<0.007 mm/min) and it is essentially insignificant, and endolymph homeostasis is distributed throughout the endolymphatic space, and local factors are more likely to cause the hydrops phenomenon. Moreover, endolymphatic hydrops may merely be an epiphenomenon that does not directly cause the symptoms of MD or degradation in inner ear function.[49]

There is much evidence for immune-mediated inflammation in MD. Anti-endolymphatic sac antibodies, endolymphatic IgG deposits, and circulating autoantibodies in MD patients have all been described. Association with inhalant and food allergy has been described as well. The previous notion of the inner ear as an immunoprivileged area has been refuted by various studies, which have demonstrated lymphatics and immune cells in association with the endolymphatic space.

Clinical Evidence for Efficacy of Steroids in MD

Despite the theoretical advantage of the anti-inflammatory effects of steroids in the treatment of MD, clinical trials have not proven efficacy of either systemic or topical steroids. To date, there are no randomized, controlled clinical trials investigating systemic steroids in the treatment of MD. However, some clinical trials have shown positive results of IT steroid therapy in MD.

Garduno-Anaya et al[50] investigated the efficacy of dexamethasone (4 mg/ml) daily IT injection over 5 consecutive days in the treatment of MD. 22 patients were enrolled in this randomized controlled trial (11 in treatment arm, and 11 in placebo arm). They reported 82% versus 57% Class A vertigo control at 2-year follow-up. They also reported subjective improvements in tinnitus, hearing loss, and aural fullness. Silverstein et al[51] in a similarly constructed RCT, did not find benefit from IT dexamethasone perfusion.

Numerous retrospective uncontrolled studies have reported promising results in controlling vertigo, hearing loss, and tinnitus with IT steroids in MD.[52]

Given the fluctuating nature of Ménière's disease symptoms and hearing changes, constructing well-controlled, prospective, randomized trials with sufficient power remains difficult. Furthermore, given the disabling nature of vertigo and variety of alternatives with high control rates placebo-controlled studies are hard to justify. Thus, evidence class B data are likely the best that can be expected in the future. At present there are very limited data to support its use. Yet, given the relative safety in regards to hearing preservation many clinicians have adopted IT steroids over gentamicin as their next step after medical therapy has failed and before moving on to surgical intervention to control vertigo.

Recommendations for Clinical Use

IT steroid can be considered as treatment for recurrent vertigo from Ménière's disease. The injection method is the same as that given previously for gentamicin. Although theoretic considerations for or against methylprednisolone or other steroids exist, dexamethasone is the best tolerated in the middle ear (the others giving an intense inflammatory response). As a result, decadron is the most commonly used and typically in the commercially available 10mg/ml dosage. Given the relative concentration gradients across the round window membrane higher or lower concentrations will have little impact on the final concentration within the perilymph. Once again, 0.3 to 0.5 mL is sufficient to fill the middle ear and the patient is asked to remain supine for 20 minutes to allow the solution to bath the round window. Typically, 3 injections are given spaced 2 weeks apart with another 4 weeks given after the last injection to determine effect.

Tinnitus

Sakata and colleagues[53] first reported on the use of IT steroid in the treatment of tinnitus in 1982, and subsequently published their clinical experience of IT steroid therapy for tinnitus in 1,214 patients. In this uncontrolled retrospective study, the authors reported good tinnitus control in 77% of patients immediately after treatment, and in 68% of patients at 6 months after treatment. Modulation of disturbances in cochlear blood flow is the most commonly cited mechanism for IT steroid having a beneficial effect on tinnitus. Given that chronic tinnitus is centrally mediated, it seems unlikely that a peripherally acting therapy would be of much benefit. For new onset tinnitus of peripheral origin there may be some merit to investigating its use. Clinical trials investigating IT steroid in the treatment of tinnitus have been limited. Uncontrolled trials have shown good results, but at least one controlled trial investigating IT dexamethasone for severe debilitating tinnitus showed no benefit over placebo.[54] Given the high rate of placebo effect (up to 60% positive response) in drug trials for tinnitus there is little evidence to support the use of IT steroid as a therapy for idiopathic tinnitus.[55]

CONCLUSION

Given the ease and relative safety of intratympanic medication administration to treat disorders of the inner ear such as Ménière's disease, sudden hearing loss, or tinnitus this method of therapy has gained popularity in clinical practice. Multiple studies from case reports to the rare randomized clinical trial abound in the literature. In each disease our confidence in IT drug therapy is tempered by the relative lack in understanding of the basic pathophysiology underlying each of these disorders. For Ménière's disease IT drug administration offers either a nondestructive alternative (steroid) before more invasive/destructive alternatives or a noninvasive alternative to other well-documented beneficial therapies. In the case of SSNHL, IT steroid offers yet another option given the lack of alternative therapies with proven benefit. In either case, the transtympanic route to administer medications to the inner ear offers promise of better, more targeted therapies in the future as our understanding of these disease processes improves.

REFERENCES

1. Fowler EP. Streptomycin treatment of vertigo. *Trans Am Acad Ophthalmol Otolaryngol.* 1948;52:239–301.
2. Beck C, Schmidt CL. 10 years of experience with intratympanally applied streptomycin (gentamicin) in the therapy of morbus Meniere. *Arch Otorhinolaryngol.* 1978; 221(2):149–152.
3. Nedzelski JM, Chiong CM, Fradet G, et al. Intratympanic gentamicin instillation as treatment of unilateral Ménière's disease: update of an ongoing study. *Am J Otol.* 1993;14(3):278–282.
4. Magnusson M, Padoan S. Delayed onset of ototoxic effects of gentamicin in treatment of Ménière's disease. Rationale for extremely low dose therapy. *Acta Otolaryngol.* 1991;111(4):671–676.
5. Blakley BW. Clinical forum: a review of intratympanic therapy. *Am J Otolaryngol.* 1997;18(4):520–526.
6. Chia SH, Gamst AC, Anderson JP, Harris JP. Intratympanic gentamicin therapy for Ménière's disease: a meta-analysis. *Otol Neurotol.* 2004;25:544–552.
7. Williams SE, Zenner H, Schacht J. Three molecular steps of aminoglycoside ototoxicity demonstrated in outer hair cells. *Hearing Res.* 1987;30:11–18.
8. Schact J. Biochemical basis of aminoglycoside ototoxicity. *Otolaryngol Clin North Am.* 1993;26:845–853.
9. Atlas J, Parnes LS. Intratympanic gentamicin for intractable Ménière's disease: 5-year follow-up. *J Otolaryngol.* 2003;32(5):288–293.
10. Hoffer ME, Allen, K, Kopke RD, Weisskopf P, Gottshall K, Wester D. Transtympanic versus sustained-release administration of gentamicin: kinetics, morphology, and function. *Laryngoscope.* 2001;111(8):1343–1357.
11. Becvarovski Z, Bojrab DI, Michaelides EM, et al. Round window gentamicin absorption: an in vivo human model. *Laryngoscope.* 2002;112(9):1610–1613.
12. Plontke SK, Mynatt R, Gill RM, Borgmann S, Salt AN. Concentration gradient along the scala tympani after local application of window membrane. *Laryngoscope.* 2007;117(7):1191–1198.
13. Balough BJ, Hoffer ME, Wester D, et al. Kinetics of gentamicin uptake in the inner ear of Chinchilla langier after middle-ear administration in a sustained-release vehicle. *Otolaryngol Head Neck Surg.* 1998;119(5):427–431.
14. Hoffer ME, Kopke RD, Weisskopt P, et al. Use of the round window microcatheter in the treatment of Ménière's disease. *Laryngoscope.* 2001;111(11):2046–2049.
15. Salt AN, Gill RM, Plontke SK. Dependence of hearing changes on the dose of intrtympanically applied gentamicin: a meta-analysis using mathematical simulations of clinical drug delivery protocols. *Laryngoscope.* 2008; 118(10):1793–1800.
16. Plontke SK, Salt AN. Simulation of application strategies for local drug delivery to the inner ear. *ORL J Otorhinolaryngol Relat Spec.* 2006;68:386–392.
17. Plontke SK, Wood AW, Salt AN. Analysis of gentamicin kinetics in fluids of the inner ear with round window administration. *Otol Neurotol.* 2002;23(6):967–974.
18. Monsell EM. New and revised reporting guidelines from the Committee on Hearing and Equilibrium. American Academy of Otolaryngology-Head and Neck Surgery Foundation, Inc. *Otolaryngol Head Neck Surg.* 1995;113(3): 176–178.
19. Beck C, Schmidt CL. 10 years of experience with intratympanally applied streptomycin (gentamicin) in the therapy of morbus Meniere. *Arch Otorhinolaryngol.* 1978; 221:149–152.
20. Harner SG, Driscoll CLW, Facer GW. Long-term follow-up of transtympanic gentamicin for Ménière's syndrome. *Otol Neurotol.* 2001;22:210–214.
21. Hoffer ME, Kopke RD, Weisskopf P, Gottshall K, Allen K, Wester D. Microdose gentamicin administration via the round window microcatheter. *Ann N Y Acad Sci.* 2001; 942:46–51.
22. Diamond C, O'Connell DA, Hornig JD, et al. Systematic review of intratympanic gentamicin in Ménière's disease. *J Otolaryngol.* 2003;32(6):351–361.
23. Huon LK, Fang TY, Wang PC. Outcomes of intratympanic gentamicin injection to treat Ménière's disease. *Otol Neurotol.* 2012 Jul;33(5):706–714.
24. Coelho DH, Lalwani AK. Medical management of Ménière's disease. *Laryngoscope.* 2008; 118(6):1099–1108.
25. Kaylie DM, Jackson CG, Gardner EK. Surgical management of Ménière's disease in the era of gentamicin. *Otolarygol Head Neck Surg.* 2005;443–450.
26. Sakata E, Itoh A, Ohtsu K, Nakasawa H, Iwashita N. Pathology and treatment of cochlear tinnitus by blocking with 4% lidocaine and decadron infusion. *Pract Otol (Japan).* 1982;75:2525–2535.
27. Sakata E, Kitago Y, Murata Y, Teramoto K. Treatment of Ménière's disease. Middle ear infusion with lidocaine and steroid solution. *Auris Nasus Larynx.* 1986;13:79–89.
28. Doyle KJ, Bauch C, Battista R, et al. Intratympanic steroid treatment: a review. *Otol Neurotol.* 2004;25:1034–1039.
29. Hamid M, Trune D. Issues, indications, and controversies regarding intratympanic steroid perfusion. *Curr Opin Otolaryngol Head and Neck Surg.* 2008;16(5):434–440.
30. Nin F, Hibino H, Doi K, et al. The endocochlear potential depends on two K+ diffusion potentials and an electrical barrier in the stria vascularis of the inner ear. *Proc Natl Acad Sci USA.* 2008;105:1751–1756.
31. Nagura M, Iwasaki S, Wu R, Mizuta K, Umemura K, Hoshino T. Effects of corticosteroid, contrast medium and

ATP on focal microcirculatory disorders of the cochlea. *Eur J Pharmacol*. 1999;366(1):47–53.
32. Banerjee A, Parnes LS. The biology of intratympanic drug administration and pharmacodynamics of round window drug absorption. *Otolaryngol Clin North Am*. 2004; 37:1035–1051.
33. Parnes LS, Sun AH, Freeman DJ. Corticosteroid pharmacokinetics in the inner ear fluids: an animal study followed by clinical application. *Laryngoscope*. 1999;109:1–17.
34. Plontke SK, Biegner T, Kammerer B, et al. Dexamethasone concentration gradients along scala tympani after application to the round window membrane. *Otol Neurotol*. 2008;29:401–406.
35. National Institute of Health. *Sudden deafness*. Bethesda, MD: Author; 2000. NIH publication 00-4757.
36. Wilson WR, Byl FM, Laird N. The efficacy of steroids in the treatment of idiopathic sudden hearing loss. *Arch Otolaryngol*. 1980;106:772–776.
37. Cinamon U, Bendet E, Kronenberg J. Steroids, carbogen or placebo for sudden hearing loss: a prospective double-blind study. *Eur Arch Otorhinolaryngol*. 2001;258:477–480.
38. Wei BPC, Mubiru S, O'Leary S. Steroids for idiopathic sudden sensorineural hearing loss. *Cochrane Database of Systematic Reviews*. 2006, Issue 1. Art. No.: CD003998. DOI: 10.1002/14651858.CD00398.pub2.
39. Stachler RJ, Chandrasekhar SS, Archer SM, et al.; American Academy of Otolaryngology-Head and Neck Surgery. Clinical practice guideline: sudden hearing loss. *Otolaryngol Head Neck Surg*. 2012 Mar;146(3 suppl):S1–35.
40. Ho HG, Lin HC, Shu MT, Yang CC, Tsai HT. Effectiveness of intratympanic dexamethasone injection in sudden deafness patients as salvage treatment. *Laryngoscope*. 2004;114:1184–1189.
41. Ahn JH, Han MW, Kim JH, et al. Therapeutic effectiveness over time of intratympanic dexamethasone as salvage treatment of sudden deafness. *Acta Otolaryngol*. 2007:1–4.
42. Alles MJ, der Gaag MA, Stokroos RJ. Intratympanic steroid therapy for inner ear diseases, a review of the literature. *Eur Arch Otorhinolaryngol*. 2006;263:791–797.
43. Conlin AE, Parnes LS. Treatment of sudden sensorineural hearing loss: I. a systematic review. *Arch Otolaryngol Head Neck Surg*. 2007;133:573–581.
44. Conlin AE, Parnes LS. Treatment of sudden sensorineural hearing loss, II: a meta-analysis. *Arch Otolaryngol Head Neck Surg*. 2007;133:582–586.
45. Rauch SD, Halpin CF, Antonelli PJ, Babu S, Carey JP, Gantz BJ, Goebel JA, Hammerschlag PE, Harris JP, Isaacson B, Lee D, Linstrom CJ, Parnes LS, Shi H, Slattery WH, Telian SA, Vrabec JT, Reda DJ. Oral vs intratympanic corticosteroid therapy for idiopathic sudden sensorineural hearing loss: a randomized trial. *JAMA*. 2011 May 25; 305(20):2071–2079.
46. Battaglia A, Burchette R, Cueva R. Combination therapy (intratympanic dexamethasone + high-dose prednisone taper) for the treatment of idiopathic sudden sensorineural hearing loss. *Otol Neurotol*. 2008;29(4):453–460.
47. Kopke RD, Hoffer ME, Wester D, O'Leary MJ, Jackson RL. Targeted topical steroid therapy in sudden sensorineural hearing loss. *Otol Neurotol*. 2001;22:475–479.
48. Salt AN, Ma Y. Quantification of solute entry into cochlear perilymph through the round window membrane. *Hear Res*. 2001;154(1–2):88–97.
49. Semaan MT, Alagramam KN, Megerian CA. The basic science of Ménière's disease and endolymphatic hydrops. *Curr Opin Otolaryngol Head Neck Surg*. 2005;13:301–307.
50. Garduno-Anaya MA, Couthino DT, Hinojosa-Gonzalez R, et al. Dexamethasone inner ear perfusion by intratympanic injection in unilateral Ménière's disease: a two-year prospective, placebo-controlled, double-blind, randomized trial. *Otolaryngol Head Neck Surg*. 2005;133:285–294.
51. Silverstein H, Isaacson JE, Olds MJ, et al. Dexamethasone inner ear perfusion for the treatment of Ménière's disease: a prospective, randomized, double-blind, crossover trial. *Am J Otol*. 1998;19:196–201.
52. Shea JJ Jr, Ge X. Dexamethasone perfusion of the labyrinth plus intravenous dexamethasone for Ménière's disease. *Otolaryngol Clin North Am*. 1996;29:353–358.
53. Sakata E, Itoh A, Itoh Y. Treatment of cochlear tinnitus with dexamethasone infusion into the tympanic cavity. *Int Tinnitus J*. 1996;2:129–135.
54. Araujo MF, Oliveira CA, Bahmad FM Jr. Intratympanic dexamethasone injections as a treatment for severe, disabling tinnitus: does it work? *Arch Otolaryngol Head Neck Surg*. 2005;131(2):113–117.
55. Patterson MJ, Balough BJ. Review of pharmacological therapy for tinnitus. *Int Tinnitus J*. 2006;12(2):149–159.

CHAPTER 21

Benign Paroxysmal Positional Vertigo

Gerard J. Gianoli

INTRODUCTION

Benign paroxysmal positional vertigo (BPPV) is a very common entity representing 15 to 40% of patients presenting to a dizziness clinic. BPPV often has a self-limited course, but can be chronic and recurrent, possibly being the most common cause of recurrent vertigo. The pathophysiology involves dislocated otoconia, from the utricle, typically migrating into the posterior semicircular canal causing abnormal stimulation. The classic syndrome is described as short-lived bursts of vertigo brought on by certain positional changes. It is less commonly known that this disorder can also be the cause of chronic, ill-defined disequilibrium. It is also frequently found in association with other inner ear disorders (Ménière's disease, vestibular neuritis, and labyrinthine concussion). Although, this has been traditionally thought of as a "benign" and self-limiting disorder, it can cause significant impairment in the quality of life and can persist for many years. The diagnosis can be made on physical exam with the Dix-Hallpike maneuver. Approximately 80 to 85% of patients can be successfully treated with a single office procedure (canalith repositioning) that results in almost immediate relief of symptoms. The remaining 15 to 20% of patients may require a second repeat procedure, treatment of associated pathology, or surgery. Cases refractory to these simple in-office procedures have been successfully treated with surgical occlusion of the posterior semicircular canal. A newer approach has come with the institution of the Epley Omniax multiaxial repositioning device.

PHYSIOLOGY AND PATHOPHYSIOLOGY

The vestibular system senses angular and linear acceleration by means of the semicircular canals and otolithic organ sensors. The semicircular canals are oriented in 3 perpendicular planes with each canal having an enlarged or ampullated end. The nerve receptor area is found in the ampulla. The cupula, a gelatinous mass, sits atop the sensory cells in the ampulla and acts as an impermeable barrier across the lumen of the semicircular canal. The cupula acts essentially weightless in that it is of the same specific gravity of the surrounding endolymph. Consequently, movement of fluid within the semicircular canal deflects the cupula and causes stimulation or inhibition of the end organ. Deflection of the cupula in the direction of the ampulla (ampullopetal) causes inhibition and away from the ampulla (ampullofugal) causes stimulation of the posterior and superior canals whereas the reverse is true of the horizontal canal. The otolithic organs, which include the saccule and utricle, have a similar gelatinous mass as the cupulae of the semicircular canals but also contain calcium carbonate crystals. These crystals detect gravity and linear acceleration.

The proposed pathophysiology of BPPV may be caused by dislocated otolithic crystals floating in the semicircular canals (canalithiasis) or adhering to one of the semicircular canal cupulae (cupulolithiasis). The cupulolithiasis theory was first proposed by Schuknecht in 1962 with the identification of basophilic particles attached to the posterior canal cupula noted on temporal bone histology specimens of patients with BPPV.[1] He theorized that the particles caused the cupula to be sensitive to the force of gravity resulting in the abnormal stimulation. The canalithiasis theory (free-floating particles within the semicircular canal) was first reported by Hall in 1979.[2] This was later confirmed in vivo by Parnes and McClure in 1992.[3] The free-floating particles typically migrate to the posterior semicircular canal (although migration to the other canals is possible) as it is the most dependent portion of the labyrinth and get trapped in the canal due to the cupula acting as a barrier at the ampullated end of the canal.

These canalith are thought to cause minimal problems until a critical mass is reached. At that point the movement of the mass of canaliths causes a hydrodynamic drag of the endolymph in the posterior semicircular canal. The abnormal stimulation by either abnormal endolymphatic flow or abnormal weighting of the semicircular canal cupulae results in the aberrant stimulation of the vestibular system resulting in the clinical symptoms of BPPV. Whereas cupulolithiasis generally causes immediate stimulation upon placing a patient in the provocative position, canalithiasis requires a short time delay, or latency, before the onset of stimulation. Although pure forms of cupulolithiasis and canalithiasis occur, both can also occur concurrently rendering a more atypical clinical presentation. Similarly, although in the vast majority of cases the posterior semicircular canal is affected, the horizontal semicircular canal has been estimated to be involved in 5 to 30% of the time. Obviously, studies of the prevalence of horizontal BPPV are greatly affected by selection bias of the individual clinics involved. Anterior canal involvement has been reported to be rare, but the author notes this is more common than reported due to selection bias. Anterior canal BPPV is not adequately assessed via the traditional Dix-Hallpike maneuver. A prone, head forward maneuver is more apt to elicit responses of anterior canal involvement, but is simply not performed routinely in clinical practice.

Cupulolithiasis is felt to be the predominate pathophysiology for horizontal canal BPPV and canalithiasis the predominate pathophysiology for posterior canal and anterior canal BPPV. Multiple canal involvement has also been reported and results in atypical findings during exam.

BPPV affecting the posterior canal, as mentioned, is by far the most common variant of BPPV. This is likely due to the dependent nature of the posterior canal, especially while lying supine sleeping at night. Very likely, free-floating crystals migrate into the posterior canal due to the effects of gravity; particularly at night while the upper limb of the posterior canal most easily can be accessed. Once in the posterior canal and the patient arises, the crystals are likely to continue their migration down the posterior canal and become trapped by the cupula at the ampullated end of the canal. At this point the crystals can either migrate further and become attached to the cupula causing cupulolithiasis or once a critical mass of crystals have formed in the posterior canal, canalithiasis may predominate. With canalithiasis, this critical mass of crystals will move cephalad within the canal when placed in the most provocative position (Dix-Hallpike position). However, there is a short time delay before this migration occurs resulting in the latency before symptoms appear. Once movement occurs, there is a hydrodynamic drag, which causes an ampullofugal deflection of the posterior canal cupula, which is excitatory. This results in the symptoms of vertigo and a torsional-type nystagmus in the plane of the posterior canal. The nystagmus would beat clockwise in the left Dix-Hallpike position for a left ear BPPV and counterclockwise in the right Dix-Hallpike position for a right ear BPPV.

A right Dix-Hallpike maneuver should result in no symptoms or nystagmus for a left ear BPPV and the converse is true for a right ear BPPV. The nystagmus ceases once the mass of crystals stops moving and the cupula returns to a neutral position, which is typically 15 to 30 seconds duration. When the patient is brought back to an upright position, the canaliths will move in the opposite direction back down the limb of the posterior canal resulting in an ampullopetal deflection of the cupula. The nystagmus associated with this is in the reverse of the direction associated with the Dix-Hallpike maneuver and is of a lesser magnitude since this is an inhibitory stimulation of the posterior canal. After repeated maneuvers the nystagmus response will fade and is said to be fatigable. This is likely due to the eventual dispersion of the crystals and loss of the critical mass of canaliths.

The horizontal canal is less commonly involved in BPPV likely due to its up-sloping anatomy with the cupula at the upper end of the canal as opposed to the inferior limb like the posterior canal. Hence, canaliths most likely will not enter the horizontal canal and, if they do enter, will migrate out of the horizontal canal during normal daily head movement. Consequently, cupulolithiasis is a more frequently proposed entity with horizontal canal BPPV. In horizontal canal BPPV, a lateral head position is the most provocative position and, unlike the case of posterior canal BPPV, this will cause stimulation for either the right or left ear-down position with just one ear involvement. Cupulolithiasis of the right ear will cause ampullopetal deflection (inhibitory stimulation) in the right-ear-down position and ampullofugal deflection (excitatory stimulation) in the left-ear-down position. This results in an ageotropic (away from ground) horizontal nystagmus, which is stronger in the left-ear-down position (excitatory position). Conversely, canalithiasis of the right ear will cause an opposite pattern. Migration of the canalith mass in the right-ear-down position will cause ampullofugal deflection (excitatory stimulation) and ampullopetal deflection (inhibitory stimulation) in the left-ear-down position. This results in a geotropic (toward ground) horizontal nystagmus, which is stronger in the right-ear-down position (excitatory position). When viewed from the clinician's standpoint, ageotropic horizontal nystagmus is viewed as cupulolithiasis and geotropic horizontal nystagmus is viewed as canalithiasis. The stronger beating nystagmus is noted on the same side as the affected ear in canalithiasis and in the contralateral ear in cupulolithiasis (Table 21–1). One way of remembering which ear is affected in horizontal canal BPPV is that the stronger nystagmus points to the affected ear, regardless of whether it is cupulolithiasis or canalithiasis. So, if the stronger beating nystagmus is going to the left, then the left ear is the pathologic ear.

Table 21–1. Horizontal Canal BPPV Etiology and Location According to Nystagmus Associated with Lateral Ear Position

Strongest Intensity of Nystagmus	Geotropic Nystagmus	Ageotropic Nystagmus
Left	Left Canalithiasis	Right Cupulolithiasis
Right	Right Canalithiasis	Left Cupulolithiasis

ETIOLOGY

BPPV is considered to be either primary or secondary. Primary BPPV is more commonly seen in the elderly population where one study identified unrecognized BPPV in 9% of a large inner city geriatric cohort.[4] Primary BPPV is the most commonly reported type, representing as much as 50 to 70% of BPPV cases. Secondary BPPV can be divided among the differing antecedent conditions and concomitant pathologies. The most commonly recognized of these is head trauma and whiplash injuries. However, many other commonly recognized conditions associated with BPPV have been noted Table 21–2.

It seems much more common to find BPPV among patients who have another pathology of the same inner ear.

DEMOGRAPHICS

BPPV has been reported in virtually all age groups but is more common with increasing age and is especially common among the elderly. There is a gender predilection for afflicting females overall, but the gender distribution appears to be essentially balanced

Table 21–2. Possible Causes of BPPV

Head trauma, whiplash
Viral labyrinthitis, vestibular neuritis
Ménière's disease
Migraine
Ear surgery and nonear surgery
Chronic otitis media
Otosclerosis
Dental manipulation
Acoustic neuroma and other posterior fossa tumors
Viral URI

among younger and post-traumatic patients. There is limited information regarding racial distribution/affinity, but BPPV appears to be common among all ethnic/racial groups.

SYMPTOMS/HISTORY

There are essentially two categories of presentation for BPPV: classic and nonclassic. Additionally, a mixture of these two presentations is not uncommon.

Classic History/Symptoms

In the classic presentation of BPPV, the patient will describe a sudden onset of whirling vertigo spells that are induced by very specific head positions or movements. The most common provocative position is with the offending ear in a more dependent position such as when rolling over in bed to one side. This position places the posterior canal in the vertical position, which will allow for the largest magnitude of cupular deflection. Other provocative positions include looking up ("top shelf syndrome"), bending over, and arising from a supine position. The patients will also note that putting themselves in the provocative position does not always produce vertigo; this is due to fatigability. The severity of the vertigo can vary significantly but is often very severe and violent. The duration of the vertigo is typically less than 30 seconds but may be described by patients as lasting much longer. This is probably due to an overestimation of the time because it is such a noxious stimuli. In patients with classic BPPV, they do not have any symptoms of vertigo or dizziness in between these discrete spells. Occasionally, a patient will report constant vertigo, but often when they are questioned very closely, they relate that whenever they move their head they feel vertiginous, but as long as their head is still they have no symptom.

Nonclassic History/Symptoms

Many patients will complain of other symptoms that have not traditionally been attributed to BPPV and not complain of the classic symptoms. It is felt that the severe classic symptoms of BPPV are often avoided by the patient, either consciously or unconsciously avoiding the provocative position. When questioning patients with nonclassic symptoms they may not report vertigo but you may also find that they never put their head back. By avoiding these certain positions, the severe rotary vertigo is avoided, but the patients will continue to note other symptoms associated with abnormal (but lesser magnitude) stimulation of the posterior semicircular canal. This abnormal stimulation is brought on by linear movements, which should not normally provoke any stimulation of the semicircular canals. The nonclassic symptoms include dizziness associated with:

1. *Arising.* The posterior semicircular canal is stimulated by an abnormal weight (misplaced otoconia) on the cupula that would otherwise not be there. Consequently, the posterior semicircular canal is stimulated when arising. This results in confusing angular input with linear input. These patients can often be confused with patients suffering with postural hypotension. The two main distinctions are normal blood pressure and pulse, and the presence of a spinning sensation. Note that postural hypotension can make a patient feel woozy and lightheaded, but it will not make them have a sensation of spinning.
2. *Leaning forward.* This, too, causes input from an angular accelerometer (posterior semicircular canal) to be confused with linear acceleration (gravity) input. In essence, leaning forward is the inverse of the provocative position (Dix-Hallpike position).
3. *Linear acceleration/deceleration.* Although this motion does not cause maximal stimulation, the effects of gravity and acceleration of the canaliths or cupuloliths will cause mild abnormal stimulation. Instead of the anticipated linear acceleration input, the vestibular organ presents a combination of linear and angular acceleration input.
4. *Vertical oscillation.* Similarly, the effects of gravity on the crystals will cause inappropriate sensation of gravity by the semicircular canal.
5. *Morning dizziness.* Typically, patients will describe mornings to be the worst time of the day for their symptoms. It has been theorized that through-

out the night the canaliths gather into and form a critical mass in the posterior canal while the patient is supine, relatively still and sleeping. Upon arising in the morning, the motions of the canaliths cause the dizziness. With repeated head movements throughout the day, the canaliths disperse and do not cause significant stimulation and hence symptoms lessen.

6. *Head rotation.* Dizziness with head rotation, especially fast head movement, is felt to be secondary to either the inertia of the canaliths or due to their gravitary pull resulting in aberrant stimulation.

PHYSICAL EXAM

The physical examination of the patient with BPPV should be focused on identifying any comorbid ear pathology although frequently the physical exam is unremarkable with the exception of the Dix-Hallpike maneuver. The Dix-Hallpike maneuver is the diagnostic test for posterior canal BPPV. The Dix-Hallpike maneuver is accomplished by placing the patient in a sitting position on the examining table and, with one movement, turning their head 45 degrees to one side and lowering the patient to a supine position. The head is extended 30 degrees below the plane of the examining table if neck mobility allows. It is probably prudent to check for neck mobility and to auscultate the carotid arteries in at risk patients prior to the Dix-Hallpike maneuver. When the head is in the down position, the eyes are examined for nystagmus and the patient s questioned for symptoms of vertigo. Nystagmus and vertigo should coincide.

Examination of the eyes could be done with simple visual inspection but due to overriding visual fixation, lesser degrees of BPPV would be missed. Consequently, a means of eliminating visual fixation is recommended, such as with Frenzel lenses or, even better, infrared video goggles. These methods enhance the sensitivity of the Dix-Hallpike maneuver. Relying on ENG or VNG tracing for evaluation will lead to many missed diagnoses of BPPV as the torsional nature of the nystagmus is not captured on these tracings. Although the Dix-Hallpike maneuver is very specific for the diagnosis of posterior canal BPPV, the sensitivity is somewhat lacking due to the fatigable nature of BPPV. In other words, a negative Dix-Hallpike maneuver does not necessarily mean that the patient does not have BPPV.

Dix and Hallpike describe the classic signs of BPPV[5]:

1. *A critical provocative position.* The episodes of rotary vertigo are often produced when the patient places their head with a particular ear directed downward.
2. *Characteristic nystagmus.* During the vertiginous attack, the eyes of the subject can be seen to produce a very specific nystagmus pattern. For BPPV affecting the right ear, the nystagmus would be a torsional movement with the fast phase in the counterclockwise direction. For BPPV affecting the left ear, the nystagmus is characterized by a torsional movement with the fast phase in the clockwise direction
3. *Latency.* This is typically 2 to 5 seconds in canalithiasis but can be delayed by as much as 30 seconds. Latency may be absent in cupulolithiasis.
4. *Limited duration.* Duration is typically less than 30 seconds in canalithiasis but may be persistent in cupulolithiasis.
5. *Reversal nystagmus.* Reversal of the characteristic nystagmus is frequently noted when bringing the patient back to the upright position after a Dix-Hallpike maneuver. However, this is usually much less in magnitude and is not always discernible.
6. *Fatigability.* Repeat testing results in diminished or absent response.

Evaluation for horizontal canal BPPV is accomplished by having the patient lie supine. While tucking the chin in slightly in order to bring the horizontal canal into a vertical plane (approximately 30 degrees ventrally), the head is quickly turned toward the test side. The eyes are examined for nystagmus and the patient questioned about vertigo. The nystagmus of horizontal canal BPPV has a shorter or absent latency and is horizontal in nature. In unilateral horizontal canal BPPV, nystagmus will typically be present with testing on either side. As detailed in Table 21–1, the direction and magnitude of the nystagmus can elucidate the mechanism of BPPV and the affected ear.

EVALUATION

The Dix-Hallpike test is the gold standard for diagnosis of posterior canal BPPV. Virtually no other pathology will mimic the characteristic nystagmus and clinical symptoms of posterior canal BPPV. Beyond the Dix-Hallpike and the positional testing for horizontal canal involvement, there are no required tests for diagnosing BPPV. However, concomitant pathology of the inner ear or skull base (such as cerebellopontine angle masses or Ménière's disease) may dictate further evaluation.

The indications for these additional studies would be based on clinical findings that do not fit under the classic presentation of BPPV. Most ancillary vestibular tests do not demonstrate any abnormality with straightforward BPPV (with the exception of the Dix-Hallpike test and positional testing). However, caloric testing, vestibular autorotation testing and posturography may show abnormalities with routine BPPV cases. Some have reported abnormal caloric results in horizontal canal BPPV speculating that the canaliths interfered with normal thermally induced endolymphatic flow or cupular deflection during caloric testing. Similarly, vertical VOR testing in vestibular autorotation testing has been shown to result in phase abnormalities in BPPV. This is likely due to a similar mechanism but due to involvement of the posterior canal. Computerized dynamic posturography, although typically normal in BPPV cases, has been shown to produce reduced stability in SOT conditions 5 and 6, the classic vestibular deficit pattern, particularly in the elderly. This has been noted to improve after successful treatment of BPPV.

DIFFERENTIAL DIAGNOSIS

Very few disorders can replicate the findings of BPPV, but there are several that can produce positional nystagmus and dizziness. Although these disorders can produce positional vertigo and nystagmus, they do not typically produce the characteristic nystagmus found with BPPV. Some of these include posterior fossa masses, craniovertebral junction abnormalities, cervical vertigo, vascular loop compression syndrome, alcoholic intoxication, and vertebrobasilar vascular insufficiency. BPPV has been implicated as a secondary pathology to a number of entities including those listed here. However, BPPV is so prevalent that coincidental occurrence of BPPV with other disorders can also be expected.

TREATMENT

Traditionally, the treatment of BPPV has been benign neglect since most cases are suspected to resolve spontaneously. Consequently a period of deferred treatment seems reasonable if the symptoms have recently occurred. Medical treatment for BPPV has been largely ineffectual, with limited response to vestibular suppressants and antiemetics. Canalith repositioning maneuvers (CRM) have been the mainstay of treatment for BPPV. These have included the Epley and Semont maneuvers for posterior canal BPPV. For horizontal canal BPPV, forced prolonged positioning and barrel roll maneuvers typically have been favored. CRM are based on the idea of moving the canalith through the offending semicircular canal and back into the area of the utricle in order to eliminate the aberrant stimulus.

Although it wasn't until 1992 that Epley[6] first published his report of the canalith repositioning procedure (CRP), he had been performing and teaching CRP in his private practice since 1979. Prior attempts to publish his findings met with rejection due to skepticism that such a simple maneuver would alleviate vertigo. In fact, skepticism ran so high that early in his career, complaints by fellow physicians were brought to the hospital committee in order prevent him from using CRP (J. Epley, personal communication, July 2008). The "Epley maneuver," or a variation thereof, appears to be the most popular maneuver by clinicians in treating posterior canal BPPV. The maneuver (Figure 21–1) based on the canalithiasis theory, is accomplished by: (1) Starting in a sitting position, (2) Placing the patient in the Dix-Hallpike position (of the offending ear) while observing for nystagmus, (3) Rotate the head 90 degrees to the contralateral Dix-Hallpike position, (4) Have the patient roll into a lateral decubitus position with the head 90 degrees further (with

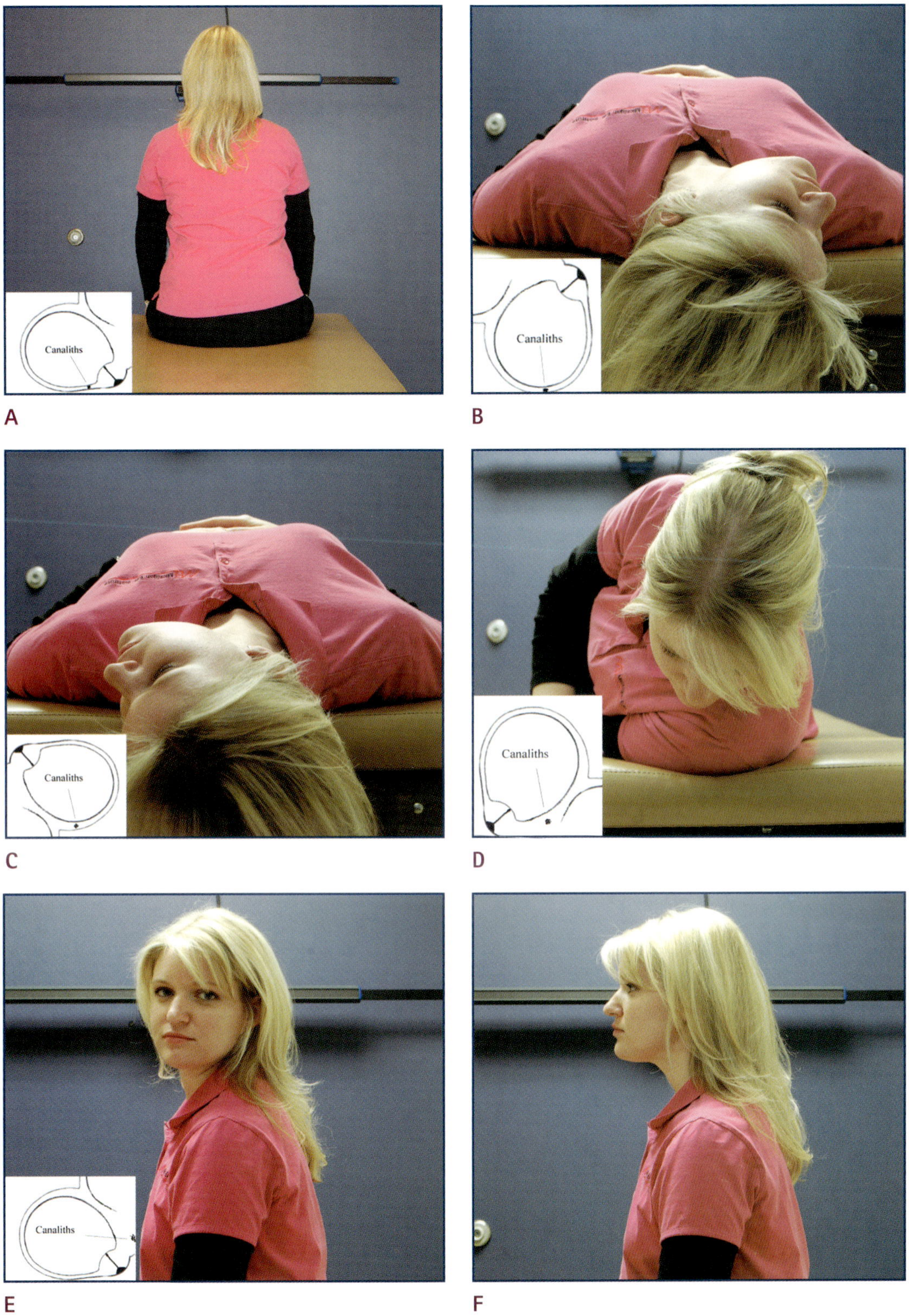

Figure 21–1. The canalith-repositioning maneuver (for right ear posterior canal BPPV) with corresponding posterior semicircular canal position and canalith position. **A.** Starting in a sitting position. **B.** Placing the patient in the Dix-Hallpike position (of the offending ear) while observing for nystagmus. **C.** Rotate the head 90 degrees to the contralateral Dix-Hallpike position. **D.** Have the patient roll into a lateral decubitus position with the head 90 degrees further (with the plane of the nose pointing 45 degrees below the horizon). **E.** Bring the patient to an upright sitting position with their head still turned away. **F.** While sitting turn the head back to midline.

the plane of the nose pointing 45 degrees below the horizon), (5) Bring the patient to an upright sitting position with their head still turned away, and (6) While sitting turn the head back to midline.

The "Semont maneuver" or liberatory maneuver was first described in 1988 and is based on the cupulolithiasis theory.[7] The patient is seated on the exam table with the head turned away from the affected side. Quickly, the patient is brought into a side-lying position on the affected side with the head turned upward. After 5 minutes, the patient is then rapidly brought to the contralateral side-lying position with the head facing downwards. After another 5 minutes, the patient is then brought back up to the sitting position. The maneuver is based on the idea that the rapid change in position would free the canaliths attached to the cupula and allow them to migrate out of the posterior canal. Although demonstrated to be an effective maneuver, the rapid changes in body position are difficult for some patients (especially the elderly and those with mobility problems) compared to the Epley maneuver.

A simple treatment of horizontal canal BPPV is forced prolonged positioning.[8] In this technique the patient is instructed to lie with the affected ear in the uppermost position for 12 hours, or nightly for several nights in a row. This has been reported to be effective for both canalithiasis and cupulolithiasis, but appears to be more effective with the former. Another treatment option is a barrel roll or barbeque roll maneuver. In the maneuver, the patient starts off supine with the head turned toward the affected ear. The patient is then rolled 360 degrees, in 90-degree increments, while keeping the horizontal canal perpendicular to the ground.

The use of mastoid vibration during CRM has been controversial. Adding mastoid vibration to CRM was first reported by Li[9] to significantly improve successful outcome, but additional studies have not replicated these findings. It may be that mastoid vibration makes the most impact in cases of cupulolithiasis. After CRM, many clinicians restrict the patient's head position for 24 to 72 hours postmaneuver. Studies evaluating postmaneuver restrictions have been mixed with most demonstrating no difference in treatment and control groups.

Surgery for BPPV is limited to only the rare cases that have frequent and multiply recurrent BPPV after CRM. The first surgical procedure directed to treatment of posterior canal BPPV was singular neurectomy (posterior ampullary nerve section), which was popularized by Gacek in the 1970s.[10] Although effective, the technically demanding nature and the high incidence of sensorineural hearing loss significantly reduced its popularity. Posterior canal occlusion was introduced by Parnes and McClure in 1990.[11] This procedure, done through a mastoidectomy approach, results in occlusion or blockage of endolymphatic movement in the posterior semicircular canal and effectively locks the cupula in place and eliminates posterior canal stimulation. Effective and technically easier than singular neurectomy, this has become the most common surgical treatment for BPPV refractory to CRM.

COMPLEX AND MIXED CANAL BPPV

Since the introduction of CRM, many clinicians have noted the presence of multiple canal involvement BPPV—mixed horizontal/posterior, bilateral BPPV, and anterior canal BPPV. In one study the incidence of multiple canal involvement was 20% and bilateral BPPV at over 10%. The nystagmus generated by multiple canal involvement can significantly complicate the diagnostic and treatment paradigm. The most prudent approach has been to treat the most suspicious ear or the posterior canal component first and then evaluate the patient 2 to 3 weeks later. At that point the clinical picture is often much clearer.

The Epley Omniax multiaxial positioning device (Figure 21–2) appears to be a very effective and useful alternative for both the diagnosis and treatment of complex/atypical BPPV.[12] Developed by Vesticon, the Omniax received FDA approval in 2008. With the Omniax, the patient is seated and harnessed in a chair that allows for 360-degree rotation in any direction while monitoring eye movement with infrared videography. The chair is controlled by the accompanying computer that records video, eye tracings and position. Although many standard maneuvers are programmed into the Omniax (eg, Epley, Barrel roll, Dix-Hallpike, etc), many less commonly used maneuvers and a free-style component are included.

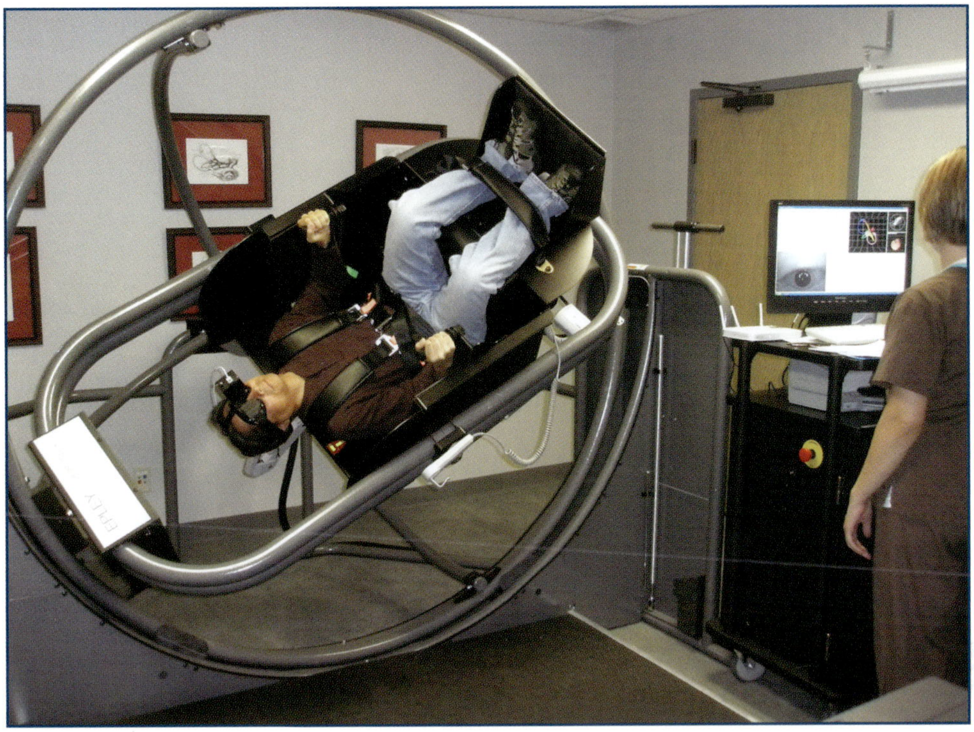

A

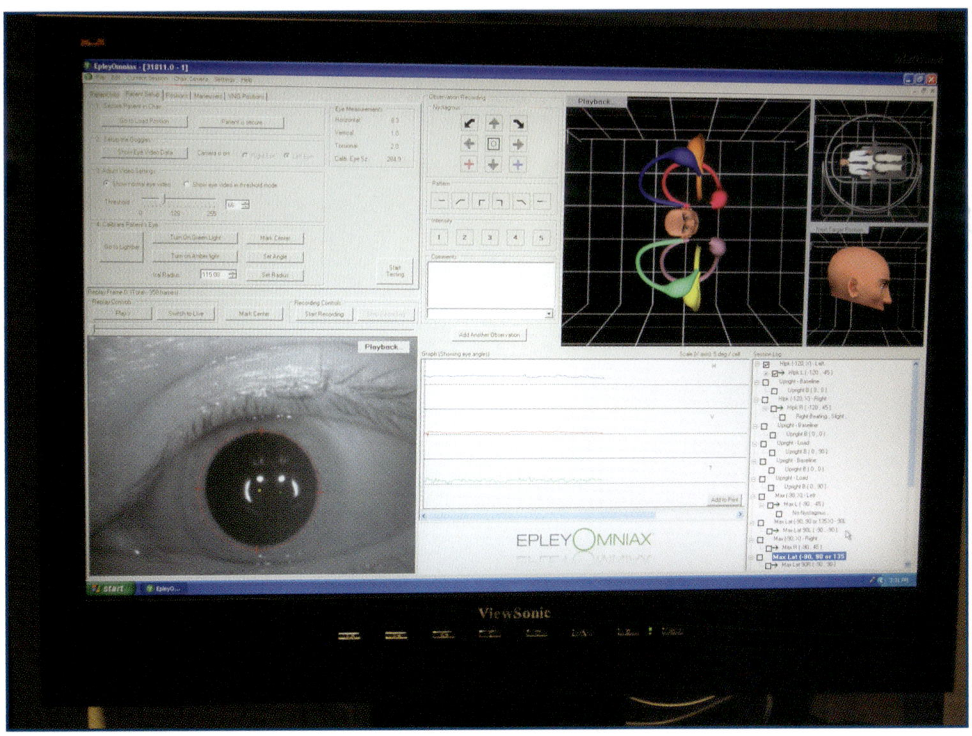

B

Figure 21–2. Epley Omniax device. **A.** Epley Omniax multiaxial positioning device. **B.** Screenshot of Epley Omniax computer control module.

The Omniax has been shown effective in the treatment of routine case of BPPV but in the author's opinion, it is most useful in the tertiary care diagnosis and treatment of complicated BPPV.

REFERENCES

1. Schuknecht HF. Cupulolithiasis. *Arch Otolaryngol*. 1969; 90:765.
2. Hall SF, Ruby RR, McClure JA. The mechanics of benign paroxysmal vertigo. *J Otolaryngol*. 1979;8(2):151.
3. Parnes LS, McCLure JA. Free-floating endolymph particles: a new operative finding during posterior semicircular canal occlusion. *Laryngoscope*.1992;102(9):988–992.
4. Oghalai JS, Manolidis S, Barth JL, Stewart MG, Jenkins HA. Unrecognized benign paroxysmal positional vertigo in elderly patients. *Otolarygol Head Neck Surg*. 2000; 122(5):630–634.
5. Dix MR, Hallpike CS. The pathology symptomatology and diagnosis of certain common disorders of the vestibular system. *Proc Roy Soc Med*. 1952;45(6):341–354.
6. Epley JM. The canalith repositioning procedure: for treatment of benign paroxysmal positional vertigo. *Otolaryngol Head Neck Surg*. 1992;107:399–404.
7. Semont A, Freyss G, Vitte F. Curing the BPPV with a liberatory maneuver. *Adv Otorhinolaryngol*. 1988;42:290–293.
8. Vanuhhuchi P, Giannoni B, Pagnini P. Treatment of horizontal semicircular canal benign paroxysmal positional vertigo. *J Vestib Res*. 1997;7:1–6.
9. Li JC. Mastoid oscillation: a critical factor for success in canalith repositioning procedure. *Otolaryngol Head Neck Surg*. 1995;112:670–675.
10. Gacek RR. Further observations on posterior ampullary nerve transaction for positional vertigo. *Ann Otol Rhinol Laryngol*. 1978;91:469–473.
11. Parnes LS, McClure JA. Posterior semicircular canal occlusion for intractable benign paroxysmal positional vertigo. *Ann Otol Rhinol Laryngol*. 1990;99:330–334.
12. Nakayama M, Epley JM. BPPV and variants: improved treatment results with automated, nystagmus-based repositioning. *Otolaryngol Head Neck Surg*. 2005;133(1): 107–112.

CHAPTER 22

Superior Canal Dehiscence Syndrome

Gerard J. Gianoli

INTRODUCTION

Superior semicircular canal dehiscence (SSCD) has been defined as the absence of bone overlying the superior semicircular canal facing toward the dura of the middle cranial fossa.[1] SSCD has been implicated as the cause of a variety of inner ear symptoms including Tullio's phenomenon, pressure induced vertigo, aural fullness, autophony, conductive hearing loss mimicking the presentation of otosclerosis, and fluctuating or progressive sensorineural hearing loss. Additionally, SSCD has also been reported to be asymptomatic. In the past, many patients with SSCD had been misdiagnosed as having otosclerosis, patulous eustachian tubes, middle ear perilymphatic fistulas, or Ménière's disease. Identification of this entity requires a high degree of suspicion, appropriate findings on physical exam, lab testing, and confirmation on high-resolution CT scan. Surgical repair of the SSCD or occlusion of the superior canal has been reported with a high degree of symptom resolution.

INCIDENCE AND ETIOLOGY

The prevalence of SSCD has been found to be much higher in series of analyzed CT scans than on temporal bone histology. Carey et al identified complete absence of bone over the superior canal histologically in 0.5% of 1000 vertically sectioned adult temporal bones.[2] There was an additional 1.4% with very thin (<0.1 mm) bone covering the superior canal. Added together, the prevalence of thin or dehiscent superior canals approached 2%. This study also reported that 50% of the SSCD cases had bilateral involvement.

Carey and colleagues[2] also analyzed 36 infant temporal bones and concluded that the thickness of the bone overlying the superior canal was consistently thin. The thickness of the bone covering the superior canal gradually thickened with age, reaching adult levels by age 3 years. They theorized that the anatomic finding of SSCD was a developmental anomaly, but since clinical symptoms were typically not noted until later in life, a second event such as head trauma or sudden change in intracranial pressure was required to propagate the symptoms found in SSCD patients.

Roberto et al[3] used tetracycline staining to investigate the deposition of bone in the dog model at 10, 25, and 50 days of age. This study demonstrated progressive deposition of endochondral and endosteal bone at the superior semicircular canal postnatally. The bone deposition decreased with age. These findings are in agreement with the observations in the study by Carey et al. In a related study, Hirvonen and colleagues[4] reported a CT study of the thickness of the superior canal in a group of patients with SSCD and those without SSCD. Among those with SSCD, the contralateral superior canal bone was thinner (or dehiscent), compared to those patients without SSCD. This finding supports the notion of

SSCD as a developmental anomaly related to bony deposition in early life.

Several observations point to a "second event" required to produce symptoms from SSCD. Among these observations are:

1. The above studies demonstrating development of bone over the superior semicircular canal occurring later (postnatally) than other parts of the inner ear.
2. The clinical observation of the presence of asymptomatic SSCD noted during intraoperative exploration of the middle cranial fossa for encephalocele repair.
3. Symptoms from SSCD do not generally present in the pediatric population.

These observations support the notion that a second event is required in addition to the congenital anomaly of thin or absent superior canal bone in order to produce clinical symptoms. Roughly half of patients report an event they attribute to symptom onset for SSCD. This "second event" is typically noted to be either head trauma or a Valsalva type episode.

CLINICAL PRESENTATION

SSCD was first reported by Minor et al[1] in 8 patients who exhibited the symptoms of short-lived vertigo spells in response to certain sounds or activities that would cause transient increases in intracranial or middle ear pressure (Valsalva, coughing, sneezing, nose-blowing, autoinsufflations). These activities would produce a torsional nystagmus, which directly implicated stimulation of the superior semicircular canal. Activities causing increased middle ear pressure (sound, positive pressure in the ear canal, autoinsufflations) induce nystagmus with the slow phase upward and the superior pole of the eye directed *away* from the affected ear. Activities causing a transient elevation in intracranial pressure (Valsalva against a closed glottis, jugular venous compression) or negative pressure in the ear canal resulted in the slow phase of nystagmus directed downward and the superior pole of the eye torquing *toward* the affected ear. The clinical findings of Tullio's phenomenon and pressure inducing nystagmus associated with SSCD has been termed Minor's syndrome. Although the vertigo caused by SSCD is most characteristically reported as short-lived, other characterizations of vestibular symptoms have been reported as well, including more prolonged vertigo spells, chronic disequilibrium, and drop attacks.

Since the first identification of SSCD as a cause for Minor's syndrome, other symptoms and clinical presentations have been identified.[5] In a recent review of their experience with SSCD, Zhou et al[6] described SSCD as a "great otologic mimicker" because of the variety of presentations and the variety of other diagnoses from which SSCD can be confused. SSCD can present with a variety clinical findings that can make distinction from other otologic entities a challenge. Among the otologic entities of which SSCD is most frequently misdiagnosed are Ménière's disease, otosclerosis, perilymphatic fistula, and patulous eustachian tube.

Symptoms noted with SSCD, include vertigo/dizziness induced by sound stimuli or pressure altering activity. Some patients may find no specific exacerbating stimuli. Another symptom is autophony, or hearing one's own voice and breathing. Other symptoms include hearing loss, aural fullness, and tinnitus (pulsatile and nonpulsatile).

PATHOPHYSIOLOGY

The "third mobile window theory" has been proposed to explain the symptoms accompanying SSCD.[7] This theory proposes that the flexible nature of the SSCD allows for egress of endolymph out of the superior canal resulting in abnormal stimulation of the superior canal cupula. Additionally, low frequency sound energy transmitted through the inner ear is allowed to dissipate through this bony defect resulting in the conductive gap noted in some SSCD patients. Merchant and Rosowski[8] proposed that SSCD could be classified among a number of lesions that produce a third mobile window on the scala vestibuli side of the cochlea. Included among these are lateral or posterior canal dehiscence, enlarged vestibular aqueduct, dehiscence of the internal auditory canal, carotid dehiscence (into the cochlea), diffuse dehiscence (such as in Paget's disease), and other congenital anomalies of the inner ear. The hearing loss in these pathologic third mobile window cases exhibits poor air conduction thresholds and good bone conduction thresholds.

The above theories do not completely explain all of the findings of SSCD. Among these is the presence of asymptomatic patients, the presentation of patients with only auditory and no vestibular findings or vice versa, Ménière's-type vertigo spells, and the absence of symptoms in the pediatric population. It has been proposed that a second event such as trauma or a major pressure-altering event (Valsalva-type maneuver) causes a disruption of very thin bone over the superior canal thus creating an SSCD. However, this only explains adult onset of symptoms and not the other findings, nor does it explain a true dehiscence in an asymptomatic patient. Gianoli and Soileau[9] proposed the theory that alteration of intracranial pressure resulted in increased compliance at the round and oval windows and, if pressure changes were extreme, potential disruption of the windows resulting in a frank middle ear perilymph fistula. This theory could explain the above exceptions to the third mobile window theory and also explain why round window reinforcement has been noted to resolve SSCD symptoms (at least temporarily) in many patients. They further proposed a grading system for SSCD as listed in Table 22–1.

Table 22–1. Staging System for SSCD

Stage 1: Asymptomatic SSCD—anatomic dehiscence with no inner ear symptoms.
Stage 2: Minor's syndrome—Tullio's phenomenon and Valsalva induce vertigo, correlating with an increased compliance of the inner ear system.
Stage 3: Ménière's syndrome—vertigo and hearing loss mimicking Meniere's disease, correlating with a frank oval or round window fistula.
Stage 4: End stage—profound hearing loss or vestibular areflexia, reflecting an end stage to the damage from stage 3.

EVALUATION

In SSCD, the hearing loss most frequently cited is a conductive hearing loss resembling that of otosclerosis. SSCD can be differentiated from otosclerosis by impedance testing and pure tone testing at lower sensation levels than routine testing.[8] Often, if tested for, the SSCD patients are noted to have sensorineural scores with sensation levels much better than the norm (eg, −5 or −10 dB). Additionally, impedance testing reveals that the acoustic reflexes are intact among SSCD patients, which is in contradistinction to the otosclerotic patient whose acoustic reflexes should be absent. Although most papers regarding patients with SCCD report normal hearing or a low frequency conductive hearing loss, there are some reports of sensorineural hearing loss.

Impedance testing can also be helpful in excluding eustachian tube dysfunction and patulous eustachian tube as the etiology for autophony or aural fullness in SSCD patients. Additionally, the absence of TM excursion with respiration would tend to exclude patulous eustachian tube as the diagnosis.

Examination of the eyes with various manipulations (preferably with means of magnification and prevention of fixation such as with infrared video goggles) can often produce the above-mentioned characteristic nystagmus found in SSCD. Testing with loud sounds in the affected ear (Tullio's phenomenon) appears to be a specific but not very sensitive finding in SSCD. Characteristic nystagmus associated with either autoinflation, Valsalva with a closed glottis or traditional fistula testing (applying both negative and positive pressure) appears to be more commonly present in SSCD patients.

Additional testing that has been useful in the confirmation of SSCD is Vestibular Evoked Myogenic Potentials (VEMP).[6,10] Several studies have identified abnormally low thresholds on VEMP testing in cases of SSCD (defined as ≤65 dB). According to one study this appears to be a more sensitive test for SSCD than the previously mentioned tests and the authors reported 91.4% sensitivity and 95.8% specificity for the diagnosis of SSCD.

Another proposed screening test included suboccipital vibration, reported by White and colleagues.[11]

In their study of 8 SSCD patients, application of 100-Hz vibration to the ipsilateral suboccipital region produced vertical/torsional nystagmus in all 8 patients. Although, this appears to be a very sensitive the specificity may be lacking since vibration induced nystagmus is present in many peripheral vestibular disorders.

IMAGING

Although SSCD is suspected by history, physical findings, and testing, radiographic imaging is required to confirm its presence. High-resolution CT scan has been the imaging modality of choice. Sub-millimeter cuts are required for adequate imaging. Cuts of 1.0 mm or larger are inadequate and will lead to an overly high false-positive rate of diagnosis. Among reports of CT scan findings of SSCD, Williamson et al[12] identified SSCD in 9% of coronal CT scans with 1.0 mm collimation performed at their institution over a 2-year period. Cloutier et al[13] found a 4% incidence of SSCD findings on CT scans with 0.55 mm collimation and reformatting in the plane of the superior canal among 581 temporal CT scans performed over a one-year period. Consistent with these findings, Belden et al[14] found an improved positive predictive value for SSCD with 0.5 mm collimation compared to 1.0 mm collimation. Both of the above mentioned studies of SSCD incidence are much higher than the 0.5% of histologically identified SSCD by Carey et al. The discrepancy of SSCD findings between 1.0-mm and 0.5-mm scans can be accounted for by averaging artifact. However there is still a significant difference between incidence of SSCD on the 0.5-mm CT study and on the histologic study. This is likely due to a combination of the averaging artifact in patients with very thin bone and study selection bias. When evaluating temporal bone CT scans for SSCD it is prudent to ensure the presence of the dehiscence on more than one image series (Figure 22–1).

Consequently, the finding of SSCD on temporal bone CT by itself does not necessarily implicate SSCD as the cause for the patient's symptomatol-

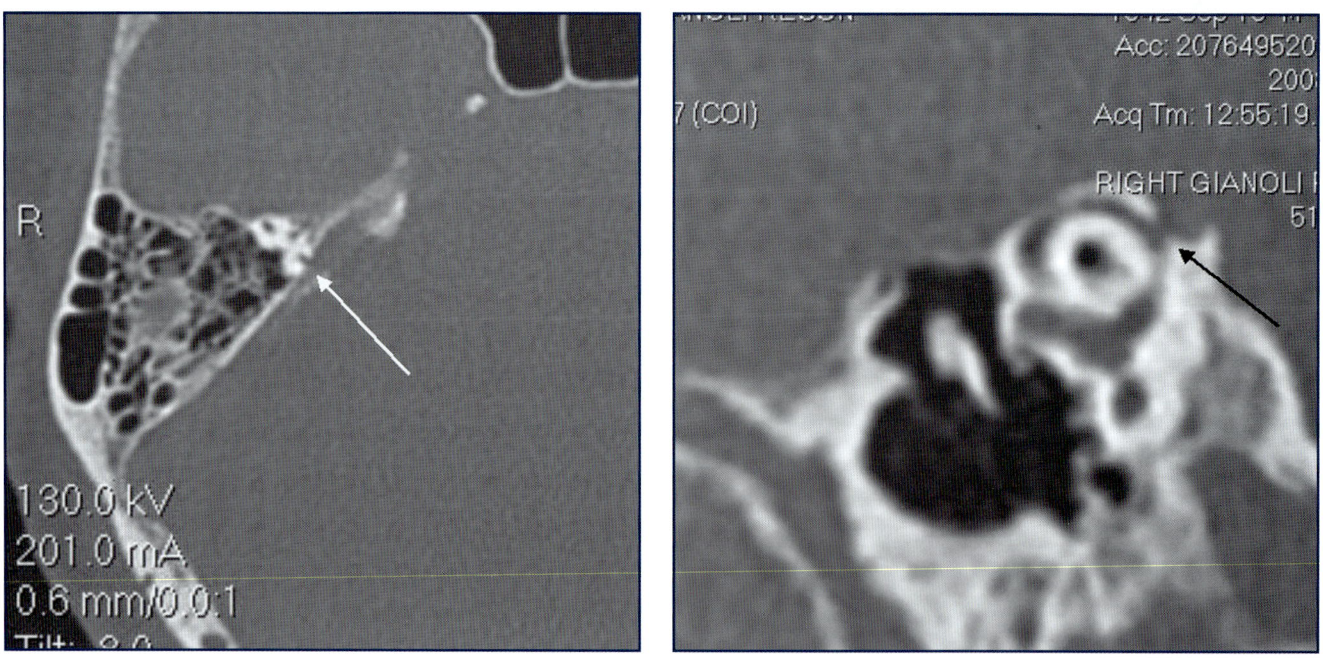

A B

Figure 22–1. A. Axial CT demonstrating SSCD at the site of the superior petrosal sinus. **B.** CT reconstruction in the plane of the superior canal demonstrating the corresponding dehiscence at the superior petrosal sinus.

ogy. Even with currently available technology, there is still a small false positive rate for SSCD diagnosis. Additionally, SSCD has been reported as an asymptomatic entity. In order to presume a causative role for SSCD in the patient's inner ear pathology, corroboration with an appropriate history, physical examination, and vestibular testing is mandatory. It should also be noted that dehiscence of the posterior semicircular canal can cause clinical symptoms very similar to SSCD, so the posterior canal integrity should be assessed during temporal bone imaging in suspected SSCD cases.

With the current multislice scanners, the images can be reformatted to slice into virtually any plane the examiner wishes. The author finds that planar cuts parallel and perpendicular to the superior canal very helpful. However, cuts that are radially sent out like wheel spokes from a central point located at the arcuate artery are probably the most useful, as all the images are always roughly a perpendicular cut through the superior canal (Figure 22–2). It should be noted that a contralateral SSCD is present in approximately 50% of patients and that the superior canal bone is often very thin in the rest of the patients.

The concept of the "dehiscent middle fossa" has been put forward with regard to more global anomalies of the middle fossa in patients with SSCD.[15] The

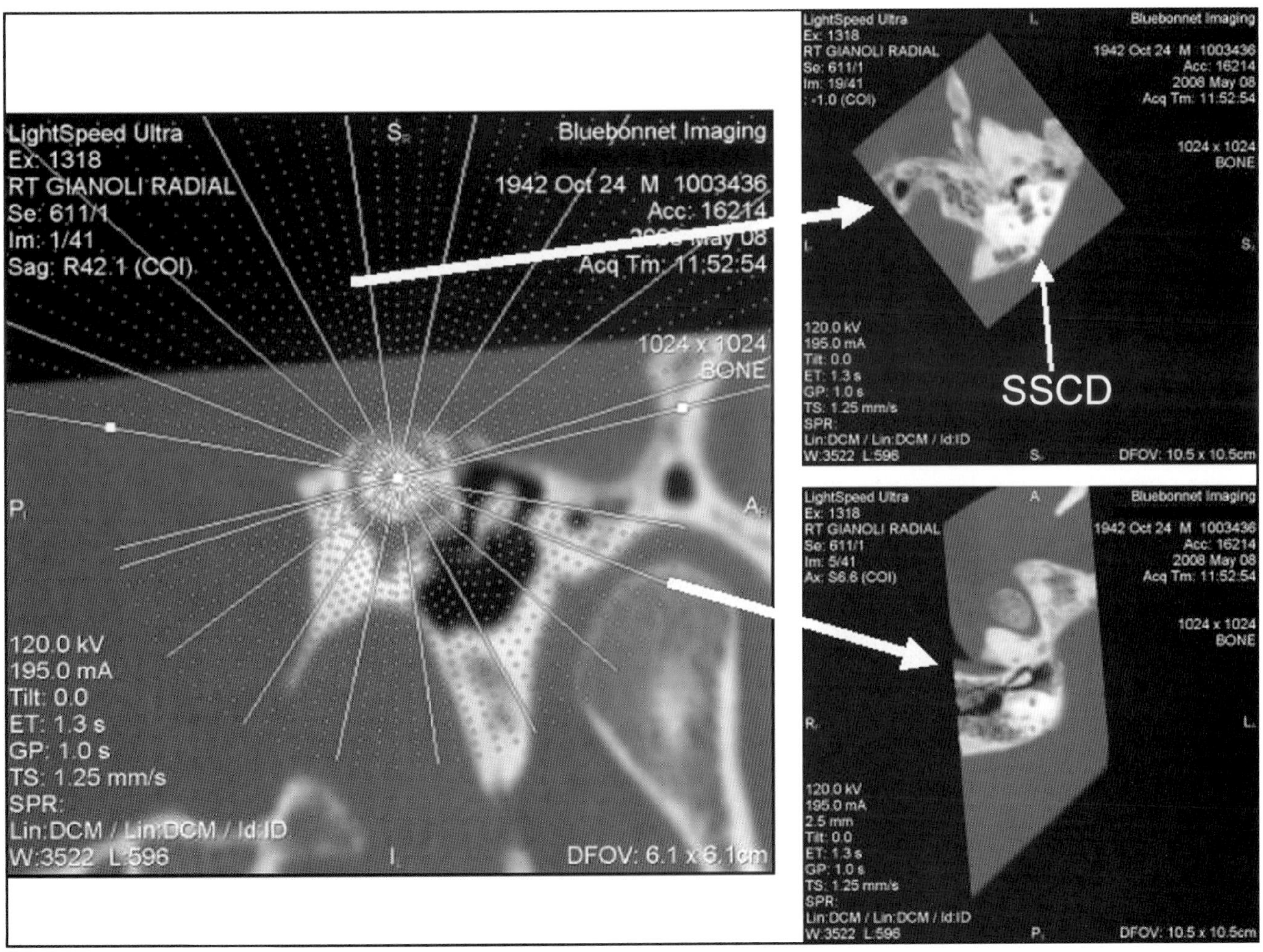

Figure 22–2. On the left, scout of CT reconstructions performed in a radial manner centered on the subarcuate artery. On the right are two corresponding slices from this construct.

constellation of findings in the dehiscent middle fossa includes SSCD, multiple tegmen defects, geniculate ganglion dehiscence, and encephaloceles. Even a case of bilateral dehiscent internal auditory canals has been seen by this author. The incidence of multiple tegmen defects is normally about 20% among random temporal bones studied. However, multiple tegmen defects are present in roughly 80% of patients with SSCD. With a higher incidence of multiple tegmen defects, encephaloceles are encountered more frequently in this patient population. Consequently, CT imaging in cases of temporal bone encephaloceles should include scrutiny of the superior canal for dehiscence since this would be important for surgical planning (Figure 22–3). Similarly, bony dehiscence of the geniculate ganglion is found in 5 to 15% of random temporal bones but has been found in 53% of SSCD temporal bones (Figure 22–4). This obviously has implications for surgical planning.

TREATMENT

Although surgical repair or occlusion has been the thrust of almost all reports to date regarding SSCD, it should be noted that many patients with SSCD do not require any intervention. Surgical intervention is generally reserved for patients who have significant symptoms who cannot be managed with supportive medical care. Surgical options include repair of the SSCD or occlusion of the superior canal through either a middle fossa craniotomy approach or a transmastoid approach, transcanal reinforcement of the oval and round windows and, lastly, a combination of oval/round window repair with repair of the SSCD.

Most of the reports in the literature describe the middle fossa approach for either repair or occlusion (Figure 22–5). With this approach, a standard middle fossa craniotomy is performed. During temporal

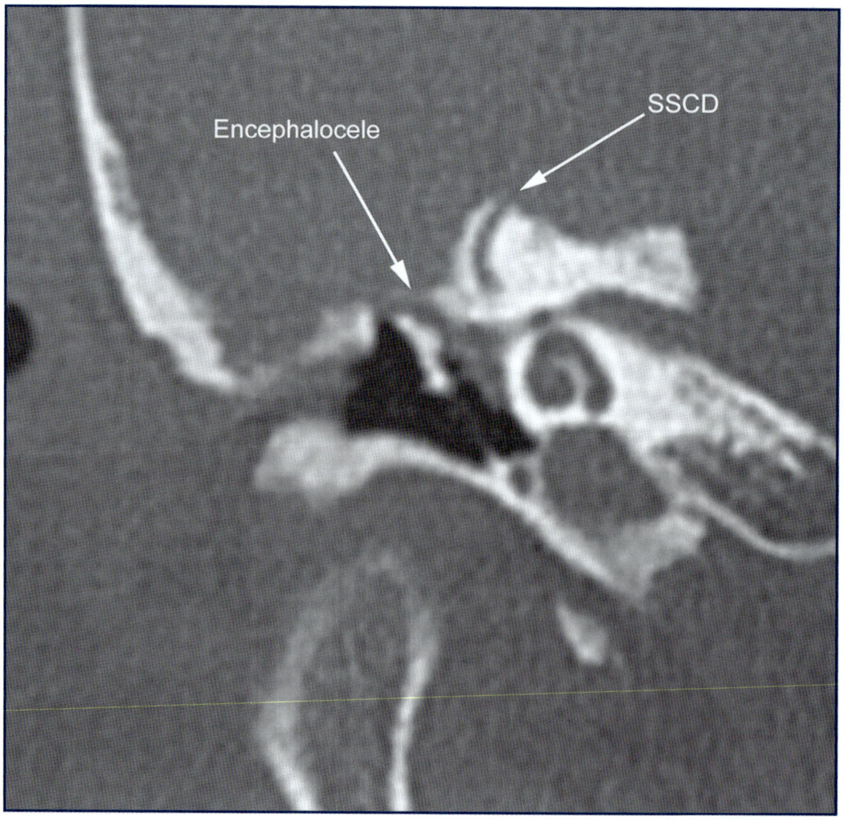

Figure 22–3. Coronal CT scan in a case of an encephalocele with concomitant SSCD.

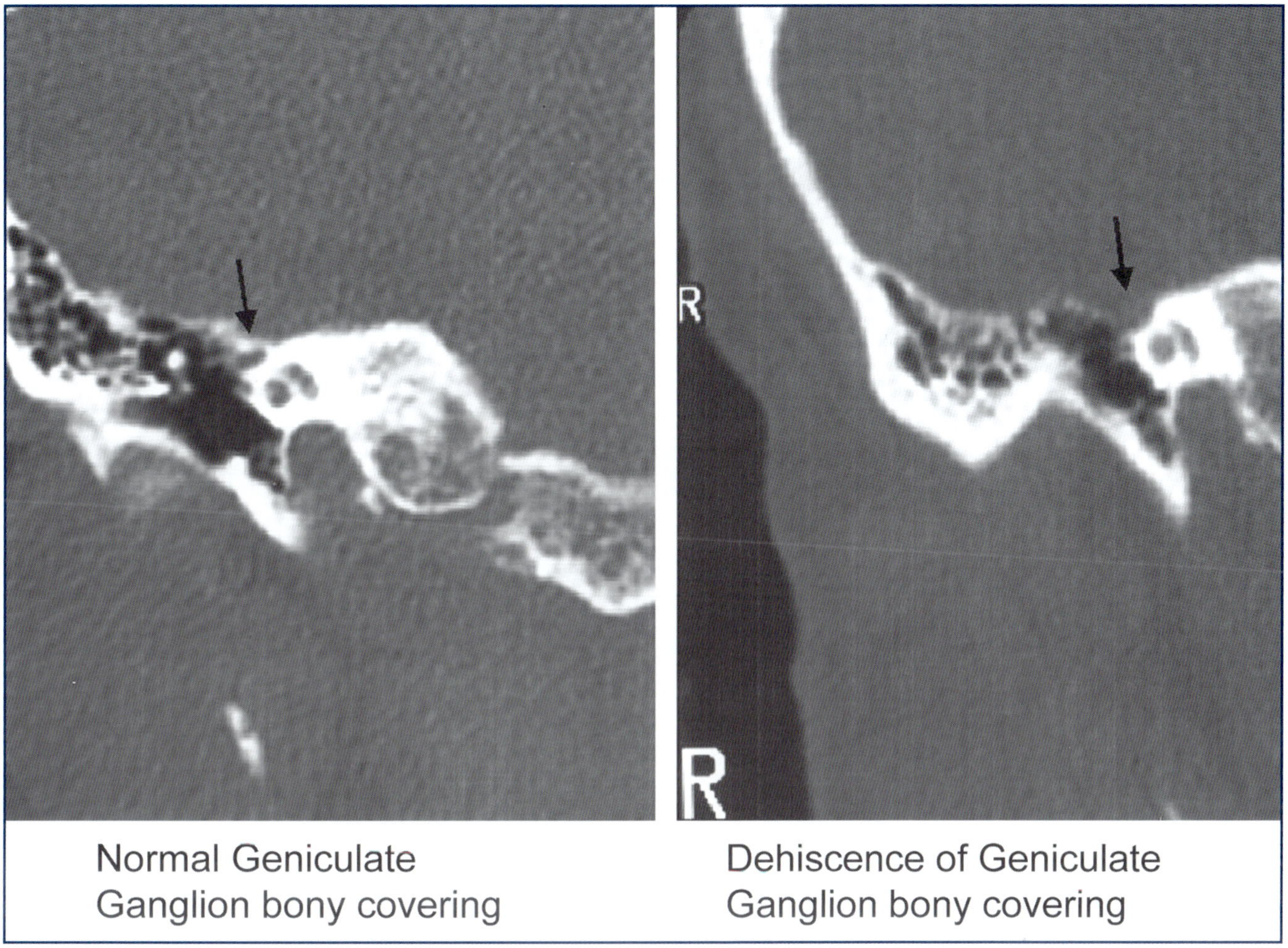

Figure 22–4. Coronal CT scans of normal bony covering of the geniculate ganglion in a non-SSCD patient (*left*) and a dehiscent geniculate ganglion in an SSCD patient (*right*).

lobe retraction care is taken to not inadvertently suction or otherwise breach the SSCD. Localization of the SSCD can sometimes be difficult due to multiple dehiscences of the tegmen that are frequently seen in this patient population. In these cases, image guided navigational systems have proven helpful. Additionally, due to the greater incidence of dehiscence of the geniculate ganglion, it is recommended that dissection proceed with facial nerve monitoring and facial nerve stimulating dissectors. Once the dehiscence is identified, repair or occlusion may be performed. Occlusion can be performed with bone wax or fascia. The author favors repair of the defect with a small piece of calvarial bone obtained from the craniotomy flap, which is fixed into place with hydroxyapatite bone cement (Figure 22–6).

In transmastoid occlusion of SSCD, a standard mastoidectomy is performed. Dissection is carried superior to the horizontal canal and the superior canal is identified at its anterior limb. The superior canal can then be blue-lined and opened for occlusion. Occlusion of the superior canal in this case proceeds similarly to a posterior canal occlusion surgery for intractable BPPV. However, it should be noted that the anatomy of many SSCD patients is such that the tegmen is particularly low-lying. This makes transmastoid occlusion technically more challenging in these patients.

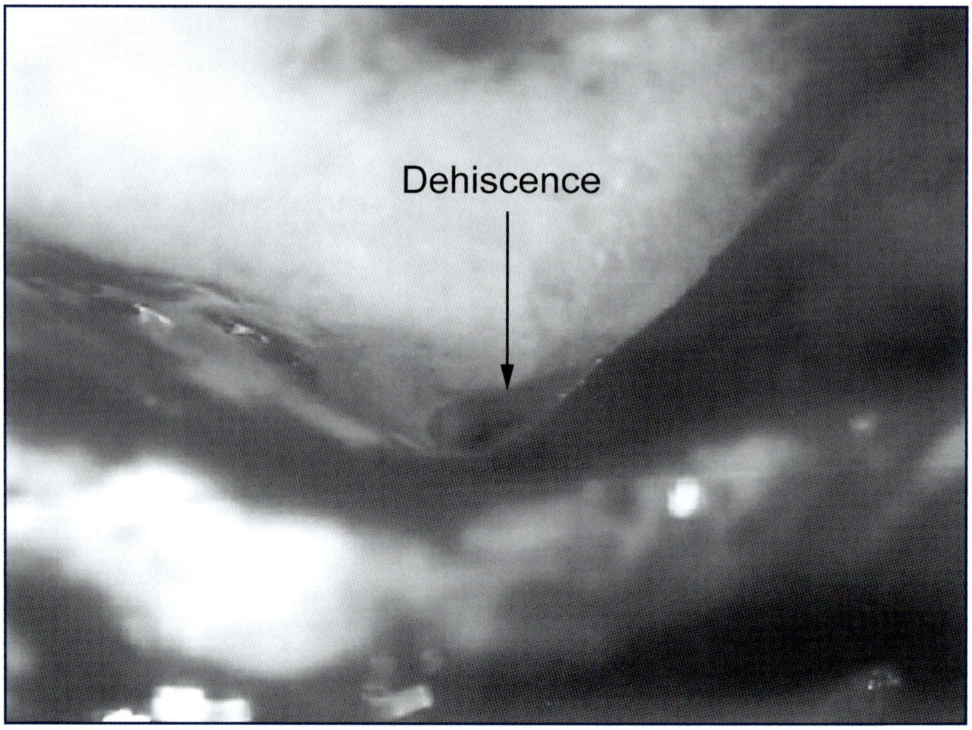

Figure 22–5. Intraoperative photograph of an SSCD as seen through the middle fossa approach.

As advocated by Kartush,[16] the transcanal approach to reinforce the oval and round windows is based on the idea of limiting the compliance of the inner ear system by reducing the mobility of the middle ear windows. This procedure was first performed for SSCD unknowingly by surgeons attempting to repair oval/round window perilymphatic fistulas. In some patients this produced long-lasting resolution of symptoms. However, there are no published studies to date to report overall success rate. The author and others have used this approach with selected SSCD patients. The author's impression is that the success rate is much lower than repair/occlusion but it does offer a more minimally invasive approach with significantly less risk to the patient. This procedure is virtually identical to the traditional routine oval window and round window repair for middle ear perilymphatic fistula. Some have advocated using a cartilage graft to reinforce the round window repair and others have advocated the use of fibrin glue and extensive middle ear packing with Gelfoam.

A combined approach of middle fossa repair of the SSCD and oval/round window reinforcement has been reported by Gianoli and Soileau,[9] who compared the outcomes of patients undergoing middle fossa repair and combined middle fossa repair with oval/round window repair. Although all patients had resolution of vertigo, outcome from the combined procedure was felt to be superior to middle fossa repair alone.

Surgical repair and/or occlusion have been reported to resolve vertiginous symptoms of SSCD with a high degree of reliability. In the few cases reported that have had failure of repair or occlusion, revision surgery appears to be successful. No published studies are available for the outcome of the minimally invasive oval/round window reinforcement approach. Although it appears successful in some isolated cases, the overall success in a large patient population is not known, nor is the long-term resolution rate.

Complications from the above mentioned surgeries are what one would expect from similar neuroto-

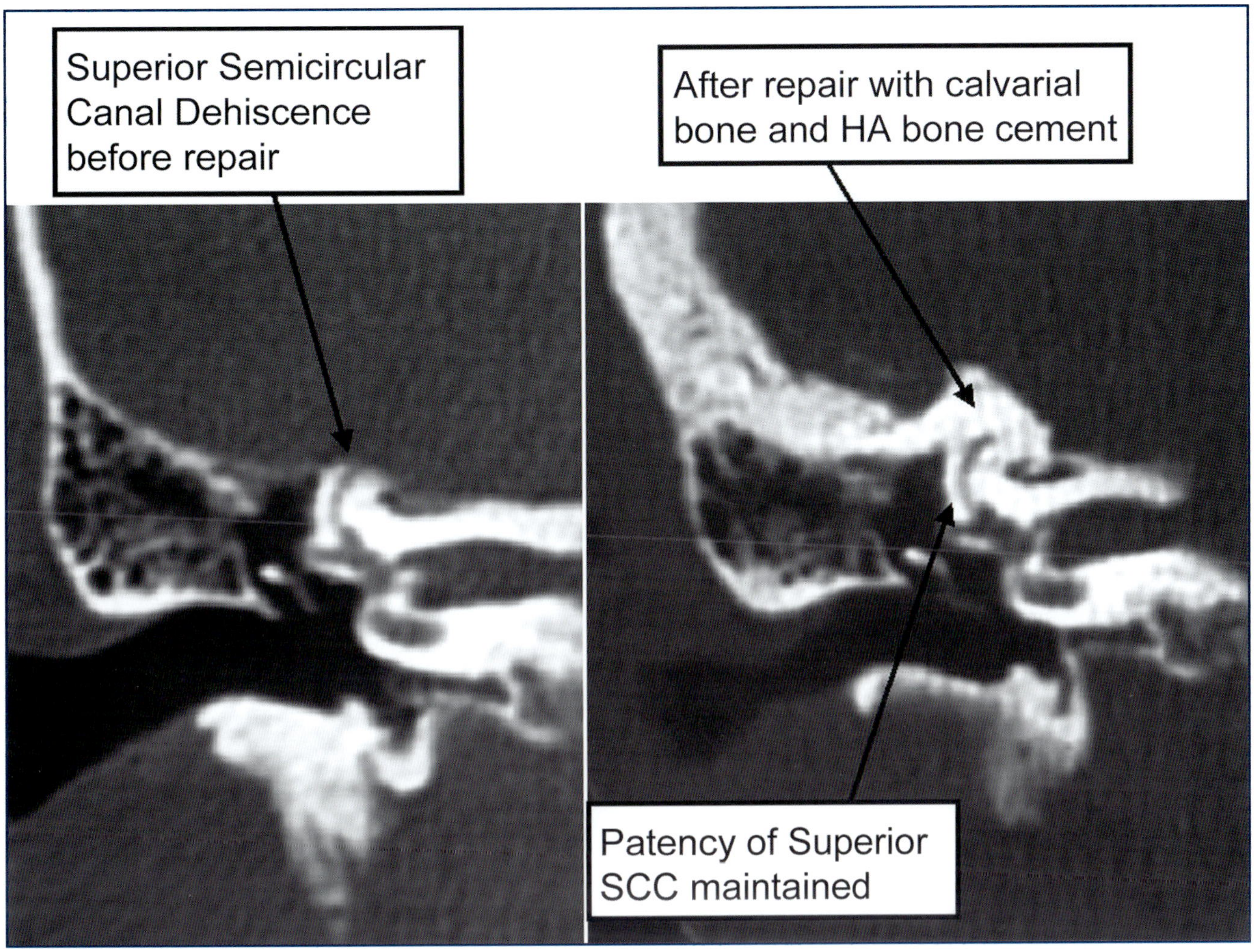

Figure 22–6. Preoperative (*left*) and postoperative (*right*) coronal CT scans in a patient who underwent middle fossa repair of SSCD with calvarial bone and HA bone cement. Note that patency of the superior canal is maintained and it is easily imaged postoperatively.

logic procedures using the same approaches. The loss of superior semicircular canal function is an expected outcome in the occlusion technique; however, loss of global vestibular function and sensorineural hearing loss has also been reported. Failure due to either misplaced bone grafts in the repair technique and inadequate plugging in the occlusion technique can occur.

REFERENCES

1. Minor LB, Solomon D, Zinreich JS, Zee DS. Sound- and/or pressure-induced vertigo due to bone dehiscence of the superior semicircular canal. *Arch Otolaryngol Head Neck Surg*. 1998;124:249–258.
2. Carey JP, Minor LB, Nager GT. Dehiscence or thinning of the bone overlying the superior semicircular canal in a temporal bone survey. *Arch Otolaryngol Head Neck Surg*. 2000;126(2):137–147.
3. Roberto M, Favia A, Lozupone E. Postnatal bone growth in the semicircular canals of the dog. *Ital J Anat Embryol*. 1998;103:27–34.
4. Hirvonen TP, Weg N, Zinreich SJ, Minor LB. High-resolution CT findings suggest a developmental abnormality underlying superior canal dehiscence syndrome. *Acta Otolaryngol*. 2003;123(4):477–481.
5. Smullen JL, Andrist EC, Gianoli GJ. Superior semicircular canal dehiscence: a new cause of vertigo. *Journal LA State Med Soc*. 1999;151:397–400.

6. Zhou G, Gopen Q, Poe DS. Clinical and diagnostic characterization of canal dehiscence syndrome: a great otologic mimicker. *Otol Neurotol*. 2007;28(7):920–926.
7. Minor LB. Superior canal dehiscence syndrome. *Am J Otol*. 2000;21:9–19.
8. Merchant SN, Rosowski JJ. Conductive hearing loss caused by third window lesions of the inner ear. *Otol Neurotol*. 2008;29:282–289.
9. Gianoli GJ, Soileau JS. *The dehiscent middle fossa: prevalence, manifestations, associated findings and results of 24 surgical explorations for superior semicircular canal dehiscence.* Presented as a Triologic thesis, publication pending. 2005.
10. Brantburg K, Bergenius J, Tribukait A. Vestibular-evoked myogenic potentials in patients with dehiscence of the superior semicircular canal. *Acta Otolaryngol (Stockh)*. 1999;119:633–640.
11. White JA, Hughes GB, Ruggieri PN. Vibration-induced nystagmus as an office procedure for the diagnosis of superior semicircular canal dehiscence. *Otol Neurotol*. 2007;28(7):911–916.
12. Williamson RA, Vrabec JT, Coker NJ, Sandlin M. Coronal computed tomography prevalence of superior semicircular cnaal dehiscence. *Otolaryngol Head Neck Surg*. 2003; 129(5):481–485.
13. Cloutier JF, Belair M, Saliba I. Superior semicircular canal dehiscence: positive predictive value of high-resolution CT scanning. *Eur Arch Otorhinolaryngol*. 2008; 265(12):1455–1460.
14. Belden CJ, Weg N, Minor LB, Zinreich SJ. CT evaluation of bone dehiscence of the superior semicircular canal as a cause of sound- and/or pressure-induced vertigo. *Radiology*. 2003;226(2):337–343.
15. Gianoli GJ. Deficiency of the superior semicircular canal. *Curr Opin Otolaryngol Head Neck Surg*. 2001;9:336–341.
16. Kartush JK. *Superior canal dehiscence syndrome symptoms resolved by reinforcement of the oval and round windows.* Unpublished data. 2002.

PART V

Surgical Dissection Guide

CHAPTER 23

Surgical Dissection of the Temporal Bone

Seilesh Babu

INTRODUCTION

The temporal bone is complicated in the sense that it contains numerous critical structures in a tight, compact area. Injury to any of the areas can lead to significant morbidity and even mortality. Practicing in the temporal bone lab is essential in order to gain familiarity and confidence with approaches to through the temporal bone. This chapter reviews drilling techniques, surgical anatomy, and procedures, serving as a guide in temporal bone laboratory dissections. A temporal bone curriculum used in our teaching course is provided in Table 23–1.

DRILL SYSTEM AND DRILLING TECHNIQUE

Drill System and Drill Burs

The most important instrument utilized in the dissection of the temporal bone is the otologic drill. The drill and the drill bits or burs play a significant role in safe, efficient technique. Modern drills either utilize gas-powered or electric powered supplies. Gas-powered drills have been more powerful, but are loud and require special equipment for their use. Electric powered drills have a rapid setup, are quieter, and recently have had a dramatic increase in power. The limiting factors for most electric drills have been their lack of speed and torque, resulting in less efficient bone removal and the amount of heat that is generated in the handpieces. Recent advances in electric motor design have overcome these limitations. They provide adequate speed and torque, water-cooled handpieces, excellent drill bits that have been modified to allow less skipping, and an ergonomic feel in surgeon's hand.

Burs or drill bits come in various shapes, cutting surfaces, and materials. The bur design is one of the most critical factors in drill usage because it is the actual interface between surgeon and bone. The flute design on the bits should allow easy removal of bone without undue force needed. Various types of burs are available, including cutting, diamond, and coarse. Cutting burs provide the most rapid removal of bone but are more likely to cause injury to surrounding tissue. Diamond burs allow delicate removal of bone without fear of easy skipping and loss of control. As they can generate heat, they must constantly be irrigated to keep the bone and facial nerve from becoming too hot. This can be used to an advantage when trying to stop bleeding from the bone.

Drilling Technique

The drill can be set to spin clockwise or counterclockwise. It is important to always check to see the cutting bur and flutes are turning in the anticipated direction. The drill will skip less, be under better control, and more efficiently remove bone when it is pulled in the opposite direction than the bur is spinning. The possibility of skipping must be kept in mind whenever drilling to make sure that no specific structure is at risk if the spinning bur were to "run in a certain unintentional direction."

Table 23–1. Temporal Bone Dissection Curriculum

The following is designed to progress through the temporal bone during practice in the temporal bone lab.
1. Examine Surface Landmarks a. Remove soft tissue off bone b. Evaluate linea temporalis, spine of Henle, mastoid tip, Macewen's triangle, zygomatic root.
2. External Auditory Canal a. Remove the skin of the external auditory canal to the level of the annulus i. May try to elevate a tympanomeatal flap but difficult in lab b. Perform canalplasty to allow visualizing of entire annulus
3. Middle Ear a. Lift the annulus between the notch of Rivinus and the 6 o'clock position. b. Identify the chorda tympani nerve, the round window niche, the promontory, the incudostapedial joint. Divide the incudostapedial joint. c. Remove the stapes and practice stapes procedure with prosthesis d. Or could remove incus and practice ossicular chain reconstruction.
4. Mastoidectomy a. Perform a simple (cortical) mastoidectomy. b. Identify middle cranial fossa dural plate, sigmoid sinus, sinodural angle, mastoid tip air cells, digastric ridge, horizontal semicircular canal, mastoid antrum, short process of incus, and mastoid antrum. c. Thin the intact external auditory canal wall.
5. Further dissection in mastoid a. Identify the facial nerve in the mastoid and remove the bone off of it. b. Expose the chorda tympani nerve. c. Open the epitympanum preserving the canal wall intact, and display the head of malleus and the body of incus. d. Dissect and identify the semicircular canals, endolymphatic sac, and retrofacial air cell tract.
6. Posterior Tympanotomy (Facial Recess) a. Open the facial recess between facial nerve and the chorda tympani to reveal the middle ear. b. Perform cochleostomy and practice electrode placement if available c. Extend the posterior tympanotomy inferiorly to divide the chorda tympani and expose the hypotympanum and round window niche.
7. Modified Radical Mastoidectomy a. Remove the posterior canal wall ensuring complete removal of the malleus head, complete exposure of the tympanic and mastoid segments of the facial nerve, and removal of the mastoid tip.
8. Labyrinthectomy a. Blue-line each semicircular canal showing the relationship of the posterior canal to the endolymphatic sac, duct, retrofacial cells, and facial nerve. b. Open and remove the horizontal, posterior, and superior semicircular canals. c. Trace openings into the vestibule. Open the vestibule and expose the second genu of the facial nerve i. Identify the spherical and elliptical recesses. ii. Using a pick, palpate the opening of the oval window from beneath.
9. Exposure of the Internal Auditory Canal a. Using the face of the vestibule as a landmark of the lateral end of the internal auditory canal, blue-line the internal auditory canal b. Without opening the internal auditory canal, blue line 180 degrees of the canal c. Identify the relationship of the jugular bulb, internal auditory canal, and cochlear aqueduct
10. Internal Auditory Canal Contents a. Open the internal auditory canal b. Note the superior and vestibular nerves. Identify the transverse crest. Gently move the vestibular nerves and identify the facial and cochlear nerve. c. Identify the vertical crest (Bill's bar).

Table 23–1. *continued*

11.	Middle Cranial Fossa Dissection a. Re-orientate the bone and remove the dura of the middle cranial fossa. b. Identify the arcuate eminence and the superior semicircular canal (or its remnant) c. Identify the greater superficial petrosal nerve and follow posteriorly d. Expose the internal auditory canal medial to the superior semicircular canal on the posterior aspect of the middle cranial fossa (60-degree angle). Blue-line the IAC e. Identify the relationship of the internal auditory canal, geniculate ganglion, greater superficial petrosal nerve, superior semicircular canal, and the cochlea. f. Remove the tegmen plate and identify the tympanic segment of the facial nerve, the tensor tympani, tendon and muscle, and the mesotympanum.
12.	Transcochlear Dissection a. Elevate the facial nerve from its bony canal between the geniculate ganglion and the stylomastoid foramen b. Dissect the medial portion of the bony canal of the facial nerve and identify the sinus tympani, the subiculum, and ponticulus. c. Open the promontory revealing the basal turn of the cochlea. d. Dissect anteriorly to show the relationship of the intrapetrous carotid artery, eustachian tube, and cochlea. e. Expose the jugular bulb and its continuity with the sigmoid sinus.

The largest cutting burs that will safely fit in the area to be drilled should be used. This allows a greater surface area so as not to put too much pressure on one area to reduce the likelihood of penetrating and damaging underlying structures. Visualization around these larger burs can be an issue and needs to be considered. Make sure to check both sides of the drill bit to prevent inadvertent damage to structures on the "other side of the bur." Also, the size of the suction-irrigation should be reduced relative to the size of drill bit that is being used as this will allow better visualization.

Drill speed is also an important variable that can be adjusted. Higher speeds work great for efficient bone removal, but at a cost of less control. When dissecting around critical structures, slowing the drill speed down will enhance control and decrease likelihood of injury. This is often forgotten in the midst of extensive procedures.

SURFACE LANDMARKS

In the temporal bone dissection lab or in the operating room, landmarks can be identified on the surface of the temporal bone after the incision and soft tissue is dissected. These should be routinely identified in order to provide a safe dissection from lateral to medial. These are each briefly described and shown in Figure 23–1.

Linea Temporalis

The linea temporalis, or temporal line, is a ridge that is easily visualized and palpated that demarcates the attachment of the temporalis muscle. It runs parallel to the zygomatic arch. It usually indicates the superior extent of the mastoid cavity and hence the level of the floor of the middle cranial fossa (tegmen).

Spine of Henle

The spine of Henle, or suprameatal spine, is a small horizontal ridge of bone located at the posterior–superior rim of the external auditory meatus. This landmark, along with the cribrose area, defines the path to the mastoid antrum, which is located about 15 mm deep to the spine of Henle.

Macewen's Triangle

Named after the Scottish surgeon, Sir William MacEwen (1864–1924), Macewen's triangle (the fossa

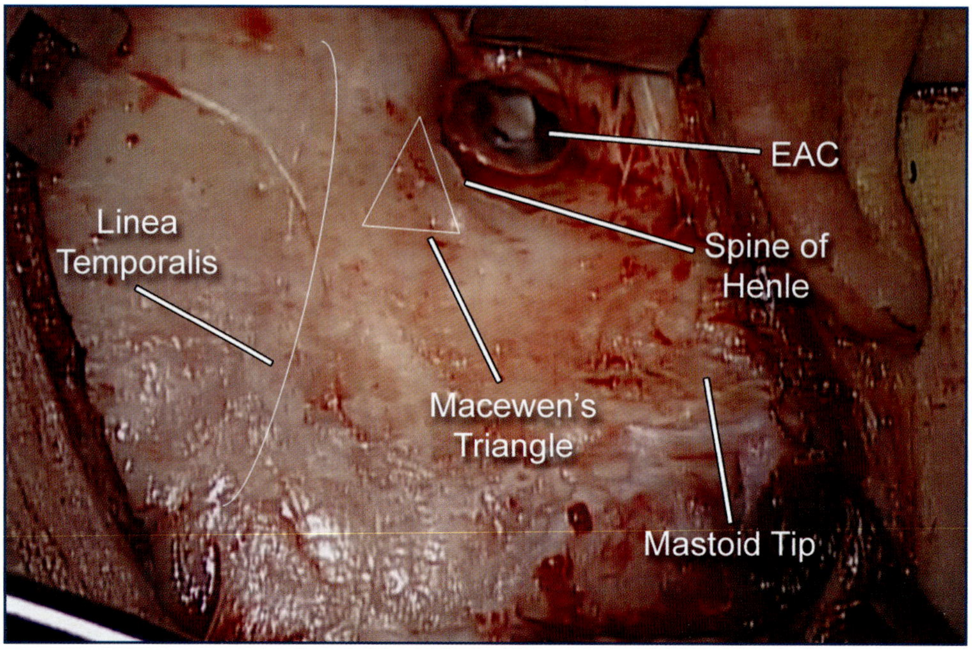

Figure 23–1. Intraoperative photograph of right temporal bone with view of surface landmarks that are labeled. Macewen's triangle is the cribrose area that demarcates the location of the antrum situated more medially. The linea temporalis is drawn in for emphasis.

mastoidea) is the name of the area delineated by the temporal line superiorly, the external auditory canal anteriorly, and a tangent to the posterior external auditory canal posteriorly. There are multiple small perforating vessels found in this area known as the cribrose area. As mentioned, this triangular depression and the spine of Henle are important to identify because the antrum sits medial to this point.

Mastoid Tip

The mastoid tip can be palpated. Dissection medial and anterior to the mastoid tip must be carefully done as the facial nerve will be found at the level of the digastric muscle, which attaches here. The tympanomastoid suture is identified along with the stylomastoid foramen. The postauricular incision needs to be carefully planned so as not to place the facial nerve at risk, especially in young children where the nerve can be more laterally located. Cautery in this area may pose increased risk to the facial nerve and must be used with caution.

Inion (External Occipital Protuberance) and Asterion

This inion is a surface landmark that usually is not visually identified, but rather palpated through the skin as a posterior bony protuberance from the occipital bone. The trapezius muscle attaches to this. This provides an idea of relationship of other structures. An imaginary line extending from the zygoma to the inion passes just superior to the external acoustic meatus and overlies the linea temporalis and asterion. The asterion is the point where three suture lines converge: the lambdoid, parietomastoid, and occipitomastoid. This point overlies the junction of the transverse and sigmoid sinuses.

Surface Landmarks on Tegmen

The tegmen covers the tympanic cavity (tegmen tympani) and the mastoid cavity (tegmen mastoideum). There is a suture, the petrotympanic suture, that delineates this division. Medial to this suture is the facial hiatus, which transmits the greater superficial petrosal nerve (GSPN) to the geniculate ganglion. The lesser petrosal nerve is in the petrosquamous suture which is also known as the superior tympanic canaliculus. The arcuate eminence, which sometimes is difficult to identify, approximates the position of the superior semicircular canal (SSCC) and is a key landmark in middle cranial fossa surgery.

Several foremen are noted along the junction of the temporal bone, the greater wing of the sphenoid, and the basiocciput. The foramen lacerum is a false foramen that is filled with fibrous connective tissue and that forms the roof of the carotid canal, which runs parallel to the petrous ridge. It is not a true foramen, as the carotid artery does not actually traverse it. The anterior temporal bone is bordered by the medial foramen ovale (transmits CN V3) and lateral foramen spinosum (transmits middle meningeal artery).

SIMPLE MASTOIDECTOMY

All otolaryngologists must learn the simple mastoidectomy and be able to access the antrum in order to manage certain disease processes and emergency complications that may arise. The goal of this procedure is to remove bone in order to visualize the antrum, the horizontal semicircular canal, and the incus. More times than not, this is adequate to treat simple ear disease. The key to the drilling the mastoid is to keep the walls of the cavity sloping so that you can see the point of your instrument as you progress medially. Beginners tend to drill down a narrow cavity with vertical walls preventing a view of the business end of their instrument (Figure 23–2).

The mastoidectomy is performed with the largest cutting bur available. Firm, steady strokes are started along a line parallel to the temporal line. This cut should approximate the superior limit of dissection and floor of the middle fossa (tegmen). The next stroke should be perpendicular to this one going parallel to the external auditory canal. All aerated bone can be removed as one progresses medially through the mastoid. The ear canal must be thinned, but not destroyed. A thin ear canal is essential in order to maintain a safe dissection as it will allow easier identification of the antrum, incus, and facial recess. Most beginning surgeons leave the ear canal too thick and making medial identification of structures more difficult. The ear canal can be followed inferiorly and the bone posterior to it can be removed.

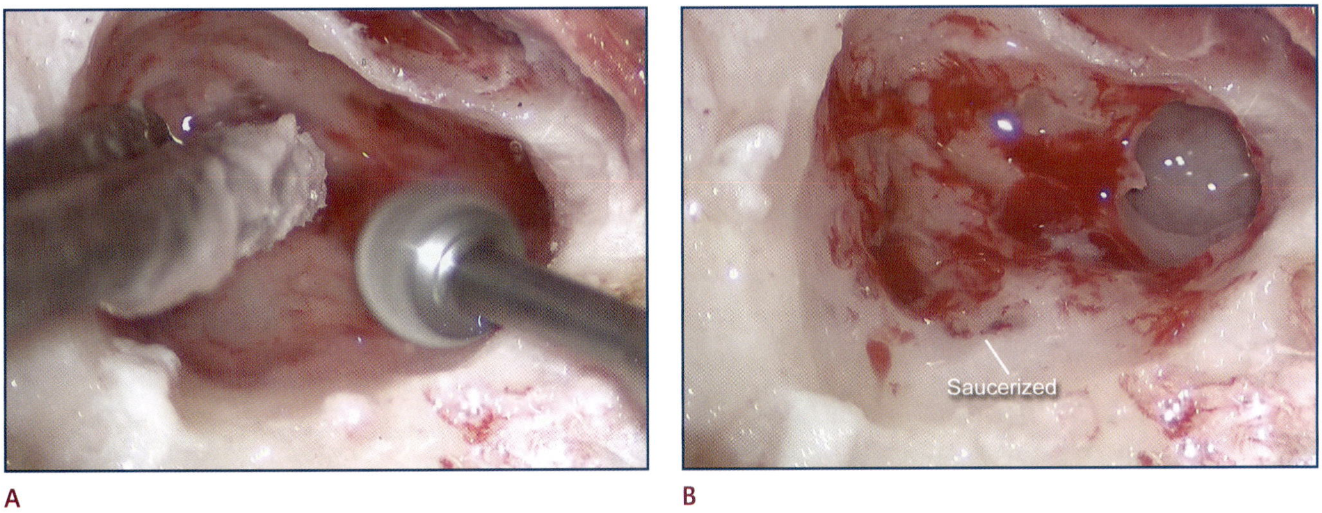

Figure 23–2. A. Intraoperative photograph of right mastoid cavity being drilled that does not have adequate "saucerization" of the edges. They are too vertical and will limit views as deeper dissection continues. **B.** Cavity with better posterior widening of edges to allow better illumination and visualization. The superior edge is still too vertical and will need to be saucerized more.

The tegmen is identified and left intact. Small amounts of bleeding and a change in the pitch of the drill will be noted as the tegmen is approached. The sigmoid sinus is identified as it courses in the posterior aspect of the mastoid bone. It is located more laterally near the transverse sinus and dives more medially and anteriorly as it heads toward the jugular bulb. The sinodural angle (Citelli's angle) is identified and marks the posterior limit of mastoid dissection (Figure 23–3). The edges of the bone must be smoothed and widened ("saucerized") so that better lighting is allowed deeper in the cavity and for easier use of instruments in the cavity.

As deeper dissection is performed, a thicker area of bone is identified, which is the petrosquamous suture (Koerner's septum) (Figure 23–4). After this is removed, the antrum is identified and a 4 mm bur is used to dissect the antrum further. Another important reminder is to change the size of the suction-irrigation tip to a similar size as the drill bit to allow enough room to work. Once into the antrum, drilling anteriorly with a 2-mm bur will allow view of the epitympanum.

The tegmen will dip inferiorly at this level, but dissection along the tegmen is the safest approach. The change in bone will be noted from cancellous,

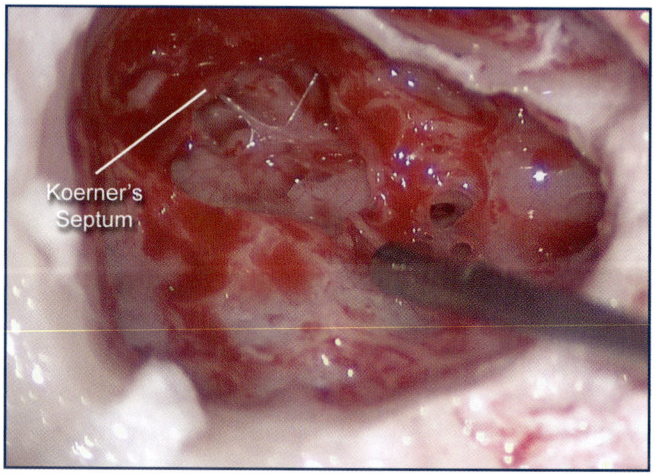

Figure 23–4. Intraoperative photograph of right mastoid cavity with numerous air cells. Koerner's septum is visualized. This bone must be removed in order to gain access to the antrum.

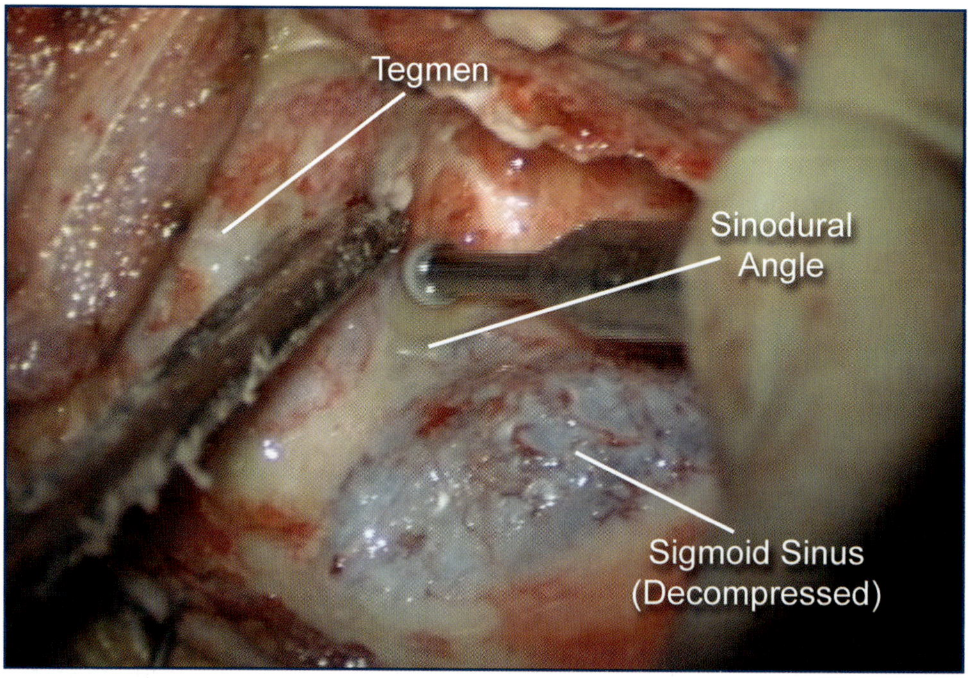

Figure 23–3. Intraoperative photograph of right mastoid cavity with drilling at sinodural angle.

airy bone to the dense endochondrial bone of the horizontal semicircular canal. Once the horizontal canal is identified, the incus reflection will be noted in the irrigation water. Careful removal of bone at the anterior edge of the antrum with a diamond bur will expose the incus. Care must be taken to avoid drill injury or trauma to the incus. The facial nerve will be at the level of the horizontal canal and the short process of the incus points to the facial recess.

Facial Recess Approach

The facial recess approach allows exposure into the middle ear space for dissection and removal of disease and placement of cochlear implants. The boundaries of facial recess are facial nerve medially, the chorda tympani nerve laterally, and the fossa incudis superiorly. The fossa incudis is merely the space that the incus occupies. A small diamond bur is used for this dissection, unless experience allows use of a cutting bur for faster removal of bone. Drilling inferior to the short process of the incus and in a direction parallel to the incus will allow safe identification of the facial nerve in its fallopian canal because the nerve is more medial (Figure 23–5). The facial nerve is carefully dissected and followed inferiorly until the chorda tympani nerve is identified at the iter chordae (where the chorda tympani nerve joins the facial nerve) heading in a superior, medial direction. Care must be taken that heat is not generated near the nerves.

An air cell can be usually found along this dissection that can be widened and allow access into the tympanic cavity usually at the level of the pyramidal eminence. The fibrous annulus of the tympanic membrane, stapes, long process of the incus, oval, and round windows can be visualized. It must be noted that the sinus tympani is still not easily visualized through the facial recess approach as it is deep (medial) to the facial nerve.

At times, the chorda tympani nerve is sacrificed to increase exposure inferiorly into the hypotympanum and this is termed an extended facial recess approach. The chorda tympani is transected at the level of the facial nerve and the space between the facial nerve and the tympanic membrane annulus is carefully widened with small diamond burs from a superior to inferior direction.

A cochleostomy is performed by drilling at the lip of the round window niche to remove the bony overhang and exposing the round window membrane completely. Once exposed, drilling can be performed on the anterior, inferior region to gain access to the scala tympani (Figure 23–6). If a dummy cochlear implant electrode is available, this can be

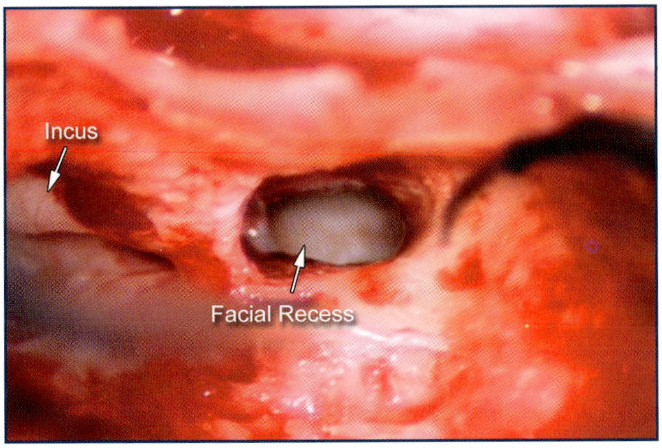

Figure 23–5. Intraoperative photograph of right mastoid cavity and facial recess. Incus is labeled and facial recess boundaries are chorda tympani nerve laterally, facial nerve medially, and fossa incudis superiorly.

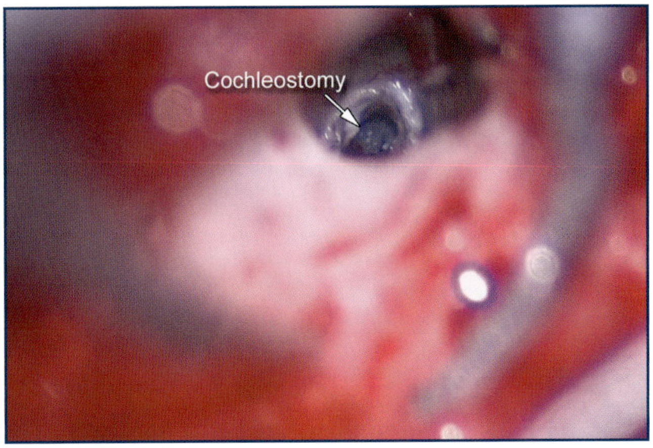

Figure 23–6. Intraoperative photograph of right facial recess with cochleostomy drilled into scala tympani at anterior/inferior region of round window.

placed. Round window insertion may be performed as well by making an incision in the round window membrane and placing the implant.

Epitympanic and Attic Dissection

The epitympanic region or attic is defined by the area superior to the level of the tympanic membrane and it leads to the aditus ad antrum, which connects to the mastoid system. It houses the head of the malleus and the body of the incus and is limited by the external auditory canal inferiorly and the tegmen superiorly. The cog, a bony projection from the tegmen superior to the cochleariform process, separates the anterior epitympanic space (the supratubal recess) from the remainder of the epitympanum.

Access to this attic is accomplished either with an atticotomy or with anterior extension from the mastoid antrum toward the root of the zygoma. The atticotomy is performed to expose the superior aspect of the ear canal. A 3-mm bur may be used to remove the bony ear canal superiorly until the tegmen tympani is identified. Medial dissection is performed until disease and ossicles are identified. If the mastoid antrum is followed anteriorly, the ossicles will be identified and if even more anterior exposure is necessary, the incus and head of the malleus can be resected. The incus is removed by separating the incudostapedial joint sharply. The head of the malleus can be carefully drilled with a diamond bit or sharply cut. The tympanic segment of the facial nerve can be easily visualized now.

ENDOLYMPHATIC SAC IDENTIFICATION AND DECOMPRESSION

Continued dissection is performed to remove the air cells around the horizontal semicircular canal, the sigmoid sinus to the jugular bulb, and the facial nerve. The bone overlying the sigmoid sinus and posterior fossa dura is removed. The sigmoid sinus can be decompressed by removing the bone completely from it with a large diamond bur (Figure 23–7).

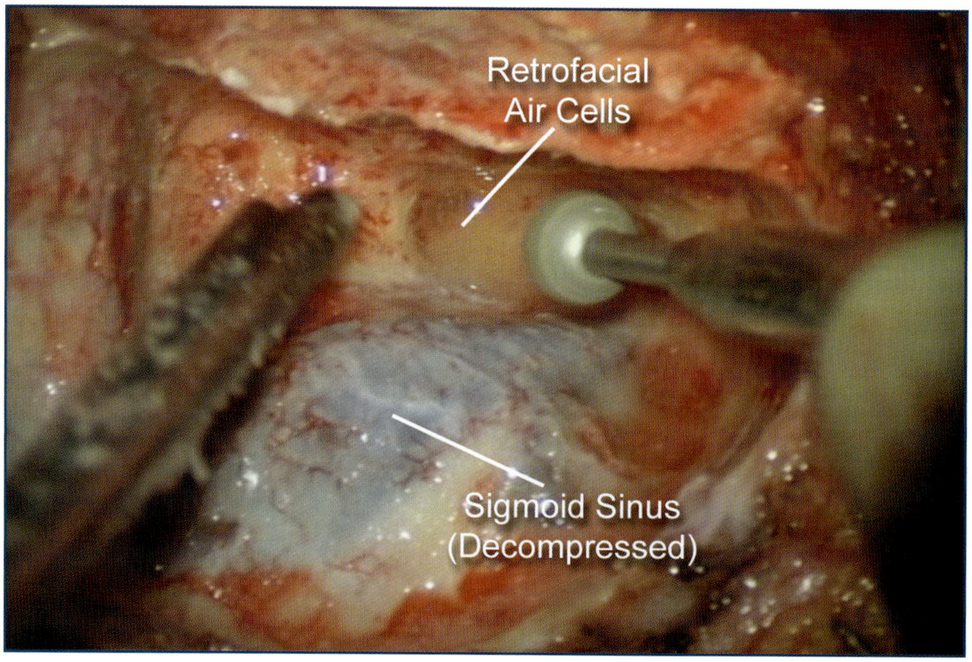

Figure 23–7. Intraoperative photograph of right mastoid cavity with sigmoid sinus being decompressed with use of large diamond bur. The facial nerve will come in close contact to the facial nerve as it courses near the jugular bulb. Retrofacial air cell tract can be followed.

Another technique involves leaving some bone in the central area of the sigmoid sinus (Bill's island named after Dr. House) as an island to allow some protection for the vein. After the sinus is decompressed, the posterior fossa dura is decompressed in a between the sigmoid sinus and the posterior semicircular canal. The endolymphatic sac can be found inferior to Donaldson's line (which is drawn along the long axis of the horizontal canal, bisecting the posterior semicircular canal (PSC) (Figure 23–8). It is a thickened area of the posterior fossa dura (Figure 23–9). The endolymphatic sac may be incised and a Silastic drain may be inserted as well. This is difficult to accomplish in the temporal bone lab as desiccation occurs.

POSTERIOR CANAL OCCLUSION

The horizontal and posterior canals are identified as the cortical bone is removed around them. The horizontal canal (HSC) is easily identified and is critical in finding other structures including the PSC and facial nerve. The HSC and the PSC are perpendicular to each other. The PSC occlusion procedure is performed to treat intractable benign paroxysmal positional vertigo (BPPV).

A diamond bur is used to drill along the PSC until the endochondrial bone is dissected and the membranous labyrinth is identified (Figure 23–10). Care must be taken not to injure and suction the fluid in the membranous labyrinth as this may lead to deafness. Bone pate, bone dust mixed with fibrin glue and/or fascia, can be used to pack the open ends of the PSCC. The CO_2 laser may be used to make the final cut of the membranous labyrinth. Fascia may be placed over the defect of the PSCC.

CANAL WALL-DOWN MASTOIDECTOMY

To convert a simple (cortical) mastoidectomy into a modified radical one, the posterior and superior walls of the external auditory canal (EAC) have to

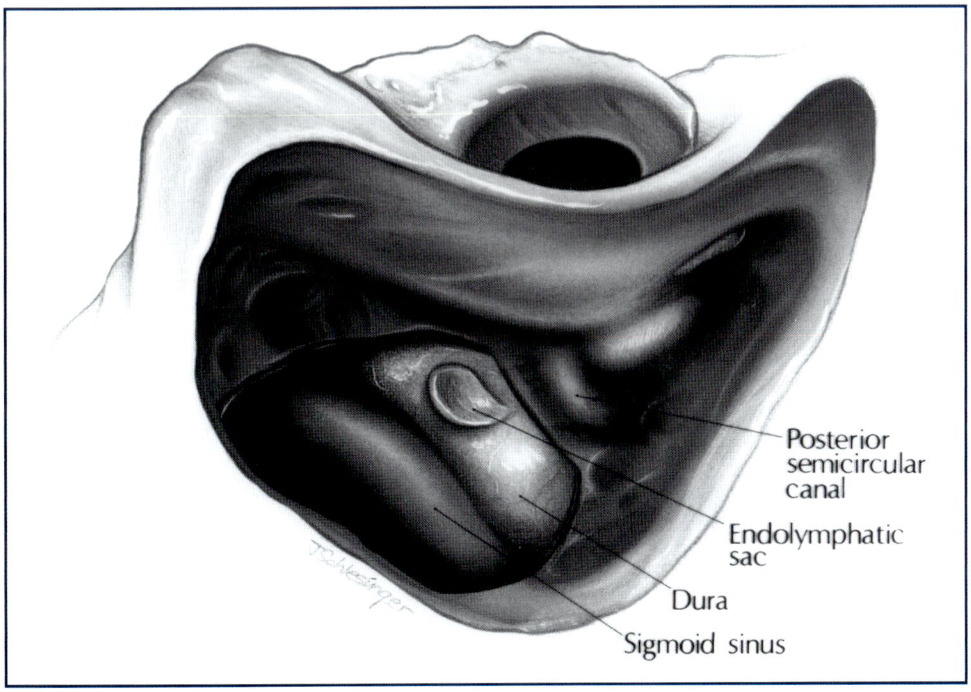

Figure 23–8. Depiction of left mastoid cavity with identification of endolymphatic sac inferior to Donaldson's line (from horizontal canal to sigmoid sinus) along posterior fossa dura.

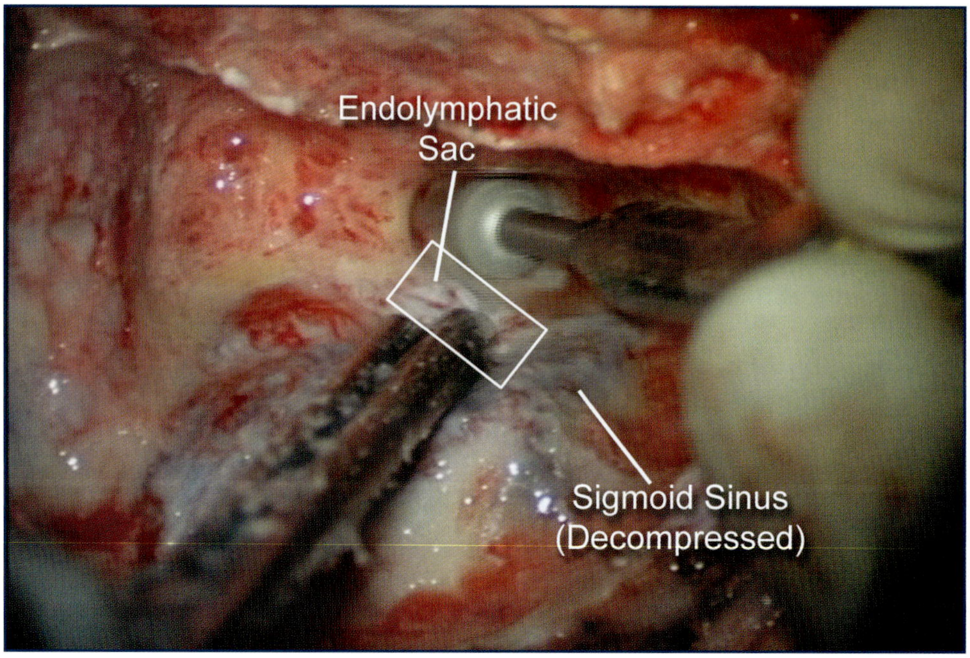

Figure 23–9. Intraoperative photograph of right mastoid cavity with endolymphatic sac being decompressed. The sigmoid sinus and posterior fossa dura have also been decompressed.

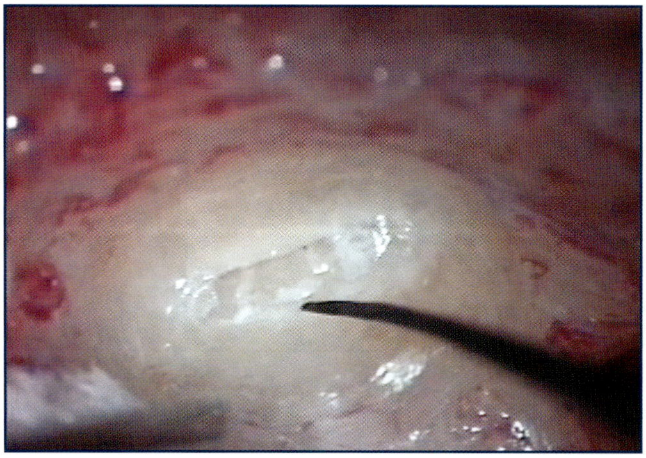

Figure 23–10. Intraoperative photograph of right posterior semicircular canal where the endochondrial bone has been removed and the membranous labyrinth is identified for occlusion. Bone pate or fascia can be used to occlude the canal.

be removed. The tympanic membrane, manubrium of the malleus, and the stapes can be left in place.

After the antrum and the facial nerve are identified, the canal wall is removed with gentle drilling from the root of the zygoma to the mastoid tip with a 5.5-mm bur. The canal wall is removed from lateral to medial down to the level of the facial nerve, called the "facial ridge." The facial ridge is lowered to the level of the annulus and the floor of the EAC. Superiorly, the medial extent of the dissection is the ossicular chain, where a thin bone is left over them and then gently removed without disrupting them. If the canal wall-down procedure is done and the middle ear space is not entered, the procedure is called a Bondy mastoidectomy. This also can be done from an endaural approach where the canal is removed from "inside" the ear canal which is widened into the mastoid cavity.

If the disease is more extensive into the middle ear, the incus may need to be removed, the chorda tympani nerve sacrificed, and a canal wall down mastoidectomy is performed. The head of the malleus may need to be removed so that the anterior epitympanum is made flush with the mesotympanum and the floor of the mastoid cavity is at the same level of the floor of the bony EAC. The mastoid tip may need to be amputated to reduce the cavity size and reduce the possibility of trapped epithelial debris.

Meatoplasty is necessary to allow adequate exposure for routine cleaning of the mastoid cavity. This is accomplished by excising the conchal cartilage.

To convert this modified radical mastoidectomy to a radical cavity,the tympanic membrane and the manubrium of the malleus are removed and the eustachian tube is plugged. The stapes can still be left in place.

LABYRINTHECTOMY AND TRANSLABYRINTHINE APPROACH TO INTERNAL AUDITORY CANAL

The semicircular canals are defined by removing the surrounding cancellous bone. Each canal should be outlined so that its endochondrial covering is easily identified. Using a medium sized drill bit, the retrolabyrinthine bone should be exposed as this is the safest area to drill. The sigmoid sinus may be decompressed and the exposure is widened until the posterior semicircular canal (PSC) is outlined.

The surgical technique for a labyrinthectomy involves blue-lining each semicircular canal: the body of the canal is gradually drilled down along the long axis of the canal until the grey or blue coloration of the lumen comes into contrast or is "blue-lined" compared to the dense, yellow bone of the canal. The HSC can be blue-lined first as it lies most lateral, followed by the PSC, whose arc is bisected by the long axis of the horizontal canal, namely, Donaldson's line. The SSC is blue-lined last, with its posterior limb discovered by following the superior limb of the PSC up to the crus communis (Figure 23–11). The superior canal is followed and blue-lined forward to its ampulla, which lies adjacent to the ampulla of the horizontal semicircular canal. Each canal lumen is then fully opened, and the otic capsule bone central to all the canals is resected, thereby exposing the vestibule.

The bone between the ampullae of the horizontal and posterior semicircular canals is removed. Careful drilling needs to be done near the ampullae of the canals as the facial nerve lies in close proximity to them. Removal of this bone resects the lateral wall of the vestibule and further bone removal will expose the fundus of the internal auditory canal. This bone lies in very close proximity to the second genu of the facial nerve, and careful removal with copious irrigation is warranted to avoid injury. In addition, undercutting the bone in this region or drilling medial to the facial nerve can lead to its injury.

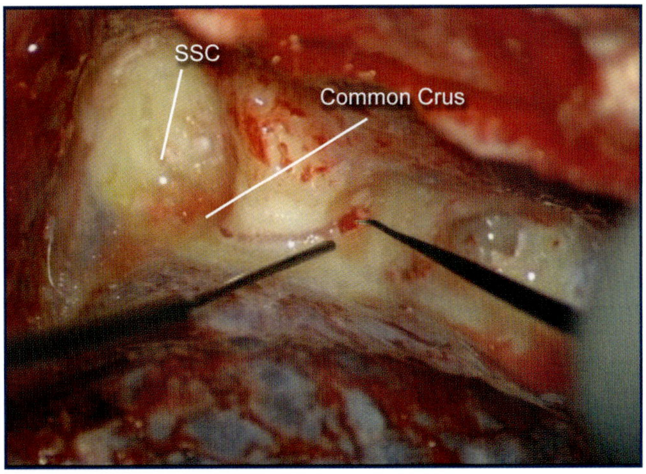

Figure 23–11. Intraoperative photograph of right labyrinthectomy being performed. The instrument is pointing to the ampullated end of the posterior semicircular canal. It can be followed to the common crus posteriorly, which connects to the superior canal. SSC = superior semicircular canal.

An alternative technique to the labyrinthectomy involves the gradual expansion of a cavity, or "Malcolm's cup" as it has become known, from the solid angle. After removal of overlying mastoid air cells and bony spiculations, the "solid angle" or "hard angle" of dense otic capsule bone that lies posterosuperior to the horizontal and posterior semicircular canals is identified. A cavity of dissection is then developed within this solid angle and gradually expanded in all directions. The posterior and middle fossa dural plates and sinodural angle denote the limits of dissection posterosuperiorly. Malcolm's cup is expanded anteroinferiorly to follow the lumina of the posterior and horizontal canals, and it is expanded deep to outline the superior semicircular canal lumen. The ampullae of each semicircular canal mark the anterior and inferior ends of dissection, as the facial nerve lies in very close proximity to each ampulla. The elliptical and spherical recesses can be identified in the vestibule that houses the utricle and saccule, respectively (Figure 23–12). In a

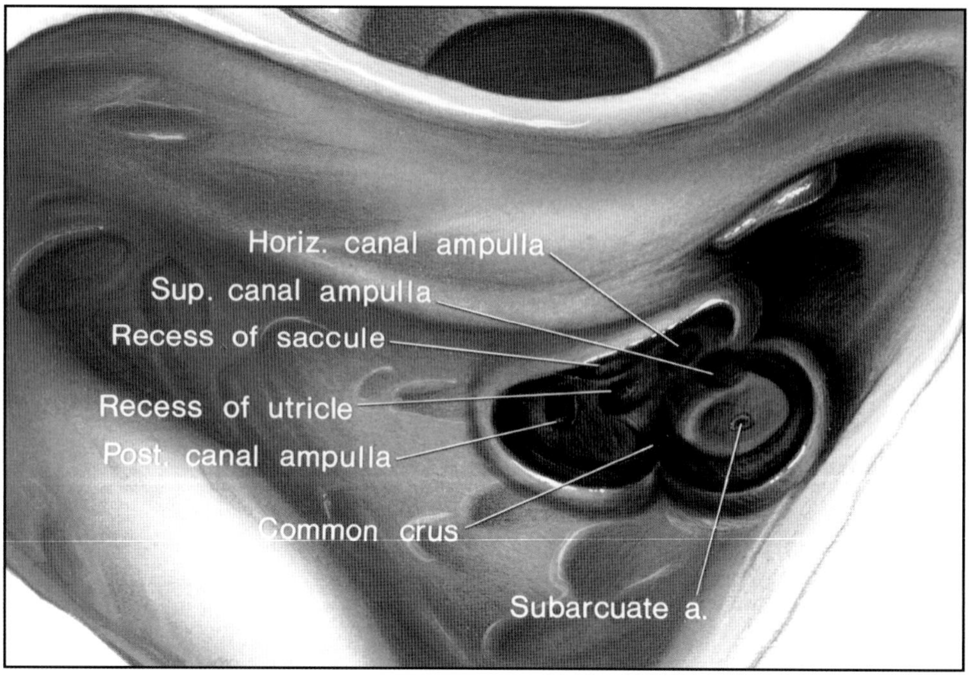

Figure 23–12. Depiction of left labyrinthectomy with each semicircular canal exposed into vestibule. The spherical and elliptical recesses are seen. Note the close relationship to the facial nerve.

labyrinthectomy, neuroepithelium needs to be removed from the ampullated ends of the three canals as well as the utricle and saccule.

The lateral wall of the vestibule is again taken down until the fallopian canal is skeletonized. During labyrinthectomy, usage of cutting burs instead diamond burrs prevents bone dust from plugging canal lumina and aids in positive identification of the canal lumina out to the vestibule and ampullae. Maintaining dissection within the confines of a recessed cup or cavity also enhances safety of cutting burr usage at this stage.

The internal auditory canal is embedded within the remaining dense bone of the posterior petrous apex. Skeletonization of the internal auditory canal begins with exenteration the bone inferior and superior to its estimated position. The inferior bone is removed until the jugular bulb is skeletonized inferiorly and the lower border of the internal auditory canal skeletonized superiorly. The dissection is carried medially until the cochlear aqueduct is identified, sometimes with egress of CSF. The superior bone is removed until the superior border of the internal auditory canal is skeletonized inferiorly, while maintaining thin bone over the superior petrosal sinus. Because of the tangential inclination of the internal auditory canal from the translabyrinthine perspective, the bone removal is deeper medially around the porus acousticus and more superficial laterally around the fundus.

Final exenteration of the superior bone is performed carefully, as the labyrinthine segment of the facial nerve curves upward superior to the level of the internal auditory canal. Medial facial nerve decompression of the labyrinthine segment can be performed by removing the eggshell-thin bone near the meatal foramen as the nerve enters the temporal bone.

The bone overlying the lateral face of the internal auditory canal is drilled down until eggshell thin similarly to the inferior and superior faces of the internal auditory canal. This amount of dissection provides 270 degrees of exposure of the internal auditory canal. The eggshell thin bone of the internal auditory canal is then elevated and removed.

Bony removal is carried further laterally to the macula cribrosa superioris, or Mike's dot, which localizes the bony perforation along the medial wall of the elliptical recess through which pass the fibers of the superior vestibular nerve supplying the utricular macula. Lateral dissection to the level of Mike's dot verifies the location of the internal auditory canal to fully expose the fundus. Mike's dot is unroofed, beneath which lies the superior vestibular nerve and internal auditory canal fundus. Just inferior to Mike's dot is the crista falciformis, or horizontal crest, further confirming dissection to the fundus.

Complete exposure of the fundus exposes the superior vestibular nerve lies separated from the facial nerve by a vertical bony crest, or Bill's bar. Gentle palpation and dissection of the superficially located superior vestibular nerve allows for a natural dissection plane to be formed between the superior vestibular nerve and the facial nerve, which lies deep to Bill's bar. This dissection plane can then be developed in a lateral to medial direction, enabling efficient and safe dissection of the superior vestibular nerve from underlying facial nerve. The superior vestibular nerve is avulsed and the facial nerve can be visualized. Inferior to the facial nerve is the cochlear nerve, medial to the inferior vestibular nerve. The facial nerve can be dissected from the IAC into the meatal foramen toward the geniculate ganglion. The nervus intermedius (Wrisberg's nerve) can be seen traveling just inferior and posterior to the facial nerve.

TRANSCOCHLEAR APPROACH

All the above steps are followed and the facial nerve is elevated out of the bony fallopian canal, fully mobilized from the brainstem to the stylomastoid foramen, and transposed posteriorly to rest on the cerebellum.

With the facial nerve completely transposed, the cochlea can be resected. The anterior petrous apex to the clivus can be resected, and the anterior limit of dissection becomes the petrosal internal carotid artery. Through this approach, the entire lateral and ventral aspects of the brainstem, the clivus, and the prepontine cistern are directly visible with minimal or no cerebellar retraction. The transotic approach is similar without transposition of the facial nerve.

MIDDLE FOSSA APPROACH

During dissection of the mastoid bone, time should be made to evaluate the bone from a superior approach to appreciate anatomic relationships. The temporal bone needs to be positioned in a manner that mimics the surgical approach to the middle cranial fossa after a craniotomy is performed with the mastoid tip pointing away from the surgeon.

Dura is elevated in from posterior to anterior to avoid avulsing the GSPN and/or geniculate ganglion which may be exposed. Surface landmarks and anatomic relationships are critical for identification of deeper structures. If the GSPN is identified along the petrous ridge, it can be followed posteriorly to the geniculate ganglion and further posteriorly to the SSC, which will be 5 mm medial and 10 mm posterior. The petrous ridge and the SSC form a right angle. The SSC may share a relationship with the arcuate eminence, although this is not an exact relationship. Careful drilling over the SSC should be done to confirm its location. The IAC can be approximated by a 60-degree angle from the SSC.

One must remember that the position and orientation of the internal auditory canal roughly approximates the axis of the external auditory canal extended medially. This axis can be further refined by removing the lateral middle fossa floor or tegmen tympani, exposing the epitympanic space and ossicles which lie directly between the external auditory canal and internal auditory canal.

The axis of the internal auditory canal can be best estimated by bisecting the angle subtended by the long axis of the arcuate eminence and the long axis of the greater superficial petrosal nerve and extending this line onto the meatal plane.

If the greater superficial petrosal nerve is identified, it can be followed in a retrograde fashion to the geniculate ganglion, uncovering the meatal foramen from which the labyrinthine segment of the facial nerve can be followed medially to the fundus of the internal auditory canal. The internal auditory canal can be skeletonized medially to the petrous ridge.

The internal auditory canal lumen can be estimated to be approximately 10 mm anteriomedial to the apex of the superior semicircular canal in a direction parallel to the petrous ridge and superior petrosal sinus. The location of the geniculate and cochlea can be estimated by locating the apex of the superior semicircular canal and measuring 5 mm anterolaterally perpendicular to the axis of the greater superficial petrosal nerve and 10mm anteromedially parallel to the axis of the greater superficial petrosal nerve.

The medial, thick bone of the petrous ridge needs to be thinned as this is the safest area for dissection initially. As the contour of the internal auditory canal is developed medially, dissection can be extended slowly laterally, taking into consideration the relative locations of the vestibule posteriorly and cochlea anteriorly. Once the bone over the IAC is thinned, it may be carefully removed with a pick. The lateral aspect of the IAC, or fundus, is dissected and the vertical crest is identified. The facial nerve is identified in its anterior location and the superior vestibular nerve is posteriorly located.

Index

Note: Page numbers in **bold** reference non-text material.

B

C

D

E

F

G

H

I

N

P

Q

R

S

T

U

V

W

X

Y